OXFORD MEDICAL PUBLICATIONS

Oxford Handbook for
Medical School

Published and forthcoming Oxford Handbooks

Oxford Handbook for
Medical School

Editor-in-Chief

Kapil Sugand
Trauma and Orthopaedics Specialist Trainee
and Surgical Research Fellow,
Imperial College London, UK

Edited by

Miriam Berry
Consultant Nephrologist, University Hospitals
Birmingham, Birmingham, UK

Imran Yusuf
Ophthalmology Specialist Trainee and
MRC Research Fellow, Oxford University, UK

Aisha Janjua
Obstetrics and Gynaecology Specialist Trainee
and NIHR Clinical Lecturer,
Warwick University, UK

Chris Bird
Consultant in Paediatric Emergency Medicine,
Oxford, UK

Consultant Editors

David Metcalfe
Clinical Research Fellow in Musculoskeletal Trauma,
Oxford University, UK

Harveer Dev
Urology Specialist Trainee and Wellcome Trust PhD
Fellow, Cambridge University, UK

Sri Thrumurthy
General Surgical Specialist Trainee,
University College London Hospitals, UK

OXFORD
UNIVERSITY PRESS

OXFORD
UNIVERSITY PRESS

Great Clarendon Street, Oxford, OX2 6DP,
United Kingdom

Oxford University Press is a department of the University of Oxford.
It furthers the University's objective of excellence in research, scholarship,
and education by publishing worldwide. Oxford is a registered trade mark of
Oxford University Press in the UK and in certain other countries

Published in the United States of America by Oxford University Press
198 Madison Avenue, New York, NY 10016, United States of America

British Library Cataloguing in Publication Data

Data available

Library of Congress Control Number: 2018954692

ISBN 978–0–19–968190–7

Printed and bound in China by
C&C Offset Printing Co., Ltd.

Dedication

We would like to wholeheartedly thank the following people for their constant support, efforts, and faith in us, in helping to realize this handbook after 7 years.

Sincere and heartfelt thanks to the following:

- The publishing team from Oxford University Press, especially Mr Michael Hawkes (Senior Assistant Commissioning Editor for Medical Books) for his patience, negotiation, and expertise. You have been there every step of the way and your efforts are very much appreciated.
- All members of the editorial team and the consultant reviewers for giving up so much of their personal time to assist the contributors and ensuring quality control of the content. Thank you for working so well as a team and bringing such superb ideas to the table.
- Our plethora of devoted contributors and educators from every field of medicine and surgery. Thank you for submitting work of such high calibre, your insights, and expert advice.
- Our colleague publishing houses for offering permission to use their images.
- Our internal reviewers for taking the time out to review, critique, and appraise our entire book and offering your constructive criticisms to improve the content.
- Our families for their love, encouragement, and motivation. Thank you for compromising and sacrificing quality time with us, once again, so that we could write this handbook for every medical student everywhere. Needless to say, we will be striving to make up for the lost time.
- Our international audience for wanting a book like this and supporting the project from the very beginning. This handbook has been written for you. We all hope that it will serve as a useful companion throughout your exciting time at medical school that will ultimately lay the strong foundations for a lifetime of clinical practice.

Foreword

This superb guide to the neophyte doctor ranges from one's first approach to medical school and how to cope with such a complex process right through to a doctor's decision on which specialty career to follow eventually. As always this Oxford Handbook covers a vast range of useful, relevant material, and this particular one will be of great value to anyone seriously considering medical school for their future career choice.

The contributors are a talented group of doctors whose expertise and interests span many different clinical specialties as well as having, between them, a vast experience in clinical academic research as well as a huge commitment in the modern complex process of medical education.

I am sure this book, where the nuts and bolts of virtually every specialty are most clearly laid out, will be a most useful guide worldwide for those not only considering a career in the medical profession but even those midway through their medical careers.

Peter Abrahams MBBS FRCS(ED) FRCR DO(Hon) FHEA
Prof. Emeritus of Clinical Anatomy
Warwick Medical School, Gibbet Hill
National Teaching fellow 2011–14
Life fellow, Girton college, Cambridge
Visiting Professor LKC School of Medicine NTU Singapore

Preface

Medicine is a huge undertaking, both to study as an undergraduate and subsequently to practise as a doctor. During your preclinical studies, you are expected to learn anatomy, physiology, and biochemistry but also genetics, pharmacology, pathology, microbiology, the history of medicine, psychology, sociology, law, ethics, epidemiology, and statistics. The list is never-ending! These are vast disciplines in their own right and medical students often struggle to understand what *exactly* they are expected to learn. The course objectives are frequently vague: 'students should be able to identify the important anatomical structures of the pelvis and lower limbs'. You are also bound to see a course handbook state: 'students may be assessed on any material from the lectures, group work, recommended reading, and *anything else that the examiners feel students should know at this stage*'. A common complaint of all medical students is that the material tested in exams feels disconnected from the topics taught. This is very different from the situation at secondary school in which core knowledge is tightly defined by a course syllabus. You would not be alone in becoming frustrated by the seemingly unpredictable, if not unlimited bounds of knowledge that appear to be expected by examiners.

Furthermore, the clinical years bring their own particular challenges. You are thrust into unfamiliar environments in which busy and overworked staff are trying to manage complex tasks with little time set aside to teach students, due to constant understaffing and lack of resources. The material that you painstakingly learned during the preclinical years somehow seems irrelevant to—or at least wholly insufficient to understand—what is going on in a practical and clinical setting. There are hierarchies, conflicts, and unwritten rules that you will navigate with varying degrees of success. You will never quite overcome the feeling of always being 'in the way'. The overwhelming burden of boundless learning returns as you wrangle with over 60 different branches of medicine and surgery, from anaesthetics to urology. The knowledge expected of you by a cardiologist in a heart failure clinic will differ wildly to that expected by a skull base neurosurgeon in the operating theatre.

Hence, this handbook was conceived as a partial solution to the complexities of learning medicine in the twenty-first century. Sir William Osler famously wrote, 'he who studies medicine without books sails an uncharted sea'. This handbook should serve as your map through the countless obstacles that you must overcome on your journey to qualifying as a doctor. First, it will help define the core knowledge that is expected of *all* medical students, which is often distinct from the niche interests of individual teachers. Second, it will identify 'high-yield' information and suggest what you should know (and so are likely to be asked) in any given clinical setting. Besides serving as a quick reference guide, this handbook introduces core topics to help guide you with further reading in your own time. It will also help you to prepare for some of the unfamiliar settings (such as etiquette and conduct in the operating theatre, on wards, and in the emergency department) where you are likely to find yourself over the next few years until retirement.

The *Oxford Handbook for Medical School* will provide you with succinct, precise, and accurate facts about medicine and surgery that are bound to come up on a daily basis whether in or out of your time in hospital. The core motivation was to bequeath all the important lessons about the medical course and subject matter to the next generation of NHS leaders, pioneers, and consultants as well as to reflect on what we would like to have known back when we were medical students. Whether you are in the cardiology clinic, on the surgical wards, in theatre, or witnessing emergency care, this handbook includes carefully selected clinical scenarios that will explain the logic behind the management plans as well as improve your confidence in explaining it to your examiners. With aide-memoires, mnemonics, pictures, and seminal research accompanied by concise text you will be able to easily deconstruct abstract principles into digestible and memorable information. Since medical school is not only about clinical attachment as it encroaches into your personal life too, there is plenty of useful information on managing finances, health issues, planning electives, and career guidance to improve your chances of professional success from an early stage. Not many other books, at least known to us, can say the same. We have also ensured that the handbook does not preach or lecture but communicates with its audience on an informal and conversational level.

Needless to say, writing this compendium has been one of the biggest professional challenges to the editorial team but if it means that we manage to improve the quality of medical education globally, uplift the competence of medical students in all corners of the world, and give you another reason to fall in love with this vocation, then all the personal sacrifices, compromises, and struggles will have been all the more worthwhile. Medicine is obviously voluminous and it is sometimes discouraging when the sudden realization dawns on you that there is much work to be done in order to carry out the responsibilities for your vulnerable patients. Hopefully the *Oxford Handbook for Medical School* will serve as a friendly companion to ease your stress throughout your studies as well as introduce you to other speciality-specific Oxford Handbooks for further information with our cross-referencing style.

The *Oxford Handbook for Medical School* is the result of efforts from eight doctors from a range of specialities to offer a one-stop survival guide for every medical student to make the most of their course from the very first day to the very last. There was a vision and intention to pose the commonest clinical scenarios, how to excel at medical school, and improve career potential early on. There are clearly many textbooks available on the market with too little or too much information, written formally as if you were being lectured, and with dense data that risk losing your attention. This survival guide synthesizes advice from over 100 doctors. It has been said that 'you should learn from the mistakes of others as you do not have time to make them all yourself'. The time you spend reading this handbook could well be one of the best investments you make at medical school.

Finally, on behalf of the editorial team, we would like to take this opportunity to wholeheartedly thank everyone involved in the success of this handbook. We welcome your feedback to constantly improve the content of this handbook in subsequent editions and we hope that the *Oxford Handbook for Medical School* will serve you well.

David Metcalfe and Kapil Sugand
Members of the Editorial Team
Oxford Handbook for Medical School
May 2018

Contents

Part 5 **Assessments and examinations**

Part 6 **Career planning**

Contributors

John R. Apps
(Chapter 54: Getting ahead)
Paediatric Specialist Oncology Trainee, Birmingham Women's and Children's NHS Foundation Trust. Birmingham, UK, Honorary Research Associate, UCL Great Ormond Street Institute of Child Health, University College London, London, UK

Bilal Azhar
(Chapter 42: Upper gastrointestinal and hepatopancreatobiliary surgery)
Vascular Surgery Specialist Registrar, London Deanery, London Postgraduate School of Surgery, UK

James R. Bentham
(Chapter 26: Paediatrics)
Assistant Professor and Consultant Paediatric and Adult Interventional Cardiologist, Department of Paediatric Cardiology, Leeds General Infirmary, UK

Miriam Berry
(Chapter 3: Preclinical medicine; Chapter 5: Intercalated degrees and special study modules; Chapter 21: Nephrology; Chapter 48: Clinical assessments; Chapter 50: Clinical examinations; Chapter 54: Getting ahead)
Consultant Nephrologist, University Hospitals Birmingham, Birmingham, UK

Chris Bird
(Chapter 3: Preclinical medicine; Chapter 6: Going clinical; Chapter 26: Paediatrics; Chapter 45: Practical procedures; Chapter 46: Basic investigations)
Consultant in Emergency Paediatric Medicine, Birmingham Children's Hospital, UK

Lesley Black
(Chapter 17: Genitourinary medicine)
GP Specialist Registrar, Severn Deanery, Bristol, UK

Deborah Bowman
(Chapter 47: Ethics and law)
Professor of Bioethics, Clinical Ethics and Medical Law at St George's, University of London, UK

Lois Brand
(Chapter 53: Making decisions)
Consultant in Emergency Medicine, John Radcliffe Hospital, Oxford, UK

Elsa Butrous
(Chapter 54: Getting ahead)
GP Specialist Registrar, Oxford Deanery, UK

James Butterworth
(Chapter 34: Colorectal surgery)
Surgical Specialist Registrar, Clinical Research Fellow, Department of Cancer and Surgery, Imperial College London, London, UK

William Butterworth
(Chapter 34: Colorectal surgery)
Core Surgical Trainee, General Surgery, Princess Royal University Hospital, London, UK

Nandini Datta
(Chapter 6: Going clinical)
Senior Resident Medical Officer, Emergency Department, Gosford Hospital, Central Coast Local Health District, Australia

Fungai Dengu
(Chapter 42: Upper gastrointestinal and hepatopancreatobiliary surgery)
ST5 General Surgery Registrar Oxford Deanery, Clinical Research Fellow in Transplant Surgery, Nuffield Department of Surgical Sciences, University of Oxford.

Harveer Dev
(Chapter 3: Preclinical medicine; Chapter 8: Cardiology; Chapter 41: Vascular surgery; Chapter 43: Urology)
Urology Specialist Trainee and Wellcome Trust PhD Fellow, Cambridge University Hospitals NHS Trust, UK

Kate Drysdale
(Chapter 14: Gastroenterology)
Hepatology Clinical Research Fellow, Queen Mary University of London, London, UK

Tegwen Ecclestone
(Chapter 56: Career planning)
Core Trainee, Northern Deanery, UK

Daniel Fitzgerald
(Chapter 56: Career planning)
Medical Doctor, Médecins Sans Frontières, Operational Centre Paris, France

Neil Gupta
(Chapter 44: Radiology)
Consultant Interventional Radiologist, Joint College Tutor for Clinical Radiology, Radiology Fellowship Program Director, University Hospital Coventry & Warwickshire, Coventry, UK

Ruofan Connie Han
(Chapter 49: Preparing for clinical examinations)
Specialist Registrar in Ophthalmology, Oxford Eye Hospital, John Radcliffe Hospital, UK

Adam Handel
(Chapter 50: Clinical examinations)
Clinical Lecturer in Neurology, Nuffield Department of Clinical Neurosciences, University of Oxford

Ayad Harb
(Chapter 39: Plastic surgery)
Consultant Plastic Surgeon, University Hospital North Midlands NHS Trust, UK

Amy Hawkins
(Chapter 55: Electives)
Specialist Registrar in Palliative Medicine, London, UK

Fiona Hayes
(Chapter 31: Rheumatology)
Consultant in Rheumatology and Acute Medicine Southend University Hospital NHS Trust, UK

Catherine Hearnshaw
(Chapter 50: Clinical examinations)
Specialist Registrar Paediatrics, Royal Derby Hospital, UK

Alexander J Hills
(Chapter 37: Oral and maxillo-facial surgery)
Specialist Registrar, Oral and Maxillofacial Surgery, Queen Victoria Hospital, East Grinstead, Sussex, UK

Thiagarajan Jaiganesh
(Chapter 12: Emergency medicine)
Consultant in Adult and Paediatric Emergency Medicine, Emergency Department, St George's, University of London, UK

Aisha Janjua
(Chapter 23: Obstetrics & Gynaecology
Chapter 50: Clinical examinations;
Chapter 51: Written exams)
Obstetrics and Gynaecology Specialist Registrar and NIHR Clinical Lecturer, Warwick University, UK

Mhairi Jhugursing
(Chapter 9: Critical care)
Consultant Anaesthetist, West Middlesex Hospital, London, UK

Irfan Jumabhoy
(Chapter 2: Studying at medical school; Chapter 54: Getting ahead)
Core Surgical Trainee, Plastic and Reconstructive Surgery, Nottingham University Hospital NHS Trust, Nottingham, UK

Raghunath Kadiyala
(Chapter 13: Endocrinology and diabetes)
Consultant in Diabetes and Endocrinology, Stoke Mandeville Hospital, Buckinghamshire Healthcare NHS Trust, Aylesbury, UK

Sheirin Khalil
(Chapter 52: Other assessments)
GP Specialist Registrar, James Paget University Hospital, Great Yarmouth, UK

Harry Krishnan
(Chapter 50: Clinical examinations)
Specialist Trainee, Trauma and Orthopaedics, Northwest Thames Rotation, UK

Kar-Hung Kuet
(Chapter 10: Dermatology)
Specialist Registrar, Dermatology, Royal Hallamshire Hospital, Sheffield, UK

Mong -Loon Kuet
(Chapter 35: Ear, nose, and throat surgery)
Specialist Registrar, Ipswich Hospital NHS Trust, Ipswich, UK

Suhas S. Kumar
(Chapter 7: Anaesthetics)
Consultant, Department of Anaesthesia and Critical Care, Norfolk and Norwich University Hospital, Norwich, UK

Lily XLi
(Chapter 40: Trauma and orthopaedic surgery)
Orthopaedic Specialist Registrar, North West London rotation, UK

Firas Maghrabi
(Chapter 20: Infectious diseases and tropical medicine)
Clinical Research Fellow in Infectious Diseases, The National Aspergillosis Centre, Manchester University NHS Foundation Trust, Wythenshawe Hospital, Manchester, UK

David Metcalfe
(Chapter 8: Cardiology;
Chapter 30: Respiratory medicine;
Chapter 41: Vascular surgery)
Clinical Research Fellow in
Musculoskeletal Trauma,
University of Oxford, UK

Yasmeen Mulla
(Chapter 4: Preparing for
preclinical exams)
GP Specialty Trainee, Thames
Valley Deanery, Buckinghamshire
Healthcare Trust, UK

Biplab Nandi
(Chapter 38: Paediatric surgery)
Lecturer in Paediatric Surgery,
College of Medicine, University
of Malawi; Consultant Paediatric
Surgeon, Kamuzu Central
Hospital, Lilongwe, Malawi

Fiona Napier
(Chapter 3: Preclinical medi-
cine; Chapter 7: Anaesthetics;
Chapter 13: Endocrinology and dia-
betes; Chapter 14: Gastroenterology;
Chapter 21: Nephrology;
Chapter 22: Neurology)
Consultant, Emergency
Department, Derriford Hospital,
Plymouth, UK

Arjun Odedra
(Chapter 5: Intercalated de-
grees and special study modules;
Chapter 54: Getting ahead)
GP Specialist Registrar, Royal
Surrey County Hospital,
Guildford, UK

Nicola Okeahialam
(Chapter 6: Going clinical)
Specialist Registrar, Obstetrics
and Gynaecology, Chelsea
& Westminster Hospital,
London, UK

Vishal Patel
(Chapter 32: Breast surgery)
Breast and General
Surgery Specialist Registrar,
North West London
Deanery, UK

Benjamin Pinkey
(Chapter 6: Going clinical)
Consultant Paediatric
Radiologist, Department
of Radiology, Birmingham
Children's Hospital,
Birmingham Women's and
Children's NHS Foundation
Trust, UK

Emma Prower
(Chapter 11: Elderly care)
Intensive Care Specialist
Registrar, Kings College Hospital,
London, UK

Tasneem Rahman
(Chapter 19: Immunology and
allergies)
Specialist Registrar
in Immunology and
Allergy, Department of
Immunopathology,
Royal London Hospital,
London, UK

Fatimah Ravat
(Chapter 2: Studying at medical
school)
Postgraduate MSc Student,
Deanery of Biomedical Sciences,
University of Edinburgh,
Edinburgh, UK

Imran Raza
(Chapter 34: Colorectal surgery)
Specialist Registrar in
Colorectal and general surgery,
University College Hospital,
London, UK

Isabel Rodriguez-Goncer
(Chapter 20: Infectious diseases
and tropical medicine)
Senior Clinical Fellow in
Infectious Diseases, The National
Aspergillosis Centre, Manchester
University NHS Foundation
Trust, Wythenshawe hospital,
Manchester, UK

Shahbaz Roshanzamir
(Chapter 11: Elderly care)
Consultant Geriatrician and
General Physician, Department
of Ageing and Health, Guy's & St
Thomas' Hospital, London, UK

Hazim Sadideen
(Chapter 39: Plastic surgery)
Department of Surgery and
Cancer, Imperial College
London, London, UK

Ahmed-Ramadan Sadek
(Chapter 36: Neurosurgery)
Senior Neurosurgical
Registrar, Jason Brice Fellow
in Neurosurgical Research,
Department of Neurosurgery,
Wessex Neurological
Centre, University Hospital
Southampton, UK

Ashraf Sanduka
(Chapter 28: Pathology)
Consultant, Department of
Histopathology, West Suffolk
Hospital, Bury St Edmunds,
Suffolk, UK

Guy Schofield
(Chapter 27: Palliative medicine)
Specialist Registrar in Palliative
Medicine, Wellcome Trust
Society and Ethics Fellow,
Centre for Ethics in Medicine,
University of Bristol, UK

Katherine Schon
(Chapter 16: Genetics)
Specialist Registrar and
Academic Clinical Fellow,
Department of Clinical
Genetics, East Anglian
Medical Genetics Service,
Addenbrooke's Hospital,
Cambridge, UK

Eshan Senanayake
(Chapter 33: Cardiothoracic
surgery)
Specialist Registrar,
Department of Cardiothoracic
Surgery, University
Hospitals Birmingham
NHS Foundation Trust,
Birmingham, UK

Stephanie Slater
(Chapter 51: Written exams)
Senior House Officer,
Acute Medicine, Croydon
University Hospital, UK

Carmel Stober
(Chapter 31: Rheumatology)
Locum Consultant in
Rheumatology, Department
of Rheumatology, Cambridge
University Hospitals
NHS Foundation Trust,
Addenbrooke's Hospital,
Cambridge, UK

Amit Sud
(Chapter 18: Haematology)
Clinical Research Fellow, The
Institute of Cancer Research/
The Royal Marsden NHS
Foundation Trust, London, UK

Kapil Sugand
(Chapter 1: Starting as a medical student; Chapter 3: Preclinical medicine; Chapter 5: Intercalated degrees and special study modules; Chapter 8: Cardiology; Chapter 12: Emergency medicine; Chapter 15: General practice; Chapter 30: Respiratory medicine; Chapter 34: Colorectal surgery; Chapter 40: Trauma and Orthopaedics; Chapter 41: Vascular surgery; Chapter 43: Urology; Chapter 49: Preparing for clinical examinations; Chapter 50: Clinical examinations; Chapter 53: Making decisions; Chapter 54: Getting ahead)
Editor-in-Chief for OHMS, Trauma and Orthopaedics Specialist Registrar and Surgical Research Fellow, Imperial College London, UK,

Quen Tang
(Chapter 40: Trauma and orthopaedic surgery)
Specialist Registrar in Trauma and Orthopaedics, North West Thames Rotation, Department of Trauma and Orthopaedics, Chelsea and Westminster Hospital, London, UK

Hannah Tharmalingam
(Chapter 24: Oncology)
Oncology Registrar, Department of Oncology, Mount Vernon Cancer Centre, Northwood, UK

Jemma Theivendran
(Chapter 29: Psychiatry)
Specialist Registrar in Child and Adolescent Psychiatry, South West London and St George's Mental Health Trust; Honorary Clinical Lecturer, St George's, University of London, UK

Sri Thrumurthy
(Chapter 8: Cardiology; Chapter 30: Respiratory medicine; Chapter 41: Vascular surgery)
General Surgical Specialist Trainee, University College London Hospitals NHS Trusts, UK

Alex Tsui
(Chapter 22: Neurology)
Specialist Registrar, Clinical Research Fellow, MRC Unit for Lifelong Health and Ageing, University College London, UK

Laura Watson
(Chapter 15: General practice)
GP, Emergency Department, John Radcliffe Hospital, Oxford

Imran Yusuf
(Chapter 1: Starting as a medical student; Chapter 2: Studying at medical school; Chapter 6: Going clinical; Chapter 25: Ophthalmology; Chapter 50: Clinical examinations; Chapter 56: Career planning)
Ophthalmology Specialist Registrar and MRC Research Fellow, Oxford University, UK

Symbols and abbreviations

~		approximately
➔		cross-reference
↓		decreased
↑		increased
→		leading to
↔		normal
♫		website
±		with or without
2D		two-dimensional
3D		three-dimensional
5HT		5-hydroxytryptamine (serotonin)
AAA		abdominal aortic aneurysm
AAGBI		Association of Anaesthetists of Great Britain and Ireland
ABG		arterial blood gas
ACEI		angiotensin-converting enzyme inhibitor
ACJ		acromioclavicular joint
ACL		anterior cruciate ligament
ACR		albumin:creatinine ratio
ACS		acute coronary syndrome
ACTH		adrenocorticotropic hormone
ADP		adenosine diphosphate
ADPKD		autosomal dominant polycystic kidney disease
AF		atrial fibrillation
AFP		Academic Foundation Programme
AIDS		acquired immunodeficiency syndrome
AKI		acute kidney injury
ALF		Access to Learning Fund
ALP		alkaline phosphatase
ALS		advanced life support
AMD		age-related macular degeneration
ANA		antinuclear antibody
AP		anteroposterior
APTT		activated partial thromboplastin time
ARB		angiotensin receptor blocker
ARDS		acute respiratory distress syndrome
AS		aortic stenosis *or* ankylosing spondylitis

ASA	aminosalicylic acid
aSAH	aneurysmal subarachnoid haemorrhage
ASCT	allogenic stem cell transplant
ASIS	anterior superior iliac spine
AST	aspartate transaminase
ATLS®	Advanced Trauma Life Support®
ATN	acute tubular necrosis
AV	atrioventricular
AXR	abdominal X-ray
BAL	bronchoalveolar lavage
BCC	basal cell carcinoma
BCG	bacillus Calmette–Guérin
BMA	British Medical Association
BMedSci	Bachelor in Medical Sciences
BMI	body mass index
BNF	*British National Formulary*
BNFC	*British National Formulary for Children*
BNP	B-type natriuretic peptide
BP	blood pressure
BPH	benign prostatic hyperplasia
bpm	beats per minute
BPPV	benign paroxysmal positional vertigo
BSc	Bachelor of Science
BTS	British Thoracic Society
CABG	coronary artery bypass graft
CBD	common bile duct
CBT	cognitive behavioural therapy
CCT	certificate of completion of training
CD	Crohn's disease
CGA	comprehensive geriatric assessment
CHD	congenital heart disease
CJD	Creutzfeldt–Jakob disease
CK	creatine kinase
CMV	*Cytomegalovirus*
CNS	central nervous system
CO	cardiac output
COPD	chronic obstructive pulmonary disease
COX	cyclooxygenase
CPAP	continuous positive airway pressure
CPR	cardiopulmonary resuscitation

CRB	Criminal Record Bureau
CREST	calcinosis, Raynaud's phenomenon, (o)esophageal dysmotility, sclerodactyly, and telangiectasia
CRP	C-reactive protein
CS	caesarean section
CSF	cerebrospinal fluid
C-spine	cervical spine
CT	computed tomography
CTPA	computed tomography pulmonary angiogram
CV	curriculum vitae
CVA	cerebrovascular accident
CVC	central venous catheter
CVP	central venous pressure
CVS	cardiovascular system
CXR	chest X-ray
D&V	diarrhoea and vomiting
DC	direct current
DHx	drug history
DIC	disseminated intravascular coagulation
DIPJ	distal interphalangeal joint
DKA	diabetic ketoacidosis
DM	diabetes mellitus
DMARD	disease-modifying anti-rheumatoid drug
DPhil	Doctor of Philosophy
DRE	digital rectal examination
DSM	Diagnostic and Statistical Manual of Mental Disorders
DTaP	diphtheria, tetanus, and pertussis
DVLA	Driver and Vehicle Licensing Agency
DVT	deep vein thrombosis
EBV	Epstein–Barr virus
ECG	electrocardiography/electrocardiogram
ED	emergency department
EEG	electroencephalography/electroencephalogram
ELISA	enzyme-linked immunosorbent assay
EMQ	extended matching question
EPO	erythropoietin
ERCP	endoscopic retrograde cholangiopancreatography
ERV	expiratory reserve volume
ESR	erythrocyte sedimentation rate
ETOH	alcohol

ETT	endotracheal tube
EUS	endoscopic ultrasound
EVAR	endovascular aneurysm repair
FACS	fluorescence-activated cell sorting
FBC	full blood count
FEV_1	forced expiratory volume in 1 sec
FHx	family history
FISH	fluorescent *in situ* hybridization
FNA	fine-needle aspiration
FNAC	fine-needle aspiration cytology
FRC	functional residual capacity
FVC	forced vital capacity
FY1	Foundation Year 1
G6PD	glucose-6-phosphate dehydrogenase
GA	general anaesthesia
GC	gonorrhoea
GCA	giant cell arteritis
GCP	Good Clinical Practice
GCS	Glasgow coma scale
GHJ	glenohumeral joint
GI	gastrointestinal
GMC	General Medical Council
GORD	gastro-oesophageal reflux disease
GP	general practitioner
GTN	glyceryl trinitrate
GUM	genitourinary medicine
HAART	highly active antiretroviral therapy
Hb	haemoglobin
HbA1c	glycated haemoglobin
hCG	human chorionic gonadotropin
HD	Huntington disease
HDU	high dependency unit
HiB	*Haemophilus influenza* type B
HIV	human immunodeficiency virus
HL	Hodgkin lymphoma
HNPCC	hereditary non-polyposis colorectal cancer
HPB	hepatopancreatobiliary
HPC	history of presenting complaint
HPV	human papilloma virus
HR	heart rate

HSV	herpes simplex virus
IBD	inflammatory bowel disease
IC	inspiratory capacity
ICD	International Classification of Diseases
ICE	ideas, concerns, and expectations
ICP	intracranial pressure
Ig	immunoglobulin
IHD	ischaemic heart disease
IM	intramuscular
IMA	inferior mesenteric artery
INR	international normalized ratio
IOL	intraocular lens
IPJ	interphalangeal joint
IPPA	inspection, palpation, percussion, and auscultation
IPV	inactivated polio vaccine
IRV	inspiratory reserve volume
ITU	intensive therapy unit
IV	intravenous
IVDU	intravenous drug user
IVF	*in vitro* fertilization
JVP	jugular venous pressure
KUB	kidneys, ureters, and bladder
LCL	lateral collateral ligament
LDH	lactate dehydrogenase
LFT	liver function test
LIF	left iliac fossa
LMA	laryngeal mask airway
LMP	last menstrual period
LMWH	low-molecular-weight heparin
LP	lumbar puncture
LRTI	lower respiratory tract infection
LUQ	left upper quadrant
LV	left ventricular
MAP	mean arterial pressure
MC&S	microscopy, culture, and sensitivity
mcg	microgram
MCL	medial collateral ligament
MCPJ	metacarpophalangeal joint
MCQ	multiple-choice question
MCV	mean corpuscular volume

MDDUS	Medical Doctors and Dentists Defence Union of Scotland
MDT	multidisciplinary team
MDU	Medical Defence Union
MEN	multiple endocrine neoplasia
MHC	major histocompatibility complex
MI	myocardial infarction
MMR	measles, mumps, and rubella
MMSE	Mini–Mental State Examination
MoCA	Montreal Cognitive Assessment
MPS	Medical Protection Society
MR	mitral regurgitation
MRC	Medical Research Council
MRCP	magnetic resonance cholangiopancreatography
MRI	magnetic resonance imaging
MS	multiple sclerosis
MSk	musculoskeletal
MSU	midstream specimen of urine
MTPJ	metatarsophalangeal joint
MV	mitral valve
N&V	nausea and vomiting
NAFLD	non-alcoholic fatty liver disease
NAI	non-accidental injury
NASH	non-alcoholic steatohepatitis
NF1	neurofibromatosis type 1
NG	nasogastric
NHL	non-Hodgkin lymphoma
NHS	National Health Service
NICE	National Institute for Health and Care Excellence
NIHSS	National Institutes of Health Stroke Scale
NIV	non-invasive ventilation
NSAID	non-steroidal anti-inflammatory drug
NSTEMI	non-ST elevation myocardial infarction
O&G	obstetrics and gynaecology
OA	osteoarthritis
OGD	oesophagogastroduodenoscopy
OGTT	oral glucose tolerance test
OHFP2	*Oxford Handbook for the Foundation Programme*, second edition
OMFS	oral and maxillofacial surgery
OSCE	objective structured clinical examination

PA	posteroanterior
PBC	primary biliary cholangitis
PBL	problem-based learning
PC	presenting complaint
PCA	patient-controlled analgesia
PCI	percutaneous coronary intervention
PCL	posterior cruciate ligament
PCOS	polycystic ovarian syndrome
PCR	polymerase chain reaction
PE	pulmonary embolism
PEFR	peak expiratory flow rate
PEP	post-exposure prophylaxis
PET	positron emission tomography
PhD	Doctor of Philosophy
PICC	peripherally inserted central catheter
PID	pelvic inflammatory disease
PIPJ	proximal interphalangeal joint
PMHx	past medical history
PMR	polymyalgia rheumatica
PNS	peripheral nervous system
PO	orally
PPI	proton pump inhibitor
PR	*per rectum* (rectally)
PSA	prescribing skills assessment
PSC	primary sclerosing cholangitis
PTH	parathyroid hormone
PV	*per vaginam* (vaginally)
PVD	peripheral vascular disease
RA	rheumatoid arthritis
RAPD	relative afferent pupillary defect
RAS	renin–angiotensin system
RBC	red blood cell
Rh	rhesus
RIF	right iliac fossa
ROM	range of movement
RRT	renal replacement therapy
RSM	Royal Society of Medicine
RTC	road traffic collision
RUQ	right upper quadrant
RV	residual volume
SAH	subarachnoid haemorrhage

SAQ	short answer question
SBA	single best answer
SC	subcutaneously
SCC	squamous cell carcinoma
SCJ	sternoclavicular joint
SDH	subdural haematoma
SHO	senior house officer
SHx	social history
SIADH	syndrome of inappropriate antidiuretic hormone secretion
SIRS	systemic inflammatory response syndrome
SJS	Stevens–Johnson syndrome
SJT	situational judgement test
SLE	systemic lupus erythematosus
SMA	superior mesenteric artery
SOB	shortness of breath
SSc	systemic sclerosis
SSM	special study module
SSRI	selective serotonin reuptake inhibitor
stat	immediately
STEMI	ST elevation myocardial infarction
STI	sexually transmitted infection
STJ	scapulothoracic joint
SVC	superior vena cava
SVT	supraventricular tachycardia
T3	triiodothyronine
T4	thyroxine
TB	tuberculosis
TBI	traumatic brain injury
TCA	tricyclic antidepressant
TEN	toxic epidermal necrolysis
TIA	transient ischaemic attack
TLC	total lung capacity
TLS	tumour lysis syndrome
TNF	tumour necrosis factor
TOE	transoesophageal echocardiography
TSH	thyroid-stimulating hormone
TTE	transthoracic echocardiography
TURP	transurethral resection of the prostate
TV	tidal volume

TVF	tactile vocal fremitus
U&E	urea and electrolytes
UC	ulcerative colitis
UGI	upper gastrointestinal
URTI	upper respiratory tract infection
US	ultrasound *or* United States
UTI	urinary tract infection
V/Q	ventilation/perfusion
VC	vital capacity
VEGF	vascular endothelial growth factor
VF	ventricular fibrillation
VSD	ventricular septal defect
VT	ventricular tachycardia
VTE	venous thromboembolism
WCC	white cell count
WHO	World Health Organization

Part 1

Preclinical

Starting as a medical student

Congratulations!

Well done and congratulations on entering medical school! It has taken some blood, sweat, and possibly tears to get here, and you should feel proud of what you have achieved. You are about to enter a course of training from which you will emerge a highly skilled individual. You have tremendous potential to positively impact the lives of others, sometimes with compassionate words, other times with your intelligence or practical skills, and even through making new discoveries or forging new treatments. You are going to touch the lives of many people in a way that they will re-member and be immensely grateful for. Remember this throughout your training, especially if at times things seem tough. You should expect that your time at medical school might sometimes be challenging for all sorts of reasons. But always remember the goal, what you said in your per-sonal statement, and the immense privilege that lies in store during medical school, and after you qualify.

Medical school is a marathon instead of a sprint, so organization and time management are paramount to make the most of your course.

Before you start

Documentation
Prepare yourself for a plethora of paperwork in order to formally accept your position at medical school and begin your studies.

University acceptance package
Along with your acceptance letter, you will receive numerous important documents. Invest the time to read the contents, making a particular note of deadlines for submitting the necessary paperwork (often required many months prior to the course start date):
- Course preparation material.
- Fees and loan information.
- Occupational health questionnaire and vaccination forms.
- Disclosure and Barring Service (DBS) forms.
- Halls of residence application forms.

Student loans
Applying for student loans is a long process and any delay in submitting your form can delay your loan approval. Students studying in England, Scotland, Wales, and Northern Ireland can apply online to the Student Loans Company. You may also need to send in evidence such as proof of identity, address, household income (in case of income-assessed category), and accounting reports. Your loan, depending on your financial circumstances, will be divided into the following:
- *Tuition fees* (paid on your behalf to the university).
- *Maintenance loan* (£4375–£7675 depending on your term address).
- *Maintenance grant* (£50–£3354 depending on household income).
- *Special support grants* (in certain circumstances only).

Some important notes
- *Graduate students* are subject to different financial support.
- *Scottish students* can apply to the Students Awards Agency for Scotland and are eligible for student loans (£940–£4500) and bursaries (Young Students' Bursary, Independent Students' Bursary, and Students Outside Scotland Bursary).
- *Welsh students* are eligible for New Fee Grants and Assembly Learning Grants, in addition to the standard loans and grants.
- *Students in Northern Ireland* will be charged a maximum of £3575 per year and may be eligible to the standard loans and grants.

Living arrangements
Living at home
Approximately 20% of students opt to live at home which can contribute to significant financial savings over the years. There is a common misconception that a consequence of living at home is social isolation, but this need not be the case. University offers the first real opportunity for many students to gain their first experience of genuine independence, and can represent a golden opportunity for your personal as well as professional development.

Halls of residence

These are usually guaranteed for first-year students. You will be given a tour of the halls on open days. Preference might be given to those coming from other cities. Important considerations when ranking your preferences include:

- price per term
- distance from main campus and hospitals
- access links (e.g. walking, cycling, buses, trains, and driving)
- catering services (some may be self-catering)
- facilities (kitchen and bathroom-to-student ratio or en suite etc.)
- neighbourhood (distance to city centre, and adjacent shops/services)
- atmosphere and personality fit with current residents.

Private accommodation

(See ➔ Oxford Handbook for the Foundation Programme, second edition (OHFP2) p. 47).

Properties are listed in local newspapers, in shop windows, with estate agents, or on dedicated websites; but always see the accommodation before making your decision. If you decide to rent accommodation privately, ensure that the duration of your contract includes term time at least. All paperwork should be in order prior to starting the course including realistic estimates of water, gas, and electricity bills, and council tax. The websites listed in Box 1.1 specializing in university student accommodation may be useful.

Buying a property

Buying a property will require you to seek assistance from estate agents and mortgage advisers. Few students are in a position to consider buying a property in the region of their university, but willing parents/guardians looking for an investment opportunity might consider this option. Depending on your down-payment, mortgage loans and interest rates will vary according to your earnings and savings. Do not forget to account for associated costs including stamp duty, solicitor fees, and conveyancing fees. A fixed rate mortgage may provide some predictability regarding the repayment amount per month (versus tracker mortgages).

Box 1.1 University student accommodation websites

- Accommodation for students: ℘ www.accommodationforstudents.com
- Tiger Student Property: ℘ www.tigerstudentproperty.co.uk

The following websites may also help for both renting and buying:
- Rightmove: ℘ www.rightmove.co.uk
- Zoopla: ℘ www.zoopla.co.uk
- Prime Location: ℘ www.primelocation.com
- Student Union: the student union at your university may be a useful source of advice about accommodation.

Occupational health clearance

Since you will be handling sharps and come into contact with bodily fluids, you will not be allowed to participate in clinical training until you have submitted the following appropriate health documentation.

Vaccinations

You need to provide evidence from your general practitioner (GP) or vaccination clinics on at least:

- hepatitis B (including boosters)
- measles, mumps, and rubella (MMR)
- tuberculosis (bacillus Calmette–Guérin (BCG))
- meningitis C.

You may also be required to show records for *Haemophilus influenza* type B (HiB), polio (inactivated polio vaccine (IPV)), pneumococcal meningitis, diphtheria, tetanus, and pertussis (DTaP), hepatitis C, and varicella.

Health questionnaire

You are required to give your personal contact details and declare any medical conditions (including those that do not require treatment), mental health disorders (e.g. addictions, depression, and psychoses), duration of previous sick leave (from school or work), current medications, use of recreational drugs, and any other information you think may be pertinent to your professional practice. You may also be asked to sign a consent form for the occupational health department to contact your GP for access to relevant parts of your notes.

Most health-related concerns which could influence your practice should have already been addressed before/at the application stage of applying to medical school. It is your responsibility as a future healthcare practitioner to provide any and all relevant information which may impact the care you can provide to patients. Withholding such information will invariably lead to professional disciplinary measures, and risk jeopardizing your place at medical school before it has even begun.

Criminal Record Bureau (CRB) check

You will be required to offer your personal contact details, national insurance number, addresses for the past 5 years, and any criminal offences that you have been prosecuted for.

Enjoy your holidays

Since you will become busy with medical school, new colleagues, and extracurricular activities, make the most of your holidays with your family and friends, travelling, and pursuing your hobbies.

Top 10 things to buy

You are starting a new chapter in your life, and you may benefit from buying a few new items to help get you off to a good start.

1. *Clothes*: everyone generally adopts two styles—casual and formal. You will need comfortable smart-casual wear for lectures, tutorials, and practicals (e.g. jeans, sweaters). When on hospital firms, you are expected to look professional with a shirt and formal trousers or a skirt; avoid wearing anything too revealing.
2. *Books*: most books will be available to borrow from the library. Yet, there may not be enough to lend out the more popular texts to every student in which case it may be worth buying them (even second-hand or from your seniors). You only tend to find this out once you begin your course and see what is available, so factor these costs into your balance sheet in the first month of medical school. There is no harm in waiting until the first few weeks of medical school have passed, during which time you can ask for advice from senior students, peers, or tutors and look at copies from the library to determine the most suitable books to buy if needed.
3. *Laptop*: essential, despite good computing facilities at every medical school, the luxury of answering online questions, writing up coursework, preparing presentations, and surfing for entertainment in the comfort of your own room means this is a necessary item for most students. Note that some companies, including Apple, offer educational discounts once you have a student card, so it may be worth delaying any new purchase until then. Software licences may also be bought at a reduced rate, or free, through the university, so do ask the IT department for advice on software you are considering buying.
4. *Extra reading lights/extension cables*.
5. *Bed sheets and towels*.
6. *Stationery and rucksack*.
7. *Kitchen utensils*: there will be some basic equipment already provided, but most students tend to bring their own as well.
8. *Iron/ironing board*.
9. *Travel/railway card*: cheaper than buying single tickets and you are likely to be eligible for more discount using your student ID card
10. *White/lab coat*: for use in certain laboratory/dissection classes (typically mentioned in the introductory documentation provided by the medical school either before you begin or in your first class).

Avoid rushing at the last minute to buy everything; it will take time to settle in, but having the right extension cables, cutlery, and stationery will make the transition a lot easier.

Buying a stethoscope

Invented by René Laennec at Necker-Enfants Malades Hospital in Paris (1816), the hallmark of medicine is the stethoscope. However, there are literally hundreds of choices available. Some are internationally renowned and some are disposable and for short-term use. It is worth investing in a quality stethoscope, which, if durable, will stay with you until the day you retire. You will require a stethoscope for most clinical examinations, in order to auscultate heart, breath, and bowel sounds, blood vessels, and measure blood pressure.

- The diaphragm (larger circle in inset in Fig. 1.1) is designed for detecting high-pitched sounds with firm skin contact, while the bell (smaller circle) is intended for detecting low-pitched sounds with light skin contact.
- Shorter tubing minimizes sound loss and transmits a better sound quality.
- Pressing more firmly will enhance sound transmission.
- You can switch from diaphragm to bell by twisting the chest piece.
- The holes within the eartips should face you when inserted into your ears.

Uses

- *Auscultation* : listening to breath, heart, blood vessel, and bowel sounds (including murmurs, abnormal breath sounds, bowel obstruction/ileus, and bruits).
- *Counting*: heart and breathing rates.
- *Manually measuring blood pressure* : listening for Korotkoff sounds using a manual sphygmomanometer.
- *Hearing aid*: if you put the eartips in the patient's ears and speak into the chest piece.
- *Measuring size of the liver*: if you place the chest piece below the nipple and start scratching from the waist upwards until the sound becomes dull, this indicates the lower border of the liver.

The basics of stethoscopes

Brand

The most popular option is to buy a Littman stethoscope, but other brands include Welch Allyn, Tytan Merlin, and Reister, to name just a few.

Model

The commonest option is the 'standard' or 'classic' model. Stethoscopes can either be analogue, which is the standard choice, or digital, which are more expensive and usually reserved for specialists. By converting acoustic sounds into electrical signals, electronic stethoscopes (or stethophones) amplify volume, reduce ambient noise, differentiate between high- and low-frequency sounds, and are pressure sensitive. Many have Bluetooth compatibility to record, analyse, and store audiovisual data on your smartphone and laptop. While there are many stethoscopes available for clinical use, all that is required for your exams and clinical practice is the standard model of stethoscope with a bell and a diaphragm.

Specialist

There are dedicated stethoscopes for various medical specialities including cardiology, paediatrics, and respiratory medicine. Again, at this stage it is worth being aware of novel types of stethoscopes, to know what to avoid when purchasing your generic 'standard' model stethoscope.

Tips

- *Colour*: almost every colour is available but many consider traditional colours (e.g. black) more appropriate than fluorescent pink.
- *Engraving*: you may request an engraving when purchasing a stethoscope (e.g. name, email address/contact details if lost).
- *Offers*: you may receive a good quality stethoscope or a substantial discount when signing up to the freshers' fair. Also, look out for special offers from your medical school shop and professional bodies.
- *Price*: there is no need to buy a very expensive stethoscope that is designed for specialities (e.g. cardiology) this early on in medical school. Most doctors use the standard model for their entire careers.
- *Infection control*: it is good practice to sterilize your stethoscope after every use with alcohol wipes to prevent cross-infection between patients. Also clean the eartips regularly and avoid sharing them to prevent infection between users.

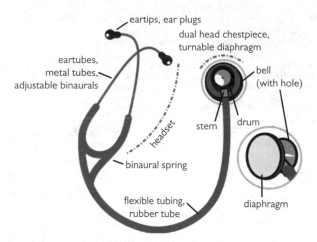

Fig. 1.1 Anatomy of a stethoscope. Reproduced from https://commons.wikimedia. org/wiki/File:Stethoscope.svg under Creative Commons Attribution-Share Alike 4.0 International license.

Paying for medical school

As one of the longest university courses, studying medicine requires effective financial planning to avoid spiralling debts. The longer course means that you will spend more by continuing to pay rent and living costs while missing out on 3 years of paid employment. You should therefore think carefully about your budget from the first day of medical school, and tally your monthly and yearly incomings and outgoings. You do not need be an accountant to make these simple estimates and avoid spending beyond your means.

Budget

It often helps to divide your outgoings into the following categories:

- Rent
- Utility bills and council tax
- Food
- Travel
- Textbooks and stationery
- Entertainment
- Clothes
- Electronic appliances (e.g. laptop)
- Miscellaneous (e.g. laundry, holidays, toiletries, and sundries).

Rent

Depends on halls of residence versus private accommodation, catering facilities, size of place, en suite, suburb, and city. This is generally a fixed cost and therefore is easy to include in your estimates of monthly expenditure.

Utility bills

May vary again depending if you live in halls of residence (usually included in fees) or private accommodation (usually excluded), number of room/flat/housemates, but on average will come to £50–£75/month. Other bills such as a TV licence, Internet connection, and landline/mobile costs also need to be taken into account. As a full-time student, you may apply for council tax exemption through your university or GOV.UK (℗ www.gov.uk). Again, this represents a fixed sum which can be accurately included in your estimates of monthly expenditure.

Food

You can still eat and drink well as a student as long as you spend sensibly. If your halls of residence have catering, you will receive breakfast and dinner included in the fees. You might consider bringing packed lunches to save money. A reasonable budget would be £30–£50/week which includes treating yourself to the odd takeaway or restaurant meal. Do not forget to find out which food outlets/restaurants offer a student discount, and be sure to register with an online voucher company for two-for-one and 50% discounts on meals (e.g. ℗ www.vouchercodes.co.uk, ℗ www.moneysavingexpert.com/deals/cheap-restaurant-deals).

Travel

Halls of residence are normally close to campus but you may need to make travel arrangements to hospitals. Universities near city centres have excellent public transport access so research your local amenities, and consider all the discounted options available, especially for regular predictable commutes e.g. travel pass, student rail card. Many students save money by choosing to cycle between sites. Occasionally, universities may offer some funding towards travel costs, particularly if you are required to travel a significant distance away from campus. For those with cars, applications for parking permits may be required for hospital sites or residential parking.

Textbooks and stationery

Most textbooks can be borrowed from the university library but popular textbooks on the recommended reading list may be worth buying. Set aside around £100 for books and stationery per year. Big savings can be made by buying used books from students in the years above or online. Universities may have online access to journals, textbooks, and databases. Be cautious about buying any scientific text that is more than a few editions old, as the material can be quite dated. Some useful websites include:

- Amazon: www.amazon.co.uk
- eBay: www.ebay.co.uk
- Used Books: www.usedbooksearch.co.uk/UK.htm
- Waterstones Marketplace: www.waterstonesmarketplace.com.

Entertainment

Work hard but also play hard. It is important to remember that while you have many years of important work ahead of you, relaxation and socializing are as fundamental to your success as learning medicine. A great deal of this should come without a price tag, as friends often make the best (and cheapest) distraction from studying. Be sure to broaden your horizons beyond the nightlife, explore the new city you have moved into, join clubs and societies at your student union, or just socialize with your new friends. You do not have to spend large sums of money to relax or enjoy yourself, and a sensible budget would be £40–£80/week depending on your location and financial circumstances.

- The National Union of Students (NUS) offer the NUS card which entitles students to a wide range of discounts from restaurants, cinemas, high street shops, electronics, and travel.
- Student Beans (www.studentbean.com) advertise the top 20 offers of the month as well as the offer of the week, saving you money on entertainment, food, clothes, and more. Surveys that pay you for participating are also advertised.

Sources of funding

Many students are financially independent and there are numerous resources available to fund your living expenses:

- Student loan
- Maintenance grants
- Bank loans
- Bank overdrafts
- Employment allowance
- Access to Learning Fund
- Hardship fund
- State benefits
- Competitions
- Scholarships
- Medical school prizes
- Charities.

Student loan and maintenance grant

All students will be entitled to a student loan (to pay for tuition) as well as maintenance loans and possibly grants. Grants are subject to a means-tested assessment (of the household income) and do not have to be paid back. If you live at home during term time then you are likely to qualify for a smaller maintenance loan. Living and studying in capital cities may also yield higher loans. International students will have different criteria since tuition fees vary.

Organizations

- Student finance section of UK government site: ℘ www.gov.uk/student-finance/overview
- Student Loans Company: ℘ www.slc.co.uk
- MoneySavingExpert.com: ℘ www.moneysavingexpert.com/students/student-loans-tuition-fees-changes
- Universities and Colleges Admissions Service (UCAS) undergraduate student loans: ℘ www.ucas.com/ucas/undergraduate/finance-and-support/undergraduate-tuition-fees-and-student-loans.

Bank loans

High street banks and building societies offer professional development loans and graduate loans specifically to university students, such as the following organizations (subject to change):

Bank	Website	Max. amount	APR
NatWest	℘ www.natwest.com	£1000–£25,000	7.7% or 8.9%
Barclays	℘ www.barclays.co.uk	£300–£10,000	5.7–9.9%
Co-operative	℘ www.co-operativebank.co.uk	£300–£10,000	9.9%

The usual repayment period is up to 5 years and there is an option to start paying after graduating and working for a few months. Make sure that you take time to read the terms and conditions and consider the outcomes of fixed versus flexible interest rates. You should think very carefully about taking on additional unnecessary debts, and never take on instant payday loans; these can be offered as 'fast cash' with ludicrous (but often very well hidden) interest rates of >1000%.

It is very rare, but not unheard of, for medical students to be declared bankrupt, often precipitated by a series of these short-term loans, with serious personal and professional ramifications. Be cautious, and seek independent financial advice wherever necessary.

Overdrafts

These are also very helpful, especially if within a student account. You may also be offered lower interest rates and other incentives such as vouchers and discounts. Again, you should think very carefully about taking on additional unnecessary debts for short-term benefits, realizing that any expenditure will need to be returned (and often with significant additional cost to yourself).

Employment

You might be able to earn a little extra with part-time employment. Consider positions in the student union, local shops, gyms, telephone centres, or tutoring. Temporary employment during long summer holidays is also a popular option. You must be careful not to stretch yourself too thinly, as medicine is a demanding course and should remain your priority.

Allowance from parents or guardians

Offers a safety net in case you need funds in an emergency. If they have agreed to provide you with some financial support, it is probably sensible to receive the money by regular standing orders or direct debits rather than infrequent lump sums, which will also help you to budget.

Access to Learning Fund (ALF)/hardship funds

These are interchangeable terms in which the finance department of your university may be able to lend you small amounts (usually a couple of hundred pounds) in an emergency or due to unseen circumstances. This help is typically reserved for students from low-income families who need financial support to remain on the course. These are usually loans (repayable) and may become grants (non-repayable) at their discretion. Applications are assessed on an individual basis. You might be asked to provide evidence of parental income and your bank statements for the past few months to see if you are eligible for fiscal support. ALF is referred to as the Financial Contingency Fund (FCF) in Wales, Support Funds in Northern Ireland, and Discretionary Funds in Scotland.

State benefits

These are available on a means-tested or non-means-tested basis to select groups including students with dependents, disabilities, or long-term illness, for instance. The following websites may be helpful:

- Turn2us: ℰ www.turn2us.org.uk
- Citizens Advice: ℰ www.adviceguide.org.uk.

Prize money

A huge arena of open competition exists for medical students to win prize money. Obviously this forms a less reliable source of regular income, but can nicely supplement your income and boost your curriculum vitae (CV).

Scholarships

These are awarded on your academic merit:
- Internal are offered by your medical school on the basis of your interview or exam performances by assessors. You may not be permitted to apply for specific ones. Ask the undergraduate medical school office for more information and to check your eligibility. Further information can also be found on your university website.
- External are offered by other organizations and are usually based on applications. You may be asked to demonstrate academic merit by sending in your CV or an essay to the board members. Ask at your undergraduate medical school office or the Medical Student Union office for more details on external scholarships. The Royal Colleges, Royal Society of Medicine, and specialty associations offer a variety of prizes specifically for medical students.

Medical school prizes

Are usually reserved for those who score the highest marks in written and clinical exams at the end of the year. Hence, no one will be able to apply for these prizes. There may be other prizes you can apply for which may be awarded for undertaking an elective abroad, contributing to the student union, or volunteering. These prizes are still competitive but less so than national contents since these are reserved for your medical school only. This information can be found on your university website as well as on the Royal College websites that run medical student competitions (e.g. elective).

Charities

May offer scholarships or educational grants to students who may have a connection with the organization, their work, location, or background. Use a search engine to find these opportunities, and consider the following publications (published annually):

- *Grants Register* by Palgrave Macmillan.
- *Directory for Grant Making Trusts* by Charities Aid Foundation.
- *Guide to Educational Grants* by Directory of Social Change.

For more general and useful information for funding undergraduate and graduate medical students, visit the following websites:

- Money 4 Med Students: ℘ www.money4medstudents.org
- British Medical Association: ℘ www.bma.org.uk/developing-your-career/studying-medicine/guide-to-medical-student-finance
- Leeds Widening Access to Medical School: ℘ www.wanttobeadoctor.co.uk
- General financial advice: ℘ www.moneysavingexpert.com.

Your first week

This will be a busy but exciting week, and you can expect to do the following:

- Moving in
- Freshers' meeting day
- Freshers' night/roadshow
- Freshers' week
- Introductory lectures
- Freshers' fair.

Moving in

This will take considerable time. If you live in the city, it would be helpful to bring your car and some (ideally willing) parents and siblings to help you. You might choose to visit beforehand to establish what amenities will be available at your accommodation, before bringing the kitchen sink!

Freshers' meeting day

This is the first time you will have a chance to meet with your year and interact with other students. This might take the form of a meet-and-greet in a large hall or over a barbeque. Use this opportunity to meet as many new faces as you can.

Freshers' night/roadshow

This is the first evening of activities for medical students where you will mingle with your classmates and your seniors, and often be adopted by a 'family'. Use this valuable resource to ask about anything that's on your mind about medical school, the course, and halls of residence—they remember what it was like to be in your shoes and you'll find everyone is eager to help and welcome you.

Freshers' week

This consists of orientation and activities planned every day for you to familiarize yourself with your surroundings and mingle with your peers. Relax, meet new people, and enjoy the festivities. You will be spending 4–6 years with your year group and will find it easier to get through the course with supportive friends and classmates.

Introductory lectures

These will be given by a group of medical students, tutors, lecturers, and possibly an influential veteran or living legend of your university. You will listen to talks given by the dean, consultants, and professors about what to expect at medical school. They will give you some advice on how to make the most of your course, juggling extracurricular activities, professional conduct on firms, and tips on scoring highly in exams. Feel free to ask anything at the end of the lecture, either in front of your colleagues or in private.

Freshers' fair

This is when every club and society that make up the student union set up a stall and recruit new members to sign up. There may also be incentives for joining for a very small fee per year (on average £5 per annum) depending on the activities offered.

There is usually a frenzy to sign up to everything that catches your eye but be realistic and ask yourself which society you will most likely end up committing the most to. Some clubs may also offer taster courses before requesting membership fees (e.g. fencing) so that you have time to make an informed decision after trying them out.

Look out for the following professional organizations and indemnity or insurance companies which can represent you for your entire career:

- *British Medical Association* (BMA; www.bma.org.uk): the political representation of doctors; offers medical students national representation, online education resources, free library loans, discounts on medical supplies, advice on electives, and monthly *Student British Medical Journal*—the first year is free.
- *Royal Society of Medicine* (RSM; www.rsm.ac.uk): an apolitical organization with national representation hosting a multitude of educational events, lectures, career advice, and competitions all year round. Other facilities include use of a bar, library, access to the *Journal of Royal Society of Medicine* (*JRSM*), and discounted accommodation in the heart of London—membership from £33.33 in your first year.
- *Medical Defence Union* (MDU; www.themdu.com): a mutual not-for-profit organization offering its members guidance, support, and defence in addressing medicolegal issues, complaints, and claims. Student membership is free and benefits include a quarterly digital journal, revision resources and situational judgement test (SJT) support, indemnity for your elective, exclusive access to The Electives Network, events sponsorship, local liaison managers, and confidential medicolegal advice.
- *Medical Protection Society* (MPS; www.medicalprotection.org/uk): offers medicolegal advice and assistance throughout the medical career. Other benefits include discounts on Oxford Handbooks and other series, regional representation, elective and career advice, event sponsorship, and free mock paper on SJTs—membership free for students.
- *Wesleyan* (www.wesleyan.co.uk): provides free income protection for medical students. Offers contact with dedicated Student Liaison Manager to assist with financial planning and sponsoring various events. Also provide Elsevier book and medical equipment discounts, free career guides on writing CVs and job interview skills, advice on electives, free RSM Student Lite membership, and tips on safeguarding financial welfare—membership free for students.
- *Medical Doctors and Dentists Defence Union of Scotland* (MDDUS; www.mddus.com): an independent mutual organization offering expert medicolegal advice and professional indemnity for doctors. Membership benefits consist of book discount, quarterly 'Summons' journal, access to online resource library, and a chance to apply for elective travel scholarship—membership free for students.

Work–life balance

It is your sole responsibility to look after yourself the best you can. As a medical student, your primary aim is to learn the theory and practice of medicine. You must also learn how to cope with a physically and emotionally demanding vocation and develop mechanisms to deal with its challenges: at times you may feel fed up, exhausted, demoralized, upset, stressed, and pushed to the limit. As a medical student, you must establish a sustainable lifestyle in which all aspects of your life can be fulfilled, in unison. By doing so, your chances of sustaining a career as a doctor—which may last 40 years or more—are greatly improved. It is very important that you register with a local GP in your first few weeks as a medical student, so that you can get help if necessary. Universities have clear lines of pastoral support which you should seek if needed.

Burnout

This is the term often given to the state of being exhausted and/or demoralized about work (lack of enjoyment, stress, physical exhaustion); it is a form of work-related depression that entails negative self-concepts, negative job attitudes, and a loss of concern about patients. Its estimated prevalence is 25–76% in doctors. Factors contributing to burnout include excessive workloads, patient pressures, lack of control, interference from managers, insecurity, reorganization, poor support, perceived threats of complaints or violence, and dysfunctional workplaces (BMA website). It is important to recognize the signs of burnout in yourself, and even in colleagues so that you can seek to address any potentially reversible causes of burnout, and identify strategies to deal with it. This applies equally to your medical student years. If you feel you may be suffering burnout, or be at risk, you may find burnout questionnaires helpful in screening for it (see ➲ 'Resources', p. 19).

Mechanisms to avoid burnout

Sleep

Requirements for sleep vary between individuals. If you are tired at the start of the working day, you are at risk of burnout. Ensure you are well rested; 7–8 hours of sleep is suggested. Consider limiting caffeine intake if you have sleep disturbance.

Friends and family

These may be among your greatest allies, and are likely to form a support network that you can access at any time. Non-medics may provide useful emotional support, and those with a medical background may provide practical advice.

Colleagues

These may face similar challenges and provide meaningful advice to challenges (peer groups or mentoring relationships). Your tutors should be the first port of call, as they may have training in helping you to deal with stressors related to your work and life outside of it. Contact them early before a problem becomes entrenched and less easily addressed.

Diet

An enjoyable meal can help in alleviating stress. It is essential you establish a balanced diet, and find times to eat and drink during the working day. This can sometimes be challenging: consider taking a flask for an accessible drink and a packed lunch.

Exercise

Aim to undertake at least four to five sessions of exercise, lasting at least 30 min, every week if possible. Indulge in forms of exercise that are accessible to you, and that you tend to enjoy. Playing a sport that you enjoy with others will provide escapism and potentially valuable sources of support. Enjoying the outdoors is important.

Hobbies

Indulge in the hobbies you enjoy: music, drawing, painting, photography, etc. Creative hobbies offer a powerful escapism from medicine, perhaps because medicine is, for the most part, minimally creative, and doctors tend to enjoy creativity.

Counselling

This is both understated and underestimated and is associated with a falsely negative stigma, especially among the younger generations. In fact, it is common practice to have a 'shrink' for successful professionals in the US, who use this sacred personal time to reflect, plan, and work through personal issues in a safe environment, without judgement and criticism, governed by a trained expert. In this way, you can feel heard and maintain firm control over your decisions and reactions without having to act out, make mistakes, and then waste time and energy performing damage control due to destructive consequences.

Resources

- BMA Burnout questionnaire: ℘ https://web2.bma.org.uk/drs4drsburn.nsf/quest?OpenForm.
- Royal College of Psychiatrists (RCPsych) guide to surviving as a doctor: ℘ www.rcpsych.ac.uk/PDF/PSS-guide-15_for%20web.pdf.
- Arnold J, Randall R, Oatterson F, et al. (2016). *Work Psychology: Understanding Human Behaviour in the Workplace* (6th edn). Pearson Education Limited.
- British Medical Association (1998). *The Misuse of Alcohol and Other Drugs by Doctors. Report of a Working Group*. BMA.

Ten responsibilities of medical students

1. *Correct declaration of occupational health questionnaire*: you will be penalized if any necessary information is withheld or falsified. You must also report to occupational health in case of needle-stick injuries when on firms for further testing.
2. *Budgeting*: stick to it and save some funds for a rainy day!
3. *Law*: you are now an adult and the law applies to you like it applies to everyone else. Any crime will question your professionalism and affect your right to work in healthcare.
4. *Meet assignment deadlines*: you must submit assessments on time since extensions are only granted in extreme, unforeseen circumstances at the discretion of the examining board. If you think you have grounds for an extension, then make an application as early as possible to allow time for deliberation.
5. *Communal chores*: you and your roommates should all chip in to complete chores out of courtesy to one another.
6. *Seek counselling when required*: recognize your limitations since there is no shame in admitting when you need additional support and guidance. Besides your university student counselling services, counselling can be provided by your friends and family, your personal tutor, and the welfare officer. You will not be a safe doctor especially if you have unresolved emotional inner conflict.
7. *Attendance*: you are expected to attend (and sign in when required) lectures, seminars, practicals, and tutorials on campus as well as your clinical firms and associated teaching sessions with doctors.
8. *Meet with personal tutor*: you must make an effort to keep in touch with your personal tutor. In the worst-case scenario, if you need your tutor to represent and defend you to the medical school, your personal tutor can only support you after having known you for a considerable amount of time.
9. *Keep up with bookwork*: amid all the joy of being a medical student, living in halls, socializing with your new friends, and pursuing your extracurricular activities, it is easy to begin to lag behind with work. If possible, try to keep chipping away at your workload, and ensure you finish off your bookwork, revision, and assignments in good time to minimize stress and so that you can enjoy the other aspects of university life.
10. *Balance*: strive to achieve a balance between keeping up with your work (studies, revision, and assignments) and play (relaxing, socializing, and hobbies). Look after yourself, eat well, and exercise. Healthy mind, healthy body. Try not to commit to too many activities (work or play) as this will spread you too thinly and reduce the quality of your contributions.

Ten tips on being a successful student doctor

1. *Bring in Oxford Handbook titles*: if you are waiting around, then prepare beforehand by reading your Oxford Handbooks. Read in advance to prepare for predictable clinical encounters (if you are going to a respiratory clinic, perhaps refresh your memory on chest examination and common respiratory disorders). This will impress your trainers.

2. *Clerking and presenting patients*: each rotation will allow practising of focused histories and detailed examinations. Aim to clerk with focused histories and thoroughly examine many patients in clinics and on the ward before presenting to your doctors. You may also be expected to present patients at ward rounds which is good practice for when you become a junior doctor.

3. *Supervision*: to ensure that you are clerking, examining, and interacting with the patient or performing a procedure competently, ask one of your seniors to supervise a consultation. This will be excellent practice for exams (see ➲ Chapter 50).

4. *Constructive feedback*: be able to handle criticism well. Any advice given to you is for your own benefit. Conversely, do not take it to heart. Learn from your mistakes; better as a student than as a doctor.

5. *Read patient notes*: it is good practice to clerk patients and then compare your findings with their notes. With time and experience, your clerking will be closer to the written notes.

6. *Observe and reflect*: see how your doctors interact with patients with respect to communication, examining for signs, and implementing the management plan. Take a step back and reflect on what you have observed. Reflection is a very important skill because it will provide you with insight to grow as a doctor. Ask yourself what you learnt, what you liked about a consultation, and what you would do differently next time.

7. *Taking initiative*: there will be long pauses during your day where you find yourself waiting. If time permits, aim to clerk and present a patient, read patient notes, or prepare for the next teaching session. With more time on your hands as a medical student, get involved with clinical research and departmental audits (see ➲ pp. 1021–1023). Your seniors will appreciate you more if they see you managing your time effectively, which will have a positive impact on your evaluation.

8. *Punctuality*: better to be 5 min early so that you do not miss out on precious teaching time or letting others wait around for you. This will also be commented on during your sign off and evaluation.

9. *Shadow multidisciplinary team (MDT) members*: holistic patient care is provided through a MDT approach. Spend time shadowing and learning about the functions of ward nurses, physiotherapists, occupational therapists, social workers, dietitians, and clinical psychologists at MDT meetings (at least weekly).

10. *Infection control*: reduce the risk of cross-infection between patients by wearing gloves/aprons and washing hands/stethoscopes.

Studying at medical school

Choosing a medical school

Location

To stay or not to stay?

An important factor to consider in choosing a university and medical school is how close you want to stay to your home. You might already know whether you want to stay close or go as far as possible! Everybody is different, but it is important to note how close your university is as well as travel costs if you plan to visit home often.

Campus or city?

Some universities are self-contained and all of their main buildings are located on campus whereas others have their buildings scattered within a city or town. Some students prefer the campus option as it provides a lovely 'university bubble' to live in during their 5 or 6 years of medical school as opposed to the hubbub of a city-based university. Keep in mind that the medical school may not always be located on campus or near the other main buildings of the university and that you may need to travel further.

These two types of university offer different kinds of lifestyle; campus universities often have all the necessities located on the campus, including shops, a gym, bookstores, and even banks, leaving little need to venture beyond university grounds with everything you could want in walking distance. This is both convenient but also restrictive in that you have little reason to go outside the bubble of campus.

Having a campus full of students is great for making friends and socializing since accommodation blocks are usually placed together, but options to go out to socialize may be limited. City and town universities have far more options, but accommodation may be at a further distance from the university buildings. They provide the benefit of being within the city centre; therefore city centre amenities are readily accessible, but not always within a close distance as on a campus university. Public transport may be your preferred option of travel rather than walking.

You would definitely be advised to visit universities on open days to get a 'feel' for which type of university you think would suit you as well as the university in general—you may be surprised!

Course

The course is possibly the most important aspect to think about when choosing a medical school. Although the content taught at each school will be similar, courses will definitely vary on a few key points.

Different teaching styles

Some medical schools place emphasis on traditional teaching, which will consist of more lectures whereas others emphasize problem-based learning (PBL), which involves a lot of self-directed learning. These styles impact the amount of contact time you receive. Some schools vary in their methods for teaching different topics—you will need to judge for yourself which teaching style will suit you best.

Length of course

Most medical courses last 5 years, but some last for 6 (with the addition of an intercalated Bachelor of Science (BSc)). Generally, courses are split into 3 years of preclinical learning, which will teach the theoretical side of medicine, with some or no clinical skills training, whereas the last 2 or 3 years are clinical placement years where you learn in a hospital or a GP practice. Although some universities offer a 5-year medical course, they do also offer the opportunity to intercalate and get an additional degree, which means one more year at university!

Content

Some aspects of modules will be different from the standard lectures; anatomy is usually either taught by performing dissections (students themselves remove tissue from a cadaver) or using prosections (anatomical structures that have already been dissected) which is something to consider if you have a preference as not all medical schools allow their students to dissect. Another aspect which differs in courses is early clinical learning—some medical schools teach their students basic clinical skills and allow students to visit hospitals and GP clinics in the preclinical years as part of their learning, whereas other courses may not introduce this until the clinical years.

Entry requirements

Awareness of the entry requirements for each medical school is very important. You want to make sure that you fit the requirements and take any necessary tests and undergo work experience before you apply.

Grades

Most medical schools will ask for three A grades at A level, often in at least two science subjects, but different universities have different specifications so it is vital that you check the entry requirements for the universities you are considering to ensure that you meet or can meet the basic grade requirement and have the right subjects. Medical schools place different emphasis on considering GCSE results, so this is also worth investigating; usually a grade B or higher is asked for in English, maths, and science subjects at GCSE.

Personal statement

This is an important part of your application—this is where you have the chance to show the admissions officer at the medical school why they should consider you. Medical schools place differing emphasis on personal statements, but use your personal statement to talk about why you want to do medicine and how you possess the qualities they are looking for in a medical student and future doctor. A good personal statement can highlight you as an ideal applicant. Display your passion and conviction for medicine and remember to check for spelling and grammar errors! Also, show your statement to your tutors who have plenty of experience.

Work experience

Medical schools are unlikely to consider applicants without any type of clinical work experience. They understand that it is not always easy to obtain work experience in a hospital or GP setting, but any kind of healthcare experience, such as volunteering in a care home for a few months, will support your application—the more work experience you have, the better, as you demonstrate that you are both committed and aware of what working in healthcare can entail.

Aptitude tests

Most (but not all) medical schools list an aptitude test in their requirements; the UK Clinical Aptitude Test (UKCAT) is the most common test and is looked at by most medical schools but the BioMedical Admissions Test (BMAT) is sometimes used instead. Medical schools place different emphasis on aptitude tests—sometimes they are used as primary criteria for consideration of an application and other times may be used to consider borderline applicants. These tests need to be completed as part of your application so it may be a good idea to research which medical schools would be most likely to accept you based on your results.

Note

More information on the UKCAT and BMAT can be found online at ✍ www.ukcat.ac.uk/ and ✍ www.admissionstestingservice.org/for-test-takers/bmat/ respectively. These websites provide information about what the tests consist of and how to book them.

Open days

You are strongly encouraged to visit the medical schools that you are considering as this can change your mind about your preferences. Open days give you the chance to attend lectures at the schools to give you more information on the courses available. They also provide the opportunity to speak to current medical students who can give you a real insight into the life of a medical student.

Learning styles

Having insight into how you learn most effectively will benefit you at medical school. As a medical student, you are expected to learn and retain vast amounts of information. The sheer volume of new 'stuff' to get to grips with can be overwhelming, which is why it is key that you start learning effectively from early on. Naturally, individuals learn in different ways and you may already have techniques that you recognize aid your learning.

Examples of different learning styles

Visuospatial learning

- When concepts and ideas are presented graphically in order to help learning, thus visual learners are generally quite good at interpreting graphs and charts.
- Ideas can be associated spatially and/or with images and shapes such as mind maps and diagrams showing relationships between ideas. Use of colour and size to emphasize key concepts is also helpful as well as highlighting, watching videos, and using flash cards.

Auditory learning

- When an individual learns through listening. This involves hearing and speaking as ways to absorb information.
- If you are fortunate, you may have lecturers that record their lectures and upload them—this is your best tool to help with ideas that you may not completely understand.
- If your lecturers do not record their lectures, you may be able to do so yourself using a voice recorder—remember to ask permission from the lecturer first though! Other ways can be to turn your notes into a chant or song, or associate particular topics with a certain kind of music. Or to come up with acronyms and a song, such as for remembering the 12 cranial nerves: OOOTTAFAGVAH '*Oh, Oh, Oh, To Touch And Feel Very Good Velvet Aah Hah*'.

Reading/writing learning

A traditional style of learning when individuals learn by reading and writing out the information. These learners benefit from reading textbooks and making notes, rewriting notes over again, condensing information through writing, rewriting ideas in their own words, and turning diagrams into words. These methods are good for cementing information in your mind. Just bear in mind that this revision method takes time, and so you will have to start earlier when making your notes to be able to revise through them again.

Kinaesthetic learning

When an individual 'learns by doing'. Kinaesthetic learners benefit from physical and tactile methods, such as doing a practical rather than reading the theory regarding a chemical reaction. Physical actions such as drawing and writing are also helpful as well as study materials that you can hold and move in your hand, such as flashcards. Role playing is also a good technique, and is particularly helpful during clinical skills practice.

Solitary and group learning

Depending on your preference, you may find it more ideal to study by yourself or with a group. Solitary learners are able to concentrate well and are good at going away and thinking through problems on their own whereas group learners benefit from discussing problems with each other. Group learning is a good way to coordinate your learning with fellow students; you can go through topics together and as individual students will have different strengths you can help each other learn—an effective way to solidify your own learning is to teach others. The risk with group learning is, of course, getting distracted! Just be sure to choose your study group wisely if you do go down this route.

Of course, individuals usually do not subscribe to just one particular style; the learning styles are not exclusive and the majority of people use different learning styles for different things.

One may find that for learning chemical processes, for instance, the tricarboxylic acid cycle, that it is easier to be able to retain the names of enzymes and the reactions they catalyse in the cycle by first drawing a diagram to visualize the process and then reciting the process out loud, emphasizing the names of the enzymes, combining both visual and auditory styles. Clinical skills such as carrying out a respiratory examination are 'hands-on' so it is effective to learn these practically rather than reading about them.

If you are unsure about how you learn, try using some of the methods described in this section and see which method(s) you find most effective.

Teaching

Teaching at university is very different from teaching at secondary school, and so is learning. At medical school, you will encounter a variety of different ways in which different parts of the course are taught.

What to expect

Responsibility for your own learning

As a medical student, you are expected to attend lectures, seminars, and practical workshops as well as going over content in your own time—organizing your own study is part of the difference between university and school. At medical school, you are the only person responsible for ensuring you complete any assignments on time and do your prep work for seminars as well as ensuring that you understand the material. If you are having difficulty completing work or understanding it, it is your responsibility to seek help. You will usually have an allocated educational supervisor who you can approach for help. Or you can contact the student support services if problems with health or family circumstances are affecting your studies.

Contact hours

You are also going to have far more hours of contact as a medical student compared to students on other courses—the nature of the medical course is intensive and this is reflected in the amount of hours you spend either in the lecture theatre or private study. You may also have a more varied schedule compared to other students, as you have more modules and placements, so your timetable will change from week to week.

Students in other faculties may not have their first academic year of assignments and exams counted towards their final graduating percentage. However, this will apply in medical school, and if you are aiming high for honours, you will need to be aiming high!

However, do not be disheartened—it is not all just work, work, work! As long as you organize your time well, you will have plenty of opportunities to take part in societies and socialize. It is well established at most universities that there is a timetable break midweek on Wednesday afternoons (usually for sports practice and society activities) although timetabling is at the discretion of your course.

Content

The first 2–3 years of medicine (preclinical years) are focused on you being taught basic medical knowledge and understanding the theory of medicine within medical school while your clinical years are spent focusing your clinical skills and being on placement, learning in a healthcare environment. You may find that during these years you are sitting with biomedical scientists, physiotherapists, and students from other health-related courses in the same lectures. It is because, naturally, your disciplines overlap in certain areas.

The medical course covers a lot of content and it can sometimes seem overwhelming. However, it is not necessary to learn everything; you will cover so much content in each of your modules that it is an important skill to learn to pick out what is relevant. Occasionally, lecturers may emphasize particular things during their lectures which can provide hints as to what they expect you to learn.

Do not expect to learn everything immediately; remember, 'slow and steady wins the race' and covering parts of your module a day at a time is far more effective than cramming a few days before your exam. We have all tried and tested that method, and trust us when we say it does not always work!

Modules

You will encounter a variety of different modules at medical school. Most modules are compulsory, but you may be allocated some optional modules. Examples of modules include the following:

Histology

Focuses on cell biology and tissue differentiation. You are also taught microscopy skills and will learn to differentiate between different types of tissue. Just be aware that for those wearing glasses, it can sometimes take a bit of getting used to when looking down a microscope! You can either take off your glasses and re-adjust the microscope viewer so you can see clearly, or try and look at samples with your glasses on!

Physiology and pharmacology

This is the study of the human body and control of systems during normal and abnormal states and the effects of drug actions on the body.

Public health

Focuses on the prevention of disease as well as the promotion of health within societies and populations, and considers health impacts at a population level.

Epidemiology

This is the study of causes and effects of disease in populations and patterns in health, and also provides the basis of public health. This module introduces various study designs and statistical analyses in reference to health in populations.

Medical biochemistry

This is the study of chemical and metabolic processes occurring in the body and the structure and function of molecules that take part in such processes, such as proteins.

Behavioural sciences

Explores patients' responses to illness and treatment and the psychological impact of social factors on health.

Human genetics

Explores heredity including the study of genetic characteristics in humans, hereditary diseases, and genetic variation. It can be quite interesting to do this module and to have a look at your own family history when drawing up a 'family tree'!

Human immunology

This is the study of the immune system within humans including looking at immunological disorders and the causes of failure of immune systems.

Microbiology

Looks at exploring the different microorganisms, bacteria, viruses, fungi, and protozoa, that are connected to health and diseases.

Haematology

This is the study of blood, clotting pathways, and diseases affecting the blood.

Embryology

Studying where life as we know it begins! This explores the ideal circumstances for conception and the development of an embryo to a newborn, and the wonders of the growth in between.

Neuroscience

Studying the nervous system including drugs affecting the system and therapeutic uses of drugs in treating neurodegenerative disorders.

Systems-based modules

These modules focus on studying some of the systems of the human body, including the anatomy of these systems. Other systems may be covered as parts of other modules:
• Cardiovascular
• Respiratory
• Neurology
• Integumentary
• Musculoskeletal (MSk)
• Endocrine
• Genitourinary
• Reproductive
• Digestive
• Immune and reticuloendothelial.

Clinical skills

This involves the teaching of both communication skills such as learning how to take patient histories as well as practical skills such as taking blood pressure or conducting respiratory examinations.

Teaching format

Lectures

These are used to introduce topics and deliver key ideas as well as to give you directions for further reading. It is a good idea to come prepared to lectures such as going over lecture notes beforehand or reading up on the learning objectives to provide you with some idea of what to expect. Most lectures are either available online or have pre-reading material on the online student portal—so remember to check that before attending. You might be tempted to transcribe everything the lecturer says, however, it is more important for you to listen and understand the content of the lecture. Being focused on making lots of notes can sometimes hinder you from paying attention to important things the lecturer may be saying. Develop an effective way of taking notes, using abbreviations, keywords, and brain maps so that important points are highlighted. You may also make notes on things that you do not understand, for follow-up questions, or annotate the handouts on things that you are interested in and want to further research. Lecturers will have different styles of lecturing. Some may prefer to have little information on handouts or slides and the main content of their lecture is spoken—it is a good idea to record these types of lecturers (remember to ask permission) as it may be difficult to go over things you do not understand later on using just the lecture materials.

Seminars

These are group sessions in which set topics can be discussed and questions asked. Seminars provide the opportunity for you to talk about subject areas in more detail, clarify things you do not understand, and both share and obtain different perspectives on subjects. They are usually led by an allocated facilitator. Preparation for seminars might involve doing some reading beforehand or completing a particular assignment. Group sessions are effective as students can often encourage each other to think differently and help each other learn. Seminars also help to develop communication as both speaking and listening skills are used. If you are anxious about speaking in front of people you are unfamiliar with, start off small and volunteer one answer or point of discussion each seminar and participate a little at a time. You may be asked to do group projects or presentations within your seminar group.

Problem-based learning

This is a method of active and student-centred learning in which students are given a problem to solve in small groups. Students gather what knowledge they have and identify knowledge they need to obtain in order to solve the problem. A tutor is also present to help guide students and facilitate the learning process. PBL is a good way of helping you to develop self-directed learning and enhance problem-solving and communication skills.

Practicals

Microscopy sessions

These sessions focus on developing your microscopy skills and may be used to aid your understanding of histology. You will learn about the different parts of a microscope, how to focus a microscope, how to stain specimens, as well as how to identify various cells and tissues by learning about particular features found on slides.

Experimental workshops

These are used to demonstrate particular concepts you have learnt about in lectures. This might involve, for instance, a neuromuscular practical to demonstrate reflex action or how to use an electrocardiogram (ECG) to enhance understanding of the electrical activity of the heart and to develop skills in interpreting an ECG.

Summary workshops

These sessions are question and answer sessions on particular topics that have been covered in lectures. They are used to summarize your understanding of lecture content as well as to provide the opportunity for you to ask questions about areas you do not understand.

Prosections

These are anatomical structures that have already been carefully dissected and are then presented to the students. Important structures are exposed and preserved for students to observe. There may be some coloured tags or pins relating to a structure (e.g. femoral nerve). You are likely to also have a worksheet to complete for the session with structures to identify and functions to deduce correctly.

Dissection

This is when students themselves remove tissue from a cadaver to identify internal structures. It is a more 'hands-on' process and can be incredibly helpful in increasing your understanding of anatomy as you learn first-hand the relationships of different anatomical structures to each other. It is an effective way of teaching anatomy as students are actively engaged with the process and what they are learning, and thus might find it easier to retain information regarding anatomy.

Dissection is not for everyone, and you do not have to be on the other end of the scalpel if you do not want to, but it might still be beneficial for you to observe your classmates dissect. Do not worry if at first you feel queasy about it—just remember that very generous individuals and families have donated their bodies so you can learn your anatomy to become a better doctor. Remember to treat that body with respect!

Assignments

You will also have assignments to complete as part of your course. They may be essays, which are used to display your understanding of a particular subject as well as develop your writing skills.

Tips for essay writing

- Plan what you are going to write in your essay before you write it.
- Make sure your essay follows a clear and logical structure—use evidence to support each point you make in order to reach a logical conclusion. If it is a practical then make sure it follows the standard format: Introduction and Aim, Methods, Results, Discussion, Conclusion, and References.
- Your essay should have points or arguments that are being emphasized or argued throughout your essay.
- Use lots of relevant evidence to back up your points—your argument or statement is more convincing this way.
- Your introduction should contain whatever point(s) you are arguing in your essay, the body of your essay should prove this point(s), and your conclusion should bring together your main points and provide a thoughtful end to your essay.
- Check your spelling, punctuation, and grammar—this can be the downfall of some potentially good essays and can look careless. Essays need to be well written, as well as well argued. You might find it helpful to ask someone to check your essay for spelling, grammar, and punctuation errors before handing it in.
- Ensure proper citation and referencing—if you have referenced another work in your essay, you must acknowledge this source or you may be at risk of plagiarizing the work of someone else. Regardless of whichever style you use, referencing should be kept consistent throughout your essay. Different universities may have referencing styles they prefer, so remember to check the requirements for your essay before submission. Common styles include Harvard and Vancouver referencing styles.
- Cite and reference as you write your essay—it is far easier and more time effective to keep track of your sources as you proceed with your essay, rather than referencing all of your sources at the end. Consider using EndNote—your library will usually have a tutorial on this or would be happy to teach you if you ask. It is a very helpful program and will serve you well during your working years too!
- If relevant and available, use a range of sources—your essay is better supported. Ideally go back to the original source rather than quote from a paper that is a review of the work done.
- Do not underestimate the value of diagrams in essays—they can be incredibly helpful in illustrating a complicated route or pathway (some universities may or may not put emphasis on these).
- Ensure that the content of your essay consists of material that is fundamental to the topic. Although some detail adds quality to your essay and showcases your understanding, too much detail will detract from the original focus of your essay. Be concise!

Coursework

You will likely have some form of coursework to complete at some point during your time at medical school. This can usually count towards a portion of one of your modules so spend time on your coursework. The best way to handle coursework is to break it down and work on it a little at a time. Time management is important so plan your work out and give yourself deadlines to meet for completing sections of your coursework. And do not forget to give yourself rewards after each milestone to keep you going!

Ask older students such as your 'medic parents' for advice on how they managed their coursework and for any tips on what the examiners are looking for. You might also want to ask them to look over your work for you to check for mistakes and ensure that your work reads well.

Plagiarism

However, be careful when sharing your work with others and avoid plagiarism, which can include not crediting sources or passing someone else's work off as your own. Universities have very strict rules regarding plagiarism, and you may have even committed plagiarism unknowingly so be sure to check and always give credit to sources if using that information in your work.

Back up

Always remember to back up your work. It may be obvious, but numerous students still fall prey to forgetting to back up important pieces of work and losing that work just before it is due. You can avoid this scenario by either copying your work onto a memory stick, emailing it to yourself, or storing it online using Google, Copy, or Dropbox cloud storage.

Lecture questions

You may be assigned 'homework' to complete before or after lectures. Questions set for completion before lectures are often preliminary questions on the topic of the next lecture to provide you with an introduction. Questions set post lectures are summary questions that are used to solidify your understanding of the lecture and test your knowledge of what you have just learned. Try not to leave these to the very end of the term before exams, as they can help with your learning as you go through a particular topic. They can also help highlight any deficiencies in knowledge, and you can seek help earlier rather than panicking a few days before the exam.

Preparation for seminars

This usually involves reading or completing a particular task for discussion during the seminar. It is important that you prepare for seminars to gain the most out of them as coming unprepared will leave you lost and unable to participate in discussions, which can hinder your learning.

Placements

Depending on your medical school, you may encounter some clinical settings from your first year. Basic clinical skills are taught in order for you to gain familiarity with them so you can perform these skills with fluency, having had plenty of practice.

Clinical learning

Your clinical learning will consist of obtaining key skills for life as a doctor. Some basic skills you may be taught in preclinical years include:

- clerking a patient
- discussing medical ethics
- performing cardiopulmonary resuscitation (CPR) on an adult, child, and baby
- first aid—treating wounds, burns, and dressing injuries
- clinical examinations
- feeling for arterial pulses
- blood pressure measurement
- conducting a peak flow examination on a patient and interpreting the result.

These are just a few of the many skills you will eventually learn. Clinical skills are practised and performed on simulated and real patients and your communication skills are also assessed. Do not disregard the marks you get for introducing yourself properly to a patient, and putting them at ease during your clinical encounter.

Clinical assessment

Objective structured clinical examinations (OSCEs)

These are clinical exams used to test your practical skills. The exam consists of a number of short tasks at different stations (such as performing CPR on a dummy at one station and taking a patient's arterial pulses at another). You are expected to perform these skills on real-life or simulated patients with an examiner observing and marking your performance.

Good preparation for your OSCE involves a lot of practice. Practise on your colleagues, friends, and family in order to gain as much experience as possible. Using a group study method for this can be very helpful. Remember that with practice, you will perform the steps of the task almost automatically. While you are on autopilot, you do not have to stop and think what to do next and are less likely to hit a mental block when you are being assessed by the examiner in the same room.

What counts as normal or baseline for people can vary—for instance, you may take a blood pressure reading for a patient and find that it is lower than what seems normal. However, this reading may be consistent with their readings in the past so rather than assuming a pathological reason, it is more likely that some people may naturally or physiologically have lower blood pressures.

GP

At some point during your degree, you will be on placement at a GP clinic. This is a place for you to observe interactions between a doctor and a variety of patients, presenting with a variety of issues. You may also have the chance to interview patients and take their histories yourself, which is a valuable way to practise your communication skills.

Dress code

It is important to keep in mind that both the GP clinic and the hospital are professional environments and as such, you will be expected to dress for this setting. This means:

- sensible shoes
- smart shirts, blouses, or dresses
- smart trousers or skirts
- no short skirts or short dresses
- no printed T-shirts
- in hospital—bare below elbows.

Your GP is also a great source of information regarding both your course and life after your degree. They are able to provide advice on how to get through the course, important things to remember for examinations, as well as what things not to worry about! Use your GP to answer questions about clinical practice and how to handle patients.

Hospital

You will also have a clinical placement at a hospital. Again, this is to hone your clinical skills and to give you experience within a hospital setting, which is different to a GP clinic in that a hospital setting has a multidisciplinary team to provide care for patients. This includes nurses, pharmacists, physiotherapists, and surgeons among others—all of whom are integral in providing different aspects of holistic patient-centred care. The benefit of a hospital setting is that you gain the opportunity to observe a variety of different wards and specialities, which are not as extensive in a GP clinic. Some of the more common specialties you may encounter during your preclinical years are medicine (acute medical or general wards), surgery, and the radiology unit. These early encounters may give you an idea of what kind of medicine you wish to pursue following your degree, and you will gain more experience of these during the clinical years of your degree and your training after your degree. However, do not set your mind on a particular field already because you will encounter a vast variety of new specialities so keep your eyes wide and your mind open.

Top ten apps for medical students

Handheld devices, such as smartphones and tablets, have allowed greater flexibility in the way in which we gather information and learn. The following applications are aimed at making learning easier and smarter, more mobile and convenient, for medical students

1. Medscape (free)

A comprehensive medical reference application, containing over 4000 conditions, 600 procedures (some with accompanying videos), as well as information on drugs and interactions, medical news, and education. Content can be downloaded for use offline, which is another handy feature. The only downside is navigating different sections of an article, which can be tricky given the detail.

2. Brainscape (free)

For those that feel more comfortable revising from notes, Brainscape is a digital flashcard system that allows you to create personalized flashcards, and then test yourself using a unique confidence-based repetition method. What's more, you can track your progress, benchmark cards for later review, and even share your cards with others.

3. Prognosis: Your Diagnosis (free)

This cartoon-based game is designed around testing your diagnostic, investigative, and treatment skills. Using over 600 specialist-vetted case scenarios across various specialties, it allows you to make decisions before a comprehensive and full breakdown is provided at the end of each scenario, allowing you to make comparisons. A fun and unique way to learn while developing key decision-making skills.

4. Daily Rounds – for Doctors (free)

A frequently updated and curated list of the latest clinical cases from medical schools, including radiology cases, this app involves a PBL approach to studying. Each grand-round style case has multiple-choice questions (MCQs) to further challenge you as you work through it, allowing for a comprehensive understanding of the case.

5. Medical Cases for Healthcare (free)

Often labelled the 'Instagram for medical doctors', this relatively new app allows users worldwide to upload medical images (while maintaining confidentiality) for discussion. Users can post questions or interesting cases and await responses from the growing community, making this a flexible, user-dependent app.

6. UpToDate (requires subscription or institutional access)

Possibly *the* authoritative, evidence-based, clinical decision support resource, this app contains updated, well-curated articles on almost all aspect of clinical medicine. Topics are long and detailed, but the interface easily allows you to skip to the relevant section and you can bookmark favourite articles for later reading. The only drawback is the high subscription costs, which are avoided if your institution has access.

7. Calculate by QxMD (free)

A concise, one-stop shop containing over 200 medical calculations and equations. This app allows you to seamlessly input patient variables into their question flow, and then derives answers with a corresponding explanation or link. It also includes various decision support tools for non-numerical stratification of patients.

8. Pocket Anatomy (£9.99)

This anatomy app is beautiful and well designed, with an intuitive user interface allowing you to browse through thousands of bodily structures. Learn by searching for individual structures, layers, or systems. The app contains concise information on each structure including clinical relevance, with space to include your own notes.

9. Read by QxMD (free)

If you find that you need to try and stay up to date with the latest primary research, Read by QxMD helps you to organize this process. You can sign up to updates from individual journals, specialties, or even review groups and be alerted when anything new arises that fits your criteria. If you have institutional access, articles can be accessed directly from the app, and PDFs saved for later reading.

10. BNF & BNFC (free)

The BNF & BNFC app is the portable, concise version of the UK drug reference books the *British National Formulary* (*BNF*) and the *British National Formulary for Children* (*BNFC*), and necessary for any medical student. It contains practical information on prescribing, including doses and contra-indications, as well as dispensing and administrating medications. There is a useful search function, it is available offline, and is regularly updated so you can stay current.

Chapter 3

Preclinical medicine

Preclinical medicine

What is preclinical medicine? Preclinical medicine comprises the basic science disciplines required for the later study and application of clinical medicine. Traditionally, preclinical medicine has been divided into individual subjects such as anatomy, biochemistry, pharmacology, physiology, and pathology. Increasingly now, medicine is taught using a systems-based approach, where one learns all of the basic science relevant to a clinical problem (such as chest pain or headache) in an interdisciplinary way. This requires medical students to integrate considerable volumes of information from an early stage.

How will I learn preclinical medicine? There are many teaching styles employed by medical schools, and it is likely that your medical school makes use of all of them to varying degrees. Since this is usually taught at the beginning and it is so different from learning in secondary school, the university will offer varying methods of teaching. Since you are now an adult learner, it is your responsibility and exciting journey to figure out which method is the best way to learn for you. Everyone learns the same way (reading, listening, etc.) but you have to find out which method is the most effective, impactful, and memorable. This will take time, practice, and patience.

Lectures

The lecture is a universal and fundamental part of learning preclinical medicine. The lecturer will provide learners with the initial introduction to a particular topic and begin the learning process. However, you must use this as a springboard for your own independent learning. For example, following a lecture on the cardiovascular system (CVS) you should then read about the physiology of cardiac myocytes, the biochemistry of cellular respiration, and the pathology of ischaemia and tissue infarction. In pursuing this approach of independently exploring and consolidating topics introduced in formal teaching, you will develop a firm theoretical foundation on which to pass your exams, and form the basis of your future clinical practice.

Laboratory practicals

Practical sessions are a vital part of anatomy (dissection), biochemistry, physiology, and pathology. They will typically require more initiative and self-guided learning than lectures or seminars. It is easy to get lost in the detail of experimental protocols so it is important to remind yourself at the end of each session what the salient learning points are. For example, in a biochemistry practical about haemoglobin electrophoresis:
- the relevant *specific* knowledge is to understand the existence of genetic mutations in the structure of haemoglobin and the functional implications of this
- the *generic* skills gained include the electrochemical principles of electrophoresis and other applications of this technique.

Small group teaching

This is often referred to as problem-based learning (PBL). Small group tutorials are often regarded as the most valuable part of preclinical education. Tutorial sessions or 'supervisions' run in parallel to lectures and practicals.

The aim is to consolidate your knowledge, and answer any outstanding questions. The facilitator or tutor will explore your theoretical understanding by asking you to apply it to new situations. Practise explaining topics to one another—the ability to explain something in simple terms is often an important measure of your own understanding. Much of the content from lectures will be reinforced with PBL in a group with your colleagues. Your tutor will present a topic from the syllabus or integrate the clinical significance in a case study for you to explore in depth together. You will be working together in a team and be set tasks to complete for the next session. You will also present your work, research, and findings to the entire group until a holistic picture is painted on a disease process from microscopic level to clinical manifestations, diagnosis, and management.

Individual study

In spite of all the lectures, practicals, and tutorials, and due to the volume of content within the curriculum, every medical student needs to develop a discipline, set aside time to revise, and commit to extra reading. It is not enough to listen to lecturers and tutors in order to absorb all that information. You are expected to direct your own learning. Since we all learn better in various ways and at our own pace, there will always be the need to learn, understand, memorize, and appreciate the learning objectives with additional background study. Medicine is a vast subject and practice, and you will find yourself studying for your entire career. You are laying the foundations of effective studying at medical school which will stay with you throughout. More importantly, never ever compare yourself to your colleagues. Some need to study more than others but everyone needs to study. All you need to focus on is doing whatever it takes to get the work done, such as writing notes, using highlighters, reciting out loud, post-it notes, flashcards, and so on.

Essays

A valuable skill to acquire is the art of writing a concise yet comprehensive account of a topic that can be reproduced in exam conditions. Where possible, you should try to write these by hand unless your final examinations are computerized. Diagrams, flow charts, and bullet points are important tools to highlight salient details. Generally speaking, the medical course requires very little essay writing compared to other academic disciplines. Yet it is a very important skill to maintain, especially during your career when it comes to higher degrees (e.g. thesis), research publications, audits, and entries of reflective experiences.

Anatomy

Human anatomy is fundamental to our understanding of disease, clinical examination, diagnosis, and treatment.

How will I be taught anatomy?

A combination of lectures and practical sessions using cadavers, prosections, or virtual tools. An effective way to learn anatomy is to visualize it and make mind maps. Make the most of your time in the dissection room and get stuck in!

What resources should I use?

Textbook

For example, Grant's, Snell's, Last's, Netter's, Gray's, and Moore & Dalley's textbooks. To be used for reference, not read from cover to cover!

Anatomy atlas

For example, McMinn's, Gray's, Netter's, as well as Acland's DVD atlas. Use these to improve your three-dimensional (3D) visualization of structures and the relationships between them.

Online resources

- ♫ www.instantanatomy.net
- ♫ www.innerbody.com
- ♫ www.getbodysmart.com
- ♫ www.ect.downstate.edu/courseware/haonline/index.htm.

Bones

Do not neglect the skeleton! There are many important relationships between the skeleton and the soft tissues (which examiners are often keen to test!).

Yourselves

Be sure to examine yourself and colleagues in order to study shape, size, position, movement, and variations in anatomy.

Top tips for studying anatomy

- *Gross topology*: in 3D and anatomical relationships (see Fig. 3.1).
- *Classify*: divide areas into smaller sections, e.g. the upper limb comprises the arm and forearm; the forearm has an anterior and posterior compartment; the anterior compartment has three separate muscle layers; and so on.
- *Principles*: establish principles over individual facts; muscles passing over the anterior surface of the elbow cause flexion, and arm flexors are innervated by musculocutaneous nerves; this is more efficient than learning the innervation of the individual muscles.
- *Relevance*: ask yourself about the practical importance each time you learn something new.
- *Surface anatomy*: use your own body as a reference.
- *Embryology*: relevant to both anatomy (e.g. dermatomes from a budding fetus) and clinical implications (e.g. congenital heart disease).
- *Radiology*: anatomy is vital in interpreting radiological images.

Important terminology

See Fig. 3.1 for anatomical planes and Table 3.1 for anatomical relationships.

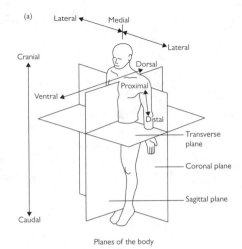

Planes of the body

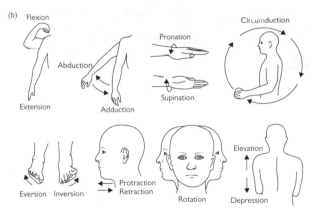

Fig. 3.1 (a) Anatomical planes and (b) movements. Reproduced with permission from Rebecca Jester, Julie Santy, and Jean Rogers, *Oxford Handbook of Orthopaedic and Trauma Nursing*, 2011; and Castledine and Close, *Oxford Handbook of Adult Nursing*, 2009, with permission from Oxford University Press.

Table 3.1 Anatomical relationships

Anterior/ventral	Closer to front, e.g. aorta anterior to spine
Posterior/caudal	Closer to back, e.g. spine posterior to stomach
Medial	Closer to midline, e.g. sternum medial to humerus
Lateral	Further from midline, e.g. thumb lateral to wrist
Superior/cranial	Closer to head, e.g. lungs superior to bowel
Inferior/caudal	Closer to feet, e.g. wrist inferior to elbow
Distal	Further from trunk, e.g. hand distal to shoulder
Proximal	Closer to trunk, e.g. thigh proximal to foot
Superficial	Closer to surface, e.g. dermis superficial to fascia
Deep	Further from surface, e.g. heart deep to sternum

Pathology

Pathology is the study of disease processes, and encompasses many fields such as immunology, haematology, microbiology, and chemical pathology.

What resources should I use?

- Cross SS. (2018). *Underwood's Pathology: A Clinical Approach*, 7th edition. Philadelphia, PA: Elsevier.
- Kumar V, Abbas AK, Aster JC. (2017). *Robbins Basic Pathology*, 10th edition. London: W.B. Saunders.

Key principles

Cellular injury and death

Mediators of cellular injury and mechanisms of apoptosis vs necrosis (including morphological features). Mechanisms of repair.

Inflammation

Acute vs chronic: *calor, rubor, tumour,* and *dolor*. Pathways → neutrophil extravasation. Outcomes are resolution (good), repair (loss of functional specialization), or chronic inflammation (bad). Role of cells (macrophages, neutrophils, mast cells, etc.), soluble mediators (complement, kinins), and cytokines (interleukin 1, tumour necrosis factor (TNF)).

Disorders of growth and differentiation

The cell cycle and controls on cell division. Hypertrophy, hyperplasia, atrophy, aplasia, atresia, metaplasia, dysplasia, and neoplasia.

Thrombosis

Virchow's triad, arterial vs venous thrombosis, aetiology, and consequences of thrombi (resolution, recanalization, propagation, or embolism). Ischaemia vs infarction vs gangrene.

Cancer

Neoplasia, hamartomas, carcinoma *in situ*, and cancer; histological features of benign and malignant lesions (e.g. adenoma vs carcinoma). Carcinogenesis, oncogenes, tumour suppressor genes, molecular genetics of adenoma–carcinoma sequence. Local effects of tumour (e.g. wheeze from bronchial obstruction) vs effects of local invasion (e.g. superior vena cava (SVC) obstruction) vs metastatic spread (liver and brain metastases) vs paraneoplasia (syndrome of inappropriate antidiuretic hormone secretion (SIADH) or neuromuscular disease).

Immunology

Immunology is the study of the immune system. You will learn about mechanisms of defence against infection and autoimmunity.

What resources should I use?

- Abbas A, Lichtman AH, Pillai S. (2015). *Basic Immunology*, 5th edition. Philadelphia, PA: Elsevier.
- Parham P. (2014). *The Immune System*, 4th edition. New York: Garland.

Top tips for learning immunology

- Conceptualize innate and adaptive immune systems as distinct but interacting, comprising a number of cell types, soluble mediators, and cytokines (see Fig. 3.2).
- Consider over- vs underactivity and the checkpoints and regulators in place to control the immune response. Immunodeficiency gives rise to recurrent and severe infection. Dysregulated immunity can cause autoimmune conditions such as multiple sclerosis (MS) and systemic lupus erythematosus (SLE).
- Mechanisms of immunomodulation, i.e. how to improve defence against infection (vaccination, immunoglobulins) vs how to reduce immune activity (immunosuppression in autoimmune disease or transplantation).

Innate

Conserved, rapid, stereotyped, and non-specific. Infectious antigen or sterile 'danger' signals sensed by pattern recognition receptors. Proinflammatory response via cytokines and neutrophil-recruiting chemokines. Neutrophil extravasation and acute inflammation.

Important clinical applications: 'collateral damage' such as systemic inflammatory response syndrome (SIRS) and septic shock syndrome (TNF alpha-mediated effects), and inherited disorders of neutrophil function.

Adaptive

More recent, slower, antigen-specific memory response. Dendritic cells present antigen to naïve T cells via major histocompatibility complex (MHC) class II. T cells have different repertoires of cytokine responses (T helper (Th)-1, Th2, and Th17). Co-stimulation. Cytotoxic CD8+ T cells. B-cell activation in lymph nodes following germinal centre reaction. Class switching between immunoglobulin subtypes. Antibody production and structure of immunoglobulin. Antibody binding to target causes either opsonization or complement-mediated cell death (see Fig. 3.3). Important clinical applications: cytotoxic T cells, diabetes, or hepatitis C infections. Memory response to vaccination. Immunotherapy for cancer.

Hypersensitivity/autoimmunity

- Immunoglobulin (Ig)-E and mast cell activation. True allergy and anaphylaxis.
- Antibody-mediated cell lysis (e.g. haemolytic disease of the newborn).
- Antigen–antibody complex deposition (e.g. vasculitis).
- Cytotoxic T cells (e.g. diabetes, tuberculosis (TB)).

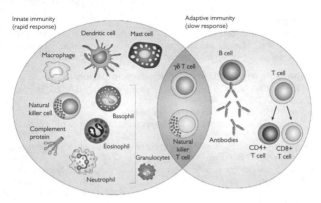

Fig. 3.2 Innate vs adaptive immunity. Reproduced with permission from Dranoff, G., *Nat Rev Cancer*. 2004; 4:11–22.

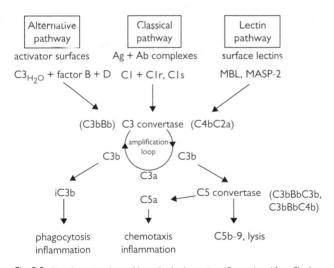

Fig. 3.3 Complement pathway. Ab, antibody; Ag, antigen. Reproduced from Skerka, C. et al, Complement factor H related proteins (CFHRs), *Mol Immunol*, 2013 Dec 15;56(3):170–80, Elsevier, under a creative commons license.

Vaccination

For both individual and herd immunity. Heat-killed antigens, live, attenuated antigens, or subunit peptide antigens. Relies on immunocompetent host (i.e. poor response in immunosuppression). Oral vs dermal route.

Important mechanisms of immunomodulation

- Non-specific: non-steroidal anti-inflammatory drugs (NSAIDs), steroids, dapsone, and plasmapheresis.
- Cell specific (to a certain degree): calcineurin inhibitors (ciclosporin, tacrolimus), and antiproliferative agents (azathioprine, mycophenolate mofetil).
- Cytokine specific: biologic agents in rheumatoid arthritis (e.g. monoclonal antibody to TNF alpha).
- Soluble component specific: e.g. eculizumab in paroxysmal nocturnal haemoglobinuria.

Specific immune deficiencies

- HIV/AIDS
- Post transplantation
- Chemotherapy
- Rare inherited causes:
  - Innate
  - Adaptive.

Microbiology

This is the study of microorganisms, including bacteria, viruses, parasites, and fungi. It is best not to treat an infection until the causative organism is known (see Table 3.2). However, if the patient is unwell and needs urgent treatment, send cultures (e.g. blood, urine, and swabs) and start broad-spectrum antibiotics. This is empirical 'blind' treatment which can be changed later to a narrow-spectrum antibiotic to lessen the risk of bacterial resistance. The local antibiotic policy should be followed and if doubt, discuss with a microbiologist.

Table 3.2 Causative organisms of conditions and treatments

Condition	Main causative organisms	Antibiotic/treatment
Meningitis	*Neisseria meningitidis, Streptococcus pneumoniae, Listeria monocytogenes*	Cefotaxime IV
Otitis media	*Strep. pneumoniae, Haemophilus influenzae, Moraxella catarrhalis*	Amoxicillin PO
Tonsillitis	Group A beta-haemolytic streptococci (80% are viral)	Phenoxymethylpenicillin (aka penicillin V) PO *or* benzylpenicillin (aka penicillin G) IV
Pneumonia	*Strep. pneumoniae, H. influenzae, M. catarrhalis*	Amoxicillin, co-amoxiclav, clarithromycin
Tuberculosis (TB)	*Mycobacterium tuberculosis*	Rifampicin + isoniazid + pyrazinamide + ethambutol (RIPE)
Endocarditis	*Staph. aureus*, viridans streptococci, coagulase-negative staphylococci (CONS)	Ampicillin + flucloxacillin + gentamicin
Gastroenteritis	• (Often viral) • *Campylobacter* • *Escherichia coli* 0157 • *Salmonella, Shigella* • *Clostridium difficile*	*Only if severe:* • Erythromycin • None • Ciprofloxacin • Metronidazole/vancomycin
Urinary tract infection (UTI)	*E. coli, Staph. saprophyticus, Klebsiella, Pseudomonas*	Trimethoprim, nitrofurantoin
• Genitourinary: • Pelvic inflammatory disease	*Chlamydia trachomatis* *Neisseria gonorrhoeae*	Azithromycin • Ceftriaxone + azithromycin • Ceftriaxone IM, then doxycycline + metronidazole
Syphilis	*Treponema pallidum*	Benzylpenicillin
Osteomyelitis	*Staph. aureus, Enterobacter,* streptococci	Clindamycin, linezolid
Cellulitis	• *Staph. aureus*, streptococci • MRSA	• Flucloxacillin, benzylpenicillin • Vancomycin

IM, intramuscular; IV, intravenous; MRSA, meticillin-resistant *Staphylococcus aureus*; PO, orally.

Pharmacology

Pharmacology is the study of drugs, consisting of pharmacodynamics (effect of drug on body) and pharmacokinetics (effect of body on drug; see Fig. 3.4).

Principles in pharmacology

Receptors: ligand-gated ion channels, G protein-coupled receptors, tyrosine kinases, steroid receptors, and their mechanisms of signal transduction, including second messenger signalling pathways; principles of antagonists, agonists, partial agonists, and inverse agonists. Cooperative and non-cooperative binding indicated by sigmoid and hyperbolic substrate concentration–velocity curves respectively.

Organ specific

- *Peripheral nerve transmission*: the mechanisms of drug action at nicotinic and muscarinic synapses at pre- and postganglionic synapses in the autonomic nervous system, and at the neuromuscular junction.
- *Cardiovascular pharmacology*: mechanisms of action of antihypertensives, digoxin, antiplatelets, antiarrhythmics, and statins.
- *Renal pharmacology*: mechanisms of action of diuretics, angiotensin-converting enzyme inhibitors (ACEIs), and angiotensin receptor blockers (ARBs). Effects of ACEIs and NSAIDs on renal autoregulation.
- *Inflammation*: immunosuppression, and the pathways involved. Common anti-inflammatories (steroids, NSAIDs, dapsone) and immunosuppression (steroids, antimetabolites, calcineurin inhibitors).
- *Cytotoxic chemotherapy*: anticancer therapies, similarities/differences. Drug action at different stages of the cell cycle.
- *Antimicrobials*: classes, mechanisms of action, and bacterial resistance. Actions of drugs in disrupting bacterial cell wall synthesis.

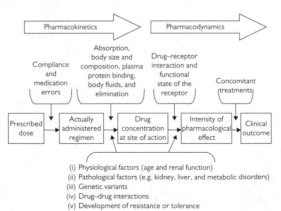

Fig. 3.4 Pharmacokinetics and pharmacodynamics. Reproduced under creative commons license from Bianca Rocca and Giovanna Petrucci, Variability in the Responsiveness to Low-Dose Aspirin: Pharmacological and Disease-Related Mechanisms, Thrombosis, Vol 2012 (2012).

Sociology

This is the study of society including some of the following:

- Relationships
- Structures
- Interactions
- Cultures.

But with increasing inequality, populations undergoing the demographic transition (see Fig. 3.5), globalization, ageing, poverty, environmental issues, and chronic illness, medical sociology is relevant.

How will I be taught sociology?

Lecture or seminar based. Sociology is a wide field so the area of study is normally limited to health and illness. Assessed by either written exams or essays as part of continuous assessment.

What resources should I use?

Ensure you have good notes from lectures—this is what you will most likely be examined on. There are several textbooks on medical sociology, e.g. *Key Concepts in Medical Sociology* by Jonathan Gabe and Lee Monaghan (2013). Read essayist Susan Sontag's *Illness as Metaphor* (1978): 'Illness is the night-side of life, a more onerous citizenship. Everyone who is born holds dual citizenship, in the kingdom of the well and in the kingdom of the sick.'

Medicalization

Where a non-medical problem becomes a medical one, e.g. alcoholism. Often linked to 'deviant' behaviour.

Ivan Illich thought medicalization by doctors and pharmaceutical companies weakens a person's ability to care for themselves. 'Illness' can be 'de-medicalized', such as homosexuality, which was listed as a psychiatric illness in the US until 1973.

The 'sick role'

The sociologist Talcott Parsons argued that for society to function, people who are ill have a duty to seek medical care while society agrees to allow them to take time off to recover. Sociologists Bloor and Horobin criticized this model, saying doctors often expect patients to know when to present (and not present with 'rubbish') and when they do present at the right time, not to question their diagnosis and treatment.[1] An Australian study demonstrated considerable accuracy in 'parental triage' when parents took their children to the emergency department (ED).[2]

Stigma

'Stigma' derives from the tattoos marking slaves and criminals in ancient Greece as social outcasts. The classic stigmatizing illness, now easily treatable and difficult to become infected with, is Hansen's disease, or leprosy. Until recently in the UK, special pre- and post-test counselling for HIV tests was obligatory because of the stigma surrounding the disease. But treating HIV testing like this was seen as a barrier to the diagnosis and treatment of patients with HIV. The British HIV Association now advises that a HIV test should be treated like any other investigation for serious illness.[3]

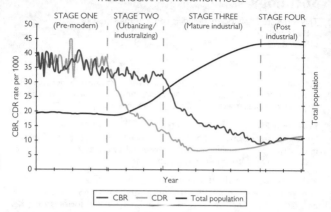

Fig. 3.5 The demographic transition. CBR, crude birth rate; CDR, crude death rate. Reproduced with permission from Montgomery, Keith. *The Demographic Transition*. http://pages.uwc.edu/keith.montgomery/Demotrans/demtran.htm

Honours

Ivan Illich was an Austrian philosopher, Catholic priest, and critic of society's 'medicalization'. He argued in his *Limits to Medicine*, that the 'physician becomes the sickening agent' as the medical establishment seeks to medicalize normal life events and deprive us of our traditional coping strategies. He described three stages of 'iatrogenesis' (from the Greek 'iatros', or 'healer', and 'genesis', or 'origin'): (1) clinical iatrogenesis, illness or death caused by a health worker; (2) social iatrogenesis, where doctors, drug companies, and others medicalize normal life stages (e.g. ageing, creating unrealistic expectations and so creating demands for their goods and services); and (3) *cultural iatrogenesis*, whereby our ability to handle illness and death are lost.[4]

References

1. Gabe J, Bury M, Elston M. (2004). *Key Concepts in Medical Sociology*. London: Sage Publications.
2. Williams A, O'Rourke P, Keogh S. (2009). Making choices: why parents present to the emergency department for non-urgent care. *Arch Dis Child* 94(10):817–20.
3. British HIV Association (2008). *UK National Guidelines for HIV Testing*. London: BHIVA.
4. Barnet RJ. (2003). Ivan Illich and the nemesis of medicine. *Med Health Care Philos* 6:273–86.

Epidemiology

Titbit
Epidemiology, *the science of health and disease in populations*, is detective work writ large and has some notable sleuths: John Snow in 1854, mapping and halting a London cholera epidemic; Bradford Hill and Richard Doll's work linking smoking and lung cancer; and the epidemiologists tackling the 2014 West African Ebola (viral haemorrhagic fever) epidemic.

How will I be taught epidemiology?
The UK's Faculty of Public Health states that all doctors should 'adopt a "population perspective" in everyday clinical practice and should consider health inequalities' (Faculty of Public Health (2014). Undergraduate Public Health Curriculum. ♪ www.fph.org.uk/uploads/PHEMS%20booklet.pdf). The faculty recommends a mix of best answer and extended matching questions, short answer questions, essays, and poster work. The London School of Hygiene and Tropical Medicine runs a mock cholera outbreak for its students (♪ www.msf.org.uk/teaching-resources-level-biology#cholera).

What resources should I use?
- Bonita R, Beaglehole R, Kjellström T. (2006). *Basic Epidemiology*, 2nd edition. Geneva: World Health Organization (♪ apps.who.int/iris/bitstream/10665/43541/1/9241547073_eng.pdf).
- The US Centers for Disease Control in Atlanta has a free online course (♪ www.cdc.gov/ophss/csels/dsepd/ss1978/index.html).
- The John Snow Society's 'Pump Handle' lectures (♪ www.johnsnowsociety.org/annual-pumphandle-lecture.html).
- Hans Rosling's ♪ www.gapminder.org, with 'bubble' visuals on population and health (the Swedish professor discovered the cause of konzo following an outbreak of the disease in Mozambique, a paralytic illness caused by high levels of dietary cyanide).

Key concepts
Defining health and disease
World Health Organization (WHO) definition of health, 1948: 'Health is a state of complete physical, mental and social well-being and not merely the absence of disease or infirmity.' All sorts of health data are collected, local to global. The first attempt to classify and thus help measure health and disease on a global scale occurred in Paris (1900) and resulted in the first *International List of Causes of Death*. Revised every 10 years, the WHO took over responsibility for this in 1948 and the system was renamed the International Classification of Diseases, or ICD. The tenth version, ICD-10, is used today and its codes must be used on UK death certificates.

Hippocrates: the first epidemiologist?
Hippocrates (470–400 BC) wrote in his essay *On Airs, Waters and Places* that the physician needs to take environmental factors into account, pointing to seasonality, the quality of the water supply, and whether the population exercised and ate healthily—or drank to excess and were 'given to indolence'.

Some jargon
- *Endemic*: the normal background rate of a disease, e.g. cases of chicken pox annually in the UK, where there is no vaccination against varicella zoster virus (VZV).
- *Epidemic*: a rise in cases of a disease above the normal background rate (epidemiologists often prefer the term 'outbreak').
- *Cluster*: a group of cases at a specific time and place.
- *Pandemic*: an epidemic/outbreak that crosses international borders.
- *Prevalence*: the proportion of people with the disease in a given population at a point in time (number of diseased/given population).
- *Incidence*: the rate of new cases of disease in a population over a given period of time (number of people who become diseased over a period of time/the total observation time of all persons).
- *Exposure*: the pathogen/protective factor being studied (e.g. cigarette smoking or olive oil consumption).
- *Mortality rate*: number of deaths for a given number of people per unit of time, e.g. crude death rate = number of deaths per 1000 people per year; under-five mortality rate (U5MR) = number of deaths of children under the age of 5 years per 1000 live births.

Analytical epidemiology
The epidemiologist is looking at the how/why of a disease in a population. Studies most commonly used are case–control studies (e.g. where people with the condition of interest are compared to those without the condition, a retrospective design used for outbreak investigations) and cohort studies (prospective, studying a population over time with the exposure of interest). These studies can establish a relationship or *association* with the exposure of interest but not *causation* (see Box 3.2).

Box 3.1 A call to Public Health
You are on-call in the ED and a 19-year-old student is triaged urgently with fever and a non-blanching rash. The following will help when you call Public Health, who will want to prevent an outbreak of meningococcal disease and give guidance on prophylaxis for close contacts, including healthcare staff.
- *Clinical case definition* (for meningococcal septicaemia): fever, petechiae, purpura, toxic patient. May have features of meningitis (e.g. headache, neck stiffness, photophobia).
- *Laboratory confirmation*: blood culture, cerebrospinal fluid (CSF) (via lumbar puncture (LP)) or polymerase chain reaction (PCR) positive for *Neisseria meningitides*.
- *Suspected case*: meets clinical case definition (but could be something else).
- *Probable case*: in opinion of team treating case, likely to be *meningococcal* disease (e.g. patient lives in university accommodation where there have been two other confirmed cases).
- *Confirmed case*: laboratory confirmation.

Box 3.2 Smoking and the Bradford Hill criteria

Sir Austin Bradford Hill (with Sir Richard Doll) established the link between smoking and lung cancer.[1] He set nine criteria for causation[2]:

1. *Strength*: the larger the association, the likelier the exposure is causal.
2. *Consistency*: different studies make the same observations.
3. *Specificity*: causation more likely in specific populations, e.g. asbestosis
   in workers in the asbestos industry.
4. *Temporality*: effect has to occur after exposure for causality.
5. *Biological gradient*: dose response, e.g. greater cigarette pack-years are
   associated with greater likelihood of lung cancer.
6. *Plausibility*: case for causation helped if thought to be biologically
   plausible but Bradford Hill qualified this, saying it depended on the
   biological knowledge of the day, quoting Sherlock Holmes: 'When
   you have eliminated the impossible, whatever remains, however
   improbable, must be the truth.'
7. *Coherence*: epidemiological and laboratory findings agree, but
   Bradford Hill said a lack of laboratory evidence does not rule out the
   epidemiological evidence.
8. *Experiment*: may strengthen case for causation, e.g. preventative
   action reduces incidence of a disease.
9. *Analogy*: the acceptance of slighter evidence, e.g. thalidomide and
   birth defects.

Descriptive epidemiology

With an outbreak of illness in a population, the epidemiologist will ask what,
where, who, when, and why, summed up by *time, place,* and *person*. Time
will look at seasonality (e.g. annual winter epidemics of RSV bronchiolitis
in infants), long-term trends (e.g. rates of dementia in the population), or
an epidemic period (e.g. number of cases during the 2014 Ebola outbreak
in Sierra Leone). Place can be anywhere from a school or hospital ward to
a continent. Age, sex, and socioeconomic status are usually included but
more specific details may be used too.

References

1. Doll R, Hill AB. (1950). Smoking and carcinoma of the lung. *BMJ* 2:739–48.
2. Bradford Hill A. (1965). The environment and disease: association or causation? *Proc R Soc Med* 58(5):295–300.

Cardiovascular system

Anatomy

Including the coronary arteries (right vs left dominant) and valves. Blood flow through heart/lungs/systemic circulation. Surface anatomy of heart and valve positions. Embryology including malformations.

Physiology

Cardiac cycle (see Fig. 3.6 and Fig. 3.7) and isovolumetric contraction (systolic ejection), isovolumetric relaxation + filling (diastole). Factors influencing stroke volume (SV) × heart rate (HR) = cardiac output (CO). Starling's law + curve. Pre-load ('venous pool' returning blood → heart) and after-load (resistance against pumping blood).

Electrophysiology

Myocardial action potentials, phases, and ion channels (Na^+ in → K^+ and Cl^- out → Ca^{2+} in and K^+ out → K^+ out → K^+ in), excitation–contraction coupling and Ca^{2+}-induced Ca^{2+} release.

Pharmacology

- Antiplatelets: aspirin (irreversible cyclooxygenase (COX) inhibitor), clopidogrel (adenosine diphosphate (ADP) antagonist).
- Anticoagulants: warfarin (vitamin K depletion), heparins (antithrombin III + factor Xa blocking), non-vitamin K antagonist oral anticoagulants (e.g. rivaroxaban).
- Beta blockers: e.g. bisoprolol → ↓contractility + HR + renin release + afterload.
- Diuretics: e.g. thiazides. Multiple mechanisms including ↓preload through salt + water excretion.
- Dilators: venous dilators (e.g. nitrates reduce pre-load), vasodilators (e.g. hydralazine reduce afterload).
- Calcium channel blockers: dihydropyridine (amlodipine) vasodilate vs non-dihydropyridine (verapamil) = antiarrhythmic.
- Digoxin: rate control in atrial fibrillation and increase in CO.
- ACEI/ARB: ↓renin/salt/water retention + improve ventricular remodelling.
- Antiarrhythmics: Vaughn Williams classification.
- Statins: HMG-CoA reductase inhibitors (cholesterol reduction).

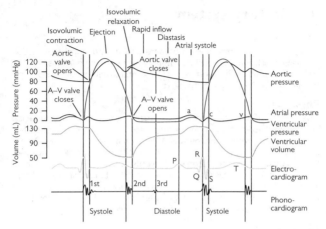

Fig. 3.6 Cardiac cycle. Reproduced with permission from Mark Kearney, *Chronic Heart Failure*, 2008, Oxford University Press.

Respiratory system

Anatomy

Passage of oxygen from the atmosphere into the pulmonary circulation through bronchial tree. Bronchopulmonary segments and relations of lobes and fissures to chest wall surface anatomy. Intercostal muscles/diaphragm for ventilation. Relation with the heart.

Physiology

Alveolar gas exchange: anatomical dead space (bronchi) vs physiological dead space (hypoperfused or hypo-oxygenated lung tissue). Role of surfactant (neonates). Ventilation/perfusion (V/Q) mismatch: higher V/Q (>1) at the apex and lower at the bases (<1). Ventilatory response to acidosis. Lung volumes: inspiratory reserve volume (IRV), tidal volume (TV), expiratory reserve volume (ERV), residual volume (RV), functional residual capacity (FRC), inspiratory capacity (IC), vital capacity (VC), total lung capacity (TLC) (see Fig. 3.8). Oxygenation: O_2–haemoglobin (Hb) dissociation curve and causes of 'shifts'; CO_2 transportation (see Fig. 3.8).

Pharmacology

- Beta-2 agonists: bronchodilatation (short-acting salbutamol, long-acting salmeterol).
- Antimuscarinics: bronchodilatation (e.g. ipratropium).
- Other bronchodilators: e.g. methylxanthine (theophylline) and leukotriene antagonists (montelukast).
- Corticosteroids: reduce airway inflammation (e.g. inhaled beclometasone or oral prednisolone).
- Mucolytics: e.g. carbocisteine and N-acetylcysteine.
- Antimicrobials: e.g. penicillins, macrolides, tetracyclines.
- Other agents: e.g. magnesium in asthma, home oxygen.

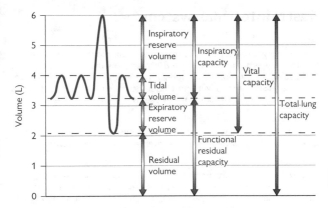

Fig. 3.7 Spirogram. Reproduced with permission from Albert RK, Spiro SG, Jett JR (eds): *Comprehensive Respiratory Medicine*. St Louis: Mosby, 1999, p 43.

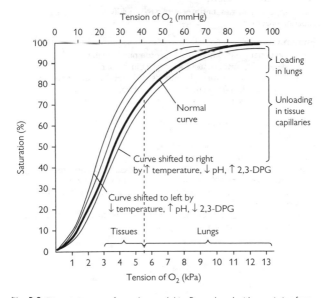

Fig. 3.8 Dissociation curve for oxyhaemoglobin. Reproduced with permission from Provan, Drew, *Oxford Handbook of Clinical and Laboratory Investigation* 3e, fig 8.1, 2010, Oxford University Press.

Gastrointestinal system

Anatomy

The luminal gastrointestinal (GI) tract spans from mouth to anus, and the hepatobiliary system (including the pancreas) joins the duodenum at D2. The coeliac artery supplies the foregut proximal to D2, superior mesenteric artery (SMA) the midgut, and inferior mesenteric artery (IMA) supplies from the distal one-third of the transverse colon to the upper rectum.

Structure of bowel wall

Mucosa, submucosa (with Meissner's parasympathetic plexus), muscularis externa (with Auerbach's autonomic myenteric plexus), and serosa.

Stomach

Chemical digestion starts with salivary amylase, and continues with gastric parietal cell HCl production and vagal stimulation of pepsin from chief cells. Additional factors such as gastrin (upregulates acid secretion and gastric motility), secretin (bicarbonate to neutralize acidic chyme), and somatostatin (globally inhibitory). Physical digestion largely mediated by neural control of gut (absent in Hirschsprung disease).

Hepatobiliary system

Produces, concentrates, and stores bile to emulsify lipids. Pancreas secretes exocrine enzymes.

Pharmacology

- Antacid tablets: e.g. omeprazole (proton pump inhibitor (PPI)), ranitidine (H2), misoprostol (prostaglandin inhibitor).
- Prokinetic drugs: e.g. metoclopramide (D2, 5HT3), domperidone (D2, D3), erythromycin (motilin), senna derivatives.
- Antimotile drugs: hyoscine (M2), loperamide and codeine (opiate receptors).
- Antiemetics: e.g. cyclizine (H1), ondansetron (5HT3), metoclopramide, domperidone.
- Portal hypertension: propranolol (beta-1 blocker), terlipressin (V1 agonist), octreotide or somatostatin.
- Immunotherapy in inflammatory bowel disease (IBD): non-specific corticosteroids, anti-inflammatories (e.g. 5-aminosalicylic acid (ASA)/ mesalazine), antimetabolite (azathioprine), biologics, e.g. anti-TNF drugs (infliximab).
- Antimicrobials: e.g. metronidazole and ciprofloxacin for Crohn's disease and traveller's diarrhoea.

Nervous system

Neuroanatomy

Central nervous system (CNS): cerebral cortex (Fig. 3.9) and functional regions (frontal, parietal, occipital, temporal); homunculus; hypothalamus and pituitary gland; basal ganglia; thalamus; lateral and medial nuclei; brainstem and cerebellum. CNS blood supply including the circle of Willis; dural venous sinuses. CNS cells are functional (neuronal) or supportive (glial). Glial cells comprise astrocytes (blood–brain barrier), microglia (macrophage like), and oligodendrocytes (myelin production).

Peripheral nervous system (PNS): links the CNS with sensory receptors and motor effectors. Also includes cranial nerves (except II!), spinal nerves, autonomic nervous system, and nerve plexus.

Physiology

Autoregulation of blood flow, cerebral blood flow vs cerebral perfusion pressure. CSF function and circulation within the ventricular system. Parasympathetic and sympathetic nervous systems, role in 'rest and digest' and 'fight and flight' respectively. Neuronal membrane and action potentials, saltatory conduction along myelinated nerve fibres: neurotransmitters. Types of nerve fibre and their structural and functional differences (e.g. conduction velocity and diameter),

Pharmacology

- Neuromuscular junction-blocking drugs in anaesthesia, and acetylcholinesterase inhibitors in myasthenia gravis.
- Anti-Parkinsonian drugs: e.g. levodopa and analogues, dopamine decarboxylase inhibitor, monoamine oxidase inhibitors.
- Antiepileptics: e.g. phenytoin, valproate.
- Immunotherapy for MS: e.g. corticosteroids (non-specific), alemtuzumab (anti-lymphocyte), fingolimod.

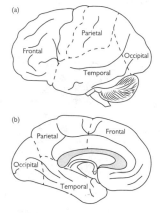

Fig. 3.9 The lobes of the central cortex. Reproduced with permission from Gelder, Michael, et al, *New Oxford Textbook of Psychiatry* 2e, 2012, Oxford University Press.

Endocrine system

Anatomy and physiology

Each endocrine system consists of an 'axis' comprising a control organ (hypothalamus or pituitary), an effector organ (e.g. thyroid or adrenal gland), and end organs (where hormones exert effects). The posterior pituitary and adrenal medullae are under neural control while the anterior pituitary and other endocrine organs are regulated by hormones.

Pituitary and hypothalamus

The posterior pituitary (neurohypophysis) produces oxytocin and ADH and has neural connections to the hypothalamus. The anterior part (adenohypophysis) is linked via a portal system to the hypothalamus, and secretes a number of hormones under hypothalamic control (see Fig. 3.10).

Parathyroids

Chief cells secrete PTH in response to falling calcium or rising phosphate concentrations. This increases the absorption of dietary calcium, the renal excretion of phosphate, and the hydroxylation and activation of vitamin D (via 1-alpha-hydroxylase in the kidney and 25-hydroxylase in the liver).

Thyroid

The thyroid hormone T3 and its prohormone T4 regulate global metabolic activity, beta adrenergy, and much more.

Kidneys

Synthesize renin which via angiotensin I and II controls salt/water retention and blood pressure. Erythropoietin (EPO) production by peritubular fibroblasts also stimulates red blood cell (RBC) production in bone marrow.

Gonads

Ovaries secrete progesterone/oestrogens and testes secrete testosterone.

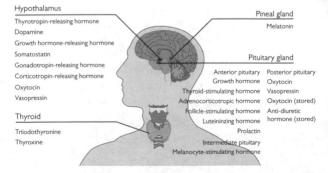

Fig. 3.10 Neuroendocrine system. Reproduced from https://commons.wikimedia.org.

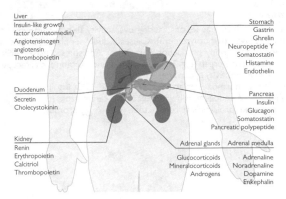

Fig. 3.11 GI endocrine system. Reproduced from https://commons.wikimedia.org.

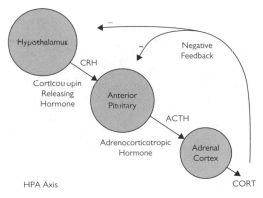

Fig. 3.12 Hormonal feedback. CORT, cortisol; HPA, hypothalamic–pituitary–adrenal. Reproduced from https://commons.wikimedia.org.

Pancreas

Alpha and beta islet cells produce glucagon and insulin respectively. Insulin mediates cellular uptake of glucose and glycogenesis. Glucagon works in reverse, by breaking down glycogen to glucose in times of stress/starvation (see ➽ p. 287). The pancreas also has a number of exocrine functions in aiding digestion. See Fig. 3.11 to appreciate the connection between the GI and endocrine systems.

Adrenals

The adrenal gland comprises cortex (steroid production) and medulla (catecholamines). The cortex is divided into GFR: zona Glomerulosa (mineralocorticoids), Fasciculata (glucocorticoids), and Reticularis (androgens). Negative feedback (see Fig. 3.12) ensures homeostasis.

Pathology

Best conceptualized as lesions causing overactivity (e.g. hyperthyroidism) or underactivity (hypothyroidism). Causes include neoplasia (Conn's syndrome), autoantibody production (Graves' or Addison's disease), infiltration of endocrine organ (e.g. TB and adrenal gland), or abnormal receptors (androgen insensitivity syndrome). Treat with:

- exogenous hormone replacement: T4, steroid, EPO, insulin
- inhibitors of endogenous hormone activity: carbimazole (thyroid), cabergoline (prolactin), spironolactone (Conn's syndrome).

Genitourinary system

Anatomy

Outer renal cortex (for filtration) and inner medulla (urine concentration) (see Fig. 3.13 and Fig. 3.14). Innermost portions of the medulla are the papillae which coalesce to form calyces which drain into the renal pelvis. This continues into the ureter which is lined by transitional epithelium before entering the bladder via the vesicoureteric junction. Each kidney contains 1 million functional units of a glomerulus (knot of blood vessels supplied by the afferent arteriole and drained by the efferent) and a nephron.

Physiology

Functions of kidney include salt and water homeostasis (and blood pressure control), acid/potassium/urea/creatinine excretion, EPO production, and calcium/phosphate balance. Maintenance of glomerular filtration rate via renal autoregulation (prostaglandins dilate afferent arteriole and renin–angiotensin system (RAS) constricts efferent).

Counter-current multiplier

Descending limb permeable to water not solute (water leaves tubule to form hypertonic urine), ascending limb impermeable to water but actively reabsorbs Na^+. Vasa recta maintains concentration gradient.

Renal pathology

- Pre renal: hypoperfusion from dehydration, low blood pressure (BP), heart failure.
- Renal: glomerulus—nephritic and nephrotic disease, diabetes. Tubulointerstitium—acute tubular necrosis from pre-renal failure, drugs (see Fig. 3.13 for overview of nephron and sites of action).
- Post renal: prostatic enlargement, renal stones, urothelial cancer.

Renal pharmacology

- *Diuretics*: block Na^+ pumps in nephron. Loop (furosemide) blocks Na-K-2Cl, thiazide (bendroflumethiazide) blocks Na^+-Cl^--cotransporter (NCC), amiloride (epithelial Na^+ channel (ENaC)).
- *Inhibitors of RAS*: ACEIs (enalapril) block AI–AII conversion. ARBs (losartan) directly block angiotensin receptor. Aliskiren directly inhibits renin (blocking angiotensinogen–AI step).
- *Mineralocorticoid antagonist*: e.g. spironolactone (K^+ sparing).
- *Drugs in renal failure*: activated vitamin D, EPO, PO_4^{3-} binders.
- *Stones*: reduce stone formation (thiazide diuretic, K^+ citrate).
- *Prostate disease*: alpha-1-adrenoceptor blockers (tamsulosin) relax bladder neck and urethra. Antiandrogen (e.g. finasteride for benign prostatic hyperplasia (BPH)).
- *Remember nephrotoxins*: NSAIDs, gentamicin, cisplatin, amphotericin, lithium.

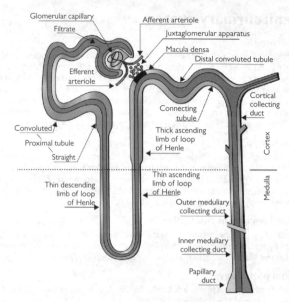

Fig. 3.13 The anatomy of the nephron. Reproduced from O'Callaghan, C (2009). *The Renal System at a Glance*, 3rd edn. With permission from Wiley-Blackwell.

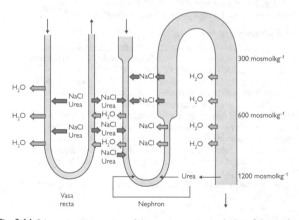

Fig. 3.14 Schematic representation of the counter-current multiplier of the renal medulla. Reproduced from G Pocock and CD Richards, *Human Physiology: The Basis of Medicine*, Third Edition, 2006, Figure 17.24, p. 369, by permission of Oxford University Press.

Musculoskeletal system

Anatomy and physiology

The musculoskeletal (MSk) system provides protection, stability, and movement to the body, and consists of bones, muscles, cartilage, tendons, and ligaments. Muscles are composed of fibres that contract and relax → movement, maintaining posture, and metabolic heat production. A joint, in which two or more bones articulate, is stabilized by ligaments and tendons. There are 300 bones in a baby which fuse to 206 by adulthood (see Fig. 3.15).

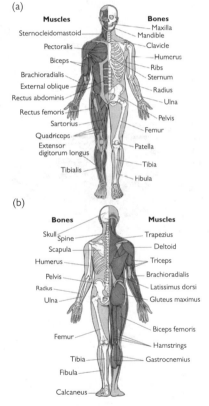

Fig. 3.15 Musculoskeletal system. Skeleton. Reproduced with permission from the *MSD Manual Consumer Version* (Known as the *Merck Manual* in the US and Canada and the *MSD Manual* in the rest of the world), edited by Robert Porter. Copyright (2018) by Merck Sharp & Dohme Corp., a subsidiary of Merck & Co, Inc, Kenilworth, NJ. Available at http://www.msdmanuals.com/consumer. Accessed (03/01/18).

Chapter 4

Preparing for preclinical exams

Preparing for preclinical exams: overview

A leap from school

The jump from A levels to preclinical medicine is a significant one. Previous revision strategies such as cramming and rote learning are unlikely to lead to success in your preclinical exams, or provide a solid foundation of medical knowledge for your future clinical career. Preclinical medicine requires a different approach to learning. The sheer volume of information in the medical disciplines (biochemistry, anatomy, etc.) may seem overwhelming at first, but you will learn how to navigate this and find what you are looking for. Graduate entry courses are similarly demanding, as the content of two preclinical years is condensed into one. You may go from being a straight A* or a first-class honours student to achieving the equivalent of B or C grades in your preclinical exams. This is normal, as you are now among a selected group of peers. Preclinical years set the foundations of medical knowledge for clinical medicine that follows; dedicate time to study during these years and the step into clinical medicine should be more natural and intuitive, and you can focus on developing your clinical skills, rather than trying to understand the subject matter of medicine.

Preclinical exams

During your preclinical years, you will be expected to learn the basic sciences: biochemistry, anatomy, pathophysiology, physiology, and pharmacology. You will also learn ethics, psychology, professionalism, communication skills, law, and sociology in the context of medicine. This knowledge is important for your clinical years and for the rest of your career. While you may look longingly at your stethoscope and wonder when you will learn how to diagnose, treat, and manage patients, it is important to learn these disciplines that underpin clinical practice. Medical schools provide both formative and summative assessments:

Formative assessments

These do not count towards your final grade. These 'mock' exams are especially useful in the first semester when you are finding your feet and familiarizing yourself with university exams. They may provide an early indication of your own progress, which will help you determine if your approach to learning in a new environment is appropriate. Some medical schools use them as progress tests to flag up any concerns to you or your tutors in case additional support is warranted.

Summative assessments

These count towards your final grades. You must pass all summative assessments to pass the year. Your medical school will have detailed information in the year handbook about how each type of assessment contributes to your overall grade. The year handbook is usually available on the medical school portal system or your medical school may give you a paper version at the start of the year.

Categories of assessment

You will be assessed using a number of methods depending on your medical school and this may change from year to year. The most common examination format is multiple choice questions (MCQs). Others include extended matching questions (EMQs), single best answers (SBAs), short answer questions (SAQs), essays, and viva oral exams. Some medical schools assess anatomy with an anatomy spotter and viva, use objective structured clinical examinations (OSCEs) in preclinical medicine, and assess group presentations for PBL.

MCQs

MCQs are often the choice of assessment for preclinical exams. Medical schools often have a bank of MCQs that they use every year, and the question bank is well protected. However, there is a range of books and websites with banks of MCQs available. It is important to read the question properly and practise your examination technique.

EMQs

EMQs present a theme: a list of structures, drugs, or receptors and ask you to select the best response to a several stems. Example EMQ:

Upper limb neuroanatomy
(a) Median nerve
(b) Ulnar nerve
(c) Axillary nerve
(d) Musculocutaneous nerve
(e) Medial cutaneous nerve of arm
(f) Medial cutaneous nerve of forearm
(g) Medial cutaneous nerve

Out of the list above, isolated injury of which nerve would cause weakness to elbow flexion and supination of the forearm?
   ANSWER D. Elbow flexion is the action which bends the arm at the elbow and supination is turning the arm so that the palms facing upwards.

Mr Smith dislocates his shoulder and experiences weakness to his deltoid muscle, select the nerve from the above list which is most likely to have been damaged.
   ANSWER C.

SAQs

SAQs are a form of written examination. Read the question and answer the question succinctly—do not simply write down everything you know. If your response is not relevant to the question then you will not gain marks and you will waste time in the exam. Here are some examples of the style of SAQs:
• Name two diseases of the basal ganglia (2 marks).
• Describe the pathophysiology of asthma. Describe and explain the pharmacological treatments for this disorder, and their mechanisms of action (8 marks).

Anatomy spotter

Some medical schools examine anatomy through anatomy spotters and/or viva examinations. You will be expected to identify structures in specimens that have been dissected, and sometimes a range of clinical images (using techniques such as computed tomography (CT)/magnetic resonance imaging (MRI)).

Essays

Your medical school may provide you with a description of the requirements to achieve each grade/percentage range. You will have written essays at school and know the basic structure of an essay (introduction, main body of argument, and conclusion). At university, your essays will need to be referenced in a formal manner and will be checked by plagiarism detection software. You will need to practise how to summarize conclusions or findings from other studies/sources and paraphrase them to avoid plagiarism. Vancouver and Harvard are types of referencing conventions that are commonly used. Consider using a reference manager program to make referencing easier for you.

Preclinical OSCEs

In the past, OSCEs were a type of examination reserved for the clinical years. However, some medical schools have introduced OSCEs in the preclinical years to bridge the gap between preclinical and clinical medicine. They are commonly used in the preclinical years to assess basic clinical skills (such as taking BP, peak flow, or doing a clinical examination in a healthy adult) and communication skills. OSCEs at this stage are helpful to practise performing in this context, especially when under pressure and with individuals watching. Tips for preclinical OSCEs include the following:

- *Time management*: while you might be unfamiliar with using a tuning fork, move on swiftly through the various components of a neurological examination. OSCEs are like driving tests, you have to exaggerate to draw attention to the boxes you are ticking. You will gain a few marks for introducing yourself, obtaining consent, and washing your hands. The majority of marks are for carrying out the required tasks in the time allocated. A few marks will be awarded for summarizing your findings. You may be asked a few questions at the end.
- *Practise* examining your flatmates and friends. This will result in a confident and well-rehearsed sequence of examination. It does not instil confidence in the examiner if you are hesitant or seem unfamiliar with devices used in the examination (such as a tuning fork). This is valid; in clinical medicine, you must instil confidence in your patients in the way you approach them.

Oral presentations

You may be asked to give a presentation as part of a summative or formative exam. Most preclinical students become increasingly confident with the use of PowerPoint, Prezi, or Keynote to create and deliver presentations.

- *Structure your presentation*: an introduction, the main body, and a summary slide is a general structure you may want to adopt.

- *Timing*: stick to your time limit. Too short suggests that you have not thoroughly researched the topic. Too long suggests that you cannot concisely present information. You must practise at least once to ensure the length of your presentation is correct—time yourself.
- *Less is more*: present the main points on the lecture slides and then elaborate on them. A slide full of text will result in your audience being disengaged and simply reading the slide with you. Images and figures are much more captivating than text, and you can talk naturally over them.

Poster presentations

Producing an academic poster and presenting it is a useful skill that some medical schools introduce in the preclinical years. If you have been in-volved in research, ask your supervisor if it is feasible to enter an abstract of the poster to a medical conference. Later, when you apply for academic foundation jobs or even specialty training, poster presentations at medical conferences will strengthen your application. Therefore, make use of the opportunities that your medical school provides.

Professional behaviour and attitudes

As a medical student, the standard of behaviour expected is different from that expected of other students at university. You will be respon-sible for patients in the near future, so it is important you instil trust with your conduct and act in a responsible manner. Most medical schools provide preclinical students with opportunities to go to hospitals or GP practices during the preclinical years. This sets the tone for how you are expected to behave. Remember to lead by example and that you have been selected to act as an ambassador for your university. The General Medical Council (GMC) has recently set out guidance for the stand-ards expected which can be found via its website (℞ https://www. gmc-uk.org/education/standards-guidance-and-curricula/guidance/ professional-behaviour-and-fitness-to-practise).

Five tips for preparing

The main challenge of preclinical exams is covering the volume of information, while identifying, understanding, and retaining the key concepts in each discipline relevant to clinical practice and commonly assessed in examinations.

Some tips include:

1. Plan

Your year handbook often has learning outcomes or objectives. These tend to be broad, such as 'understand the gross anatomy of the heart and blood vessels'. This is different to your A levels where a detailed syllabus is provided. Make a detailed plan of all you need to cover and when you are going to revise.

2. Start early

The most important strategy when revising for preclinical exams is starting early. After making a plan, you will appreciate the sheer volume of information that you are required to know for your preclinical exams. Therefore, start early in the semester and do not leave all your revision to the week before your exams.

3. Small chunks

Small chunks of information are easier to digest than attempting to learn a whole module. Try short periods of revision of 20–30 min with breaks in between to maximize your efficiency. If you spread out your revision, you will be able to manage your time effectively. This means you can still keep up with hobbies and sports and are less likely to burn out at a critical time (just before the examinations).

4. Find your learning style

Diagrams, writing bullet points, explaining a topic to a fellow student, or listening to podcasted lectures are examples of different types of learning styles. Find the one that works well for you.

5. Mnemonics

'Mnemonic' originates from the Ancient Greek word meaning memory. Some find mnemonics useful for aiding in the recall of facts, at least initially. Learning large numbers of these, simply because they exist, is unlikely to be helpful.

Examples of questions

Here are some examples of the style of questioning in preclinical exams.

Example 1. The mechanism of action of sildenafil is:

(a) vasoconstriction through inhibition of cGMP-specific phosphodiesterase type 2 (PDE2)
(b) vasoconstriction through inhibition of cGMP-specific phosphodiesterase type 3 (PDE3)
(c) vasodilation through inhibition of cGMP-specific phosphodiesterase type 3 (PDE3)
(d) vasoconstriction through inhibition of cGMP-specific phosphodiesterase type 5 (PDE5)
(e) vasodilation through inhibition of cGMP-specific phosphodiesterase type 5 (PDE5).

ANSWER E. Vasoconstriction is contraction of smooth muscle, whereas vasodilation is relaxation of smooth muscle. cGMP-specific phosphodiesterase type 5 is an enzyme. You will need to learn the mechanism of action of common drugs. In this example, knowing that sildenafil causes vasodilation can help you deduce its side effects such as headaches and flushing which will be helpful when you later consult in the clinical years; it may be the cause of a presenting complaint of headache. This example shows how basic science knowledge underpins clinical decision-making.

Example 2. Which organism is most likely to be responsible for gastro-oesophageal reflux disease (GORD)?

(a) *Helicobacter pylori*
(b) *Candida albicans*
(c) *Clostridium difficile*
(d) *E. coli*
(e) *Salmonella*.

ANSWER A. This question requires factual recall.

Tip
There is little certainty in medicine. There may be answer options which contain words such as 'always' or 'never'—these are unlikely to be correct. Answers which contain words such as 'often' and 'usually' are more likely to be correct.

Example 3. Which of the following is not one of the four Beauchamp and Childress' principles of biomedical ethics?

(a) Respect for autonomy
(b) Beneficence
(c) Non-maleficence
(d) Justice
(e) Empathy.

ANSWER E. As well as the traditional basic sciences, you will also be examined on medical ethics, medical psychology, professionalism, communication skills, medical law, and medical sociology.

Tip
Trust your instinct. Your first answer is usually the correct answer. If you overthink and imagine the examiner is tricking you, you lose marks on straightforward questions.

Example 4. What structure is not found in the cubital fossa?
(a) Median nerve
(b) Ulnar nerve
(c) Radial nerve
(d) Brachial artery
(e) Biceps brachii tendon.

ANSWER B. The radial nerve does not always run in the cubital fossa. However, the ulnar nerve is found in a groove of the posterior aspect of the medial epicondyle of the humerus, never in the cubital fossa. Therefore the answer is B. Impingement of the ulnar nerve is also known as cubital tunnel syndrome.

Tip
Remember to read the question properly. If you miss that the question stem contains the word 'not', you may select the wrong answer. Skim reading questions can lose you marks when you have done the hard work and know the answer. In dealing with these types of questions, you may find it helpful to tick all the options that you know with confidence the cubital fossa does not contain. Then decide between the options that are left. In a time-constrained examination situation, you may accidentally misread the question and select one of the structures that the cubital fossa does contain, whereas the question is asking for which one is not part of the cubital fossa.

Example 5. Which statement best describes what the Frank–Starling graph shows?
(a) Ventricular preload load in relation to end-systolic volumes.
(b) Ventricular preload load changes in relation to changes in stroke volume.
(c) Ventricular preload load changes in relation to venous return.
(d) Venous return changes on relation to end-diastolic volumes.
(e) Venous return changes on relation to end-systolic volumes.

ANSWER B. The similarity between each statement shows that you really must know your physiology and MCQs are by no means easier than written papers. These questions are sometimes called SBAs.

Tip
If you do not know the answer to the question, star or highlight the question and move on to the next. Attempt all the questions and pace yourself. You can attempt difficult questions later, with the knowledge that you have answered the easier questions first. You do not want to be left with barely seconds to answer easier questions.

Resources

Year handbook

Your medical school handbook will provide you with detailed information about the types of exams your medical school has chosen for assessment, how your preclinical exam results are used, and information about failing and extenuating circumstances.

Learning objectives/outcomes guidance

This has the closest resemblance to an A-level syllabus at university. These objectives or learning outcomes are broader than the syllabus provided for your A levels. However, they help you manage your learning and revision. It is easy to get overwhelmed when you think that you have to learn all of biochemistry, anatomy, or pharmacology. Work your way through the learning objectives during term time, ticking off objectives as you go along. This way when you get to Christmas and Easter, you will have a general idea of the depth and breadth of the modules.

Past papers

Your medical school may provide past papers on the student portal. Often medical schools have a limited bank of questions, so they are unlikely to publish large numbers of these, particularly MCQs. Moreover, your medical school may provide past questions but without mark schemes or examiner reports. Ask your undergraduate tutors or senior colleagues if you are unavailable to source them. Find all the past papers and practise completing them in the time allocated. Make your own mark scheme with your colleagues. Revisit these past questions, as it is likely the odd question may resurface in your exams. Practising using past papers will give you confidence and settle your nerves before you sit your first preclinical exams.

Books

You will have a suggested reading list and your medical school library should hopefully stock more than one copy of the recommended texts. These books are likely to be loaned out during peak times in the year. Buying all the recommended textbooks can be expensive and is usually unnecessary. You may be able to photocopy relevant pages of some textbooks, which can be annotated as you wish. The core topics such as anatomy, physiology, and pharmacology are likely to need regular reference, and a textbook in each is usually advisable. Senior students often sell their preclinical textbooks, so look out for the second-hand book sales.

Online subscriptions

There are a few MCQ question banks online. It is useful to practise questions with a simulated time limit, and feedback is often provided (score by specialty of discipline). Questions may vary from the questions that you will actually get in the exam, and factual inaccuracies in the questions do exist on occasion. If you subscribe online, their mobile app version is often free to download.

Examples of online medical question banks
- Medical Educator: ✑ www.medicaleducator.co.uk
- Multiple Choice Questions: ✑ www.mcqs.com
- Leeds Medical Student's Representative Council: ✑ www.mcqs.leedsmedics.org.uk/index.html
- BMA OnExamination: ✑ www.onexamination.com.

Lecturers/undergraduate tutors

Preclinical exams often test your ability to learn independently. However, if you are struggling to understand key concepts in the disciplines, ask your lecturers or undergraduate tutors for help. Most reply swiftly to an email when you ask a specific question. Try to refrain from asking 'Will this be on the exam?' or asking questions that are too broad. Tutors and lecturers are often passionate educators and most educators want to teach, not provide you with the minimum to simply pass exams.

Senior medical students

May provide a useful source of advice, having been through the same course and examinations. It is very likely you will meet more senior students through societies or in the library etc. Most will happily impart wisdom and provide useful practical advice and guidance. They will be well placed to recommend books and useful strategies that may be fairly specific to your medical school (e.g. there may be an influential lecturer on your course who has written a book and tends to write questions around its content).

Courses

These can offer you the reassurance that you have revised effectively. Medical societies often provide these courses taught by more senior medical students for free and will give you handy tips specific to your medical school exams. However, intense weekend courses are unlikely to give you all the knowledge you need to pass preclinical exams and they are no substitute for dedicating time to study. Basic science questions feature later in clinical exams and will form the basis of your clinical knowledge, so learning concepts thoroughly is the only advisable approach.

Mobile apps

There are a range of companies who provide MCQ or anatomy apps, in addition to online subscriptions. If you are on the train home or travelling to clinical placements in your preclinical years, these may be an efficient use of time. The *BMJ OnExamination* app provides an extensive bank of MCQs and EMQs in the basic sciences to complement its online resource. The *One2One Medicine Preclinical* app is a free app with over 500 questions. The *TeachMeAnatomy* app provides both detailed anatomical images and numerous MCQs. 3D4Medical provide a range of anatomy apps such as *Essential Anatomy*. Medical students have developed some of these apps themselves.

Dealing with poor results

Extenuating circumstances

During each semester and in the run up to your exams, you may experience bereavement, illness, or run into financial difficulties. Various terms such as extenuating or mitigating circumstances are used to describe these unforeseen circumstances. If events have affected your ability to study then you should consult the pastoral support available at your medical school. Moreover, you can discuss the impact that it has had on your studies. They may be able to offer an extension for essays or offer the option of deferring your exams. Some medical schools operate a policy of 'Fit to Sit'. If you choose to sit an exam, you have declared yourself 'Fit to Sit' at the start of the exam. Therefore, if you fail that exam, circumstances such as bereavement, will not be taken account. However, if you have a chronic illness during the semester and choose to sit the exam and fail, you cannot claim in retrospect that your chronic illness affected your ability to study. Seeking help early is a sign of professionalism that you possess insight into your health and well-being. This is important in your future medical career. It is worth discussing any such issues with your personal tutor, the welfare officer, and the occupational health service.

Failing

You may fail an examination or two during your preclinical years. This may very well be the first time you have failed something. The key thing is to pick yourself up, reflect on where you went wrong, and make a plan on how to prepare for your resit. Failing examinations can be stressful, but most people manage to persevere and pass their resit(s). Quite often, it is the sheer volume of work that has left you unprepared to sit the exams, rather than a question of intelligence. Some medical schools provide resit classes to help you pass. Make an appointment with your undergraduate tutors to discuss certain topics that you find difficult.

You will fail in some form during your medical career—whether it is passing your first professional examination such as membership exams, getting the speciality job of your choice, or publishing research. Unfortunately your patients may not recover as expected or respond to treatment even if your management was correct, possibly leading to their mortality in spite of your best efforts. Therefore it is important to learn how to cope with failures. Medical schools normally only allow *two attempts* at a preclinical exam. So take failing an exam seriously and study hard for the resit. If you fail after the third attempt, you may be required to withdraw from the course or take a year out to sort out any issues. This happens to a minority of students but the lesson here is that no one is immune to some sense of 'failure'. Leave yourself no other choice but to get back up again and try until you succeed. Do not allow one poor mark, bad experience, or obstacle at one time to define your whole career!

Uses for exam results

Intercalation

(See ➋ Chapter 5). If intercalating, all summative assessments from pre-clinical years will be used in combination with your intercalation year percentage to determine your degree classification for your intercalated degree of Bachelor of Arts (BA), BSc, or Bachelor of Medical Sciences (BMedSci):

• First-class honours degree: more than 70%.
• Upper second-class honours (2:1) degree: 60–69%.
• Lower second-class honours (2:2) degree: 50–59%.

Medicine degree

Your medicine degree (Bachelor of Medicine, Bachelor of Surgery (MBBS)) is not classified with the conventional classification of first class, 2:1, or 2:2. All summative assessments from preclinical years and the clinical years will contribute to your final grade. The top performing part of your cohort will graduate with a degree of MBBS with Honours. It varies between medical schools how they calculate Honours, so consult your year handbook or ask your undergraduate tutors for the specific percentage or merits that are required. Distinctions are usually awarded to the top 5–10% of your year. You will graduate at the end of your 4/5- or 6-year course with any of the following on your degree certificate, depending on your medical school:

• MBChB
• MBBS
• MBBCh
• MBBChir (Cantab)
• BMBCh (Oxon)
• BMBS
• MB, BCh, BAO.

Deciles

Summative assessments from both the preclinical and clinical years are usually used to determine your decile. Deciles range from first decile (top 10%) to tenth decile (bottom 10%). When you apply for junior doctor jobs in your final year, all summative examinations from year 1 to year 5 (or year 6 if you intercalated) will be used to calculate your decile. Each medical school has a unique method of calculating how you are ranked in your cohort and this method may vary from year to year. Some modules or components are deemed to carry more weight and importance than others. Most medical schools tend to put greater weight on clinical years compared to preclinical years when calculating deciles. Your medical school should provide information in your handbook.

Leaving preclinical medicine

It is estimated that approximately 8% of preclinical students drop out of medicine within the first 2 years. Some premedical students decide that they no longer hold aspirations to train as a doctor and no longer want to continue with the course. Medical schools usually offer exit qualifications at the end of at least 3 years of study. Degree qualifications with a BSc or BA are offered and the standard degree classification usually applies.

Ten tips for succeeding at your preclinical exams

1. Start early

Revising a whole module on the Sunday before the exam is impossible. However, scheduling time to learn a few metabolic pathways and the mechanism of action of a few drugs is more manageable and you are more likely to commit the detail to memory. University gives you freedom to manage your time. Do not spend all your time socializing or overcommit to any single activity. If you dedicate some time to studying early on, you will not have a pile of disjointed lecture notes to scramble through at Christmas and Easter.

2. Repetition

There are aspects of the course that require rote learning, or require you to simply memorize detail (drug names, for example). You must revisit topics more than once until you are satisfied that you have retained those details.

3. Time management

Calculate how much time you require per question. If in an exam you are struggling to answer a question, highlight the question and return later. If you spend a disproportionately long time on one question, you may not have time to answer easy questions later on in your exam.

4. Practising exam questions

There is no guarantee that the same questions will come up in the exam. Therefore, do not focus on the content of practice exam questions. However, practising exam questions will help you apply your knowledge and refine your exam technique.

5. Take a break

Exercise, play a musical instrument, or see your friends. Taking regular breaks will make you more productive. After your break, you will return with renewed enthusiasm for understanding abstract principles compared to if you had stayed at your desk staring at the same page for 2 hours.

6. Sleep

The midnight oil burns ardently for many medical students. However, it is important to take care of yourself and sacrificing sleep is counter-productive.

7. Do not get overwhelmed

At times, passing your preclinical exams may seem challenging. However, the vast majority of students make it through to the clinical years. The key strategy is to work steadily throughout the year.

8. Read the question

It can be stressful when presented with 120 MCQs to answer in 120 min and you may misread a question. You may misread the question stem that has asked you to select which statement is false and instead selected an option which is true. A handy tip is to mark each MCQ that is false with a cross and each MCQ that is true with a tick. Then read the question stem again to check you need to select an answer that is false.

9. Do not cram

You may meet some people who claim to do no revision or find preclinical exams easy. If you glance back at the example questions in the chapter, you will realize that you cannot pass your preclinical exams with cramming or doing no revision. Medical knowledge is not innate. It requires hard work, understanding of abstract concepts, and time to accumulate and commit these facts to memory, so you are able to demonstrate your knowledge in the exam.

10. Focus on yourself

Everyone learns in a different way and has different strengths. You are likely to be competitive, but comparing yourself continually to your peers is more likely to be harmful. It might take you much longer than your flatmate to learn something or you may be disappointed that your best friend beats you in every exam. Later on in your career there are more exams to come and more chances for you to excel. You have not worked this hard to compete with anyone, your greatest strength and weakness is yourself. If you look at the bigger picture, you will quickly realize that there will be many opportunities for you to hone your skills. This is where patience is a virtue.

> **Tip**
>
> Problems hit everyone! Consider discussing your issues with your personal tutor or the Welfare Officer who can offer support and guidance on behalf of the university.

Intercalated degrees and special study modules

Should I start an intercalated degree?

'Intercalating' is an opportunity to obtain a standalone qualification by taking a break from your usual medical studies. The qualification is normally a BSc degree in a medically related subject, completed in 1 year. Approximately a third of undergraduates undertake an intercalated degree in the UK. Intercalating means you will lengthen your course but qualify with two degrees.

Project

There are numerous choices available for what you want to spend months on researching, categorized into the following:

- *Laboratory projects*: involve molecular or animal research.
- *Clinical projects*: based in hospitals collecting data or samples from patients.
- *Library-based projects*: retrospective and use secondary sources to compile a report (e.g. history of medicine).
- *Clinical audit*: a quality improvement process in which you compare data you collect on patient care against explicit national guidelines and implement a change to improve service provision.
- *Grant proposal and study design*: gives you the opportunity to compile a commercial proposal to submit to an organization to obtain funding for a project.
- *Other projects*: may include a poster presentation, coursework, team assessments, and vivas, depending on your intercalated degree.

Why *should* I intercalate?

- *To explore your personal interests*: the medical curriculum covers a breadth of topics, with limited time and opportunity to delve into a particular subject. Intercalating enables you to study an area of interest in far greater depth by learning about current thinking or conducting focused research.
- *To experience a particular field*: perhaps you fancy yourself as an expedition medic, or aspire to change public policy? From global health to healthcare economics, intercalation can provide an early opportunity to discover niches outside the mainstream. A scientific degree will provide a good introduction into academia, clinical governance, and advancement of education and medical literature. A BSc is the first step to a higher degree such as a Masters and a Doctor of Philosophy (PhD/DPhil).
- *To gain new transferable skills*: all programmes will significantly enhance your ability to effectively communicate your findings, review literature, and analyse critically. These skills are invaluable throughout your career—doctors need to evaluate evidence in any branch of medicine to offer optimal patient care.
- *For careers in academic disciplines*: participation in research is becoming increasingly crucial for trainees pursuing competitive specialties, such as surgery and academic medicine. Intercalated degrees may confer an advantage to enhance your CV as an undergraduate. An intercalated degree can boost your career prospects and counts towards extra points for your job applications.

- *Academic achievement*: your research could lead to significant achievement on your CV, portfolio, and job interviews if:
  - it gets published in a peer-reviewed journal on the PubMed/MEDLINE database that can be accessed all over the world
  - it gets accepted into a regional, national, or international conference for you to present your research findings
  - it gets published as an audit in your local hospital
  - regardless of the outcome and if your work does not get published in the worst-case scenario, you will always have your thesis with your name to add to your portfolio.
- *For a hiatus*: many medics report that intercalation broke up their course with a refreshing chance to enjoy an altogether different type of study. It is a nice break from strenuous clinical studies and rotations, and a chance for you to feel rejuvenated. Also, depending on the intensity of your chosen course and research project, you will find yourself having more spare time than when on clinical rotations to pursue your extracurricular activities.
- *Post-nominals*: are a perk upon satisfactory completion of your intercalated degree (e.g. BSc Hons, Master of Science (MSc), etc.)
- *Travelling*: may become an option if:
  - you choose to do an external intercalated degree (outside your university) giving you an opportunity to spend time in another city and campus for a year making new contacts and friends
  - some universities offer you the chance to carry out your research project abroad, such as in Tanzania for infectious diseases or Japan for gastric cancer.

Why *shouldn't* I intercalate?

Since intercalation is compulsory at some universities, students elsewhere might feel compelled to follow. Do not start a perfunctory degree! Make sure you are genuinely keen to spend a year engrossed in a particular subject to enjoy the challenges and rewards a wisely chosen one brings.

- *Expectation*: your supervisor may have forgotten what it was like being a medical student and may have far too many expectations from you. You must recognize your limitations and do not hesitate to ask for help and guidance from your supervisor. You will become more comfortable with research as you gain experience.
- *Cost*: you will be charged for an additional academic year so make sure that you are able to afford your tuition fee (up to £9000), rent, and living expenses. It is wise to seek alternative sources of funding such as internal and external scholarships and bursary schemes from the National Health Service (NHS) Business Service Authority (℞ www.nhsbsa.nhs.uk).
- *Lectures*: if you did not enjoy your time in preclinical and biomedical lectures, then bear in mind that the majority of your BSc will consist of attending lectures, sometimes for the entire day. Besides didactic lectures, there will an array of other activities including tutorial discussions, seminars, and team presentations.

- *Project duration*: there is no guarantee that you will be able to complete your project within the allocated time which means that there is no guarantee of journal publication or conference presentation. However, you can always try to complete the project during your vacations afterwards and try to publish then. Under a fifth of British undergraduates submit their research to journals.
- *Extra study*: it is an additional year and will prolong your time until graduation. However, an intercalated degree will work in your favour when applying for competitive jobs.
- *Supervision*: if your supervisors are full-time clinicians, you may not be given as much dedicated time for supervision compared to those who are full-time researchers. You are expected to be dynamic, work independently for most of the time, and figure out solutions to any rate-limiting steps. It is more likely that you will complete your project in time, present your findings at conferences, and publish your thesis if you are closely monitored and effectively guided by a hands-on supervisor.
- *Funding*: if your project budget runs over, then you may need to pause your research until more funding can be arranged which is a luxury that you cannot afford in the short time allocated before the submission deadline for your dissertation.

Choosing the right intercalated degree

Hundreds of intercalated programmes are available across the UK. This might seem daunting, but degrees can be narrowed down easily to suit your preferences by systematically considering your criteria.

Location

Begin by selecting a course according to your personal circumstances. External intercalators should consider the distance from family, friends, and your medical school. It is worthwhile finding out if you are expected to return during the year, and the financial and logistical feasibility of finding new accommodation and travelling.

Subject

Completing a degree in 1 year is intensive and demanding compared with the rest of the medical course. There is greater reliance on self-directed learning, with an increased scope for original thought, and often a student-selected component or project to steer in your own direction. It is therefore worthwhile searching for a subject that you feel passionate to pore over!

Assessments

Will ultimately decide the classification of your degree, so determine which methods will be used (MCQ, essays, presentations, viva voce, dissertation) and their weightings. The overall result might depend on submitted coursework, end-of-year examinations, or a combination: play to your strengths.

Support

For independent components and projects, students are customarily assigned one or more supervisors who are university staff members or clinicians. You could be engaged in a project under their supervision for months, so finding someone with whom you can develop an effective working relationship is important. If you have found a degree subject and project that interests you, contact your potential supervisor to arrange a visit. Communication is key: if they do not seem open and approachable, you can investigate alternatives. Additionally, inquire about the welfare resources accessible at your host institution while you are intercalating. Some students occasionally suffer unforeseen events requiring mitigation, which may be complicated by living away from your familiar support network and your GP.

Master's degree

Some master's programmes leading to the award of MSc, Master of Research (MRes), etc. do accept medical students, but most require you to have completed 4 years of your main degree to be eligible or an intercalated BSc first. They often have term dates incompatible with the medical course, requiring an academic leave of absence. Beware that entitlement to future funding from Student Finance may be affected according to an equivalent level qualification rule.

Finding a programme and applying

Searching for a degree

№ www.intercalate.co.uk is a useful reference guide listing intercalated courses. It has a geographical search function and maintains a comprehensive database of individual programmes.

Alternative subjects

There is a growing number of alternative subjects to study as an intercalated BSc which are not related to the conventional specialities. Doing an intercalated degree in a non-conventional subject will showcase your talent and versatility and give you a competitive edge. A few contemporary subjects include

- health management (Imperial College London)
- healthcare ethics and law (Birmingham and King's College)
- philosophy, medicine and society (University College London).

Variations

The most common intercalated degree at medical school is a BSc. Oxford and Cambridge graduates have their traditional BA automatically upgraded to Master of Arts (MA). A BMedSci is otherwise offered at Birmingham, Edinburgh, Nottingham, Sheffield, and Queen Mary's (Barts and The London School of Medicine and Dentistry).

Internal opportunities

You will be given several lectures throughout the year about how the system works and which choices you have at your university. You will also be told about the content and modules available for each intercalated degree in more depth. Your university intranet should have a dedicated section on intercalated degree options with lectures from previous years.

External opportunities

Some may have the opportunity to undertake an intercalated degree at another institute, depending on the following:

- *Subject choice*: if your preferred subject is already offered internally, it is unlikely that you will be permitted to study that subject elsewhere.
- *External university*: select universities offer intercalated degrees to external candidates depending on spaces available, your previous exam performance, and possible interviews.
- *Permission*: your university has full discretion to grant you an academic leave of absence depending on your exam performance and professional conduct.

Your university may have internal awards available. Other organizations offer grants and bursaries—particularly Royal Colleges and charitable research organizations.

Clinical research projects

(See ➲ 'Clinical research' pp. 1024–1027). Clinical research is broadly defined as involving human subjects with the goal of understanding and improving the diagnosis, treatment, and management of disease. It aims to inform clinical guidance by generating knowledge about best practice. Such research opportunities are by no means confined to intercalated degree courses—there are many ways for motivated medical students to get involved in elective or extracurricular projects.

Why should you get involved in clinical research?

Medicine is an evidence-based profession, and conducting research will equip you with a transferable and valuable skill set, even if you are not considering an academic career. Formulating questions, appraising literature, and understanding the methodology and ethics of science are competencies expected of doctors by the GMC. Research projects furthermore provide experience in communicating results through presentations and writing. If you are passionate about a particular specialty, getting involved at the forefront of understanding will allow you to engage and network with distinguished leaders in the field. Academic clinicians are often eager to teach, inspire, or even mentor students who approach their area of interest with enthusiasm.

Successful research projects open opportunities to present your findings at conferences or achieve authorship of a journal publication. This rewarding endeavour involves a large amount of effort and a small amount of luck, but will embellish your CV, and confer additional points on application to the Foundation Programme. Prestigious scientific breakthroughs have been initiated by students of medicine throughout its history. Charles Best, a Canadian medical student, successfully treated a diabetic patient after isolating insulin from pancreatic islets, which were first identified by German medical student Paul Langerhans. Your contribution could ultimately have a far-reaching impact on patients!

Types of research

Primary medical research generates novel and original data from laboratory or healthcare settings. Laboratory projects may be classified as 'wet lab' (experimenting on biological tissue) or 'dry lab' (involving computational modelling and analytics). Secondary medical research involves gathering and analysing existing data, e.g. by systematic review and meta-analysis.

Choosing a project

Weigh up your preferences carefully as it can be quite awkward if you change your mind halfway through. You will be spending at least 3–4 months doing this day in and day out. Every researcher encounters frustrations when delving into the unknown. Browse the latest copies of journals in the library in order to appreciate examples of research currently trending in your areas of interest.

Finding a supervisor

Intercalated degree students will often be offered a list of upcoming projects in various departments and with named supervisors. Your principal supervisor will usually be the expert in their field, renowned and well published. Your principal supervisor will be the person you report to and who will sign off work. Since he or she is the head of a research department too and extremely busy, you may be given a day-to-day supervisor who will supervise you throughout the entire undertaking, from planning to publication.

Begin by searching the departmental directory of your university and teaching hospital websites for profiles of consultants and principal investigators (PIs) by area of expertise (a PI is a scientist charged to lead a particular research study). Institutions will usually maintain web pages containing their research interests, publications, and contact details. Alternatively, publication records can be sought by looking up your prospective supervisors by name on PubMed. Make a list of all those whose work is aligned to your objectives.

After identifying prospective supervisors, send a formal email to each, introducing yourself and expressing your interest in working with them. Sending multiple queries simultaneously is acceptable providing you do not promise any commitment at this stage. Follow up all positive replies by trying to arrange a face-to-face meeting at the supervisor's convenience, and otherwise offer a telephone call. If they have a personal assistant, do not hesitate to contact them to confirm your availability. Be persistent in chasing up pledges, which can easily get lost among the competing demands on researchers' time.

Prepare thoroughly before meeting supervisors for the first time: they will expect enthusiasm, knowledge about their own research, and broad ideas of what you hope to accomplish. Ensure plans remain realistic by discussing your role openly and explicitly explaining your timeframe and availability to the supervisor. Finally, request details of former students under their guidance. In turn, speak to them for recommendations, and try to find out if previous projects yielded any presentations or publications.

The only time you may be expected to find a supervisor is if you have organized a project by yourself and one that was not initially advertised through the medical school. In this case, you need to also provide a research proposal, sources of funding, and ethical approval to the medical school before starting the project. Hence, it is much easier to choose an advertised research project. It is wise to hold at least weekly meetings with your supervisor to discuss your latest research findings and so that your progress can be consistently monitored. This will also minimize the risk of straying away from a high grade.

Sources of funding

Not only do you have to account for the expenses of an additional academic year of undertaking an intercalated degree, you also have to appreciate that research does depend on available funding. If you sign up to an advertised research project, then both ethics and funding may already have been arranged by your supervisor before you start. When joining an existing project, the cost of your contribution will usually be absorbed under an existing grant. Internal scholarships may also be offered in open competition. However, securing additional funding can widen the horizon of your research, and represents a prestigious accolade in its own right. Many organizations and charitable trusts offer bursaries to competitive medical students undertaking vacation projects, electives, and intercalated degrees. Forward planning is essential since applications for these awards often open just once per year, requiring full details of your intended project as well as a written reference or input from your supervisor. Some organizations offering scholarship include the following:

- The *Association for the Study of Medical Education* (ASME) is available for students doing projects and degrees in medical education worth £300 (℗ www.asme.org.uk).
- The *British Association of Dermatologists* offer up to £3000 (℗ www.bad. org.uk).
- The *British Association of Plastic, Reconstructive and Aesthetic Surgeons* (BAPRAS) may support undergraduates with up to £500 (℗ www. bapras.org.uk).
- The *Royal College of Surgeons of England* is offering an intercalated BSc degree in surgery or surgical-related area and will review each project individually (℗ www.rcseng.ac.uk/standards-and-research/research/ fellowships-awards-grants/awards-and-grants/medical-student-awards/ intercalated-bachelor-science-degree/).
- *Amgen Scholars* provides full funding for undergraduates to participate in research opportunities at world-class institutions across the globe (℗ www.amgenscholars.eu).
- The *Wolfson Foundation* offers support for intercalation projects. Applications must be made via your institution—enquire within your medical school for more information (℗ www.wolfson.org.uk).
- The *Carnegie Trust* is open to Scottish students in their third year. Applications must be made via your institution for 2–8-week projects (℗ www.carnegie-trust.org/schemes/undergraduate-schemes/ vacation-scholarships.html).
- *Money for Med Students* is the website of the Royal Medical Benevolent Fund and is laden with research funding opportunities (℗ www. money4medstudents.org).
- The *UK Medical Student Association* (UKMSA) lists a wealth of organizations offering specific research opportunities and funding (℗ www.ukmsa.org/research/studentshipsandfunding).

Vacation studentships

Sometimes, funding can be applied for from external organizations which also offer their own research projects. In this case, supervisors and ethical approval should usually be arranged prior to your involvement. As it would be an external research placement, you ought to seek permission from your medical school and check eligibility criteria. The advertised project may start later than internal projects in which case you will have less time but be expected to produce high-quality research, a presentation, and a thesis by the set deadline regardless. The organizations in Table 5.1 may be of some help.

Table 5.1 Organizations for placements

Subject	Association	Website	Duration	Funding
Biochemistry	Biochemical Society (BiochemSoc)	www.biochemistry.org	6–8 weeks	£1600
Biomedicine	Wellcome	www.wellcome.ac.uk	6–8 weeks	£1520
Bioscience	Biotechnology and Biological Sciences Research Council (BBSRC)	www.bbsrc.ac.uk	10 weeks	£2500
Fertility	Society for Reproduction and Fertility (SRF)	www.srf-reproduction.org	8 weeks	£1520
Microbiology	British Society for Antimicrobial Chemotherapy (BSAC)	www.bsac.org.uk	10 weeks	£1800
Microbiology	Society for General Microbiology (SGM)	www.socgenmicrobiol.org.uk	8 weeks	£1880
Pathology	Pathological Society (PathSoc)	www.pathsoc.org	6–8 weeks	£1500
Physiology	Physiological Society (PhysSoc)	www.physoc.org	6–8 weeks	£1200
Science	Nuffield Foundation	www.nuffieldfoundation.org	6–8 weeks	£1440
Science	Medical Research Scotland	www.medicalresearchscotland.org.uk	6–8 weeks	£2000

Getting the most out of research projects

Whatever your chosen discipline, the independent work undertaken while intercalating can be disseminated as abstracts, presented at conferences, and even published in peer-reviewed journals. Conferences often give awards for the best poster presentation delivered by a medical student, and there are numerous prizes available for essays and original research by professional organizations representing medical and surgical specialties.

Useful reference

Stubbs TA, Lightman EG, Mathieson P. Is it intelligent to intercalate? A two centre cross-sectional study exploring the value of intercalated degrees, and the possible effects of the recent tuition fee rise in England. *BMJ Open* 2013;3:e002193.

Information governance and backup

In clinical research, you will inevitably work with health records, or information which can identify people, or which would enable their identity information to be retrieved. It may be your first time with authority to access large volumes of confidential information, and it may be tempting to save and backup your hard work as usual. Beware that clinical data is different. Retaining, copying, and transferring sensitive data (both paper and electronic) is subject to strict legal requirements as well as local trust policies, known collectively as 'information governance'. Consult your supervisor and governance department at your hospital for advice before you start.

Good Clinical Practice (GCP) training

Everyone involved in the conduct of clinical research should receive GCP training commensurate with their roles and responsibilities, to ensure the rights, safety, and well-being of participants are protected. Practically, GCP teaches the laws, frameworks, and guidelines which govern the set-up and conduct of trials, and will empower you to consent and recruit participants. You can either attend the courses or complete the online version.

Key points

- Choose a topic based on your genuine personal interests.
- Seek supervisors with a proven track record of mentoring undergraduates.
- Ask if funding is already in place for the project. This will save many headaches. If not, then apply for funding as soon as you have confirmed a project. You must appreciate that all applications do not receive funding. Additionally, there may be numerous stages of applications ahead of you which all take plenty of time!
- Diligently compile your findings soon after acquisition.

After the project

Communicating your findings: presenting posters and oral talks

Presentations serve to share information of value with others in the medical profession and scientific community. Posters and oral talks are the two most common methods for communicating your findings face-to-face. By presenting, you will receive helpful feedback from members of the audience, exchange ideas among researchers familiar with your topic, and meet like-minded potential collaborators.

Besides conferences, research can be showcased at your medical school, pitched to the faculty where it was conducted, or presented at a local hospital trust. Your CV will be enhanced by any of these activities. Conferences will invite exhibitors to submit an 'abstract' in advance (a short, written summary of your work which lets them decide if your research matches their interests).

- Organizers screen received abstracts to confirm your project is relevant to the event, in which case you may be offered a poster or an oral presentation.
- Abstracts form the beginning of published journal manuscripts.
- Abstracts are 'indexed' by libraries and databases, meaning users can search their content to retrieve relevant literature.

In every case, they are paramount to capturing attention.

Abstract writing tips

Abstracts are traditionally structured into certain headings and limited to 250–350 words or less.

Background

This section is often the shortest, and contextualizes the overall purpose of your project by introducing the rationale for investigation in as few as two sentences:

1. Summarize *what* is already known about your topic—cite previous studies as references.
2. Explain *what* is unknown and outline *how* your project adds to this existing knowledge.

You should reduce jargon to a non-technical level that your audience will understand.

Aims and objectives

States exactly what your project intends to measure and discover—bullet points are appropriate. Readers will refer to your aims when deciding if your methodology is suitable, and if your results indicate success.

Methods

An objective description of what you did to obtain your results. Not every intricacy needs to be included in this section. To decide what to exclude, list each step of your experimental process from start to finish. Now ask whether knowing each detail could affect the conclusions a reader draws from your study. For example, it may not be relevant to mention the make and model of a prosthetic heart valve for a project comparing surgical vs medical management of aortic stenosis, but it would be important if comparing outcomes from two different manufacturers. Key parameters to expand include:

- *population*—the participants and how were they selected
- *intervention/indicator*—the tests or procedures under scrutiny
- *comparator*—any controls or alternative strategies or exposures
- *outcome*—how the consequences were measured and analysed.

Results

Readers perusing an abstract will be most interested to learn about the findings of your study. Therefore, this section should comprise the longest part and quantify as much relevant detail as the word count permits. For example, '5-year mortality rates differed significantly between medical and surgical groups' is better expressed as 'The 5-year mortality rate was higher in surgical than in medical patients (15% vs 12% respectively, $p < 0.05$)'. Always provide the mean value of outcome measures and their p-values, as in this example. Test statistics need not be included for comparison studies; however, the r-value should be added in correlation studies.

Conclusion

Can be simplified to three elements:
1. Based on the results, derive take-home messages related directly to the original aims and objectives.
2. Without reiterating any numbers, highlight the implications of the outcome measure (only the results section should contain data).
3. Customarily end with an opinion or perspective on the importance of the findings for the field.

Poster presentations

A poster presentation is a visual summary of your entire project. It can be thought of as a graphical version of an abstract: designed using a computer program such as Microsoft PowerPoint, printed on A1 or A2 large-format card, then discussed face-to-face with judges at an academic event. Posters are made for exhibition at specific meetings after the organizers have approved a pre-submitted abstract of your research. There may be over 50 on display at a national conference, with prizes available for the best (scored on both your content and conversation). Make sure you check what the poster size should be before designing it, especially whether it is portrait or landscape as the conference boards will be set-up accordingly.

Tips for designing a poster

Authorship

Before creating a poster:
1. Check with your collaborators that you may present the group's shared findings and intellectual property.
2. Confirm how their names should be credited on the poster.
3. Ask if they have any conditions or suggestions for the design.

Include the names of every colleague who contributed to the project on your poster and involve them throughout the process—all co-authors must approve your submission, and may offer you use of digital diagrams and figures they have designed previously.

Specification

You must adhere to the size and orientation specified by the conference (e.g. A1 portrait). Judges may otherwise disqualify you from the competition, or organizers may altogether disallow you from presenting! Using Microsoft PowerPoint, the poster can be created on a single slide, set up by clicking on the 'Design' tab and inputting dimensions manually through 'Page Setup'.

Layout and content

Ask your supervisor to see examples previously produced by researchers in your team (see Fig. 5.1 for an example). Identify the audience and tailor your content to be as accessible as possible to delegates. For instance, conferences about a niche subject might favour a focus on the exact details of your methods, whereas an overarching explanation will benefit generalized meetings. Will the posters be marked for a competition, and by whom?

- Include a title, list of author names, and all the aforementioned sections expected in an abstract: background, aims/objectives, methods, results, and conclusion/discussion.
- Components can be laid out vertically in columns, or horizontally in rows, whichever makes your information flow most intuitively.
- Include enough text to provide a basic understanding of your project, but not so much that readers feel bored. Remember you can expand and explain further during discussion with judges.
- Dark font on a light background is most legible.
- Use abbreviations: familiarize your reader by iterating the full name on first use (with the abbreviation in parentheses).
- It is similarly acceptable to re-christen long scientific names (e.g. 'coenzyme Q10' becomes 'CoQ').
- Exploit maximum use of figures and diagrams to allow the reader to visualize concepts—a picture paints a thousand words—even your methods can be summarized in a flow diagram.
- List references and acknowledgments of funding.
- Add your email address so people can subsequently contact you with afterthought comments, questions, or proposals.

After creating a poster

Ask colleagues to review and critique your draft; friends and family without a medical or scientific background are an excellent source of feedback on aesthetics and clarity. Once you and your supervisor are happy, get the finalized version printed professionally. Printing companies will offer several options:

1. *Lamination* bonds a thin film over the paper to give a *gloss* finish (like magazine paper) or *matte* finish (which minimizes glare).
2. *Encapsulation* will protect your poster from creases, fingerprints, and scratches by encasing the paper in plastic.

Additionally, print several copies of your poster on ordinary A4 paper for interested peers to take away.

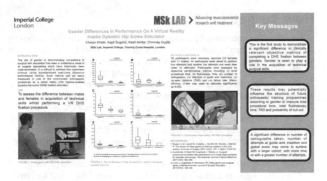

Fig. 5.1 Example presentation poster. Reproduced with permission from Dr Kapil Sugand (co-author) and MSk Lab, Imperial College London.

Tips for discussing a poster

- Practise, practise, practise presenting your poster orally to anyone who is willing to listen—usually for 5 min, with a further 5 min for questioning—keep strictly within time limits.
- If you are unsure how familiar your audience is with your subject area, ask them before you begin. It is safer to assume zero prior knowledge and an infinite capacity for intelligent thought.
- Be prepared to boil down your research in a few minutes and be able to summarize your project in one concise sentence.
- Verbal discussion may influence the judges as much as the poster.
- Invite questions from your audience at the end or throughout.
- It is not merely what you say, but how you say it. Judges will be impressed by enthusiasm while demonstrating your work.

How to get published

It is a common misconception among medical students that co-authoring primary medical research is the only way to get published. Although novel findings are attractive to many journals, secondary medical research offering novel insights into existing data are held equally dear. Most projects are worth reporting to the scholarly community of scientists and clinicians if you can devote a few hours each week to the cause.

1. After the completion of any project, strive to analyse results, draw conclusions, and contextualize the importance of findings as soon as possible. The world of research is vulnerably fast-moving and filled with breakthroughs named after investigators who communicated—not discovered—them first.

2. Conduct a thorough literature search to survey where your work fits within the landscape. The most popular resource is PubMed (℠ www.ncbi.nlm.nih.gov/pubmed/), a free website for searching MEDLINE (the National Library of Medicine database of clinical and healthcare abstracts and citations). In case MEDLINE is saturated with papers on your topic, consider writing about it from a different, unique perspective.

3. Re-read your supervisor's most recent publications to appreciate an appropriate scientific template and writing style. Proceed to compose an academic manuscript from your own project. This endeavour can be copiously time-consuming, ideally undertaken by dedicating a couple of hours each week to drafting. You might like to enlist the help of experienced PhD students for guidance.

4. In addition to your supervisor who will thoroughly understand the topic, ask another faculty member with whom you enjoy a good professional relationship to critique the draft.

5. Identify journals which are likely to accept your paper: there are currently over 5000 indexed by MEDLINE; your supervisor will be best placed to suggest the most suitable. Journals are ranked by 'impact factor': a proxy measure reflecting their relative importance within a field. Papers must be submitted to one journal at a time to be considered for publication, usually to those deemed more important, before those with lower impact factors.

6. Each potential publisher maintains a website containing instructions to prospective authors. Ensure these criteria are strictly met by formatting articles accordingly; otherwise your submission will get rejected outright. Including a cover letter can outline the importance of your article to the journal's readership. Some editors may kindly return feedback recommending improvements.

Rarely will any journal commit to publishing your finished product without recommending multiple revisions to the article. Commonly, ideas are rejected altogether. Do not be put off: present your idea to another journal—you are likely to learn from criticisms.

Notes on writing your scientific manuscript

- Always credit other people's work honestly and properly using references.
- Any article that contains personal medical information about an identifiable living patient requires their permission for publication by obtaining prior written consent.

- Ensure any images and figures are included at a high resolution of at least 300 dots per inch.
- Stringently check spelling and grammar by proof reading.
- Ensure that you abide by the in-house formatting guidelines for each journal listed on their website—otherwise the submission will be automatically rejected and sent back to you.

Once an article has been submitted, it will firstly be scrutinized for publication by an editor. Promising papers are then constructively forwarded to further editors or external peer reviewers for second opinions. If these adjudicators decide to pursue your article, they may specify alterations to be made before acceptance (see Fig. 5.2).

Acta Orthopaedica 2015; 86 (6): 695–701　　　　　　　　　　　　　　　　　　　　　　695

Training effect of a virtual reality haptics-enabled dynamic hip screw simulator

A randomized controlled trial

Kapil SUGAND[1], Kash AKHTAR[2], Chetan KHATRI[1], Justin COBB[1], and Chinmay GUPTE[1]

[1] MSk Lab, Imperial College London, Charing Cross Hospital, Fulham; [2] Blizard Institute and Department of Trauma and Orthopaedics, Barts and the London School of Medicine and Dentistry, Queen Mary University of London, and Barts Health NHS Trust, London, UK.
Correspondence: ks704@ic.ac.uk
Submitted 2014-08-20. Accepted 2015-04-14.

Background and purpose — Virtual reality (VR) simulation offers a safe, controlled, and effective environment to complement training but requires extensive validation before it can be implemented within the curriculum. The main objective was to assess whether VR dynamic hip screw (DHS) simulation has a training effect to improve objective performance metrics.

Patients and methods — 52 surgical trainees who were naïve to DHS procedures were randomized to 2 groups: the training group, which had 5 attempts, and the control group, which had only one attempt. After 1 week, both cohorts repeated the same number of attempts. Objective performance metrics included total procedural time (sec), fluoroscopy time (sec), number of radiographs (n), tip-apex distance (TAD; mm), attempts at guide-wire insertion (n), and probability of cut-out (%). Mean scores (with SD) and learning curves were calculated. Significance was set as p < 0.05.

Results — The training group was 68% quicker than the control group, used 75% less fluoroscopy, took 66% fewer radiographs, had 82% less retries at guide-wire insertion, achieved a reduced TAD (by 41%), had lower probability of cut-out (by 85%), and obtained an increased global score (by 63%). All these results were statistically significant (p < 0.001). The participants agreed that the simulator provided a realistic learning environment, they stated that they had enjoyed using the simulator, and they recognized the need for the simulator in formal training.

Interpretation — We found a significant training effect on the VR DHS simulator in improving objective performance metrics of naïve surgical trainees. Patient safety, an important priority, was not compromised.

Orthopedic training in Europe and North America has significantly changed in the past decade due to stricter regulations on working time (Philibert et al. 2002, Nasca et al. 2010). The European Working Time Directive (Department of Health 2004) was initially prepared to safeguard both patients and healthcare professionals by promoting risk reduction and increasing patient safety. With trainees taking double the time, on average, per procedure than consultants (Bridges and Diamond 1999), opportunities to train in the operating room have decreased substantially to attain greater economic efficiency—with an 80% decrease from the traditionally estimated 30,000 hours to 6,000 hours of experience before these regulations were implemented (Chikwe et al. 2004). Simulation offers a risk-free learning environment.

With 1.6 million fractures reported in Europe in the year 2000, osteoporotic fractures accounted for more disability-adjusted life years lost than common cancers with the exception of lung cancer (Johnell and Kanis 2006), and they therefore represent a significant burden of morbidity. A dynamic hip screw (DHS) simulator may provide a means of safely training surgeons to reduce the risk of failure. However, any simulation system requires validation regarding its efficacy and acceptability.

A literature search found only 3 studies using VR models for DHS fixation. Blyth et al. (2007 and 2008) reported on a simulator using conventional computer interfaces (mouse and keyboard). Froelich et al. (2011) reported their findings on construct validity of a haptics-enabled simulator using a phantom stylus that had an interface with force feedback. Pedersen

Fig. 5.2 Published journal article. Reproduced from *Acta Orthopaedica* under CC-BY-NC-ND 3.0 licence, and permission from lead author, Dr Kapil Sugand. © Nordic Orthopaedic Federation.

Laboratory research

You may get the chance to experience basic science laboratory research during a special study module, an intercalated BSc, or even as an extracurricular activity. It is an opportunity not to be missed, and offers many invaluable skills: 'wet-bench' techniques such as cell culture or Western blotting, critical and independent thinking, objective critique of scientific literature, basic statistics, etc.

Brief background

Anatomical pathology

This is the branch of pathology dealing with tissue diagnosis of disease based on gross, microscopic, molecular, chemical, and immunological examination. It encompasses the following branches:

- *Histopathology*—the study of changes in tissue caused by disease:
  - Histochemistry is the science of staining tissue sections for diagnosis.
  - Immunohistochemistry is the science of detecting the presence, abundance, and localization of antigens and proteins using antibodies.
  - Immunofluorescence tags a coloured dye molecule to an antibody.
- *Cytopathology*—the study of disease at cellular level:
  - Specimens are collected from smears or fine-needle aspirates.
- *Pathophysiology*—the study of disordered physiological processes as a result of disease.
- *Electron microscopy*—uses high-resolution magnification at cellular level.

Clinical pathology

This is the branch of pathology dealing with microscopic and macroscopic analyses of internal bodily fluids (e.g. blood, urine, and semen). It consists of the following branches:

- *Microbiology*: the study of microorganisms; can be categorized into immunology, bacteriology, parasitology, virology, and mycology. Cultures and sensitivities are also deduced.
- *Chemistry*: the analysis of serum or plasma constituents (e.g. renal function test), blood sugar, lipid profiles, protein and enzymes (e.g. liver function tests), toxicology (e.g. paracetamol overdose), and endocrinology (hormone profiles).
- *Haematology*: the analysis of red and white blood cells, platelets, and clotting function.
- *Reproduction biology*: for analysis of gametes.
- *Genetics*: the analysis of DNA and genetic data.
  - *Cytogenetics* is used to deduce a cellular karyotype.

Which lab?

This is probably more important than the actual subject matter of the project, particularly for a short placement. You are unlikely to accrue much publishable data in a matter of weeks or months, yet fostering a good working relationship leads to future opportunities.

Which supervisor?

Do not focus so hard on finding a placement with the most influential professor that you overlook the need for someone with the time to supervise you on a day-to-day basis. Being unsupervised in a new and alien environment can be a lonely and frustrating experience. If possible, visit the lab (and supervisor) before starting and find out who will be directly in charge of you. You are looking for a lab with research assistants or PhD students who will take the time to talk you through new skills rather than leaving you floundering.

Which project?

You are unlikely to have much say over this at an early stage. Often a supervisor will have a set project in mind to answer a specific question, and you will not be expected to have much creative input at the beginning. It is important, however, to have a basic grasp of the context of your work; ask your supervisor to recommend some relevant review articles to introduce you to the field. You will certainly gain expertise in the field of study if you take the initiative to conduct a short literature review. This may also act as the basis of your publication. You should also have a realistic expectation of what can be achieved in the time you have; if a technique takes 6 months to master, it may not be well suited to a shorter placement.

What outputs?

It would be unusual if a short period in the lab were to culminate in a *Nature* paper but do not let that stop you at least trying! However, it is useful to have something to show for your efforts, such as a poster presentation at a local conference or medical student forum.

What next?

You may decide that basic science is not where your future lies, which is valuable to know. Hopefully, however, you may be inspired to pursue a career in academic medicine, and your lab experience will give you some direction and useful contacts. Applications to the Academic Foundation Programme are competitive, and having spent time in a lab will stand you in good stead.

Skills in basic science

Generic skills

Essential statistics

Relevant to every quantitative technique in medical research. Selecting the correct statistical tool is imperative for meaningful data analysis. A popular and uncomplicated statistics program is GraphPad Prism which offers a free 30-day trial and reduced rates for students (℗ www.graphpad.com/demos/).

Critical appraisal of scientific literature

Make an effort to attend lab meetings and journal clubs, and do not be afraid to ask questions! Much like clinical medicine, it is best if you clear any confusion sooner rather than later, especially when you will be expected to lead the management of a patient or a research project after you graduate. If you get the chance to present a paper yourself, it is a great learning opportunity. Similarly, your department is likely to run a series of seminars, which are well worth attending however far removed from your immediate field of interest.

Presentation of data

Oral presentations (at meetings or conferences) and written communications (such as posters and submissions to journals) both require a great deal of skill. Much emphasis is put on the abstract, which should succinctly summarize both the context and content of your work. Assume your reader is an experienced scientist outside of your immediate field.

Specialist skills

Animal research

You will need a Home Office licence (℗ www.gov.uk/research-and-testing-using-animals) and local security clearance before working with live animals in research. These may prove prohibitive for a short lab placement, though postmortem work does not require a personal licence. Most animal research in the UK uses mice and rats, though other species such as primates, rabbits, fish, and farm animals are sometimes used. No investigators relish the prospect of animal research but most agree that it is a vital part of medical science. Even a brief exposure to this field will make you appreciate the measures in place to legislate and optimize the use of animals. Use common sense when discussing this outside of work.

Cell culture

This describes the techniques involved in growing and maintaining either primary cells (i.e. isolated directly from tissue) or cell lines (immortalized, genetically identical) *in vitro*. Typically, it takes days to weeks to achieve a population of cells ready for an experiment though doubling time can vary. You will become skilled at light microscopy in order to chart the progress of your cells and preparation of cell culture media and this is before your experiment has even started.

Confocal microscopy

This is a rapidly evolving technology used to optimize spatial resolution and 3D imaging of tissues. Antigens of interest within a tissue or cell population are labelled using fluorescent antibodies, and are identified by the use of fluorescent filters and detectors. Provides anatomical/spatial and dynamic data. Particularly helpful alongside 'reporter mice' which are genetically engineered so that a specific antigen or cytokine fluoresces without further labelling.

Enzyme-linked immunosorbent assay (ELISA)

This technique is used to quantify the concentration of antibody or antigen in a sample. It requires fastidious precision in pipetting and making serial dilutions for a reference curve but when used successfully provides robust and reproducible data. Gives a valuable insight into why some clinical tests take a long time to be reported!

Flow cytometry or fluorescence-activated cell sorting (FACS)

Cells can be labelled with antibodies that bind to the cell surface or intracellular antigens, which then fluoresce when excited with light of a certain wavelength. This fluorescence is detected by sensors within the flow cytometer. For example, a fraction of human leucocytes could be stained with one colour for CD3 (T cells), another for CD19 (B cells), and a third for CD15 (neutrophils). This information can be used to quantify populations within a sample, or even to separate it into its individual components (cell sorting).

Microarray and bioinformatics

The field of genomic analysis is expanding at a staggering rate, and is frequently used to evaluate gene expression in thousands of different genes simultaneously. Such large data sets mandate a sophisticated grasp of bioinformatics and familiarity with computer programs such as R and Bioconductor.

Microbiological culture

Many labs work with infectious microorganisms such as bacteria (*Salmonella, Escherichia coli*, staphylococci) and viruses (HIV, influenza). They may be studied *in vivo* (i.e. injected into animals) or *in vitro* (cell culture). Unsurprisingly, this work is carefully regulated and the risk to the law-abiding investigator is very low.

Polymerase chain reaction (PCR)

This is used to amplify a small sample of DNA allowing for subsequent identification (e.g. of a microorganism, or a gene mutation) or quantification. Thermal cycling is used to melt, anneal, then amplify the DNA sequence in question. Extremely versatile and a good example of molecular biology in practice.

Western blotting

The quintessential lab technique both eulogized by sentimental professors and loathed by struggling PhD students! This is a semi-quantitative method of analysing proteins of interest, e.g. the presence of antibodies in a clinical sample or a change in protein expression under experimental conditions. Sodium dodecyl sulfate polyacrylamide denaturing gel electrophoresis (SDS-PAGE) is a frequently used method for separating proteins by gel electrophoresis.

Ten tips on making the most of your time in the lab

1. *Have a realistic idea* of what you want to achieve in the given time. Many short projects do not end in meaningful data; this is not necessarily a reflection on you!
2. *Keep an open mind*. You will be surrounded by people from a different background, with different skills and interests to your own. Expect to learn from your non-clinical colleagues and they may do the same.
3. *Persevere*. Most experiments do not work the first time, and often a protocol needs to be repeated again and again before it is reproducible. Write fastidious laboratory notes so you can identify what worked or did not work.
4. *Be a good colleague*. If you use the last of a reagent or piece of equipment, ask someone how to replace it!
5. *Share the knowledge*. If someone takes in interest in you as a new starter, reciprocate when someone else joins the lab after you. This will clarify matters in your own mind and expose any gaps in your knowledge.
6. *Ask questions*. They are rarely as stupid as you fear they are, and often half the room is wondering the same thing!
7. *Do not take short-cuts*! If you have spent 10 days preparing a cell sample, don't compromise your experiment by a sloppy assay or analysis.
8. *Read*! You will rarely have so much time available to scour PubMed for articles of interest. Look beyond the title, think what has this paper shown for the first time, and how would I have done things differently?
9. *Have something to show for your time*. This could be a poster in the medical school or at a local meeting, or a written report summarizing your work. This is a good exercise in scientific writing. Think about how you can describe your lab experience to enhance your CV.
10. *Enjoy the freedom*. Lab time offers an unparalleled opportunity to be your own boss. This gives you a chance to organize your time in a way that is not possible in clinical medicine. Finding out how you work most effectively is a valuable life skill.

Essential statistics

'Statistics are like bikinis. What they reveal is suggestive, but what they conceal is vital.' Aaron Levenstein

It is said that with a good statistician, one could extract any desired result from a data set, and a vast array of statistical tests have been described for different conditions. As a medical student, you should have an appreciation of basic statistics, both in order to describe accurately any data that you may accrue yourself, but more importantly to understand and critique data that are presented to you.

Describing a data set
- *Mean*: sum of data divided by number of data (average). Commonly used but influenced by outliers. Appropriate in 'normally' distributed data.
- *Median*: the middle value in numerically ordered data. Better suited to skewed distributions.
- *Mode*: most frequently occurring value. Does not represent data fully.
- *Frequency*: the rate at which an event occurs over a period of time or in a given sample.

Describing the distribution of data
- *Normal distribution*: a symmetrical 'bell curve' in which the mid-point signifies median = mean = mode (see Fig. 5.3).
- *Parametric testing*: based on the assumption that the distribution of the underlying population from which the sample was taken is usually normally distributed.
- *Range*: the difference between the largest and smallest data points.
- *Standard deviation (SD)*: the spread of data from the mean (square root of variance). Very commonly used in conjunction with the mean.
- *Standard error of mean (SEM)*: how accurately SD describes the data, i.e. reduces with increasing data points.
- *Confidence interval (CI)*: a range in which 95% of data are expected to fall. Usually mean $+/- 2 \times$ SEM.
- *Interquartile range (IQR)*: a quartile divides a data set into four equally sized parts. The IQR is the difference between the first and third quartiles, and hence describes the range of the middle 50% of a data set. Not greatly influenced by outliers. Often used alongside the median.
- *Correlation*: a relationship between two or more factors.

Describing a hypothesis
- H_1: a proposed explanation requiring scientific experimentation to prove or disprove the theory
- H_0: known as a null hypothesis which states that there is no relationship between measures and that all observations occur due to chance. This is used in more widely in medical research (e.g. lung cancer is not related to smoking). The null hypothesis can never be rejected, instead it is either accepted or not accepted.

Statistical significance
- *P-value*: the probability of a result occurring by chance if the null hypothesis is true. Usually taken to be <0.05 (often represented as *). This is an arbitrary threshold liable to:
  - *Type I error (α)*: null hypothesis is incorrectly rejected or finding a result where none exists. Its rate is equivalent to the accepted significance level (5%).
  - *Type II error (β)*: when the null hypothesis is incorrectly accepted or failing to find an effect that is present.

In medicine, a type I error is considered to be more important than type II in that a positive finding is more likely to change practice than a negative; α should be less than β. This leads to:
- *Power*: probability that a test rejects the null hypothesis when the alternative is true (i.e. $1 - \beta$). Usually 80–90%. Greatly influenced by *sample size (n)*. Power calculations are done before an experiment or trial to determine what sample size will 'power' the trial to detect an effect. Hence a *p*-value <0.05 may not actually be significant if the sample size is too small. Beware that what may be statistically significant may not be biologically or clinically significant, and vice versa.
- *Positive predictive value (PPV)*: the proportion of patients with positive test results who are correctly diagnosed.
- *Negative predictive value (NPV)*: the proportion of patients with negative test results who are correctly diagnosed.

Tests of statistical significance (or how *p* is calculated)
- *Student's t-test*: probability of the difference between two data sets having arisen by chance. Can be paired or unpaired. Requires data to be normally distributed.
- *Mann–Whitney U test*: also known as Wilcoxon rank sum test. Used to detect statistical significance between data sets which are not normally distributed.
- *ANOVA* (or one-way analysis of variance): calculates differences between means of more than two groups (where multiple *t*-tests would increase type I error).

Other important terms
- *Dependence*: a relationship between two sets of data.
- *Hazard ratio*: similar to relative risk (RR) but useful when the risk information is collected at different times.
- *Odds ratio (OR)*: the odds of an outcome (e.g. lung cancer) in conjunction with a particular variable (e.g. smoking) compared to without it. If OR = 1, exposure does not affect odds of disease; if OR >1, exposure is associated with higher odds of disease; and if OR <1, exposure is associated with lower odds of disease. *Note does not imply causation!* Risk ratio or RR are crudely comparable to OR.
- *Number needed to treat (NNT)*: the number of patients required to receive an intervention in order to prevent one outcome. For example, triple therapy vs histamine antagonist in *Helicobacter pylori* eradication in peptic ulcer disease, NNT = 1.1 vs antibiotics vs placebo in prevention of infection following dog bite, NNT =16.

- *Number needed to harm (NNH)*: the average number of patients who need to be treated with an intervention for a period of time to cause one adverse outcome.
- *Absolute risk (AR)*: the probability of a specified outcome during a specified period.
- *Absolute risk reduction (ARR)*: the decrease in risk between the intervention and control cohorts as a result of activity or treatment.
- *Relative risk*: ratio of incidence of disease in exposed individuals to the incidence of disease in unexposed individuals.
- *Bias*: a systematic error that causes deviation from the true value, may it be selection, measurement, or analysis.
- *Cohort*: a group of people.
- *Continuous data*: a set of data that can be measured.
- *Ordinal data*: consists of values or observations that can be ranked or belong on a scale.
- *Nominal data*: consists of items that are categorical (e.g. a set of measurements).
- *Discrete data*: categorized into a classification based on counts.
- *Incidence*: the number of new cases of a condition occurring in a population over a specified period of time.
- *Prevalence*: the proportion of people with a finding or disease in a given population at a given time.
- *Likelihood ratio*: the probability of a test result in patients with a specified disease divided by the probability of that test result in people without that disease.
- *Stratification*: categorizes individuals with common factors (e.g. age, sex, ethnicity) into classes (or strata).
- *Sensitivity*: relates to the ability of a test identifying positive results correctly (true positives).
- *Specificity*: relates to the ability of a test identifying negative results correctly (true negatives).

Statistical software

Microsoft Excel performs simple analyses and ought to be sufficient. GraphPad, Prism, and Stata are recommended for more sophisticated tests. SPSS and R are used for large data sets or complex analyses.

Resources

These resources may be of help:

Books
- Peacock JL, Peacock PJ (2010). *Oxford Handbook of Medical Statistics*. Oxford: Oxford University Press.
- Peacock JL, Kerry SM, Balise RR (2017). *Presenting Medical Statistics from Proposal to Publication*, 2nd edition. Oxford: Oxford University Press.
- Petrie A, Sabin C (2009). *Medical Statistics at a Glance*, 3rd edition. Oxford: Wiley-Blackwell Press.

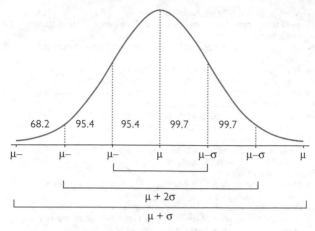

Fig. 5.3 Normal distribution curve. Reproduced from Ray, Sumantra, et al, *Oxford Handbook of Clinical and Healthcare Research*, 2016, Oxford University Press.

Journals
- *Statistics in Medicine*: ℰ www.onlinelibrary.wiley.com/journal/10.1002/(ISSN)1097-0258
- *British Medical Journal* (Endgames: Statistical Question): ℰ www.bmj.com.

Websites
- Statistics at Square One: ℰ www.bmj.com/about-bmj/resources-readers/publications/statistics-square-one
- Centre of Statistics in Medicine: ℰ www.csm-oxford.org.uk.

Part 2

Clinical medicine

Chapter 6

Going clinical

The value of the clinical experience

'In the NHS, training and the delivery of patient care are inextricably linked. It is recognised that the majority of training should take place in a service environment and that quality training leads to professionals who deliver high standards of patient care and safety.'[1]

Learning medicine in a clinical environment is very different to the mainly lecture-based years. Now you have to begin drawing parallels between pathology and the real-life experience of your patients. Contrary to popular belief, being a good doctor does not require you to be the smartest individual! Other qualities are essential, which cannot solely be learnt from a lecture, and will develop throughout your clinical experience. Meaning that if you did not excel in your pre-clinical years, do not fret, you may flourish now!

The big picture—to prepare you for your responsibilities as provisionally registered doctors: *Tomorrow's Doctors* (2009)

Tomorrow's Doctors (2009)[2] is written by the GMC and outlines the standard of practice required by a UK medical graduate. Clinical placements are an important part of this and what makes a good doctor, as they provide many opportunities to learn crucial skills that are indispensable for your future career.

Ten skills you will learn and develop through clinical experience

These skills are based on the UK Foundation Programme 'Person Specification'[3]: the UK Foundation Programme is the 2-year programme medical students embark on after graduating.

1. Knowledge
2. Good communication
3. Empathy
4. Working under pressure
5. Organization
6. Problem-solving and making a decision
7. Effective teamwork
8. Management and leadership
9. Professionalism
10. Personal development: through teaching, research, and audit.

Why students become disillusioned

Students spend their preclinical time daydreaming about finally making it into hospital. However, it does not take long for the majority of students to become disillusioned to some degree. This may be because of the following:

- Medicine is difficult, and students feel as though they do not know what is happening.
- Often it is not obvious when learning is happening; students often live for the one day when the doctor imparts a list which they can scribble down in a notebook. They may feel this is the sum total of their leaning for the day; it is not, as you will gain far more than you think.

- Healthcare professionals unrelated to medical teaching can range from disinterested to hostile. Do not be put off.
- No one is forcing you to be present, and you might leave at the first sign of hunger or tiredness.
- The environment is alien and/or frightening; you do not know what to touch, where to stand, and patients ask you to do things.
- Even the most benign consultant can appear challenging or intending to intimidate when asking questions.
- Students often feel as though they have all the time in the world to learn what they need to know for finals; but your clinical placement will only be 6 weeks and become the extent of your experience in a given speciality.
- Healthcare professionals are busy, and certainly in the early years you cannot contribute and will mostly be in the way.
- Book work is comforting, but clinical work allows you to identify gaps in your knowledge, and helps you find things you can focus on.

The value of being present

Assessment

Incorrectly or otherwise, consultants assess students based on their presence. If, on reaching the end of block assessment, you are having difficulty getting signed off, being seen by other members of the team would make your position unimpeachable.

Learning medicine is a function of time

This is why a consultant's judgement is better than that of the senior house officer (SHO); as a result of seeing more patients and working for longer. By being present you are starting on the path of absorbing the knowledge and experience that will make you a better doctor (even if it does not seem evident for large parts of the day!).

Exams

It is often apparent to assessors in clinical exams which students have seen cases for the first time in their exam. Recall the student who reaches the end of their paediatric clinical exam but does not know how to undo the baby's clothing; some things cannot be taught by textbooks.

Medicine is unpredictable

Hanging around can pay off—leaving 1 hour earlier may mean you miss the opportunity to see the cardiac arrest. You will also find yourself often waiting for things to happen or for teaching to start. This is the time to capitalize by reading around a topic and using this handbook to improve your experiences in the clinical setting. It is necessary to 'waste' time in order to benefit from these valuable clinical experiences.

Being around allows you to establish a rapport with the team

Making them more likely to interact and teach, giving them the impression of enthusiasm. Students arrive and expect to be taught, which is not always conducive with the primary function of hospitals and staff to treat patients. The more often you are around, the more likely you will be around to gain teaching opportunities. Being present on the ward allows you to learn how to interact with the rest of the team.

Focused learning
Allows you to focus your learning when off the wards, e.g. this will ensure you do not spend lots of time on Takayasu's arteritis before you understand heart failure.

Part of the team
Being consistently present allows you to be a part of the team. Students are often unreliable because of other commitments (e.g. teaching, pub lunch); this is a barrier to them becoming a regular team member who is given their own tasks/responsibilities. If you have a role as a member of the team, you will be well prepared for your first job.

Insight
Insight into your professional future makes it easier to start making clinical career decisions earlier on if you have experienced different specialties.

The middle ground is working out for yourself the useful elements of hospital medicine. Once you have been a clinical student for a short while, you start to understand what you must attend and what might be less effective. Time in a clinical environment will make you a better doctor. Visibility will get you higher grades. However, you are only a student for a few years, and you do have a lifetime of work in clinical environments ahead of you. In the current environment, you also need to focus on extracurricular activities (see ➡ 'Extracurricular activities' pp. 1012–1015). Your aim should be to work effectively, which is as much about strategizing as it is about spending as much time as possible on the wards.

If your consultant has a clinic, it makes sense to attend this. They are less likely to spend time on the wards (ward rounds excepted), which should be factored into your decision-making. The key is to plan your learning; e.g. it is probably suboptimal to attend an all-day list of inguinal hernias. However, an hour spent reading about hernias and relevant anatomy before going to theatre will ensure that you gain the most from that experience. This still means you will have the rest of the afternoon to pursue other activities.

Remaining motivated on clinical placements
- Get to know the clinical team—this will make the clinical environment feel more human.
- Read and try to anticipate questions you might be asked.
- Developing your own syllabus and/or learning objectives will help structure your time and make you feel in control of learning. The pages in this handbook will help you through each individual placement.
- Chose your clinical partner carefully. If you chose somebody who wants to attend, you will have to attend to keep pace. Negotiate with your partner, but remember you are responsible for your own learning.
- Develop a work–life balance.

Your clinical responsibilities
You have no clinical responsibilities for patients. There are two circumstances under which a responsibility arises. You are responsible for your own conduct if you volunteer for something, e.g. siting a cannula, delivering an urgent cross-match to the blood bank, where the team will be dependent on you completing this task. Secondly, general responsibilities defined by

the GMC's *Medical Students: Professional Values and Fitness to Practise*. In particular:

- only work within the limits of your competence and ask for help when necessary
- accurately represent your position and abilities
- ensure you are supervised appropriately for any clinical tasks you perform
- respect the decisions and rights of patients
- do not unfairly discriminate against patients by allowing personal views to adversely affect your professional relationship
- behave with courtesy
- report any concerns about patient safety to the appropriate person.

References

1. Temple J. (2010). *Time for Training: A Review of the Impact of the European Working Time Directive on the Quality of Training*. London: HMSO. ℘ www.mee.nhs.uk/pdf/JCEWTD_Final%report.pdf
2. General Medical Council (2009). *Tomorrow's Doctors*. London: GMC. ℘ www.gmc-uk.org/education/undergraduate/tomorrows_doctors.asp
3. The Foundation Programme. *UK Foundation Programme Commencing August 2016 (FP 2016) Person Specification*. ℘ www.foundationprogramme.nhs.uk

Your responsibilities and professionalism

For many years, doctors have been known as one of the most trusted professions. An Ipsos MORI poll in 2015 of >2000 British adults reiterated this:[1]

- Doctors remain most trusted profession: 90%.
- Teachers: 86%.
- Ordinary man/woman in the street: 62%.
- Journalists: 22%.
- Politicians: 16%.

In 2005, the Royal College of Physicians sought to define the role of medical professionalism in the twenty-first century. This report was called *Doctors in Society: Medical Professionalism in a Changing World*. They defined medical professionalism as follows:

'Medical professionalism signifies a set of values, behaviours, and relationships that underpins the trust the public has in doctors.'

To supplement this definition they also described the 'day-to-day practice' doctors are committed to, including:

- integrity
- compassion
- altruism
- continuous improvement
- excellence
- working in partnership with members of the wider healthcare team.[2]

Therefore, in order to uphold the standards of professionalism, behaviour, and care this commitment needs to begin with medical students.

Learning professionalism is important to you now and for your future, as a doctor, and so has been incorporated in most medical school curriculums. It has been suggested that there are four key ways to do this:[3]

1. Role models
2. Formal teaching
3. Experimental learning
4. Prior experiences.

Much of the GMC guidance not only applies to qualified doctors but to you as medical students. This applies even more so when in clinical years. The GMC states: 'Medical students have certain privileges and responsibilities different from those of other students. Because of this, different standards of professional behaviour are expected of them.'[4] It is important to begin thinking about your responsibilities and professionalism as a medical student and future healthcare profession.

The following points on how to maintain professionalism are stated by the GMC in the 'The doctor as a professional' section of *Tomorrow's Doctors* (2009)[5]:

1. Make the care of the patient the first concern.
2. Be polite, considerate, trustworthy and honest, act with integrity, maintain confidentiality, respect patients' dignity and privacy, and understand the importance of appropriate consent.

3. Respect all patients, colleagues, and others regardless of their age, colour, culture, disability, ethnic or national origin, gender, lifestyle, marital or parental status, race, religion or beliefs, sex, sexual orientation, or social or economic status.

4. Acquire, assess, apply, and integrate new knowledge, learn to adapt to changing circumstances, and ensure that patients receive the highest level of professional care.

5. Continually reflect on practice and, whenever necessary, translate that reflection into action.

6. Recognize your own personal and professional limits and seek help from colleagues and supervisors when necessary.

It is important to remember that we are all human and so mistakes will inevitably happen. As doctors are a highly trusted profession, at times the high expectations held by the public and patients may not always be met. This does not necessarily mean that the doctor is not committed to patient care. True professionalism is learnt and improved when mistakes are made but then reflected upon: an idea that should be instilled within medical students. This will ensure for you and for others in the future that when similar mistakes occur, the correct steps can be taken to ensure that the problem is resolved and patient care standards are upheld.

Hospitals are old-fashioned institutions that have a few unwritten rules which the uninitiated are unlikely to be aware of. Observing these rules will leave colleagues thinking that you are polite, professional, and competent. To play safe, introduce yourself to everybody in the clinical environment whom you encounter, but most importantly identify yourself to the most senior doctor and charge nurse. A confident, smiling introduction will leave a lasting impression of friendliness, enthusiasm, and effectiveness.

Although it is probably unfair, a medical student's underconfidence may be interpreted as rudeness by other healthcare professionals or patients. You should therefore make an effort to say hello and smile at everyone you encounter. Humility pays dividends. Consider starting all requests with 'I know you are busy, but I wonder if you could please help me ...'. It is important to understand that everyone in the clinical environment is overworked and resources are stretched.

Colleagues
- Respect nurses since they can make you and equally break you!
- Beware the ward receptionist/clerk's chair. Do not use or remove!
- You should never interrupt a conversation between colleagues when they are discussing a patient's management. Keep your distance, keep quiet, and keep patient until it is your time to speak.

Patients
- Most patients are nice and interested in helping medical students. They will usually agree to help if asked in the right way—be polite, humble, and professional.
- Introduce yourself appropriately by name and title.
- Always pull the curtains around the bed and wash your hands before, in between, and after examining every patient.
- If you are with a doctor, why not help by pulling the curtain around and preparing the observation chart?
- Patients have little stimulation in hospital and often spend the day asleep. This causes trouble when you have been asked to take a history and examination. Most patients may not mind being interrupted, but reconsider if a patient is clearly sleeping deeply (e.g. snoring under sheets).
- Protected mealtimes should never be interrupted. Do not underestimate the importance of nutrition as part of every treatment plan.
- Do not interrupt when patients are spending time with their relatives as this may cause them to leave prematurely.

Commitment to patient care starts with training

It is essential to remember that as a medical student your first aim is to learn how to provide good patient care, not to be the main team member responsible for providing care. So even though you are playing an active part within the healthcare team, your main role is also to learn:
- history taking
- examination
- how to interpret results
- practical procedures and skills
- prescribing
- management
- ward work.

References

1. Royal College of Physicians (2005). *Doctors in Society: Medical Professionalism in a Changing World*. Report of a Working Party of the Royal College of Physicians of London. London: RCP.
2. Ipsos MORI Trust Poll, 5 January 2015. ✆ www.ipsos-mori.com/researchpublications/ researcharchive/15/Trust-in-Professions.aspx
3. Baernstein A, Oelschlager AMA, Chang TA, Wenrich MD (2009). Learning professionalism: perspectives of preclinical medical students. *Acad Med* 84:574–81.
4. General Medical Council (2009). *Medical Students: Professional Values and Fitness to Practise*. London: GMC. ✆ /www.gmc-uk.org/education/undergraduate/professional_behaviour.asp
5. General Medical Council (2009). *Tomorrow's Doctors*. London: GMC. ✆ www.gmc-uk.org/education/undergraduate/tomorrows_doctors.asp

How to be useful

Rule #1: always make yourself useful!

When on a clinical attachment it is important to make the most of your time there and be useful to your team. Fortunately, as a student on placement, anything you do to help the team will only aid your learning, and will therefore be useful for you too. Be proactive! If you get 'stuck in' and avoid playing a passive role on the ward then the junior staff will appreciate your presence and give you more things to do.

A simple way to do this is by helping to take on some of the duties of the junior doctors. Firstly use your common sense. If you see the probably exhausted junior doctor slowly drowning in a sea of notes, drug charts, and observation charts on the ward round: help them! Many hands make light work after all. You will instantly feel more involved with the team and find yourself with more opportunities to ask questions (meaning that you will not be left feeling hidden in the background).

Other ways to help

- *Write in the notes*: different hospitals will have rules on whether medical students can write in the notes or not, so ensure you check this. Please remember: write in black ink (make sure it is legible), time and date, signature, and counter-signature from one of your seniors. If you are unsure about the format do not be afraid to just ask the junior doctor.
- *Jobs after ward round*: ask for a patient list prior to the ward round and make notes of the jobs that need to be done. After the ward round go with the team to discuss the jobs list and offer your help for simple things such as taking blood, inserting a cannula, or performing an ECG.
- *Jobs*: ask if there are any jobs from your team. They will really appreciate this, as it will free up their workload and possibly create some spare time to teach you by the bedside. However, do not work outside of your competencies. Remember to recognize your own limitations, both in knowledge and skill.
- *Clerk new admissions*: take a thorough history and examination before presenting your findings to a doctor.
- *Is it possible to be too keen?* Do not overwork yourself and take on too much, remember you still have exams to pass! If you have been shadowing the junior doctor all day, do not feel the need to stay for a late shift if you already have a lot on. The team understands that you need time to rest and to study. You will have all the time in the world to work lengthy hours once you qualify! So use your time wisely now. One of the best ways to feel motivated is to contribute to the care of the patients.

  The more tasks you take away from the ward team the more time they will have to teach you and recognize your contribution when it comes to end-of-placement sign-off/evaluation/feedback.
- *Practical procedures*: you must learn to take blood and site an IV cannula at a minimum before finishing medical school. You should also learn to place a urinary catheter and perform ABGs. The earlier in your medical school career you can perform these tasks independently, the more useful you will be to your team. Much like business, it is a bit of give and take.

- *Administrative tasks*: there are lots of tasks which occupy doctors'
  time which do not necessarily require a medical degree to complete.
  Although these will cause you much upset during the rest of your career,
  early on they create an opportunity to help the team while waiting
  for interesting things to happen. Obvious examples are printing blood
  forms, labelling blood bottles, assisting with discharge summaries (which
  should be appropriately supervised), updating the patient list, etc. If you
  are attached to the ward team for any length of time it can be helpful
  to update the ward list; this will also help you get to know patients and
  understand how their management progresses with time.
- *Assisting with the ward round*: it is easier to follow the ward round
  passively but this can give the impression of disinterest. Ward rounds
  are a team effort. This is one way of ensuring a smooth progression
  around the patients with minimal interruptions. Tasks within your skillset
  include drawing the curtains, and ensuring the observation chart and
  drugs chart are immediately available. You may be asked to document
  events of the ward round.

In an emergency situation, the following things will usually have to be
obtained:
- Crash trolley.
- Patient notes.
- Drug chart.
- Most recent blood results.
- Someone will take the ABG sample; you should only volunteer to do
  this if you are comfortable with running this sample and know where
  your ABG machines are.

Ten tips for surviving clinical medicine

1. *A little introduction goes a long way.* Apply this not only to patients, but to doctors and nurses too. Letting people around you know who you are means you are less likely to loiter in the background feeling uncomfortable and ignored.

2. *Always be on time.* Better yet early! Do not be the student who is routinely late. Make a good impression early on and your clinical attachment is more likely to run smoothly.

3. *Be polite, confident, and smile!* It can be quite intimidating entering a new ward and not knowing the ropes. Often you may feel like you are constantly in the way, but being friendly with all the healthcare team will make them more likely to help you!

4. *If you do not know the answer to a question, do not be afraid to say so.* This is often quite a daunting situation but do not worry! No one expects you to know everything; that is why you are here. If you do not know the answer just say so.

5. *No question is a stupid question.* The likelihood is that another one of your peers was too scared to ask it as well! Asking the question will only benefit all of your learning.

6. *Practise examining and taking histories from patients.* Practice makes perfect! Ask the nurses and doctors on the ward to point you in the direction of the best patients. Broaden your experience in clinical medicine, by seeing patients with many doctors; there are many approaches to history taking and examinations. Gain an understanding of the patient's clinical course and speak to others in the MDT.

7. *Get to grips with practical procedures.* Take any opportunity that arises, be it venepuncture, cannulation, and so forth. Being confident with these early on is very important and will make OSCE examinations and future employment much easier

8. *Be a team player.* Your firm and other colleagues are all in the same boat so when a learning opportunity arises: share! Often your peers can be your greatest resource.

9. *Active learning.* You are responsible for your own learning! Striking a good balance between clinical and library work is very important; although being on the wards can be exciting, remember you still need to pass your exams! Always keep assessment forms ready, to be handed to your seniors whenever you can (at the appropriate time). Reinforce your clinical exposure with further reading, including material you might anticipate encountering the next day (e.g. likely cases in clinic, or operations on tomorrow's theatre list). Set a target for every day (e.g. a single examination watched by your partner).

10. *Enjoy yourself!* Appreciate that you have worked long and hard to get to this position, so do not take it for granted. Although it is difficult to enjoy yourself with sick patients around, know that your contribution (whether administrative, procedural, or spending time with your patients) is contributing to their recovery. That ought to be your job satisfaction.

Making the most of free time

Entering clinical years may require you to make some changes to your life and schedule. But do not be scared, you can still have a life!

Medicine is only a fraction of your life, not your entire life!

Although it may seem like the free time you have is limited (and will decrease now that you are entering your clinical years), it is important that you make the most of any available time you have to enjoy yourself. The last thing you want is to regret not doing so in the future when you are working. It can be quite difficult to strike the perfect work–life balance. But it is simply a matter of time management, if you work hard and plan ahead you can definitely find time to rest, play hard, and pursue your hobbies.

Free time at home

A *three-pronged approach* can be taken to make the most of your free time at home.

1. *Use your time wisely*: get organized and make a plan of things you need to get through in the day, be that work, or extracurricular activities.
2. *Effective studying*: entering clinical years may require you to change your original, mainly lecture-based way of learning. Try and find the best way for yourself.
3. *Do other things!*: your medical school will have and will be continually creating new sport teams, clubs, and charities that you may be interested in joining. Do not forget simple things such as going to bed early, going to the gym, watching a film, going out for a drink, seeing your friends, reading a book, etc.

Remember that free time is not necessarily just your time at home but you may also be faced with the situation where you have nothing to do when on placement.

Free time on the wards

- Find a doctor who is free to teach you and your firm.
- Take a history or examine a patient.
- Ask any of the junior doctors if they need any help with any of their jobs list. Use this to practise skills such as venepuncture and cannulation.
- Become familiar with the topics in this handbook.

You do not have to be on the wards around the clock. It is always a good idea to do book work to reinforce the clinical knowledge you are picking up on the ward. The doctors were all students once and recognize the need to study.

A clinical environment is necessarily inefficient, which means lots of free times for students while waiting for scheduled events.

Ad hoc free time (e.g. a patient did not attend (DNA) in clinic or a theatre patient was delayed) can allow you to do a few useful things:

- *Reading*. Relevant pages from this handbook, the *Oxford Handbook of Clinical Medicine*, or another speciality text. You never know when your consultant will quiz you on something you have read. Consolidate knowledge about previous patients or prepare for questions about your patient/case.

- *Using people around you.* Ask anyone nearby who is also free (e.g. consultant with patient) to quiz you on a topic of their choice. Most people will respond to enthusiasm.
- *Use your partners.* You may wish to practise your examinations with your partner, or perhaps prepare questions beforehand which can serve as a longstanding competition.
- *Patient information leaflets.* Cover a multitude of conditions with a reasonable level of detail.
- *Smartphones.* These need to be used carefully to avoid offending a consultant. Make sure you inform your senior if you are using medical applications as not all may be aware of what you are doing.
- *Consider asking others before you leave* (e.g. charge nurse, junior doctor). This is considered as being courteous.

Consider the following if you have a few hours spare (e.g. consultant sends you away mid morning before a fixed commitment in the afternoon):

- *Speciality procedures.* Turn to your specialty page to see if there are any other procedures you might be able to attend instead.
- *Other clinics/theatres.* If you are interested in a specific speciality, take the opportunity if it presents itself but not at the expense of your expected commitment to your firm's activities.
- *Day surgery.* If you have a few hours, day surgery can be a nice compromise to other lists as they are more efficient and have a higher turnover of patients, allowing you to see three or four patients as opposed to one major or emergency case.
- *Practical skills.* Ask which procedures need performing (e.g. a patient needs their blood to be taken).
  - You should only attempt venepuncture/cannulation/ABGs etc. if you feel able. You might want to visit the skills laboratory if you are less confident.
- *ED.* When you are feeling more confident, ask a clinician to see a few simple cases which you can discuss.
- *Administration work.* Might include assignments, research paper, reflective practice, or audit.
- *Radiology reporting.* Go to the radiology department and ask to sit in on reporting sessions—learn patterns from the experts!
- *E-learning resources.* Working through an online *BMJ* learning module for instance.
- *Formal teaching.* Check out departmental teaching/grand rounds.

Teaching overview

Preclinical students tend to be mainly dependent learners and as they progress through clinical years become more self-directed ready to be in-dependent practitioners in the future. Teaching here is not only used to acquire and broaden knowledge but also to help you apply it to a clinical context and learn the new skills necessary to support you in your transition to working life. Teaching while on placement can happen in a wide variety of environments, and will frequently occur without you even expecting it! Long gone are the days of mostly scheduled lecture-based teaching. It al-lows you to:

- *role model*—observe, first-hand, doctors and their team on the job and learn how things should be done, e.g. things which students often neglect: writing in the notes, doing discharge summaries, referrals, investigation requesting, and prescribing
- take histories from, and examine real/simulated patients; this allows you to familiarize yourself with common presentations and signs
- observe and develop your communication skills
- interpret data and problem-solve
- practise and perform clinical skills.

There are a number of ways teaching can be delivered to you:

1. By the bedside

This has traditionally been thought the most effective way of teaching in the clinical environment as it promotes 'real' patient contact and so im-proves students' clinical and communication skills. Patient-centred teaching can happen in:

- primary care
- on the wards
- in clinics
- in theatre.

2. Protected teaching

A planned session that is not interrupted by clinical duties ('bleep-free'):

- Traditional lectures.
- Small group teaching.
- Simulated clinical skills.
- Simulation/role play sessions.
- Self-directed learning.
- Bedside teaching can also be organized as protected.

It is also important at the undergraduate level to begin developing your own teaching skills, as teaching is very important to patient care. Many med-ical schools therefore, as part of their curriculum, encourage this by having teaching modules and assessments.

How to arrange teaching

By spending time in a clinical area you will naturally pick up a lot of information. While this will broaden your knowledge base, it is essential to consolidate your leaning. An easy way to do this is to arrange teaching during your hospital attachment, in addition to the formal sessions in your curriculum.

Who can you ask for teaching?

Anyone! The GMC's *Good Medical Practice* states: 'You should be prepared to contribute to teaching and training doctors and students.'[1] Hospitals are full of professionals looking for the opportunity to teach students. All you have to do is ask. Do not think you are limited to only being taught by doctors. You may approach any healthcare professional, including nurses, pharmacists, physiotherapists, and radiographers to mention a few. You can learn from all of these different perspectives and build that knowledge in to your practice. It may seem intimidating to approach a healthcare professional to ask for teaching; however, most are more than happy to help. Do not forget that they will benefit too, as some may ask you to fill in a feedback form to use for their portfolios.

How to ask for teaching?

The best way to go about this is to spend a little time on the ward, perhaps go on the morning ward round and befriend the junior doctors. If they are looking particularly busy and stressed then it is best to leave it for another time. However, when they have a free moment do not be afraid to ask them if they could teach you something. Ideally, you should have a topic or examination in mind that you would like help with. Having a junior doctor watch you examine a patient can be an invaluable experience because they have only recently completed medical school OSCEs and know what is required of you. Most hospitals will create a 'firm' or 'team' of students and attach you to a consultant who will offer you teaching on a weekly or fortnightly basis. In this case, you may need to liaise with the consultant's secretary to ensure your teaching is going ahead. Do try your best to attend these teaching sessions, as you will learn an incredible amount from the consultants and it cannot hurt to make a good impression! You will have to be flexible with your timetable and occasionally you may reschedule but do not let this deter you.

How to arrange teaching

Before your teaching takes place, have a think about what topic you would like to cover. It is best to let the doctor know in advance so they can prepare. This will give them time to collect any interesting patients or cases to make your teaching more useful. You can also show them your learning outcomes on the university curriculum and work through each of them.

Bedside teaching

This takes place on the ward, focused on a patient. In general, this tends to be practical, where you are observed examining a patient or taking a history. You may be asked to find patients in preparation for your teaching. If you go on to the ward and ask any of the nurses or doctors they will be able to let you know who to approach. You will need to take consent from the patient before your teaching. Most will be happy for you to examine them as long as you let them know when it will be and that it would benefit your learning. If possible, try to run through the examination or topic of choice before the day. It will make the teaching more interactive and useful for you if you have a little background knowledge. You can ask the doctor to watch you examine a patient and mark you as if you are doing an OSCE. By practising in situations where you are being assessed, you will become used to the pressure and may help your exam performance.

Informal tutorials

These may take the form of a presentation or a case-based discussion. A case-based discussion is centred on a clinical scenario and can help put learning into context. In this kind of learning you will more than likely be asked questions on the subject, in order to make the teaching interactive. Therefore, it will save you some embarrassment if you do some pre-reading and are able to contribute! The important thing to remember is that this is your chance to learn what you think is important. These tutorials can be tailor-made to your learning requirements.

Teaching ward rounds

You can learn a lot from a good ward round. This is dependent on the consultant and how busy the ward round is. You will see many patients during the round, with a variety of medical conditions. This is the perfect opportunity to observe the management of these different conditions. Try to take advantage of this opportunity by listening carefully while the history is read out and ask questions. Do give honest feedback after teaching sessions. Your thoughts and comments can really help develop their teaching styles and benefit future sessions. For example, if you would like more case-based discussions then either let them know or write it down in a feedback form. That way, for the following teaching the doctor will be able to prepare a case in advance, improving your learning and making the teaching more interactive.

Reference

1. General Medical Council (2013). *Good Medical Practice*. London: GMC. ℘ www.gmc-uk.org/-/ media/documents/good-medical-practice---english-1215_pdf-51527435.pdf

Taking control of your teaching

Don't take a back seat! You are in control of your learning once you reach clinical years.

Introduce yourself

If staff members do not know who you are, they will question you and ask the purpose of your visit. Do not take this personally, as this is for patient safety. Or they may just ignore you and not share their pearls of wisdom with you—this defeats the purpose of you being present in clinical areas. You will get a lot further if you are on friendly terms with everyone.

Ward rounds

You will definitely be expected to attend ward rounds during the week. This can be a tedious experience if you are just following the group around and not engaging with the team. On some wards you will luckily have a helpful junior or middle-grade doctor who will involve you. If not, then be pro-active! Ask if you can write in the notes. Ask if you can present the patient.

Practise presenting patients

It would be much more educational for you as a future doctor and also demonstrate your proactive engaging nature if you offered to present some of the patients on the ward round that you may have seen earlier or re-view their history, examination findings, and investigation results prior to the ward round. If you see an interesting patient on the ward round then go back afterwards and examine them yourself. Compare your findings with what is documented. Remember, if you see a patient with an unusual condition then use their case for your portfolio.

Theatre

If you are on surgery, then go in early and ask if you can 'scrub in' to theatre. They may even let you assist. If you are on anaesthetics, again go in early while the patients are consented and ask the anaesthetist if they will show you how to insert airways and intubate. If you show enthusiasm they will probably let you try as well. Practising and polishing up skills such as cannulation or insertion of a catheter will only serve to help you in the long run.

Top tip

If you are particularly interested in an area then let the team know and ask if there are any audits you can get involved in. It is a good idea to start doing audits in medical school, not only because you will gain experience of how to do them but also to help with your CV in the future. A good audit poster can be submitted to a conference. A great audit may be presented at a regional and national conference, all of which will make your CV stronger for after medical school.

Shadowing the on-call team

Ask the junior doctor if you can join them for an on-call shift. There are two different types of on-calls. Ward cover is where the doctor will be in charge of most of the medical or surgical wards. They will be bleeped for any sick patients or jobs needing doing. Admissions shifts are where doctors see new patients, coming in from either the ED or via GP refer-rals. They will clerk them, order any investigations, and make management plans. Depending on what you want to get out of your time there, pick an appropriate shift.

> **Top tip**
>
> Clerking is an exciting way to learn. You will get the chance to engage all the knowledge you have to work out what is going on with your pa-tient. It is almost like being a detective! Once you have seen a patient with a specific condition, it is a lot easier to remember the management of it.

Read every day!

If you come across something you do not know much about or have not heard of before, then when you go home spend half an hour reading about it. Doing a little each day will really help you in the long run. For example, if you see a patient with chest pain then read about the causes and investi-gations you would do.

Always be professional

Even though you are not yet qualified, get into the habit of maintaining a cer-tain level of professionalism. Take note of any members of staff you think excel at this as well as ones who do not. And try and mimic the ones who do it best—that is the best way to learn these soft skills that go a long way in making you a successful clinician.

Jobs

Learn how to do all the nitty gritty jobs. Unfortunately, a large part of our job is to fill out paperwork and make phone calls. Although this does not sound very exciting, it will make your life a lot easier once you have gradu-ated if you have a little understanding of the logistical aspects of being a doctor. This means knowing how to write discharge summaries, phone the X-ray department, phone the laboratory, and chase results. Learn how to bleep. This may sound simple but it really is the main way we communicate with each other in hospital. Get used to doing it early on.

Handover

Learn how to handover a patient. This is really important for when you start working as it is a crucial part of the job. Listen to how patients are handed over on the phone and in person. Even better, ask if you can do it. For example, if the doctor you are with is handing over a patient to the specialist registrar, then ask if you can do it. Read the history carefully, look through the investigations and see what medications they are on. Try to anticipate any questions the registrar may ask you. Try using the *SBAR* method of framing critical conversations (i.e. Situation, Background, Assessment, and Recommendation; see Box 6.1) developed by the NHS Institute for Innovation and Improvement.

Share!

If you find a patient with a really good murmur, then let your colleagues know about it so they might be able to listen as well. If you find out about some teaching then let everyone know and everyone can benefit from it. Medicine is really all about being in a team and we need to look out for each other. Chances are if you help someone out they will do the same for you! The key thing to stress here is if you do not ask then you do not get. You may feel as if you are being pushy and sometimes might not get what you want. Just remember to always be polite and be sensible with what you are asking. Take an active role in your learning.

Box 6.1 SBAR tool

S: situation
- Identify yourself and the site/unit you are calling from.
- Identify the patient by name and the reason for your report.
- Describe your concern.

B: background
- Give the patient's reason for admission.
- Explain significant medical history.
- You then inform the consultant of the patient's background: admitting diagnosis, date of admission, prior procedures, current medications, allergies, pertinent laboratory results, and other relevant diagnostic results. For this, you need to have collected information from the patient's chart, flow sheets, and progress notes.

A: assessment
- Vital signs.
- Contraction pattern.
- Clinical impressions, concerns.

R: recommendation
- Explain what you need—be specific about request and time frame.
- Make suggestions.
- Clarify expectations.

Wards

What are ward rounds?

Wards rounds are when all the patients are reviewed and management plans are made for their future care. They provide the opportunity for patients to meet the consultants and vice versa. It also gives staff the chance to interact with each other and to make decisions in a multidisciplinary manner.

When do they start?

This usually depends on individual units, and timings can vary not only between specialities, but also between consultants. Depending on how many patients there are to see, they may last anywhere from 30 min up to a few hours.

Who is present on a ward round?

There will normally be a consultant who will lead the ward round, accompanied by one or two junior doctors. They may be foundation doctors to registrar level. The nurse looking after the specific bay of patients will also be on the ward round, to inform you of the progress of the patient and any salient points from the last medical review.

Who does what on the ward round?

The junior doctors will prepare the notes and give the consultant a brief summary of the patient's care to date. Then they will show the consultant any recent investigations such as blood results or scans. While the consultant reviews the patient, the juniors document the consultation in the notes.

What can you do on a ward round?

A great opportunity to learn and impress your consultant would be to go in a little bit early and prepare one of the patient's notes for the ward round. This would mean familiarizing yourself with the history and current investigations so you are able to present the case on the ward round.

Writing in notes on a ward round

You may be asked to scribe for a few patients on the round (see Box 6.2). A simple way of remembering what to include is the mnemonic **SOAP**:
- Subjective: what does the patient say? How are they feeling? How do they look to you (e.g. unwell, tired, alert, lying in bed vs sitting out)?
- Objective: what are their observations, examination findings, and investigation results?
- Assessment: what is your impression after considering the subjective and objective findings? What is the diagnosis? Is the patient on the ward clinically stable, improving, or deteriorating?
- Plan: write down all the jobs you need to do for this patient. What is going to happen in the next few days? What needs to be done to aid in the patient's discharge planning?

Top tips
1. Write the date, time, and location of the ward round.
2. Write the consultant's name who is taking the round.
3. A good habit to get into is to write a brief summary and problem list at the top of the page so that anyone seeing the patient at a later date has an idea of what is going on.
4. Try to write legibly and in shorthand.

Box 6.2 Example of ward round entry

dd/mm/yy   <u>WR DR BONES</u>
Time
Ward 2
84 ♀ admitted with: cough + SOB

Problems:
1. LRTI—CURB65 score 2
2. Confusion
3. Reduced mobility
Treated with IV clarithromycin and amoxicillin —day 3
S: Cough improved + not SOB now
O: Obs: stable and apyrexial
BP   105/86
Sats   98% on 1 L O2
RR   18
Pulse   82
Temp   36.2
Bloods: normal, blood cultures negative
O/E: looks comfortable at rest
CVS: HS 1+11+0, rad 80 bpm and regular
GI: abdo SNT, bowel sounds present, bowels opened today, catheter *in situ*
Resp: equal expansion, resonant percussion, vesicular BS + 0

Impression: resolution of LRTI
Plan:
1. Convert to oral antibiotics and monitor for 24 hours
2. Wean off oxygen and TWOC (trial without catheter)
3. PT/OT assessment, encourage mobility and sit out
4. Encourage oral intake
5. Aim home mane and GP r/v in 1 week

Ben Bloggs FY1 #1234

The team

After the ward round, the junior doctors sit down together and split up the jobs. This is a perfect opportunity for you to practise some clinical skills such as venepuncture and cannulation. If you are a bit nervous at the start it is perfectly acceptable to ask for supervision. You will be a massive help to the team by doing these kinds of odd jobs. You will meet many different people working in the team on the ward, and it will be handy to know a little about each of their roles:

- *FY1*: stands for Foundation Year 1. This doctor is the most junior in the team, in their first year post graduation. Their role in the team is to carry out jobs from the ward round and keep the patients stable. Most importantly they have to know when to escalate and ask for help.
- *SHO*: an old term that is now used broadly for the grades of Foundation Year 2 trainee up to Core Trainee/Specialty Trainee Year 2 in the specialties. They are often in the 'lower tier' of the rota. They work closely with the FY1 and are useful where senior input is required.
- *Registrar*: also an old term still in use, and can refer to anyone in training from Specialty Trainee Year 3 to 8, depending on the specialty. The registrar is usually the most senior doctor present on the ward on a day-to-day basis. They will be responsible for much of the important decision-making throughout the day. Registrars seeking additional training or who may be out of formal training are also referred to as Associate Specialists and Clinical/Research Fellows.
- *Nurses*: invaluable to the smooth running of a ward. Get on their good side and they will really help you out, e.g. they will let you know of any good patients to see or clinical skills you can practise. Your medical school may require you to get certain clinical skills signed off. Carrying out observations and setting up IV infusions and SC injections are just a few of the jobs the nurses do. If you need to get any of these skills signed off then the best person to ask for help is the nurse on the ward. You can differentiate their grade by the colour of the uniform (e.g. dark blue signifies senior nurse).
- *Pharmacist*: most wards will have a pharmacist attached to that ward who will check that correct medications have been prescribed for patients and help out with any drug queries. They can offer to give you a tutorial on a tricky subject, e.g. antibiotic prescribing.
- *Physiotherapist/occupational therapist*: in the notes for many patients it will be written to arrange an OT/PT review. This will be for patients who need help with their activities of daily living and mobilizing. They play an integral role in rehabilitating patients.
- *Ward clerk*: carries out all the administrative duties.
- *Student*: do not forget that you are also a key member of the team! Never demean yourself by saying that you are *just* a student. If you are enthusiastic and willing to get involved, you can be a great asset.

What to do on the ward in your spare time

- *History taking*:
  - Learning how to take a medical history is an important skill to master early on in your studies.
  - The ward is the perfect opportunity to practise as it will be full of patients with different presentations and conditions.
- *Practise examinations*:
  - There are several key examinations to become confident in— each specific to the placement you are on (e.g. cardiovascular, gynaecological, and neurological).
  - *Top tip*: go and examine a patient with another student. One of you can take the history and the other can examine. You can mark each other and afterwards give feedback. This is a great way to prepare for OSCEs and get used to someone observing you while you are examining a patient.
  - *Top tip*: practise identifying the positive findings on examination as this is tested in final year OSCEs. If you consciously make an effort in earlier years, it becomes easier later on. Ask FYs on the ward for any patients with positive/interesting signs.
- *Get acquainted with ECGs*:
  - ECGs are among the most commonly ordered investigations in the hospital.
  - They are also something many medical students struggle with.
  - Learn a systematic way of interpreting ECGs and get used to looking at them.
  - *Top tip*: interpret an ECG before looking at the patient's notes. Then explain your findings to one of the doctors on the ward and see if they agree with you. Afterwards, if you read through the notes it will help you build a picture about how different conditions may affect an ECG.
- *Observe any interesting procedures*:
  - If you are lucky you may observe an unusual procedure on the ward, such as lumbar punctures or chest drain insertion.
- *Clinical skills* (see ➔ Chapters 45 and 46):
  - *Venepuncture*: the ability to take blood is absolutely essential as a medical student and for the rest of your career. Even consultants are called to perform this task at times.
  - *Cannula insertion*: if you can do this you will become extremely useful on the wards, and thus gain favour with nurses and doctors, and also actively participate during an emergency!
  - *Catheterization*: nurses can perform these so if you do not have a doctor around, ask one of the nurses to show you.
  - *ABGs*: you may have access to simulated arms to perform this, which is a great way to practise. If not, request to be taught by a doctor.

Outpatient clinics

Outpatient clinic services are used for patients who need specialist follow-up but do not necessarily need to stay in hospital. They bridge the gap between primary and secondary care.

You will mainly be attending clinics during your later years of medical school where you are required to become experienced with specialist subjects. By this point, you will have definitely encountered cardiology, gastroenterology, respiratory, and neurology. It is of course important to attend clinics in these specialties as you will see conditions and treatments you would not otherwise see on the wards. However, you now also have the chance to see other sides of medicine and surgery, such as dermatology, oncology, paediatrics, and psychiatry, to name a few.

The clinic will be held in the outpatient department of the hospital. It will usually consist of the consultant or sometimes junior doctors running the clinic. Clinic appointments often run behind so patients will have had a bit of wait before going in. It is important to remember this as it can help explain why some patients may seem a little annoyed when they come in. A simple explanation and apology at the start of the consultant is usually enough.

Before the clinic

How to choose a clinic

In general, you will be assigned to a certain specialty for a length of time and will go to their clinics. It is not necessary to attend every clinic on offer, as not all of them will be relevant for you.

- *Do* try to attend general clinics, where you will get an overview of a topic. Here you will learn about management and monitoring of common conditions. Clinics are a great place to learn about chronic diseases and to see disease progression. You can sit in on specialist clinics if you have a particular interest in a topic but if you do not then it may not be very useful for you. As a medical student it is most important to cover all the basics.
- *Do* try to attend a new patient clinic. Here you will get the chance to listen to the patient's story and challenge yourself to figure out the differential diagnoses and appropriate investigations. There is great opportunity here to follow a patient's journey from diagnosis to management. Certain doctors will do teaching clinics. These clinics tend to take two or three students at a time and are designed specifically with you in mind. You will learn a great deal in these clinics as the doctors are prepared for you. In general, as only a few students are allowed in these each time, you will be assigned a time to go or have to sign up.
- *Do* know where the outpatient department is situated and with whom you are sitting in with.
- *Do* check with the outpatient reception the day before that the clinic is going ahead as scheduled.
- *Do* read the GP referral letter. GPs will write to the consultant asking them to review the patient and explaining why they need specialist follow-up. Once you read a few of the letters you will start to see what makes a good referral and what does not. The key to a good referral letter is to clearly explain the patient's history, any relevant

investigations, treatment already tried by the GP, and why they feel the patient needs to be seen.

- *Do* read up on the topic of the clinic before attending. For example, if you are going to an IBD clinic then read about ulcerative colitis and Crohn's disease beforehand. Having some background knowledge will make the clinic more interesting for you and you will not be embarrassed if the consultant starts asking you questions! Seeing the management of a condition in clinical practice will help you remember it in the future.
- *Do* read through your learning outcomes for the topic of the clinic. Then while you are there you have an idea of what you are trying to achieve. You may be asked by the consultant if there is anything specifically you would like to know and this is a perfect time to ask if you are prepared with knowing your learning objectives.
- *Do* bring your stethoscope! You will be expected to examine patients or the consultant will ask you to listen to an interesting patient's heart. Do not be caught out by forgetting your stethoscope at home.

Top tip

Be sure to arrive 10–15 min early so that you can ask the consultant's permission to sit in and make a good first impression.

During the clinic

How to make the most out of a clinic

- *Do* be proactive in clinic. Just watching the clinic run can get quite tedious after a long time. So make the most of your time there and ask if you can take the patient's history before they go in to see the consultant. Spend about 10–15 min taking a history and examining the patient. Then you can present your history and differentials or management plan to the consultant. Compare your findings with the consultant's interpretation. You could also ask if you could examine the patient; you may get the opportunity to perform a specialized examination that you may not be able to do on wards.
- *Do* bring with you any clinical skills booklet you have that needs signing off.
- *Do* ask questions! You need to understand the logic behind treatments.
- *Do* bring a textbook with you to read in quiet moments. Sometimes patients do not attend appointments so you may have a prolonged wait in which it can be useful to read up about the last patient you saw. Another option at this point includes asking for teaching on any relevant topic from the consultant or other doctors present.
- *Do* watch carefully how the consultant and patient interact. This is a time to pick up any good habits you observe. You may end up observing the consultant breaking bad news. Pay careful attention to the words used to explain the news to the patient and the tone of the conversation. This is a very important skill to learn, and patients will always appreciate the doctor who was sensitive during their difficult hour.
- *Don't* stay in a clinic if you are finding that it is not useful. You may find that at certain times your time may be better spent elsewhere, e.g. on the wards or doing some reading on another topic. Politely excuse yourself

from the clinic, asking permission from the consultant to see whether there are other opportunities such as the ward or theatre where you would be able to gain some extra experience. Similarly, if you have an appointment you must attend which falls midway through the clinic then it is a good idea to let the consultant know at the beginning what time you will have to leave. Large numbers of patients are seen in clinic every day, so the consultant may not have time to go through each patient with you or answer any questions. Unfortunately this can really hinder your learning in the clinic. If you find yourself in this position then you can either try to make it a useful experience yourself or ask to be excused. One way in which to help yourself learn in this situation is to take a notebook and document the history or consultation as it goes. Try writing as if you are actually writing in the notes and have a think of what your plan would be. Ask questions after the consultation or at the end of the clinic.

- *Don't* be offended if a patient requests that you are not present for the consultation. Consent always has to be taken to allow you to sit in clinic. Certain specialties, such as genitourinary medicine, have more sensitive subject matter than others so it is quite likely you may be asked to leave at some point. Just go out of the room and grab a cup of coffee until the patient has left.
- *Don't* act bored. You may not feel very engaged, however, do not yawn or show your boredom. Do not forget the consultation is for the patient and they are doing you a favour by letting you sit in. If you feel yourself losing interest or getting tired either excuse yourself or go grab a coffee and come back. Similarly, do not use your phone in front of patients.
- *Don't* stay in the clinic if the next patient is someone you know or another student of your university. It is possible for this situation to arise, if it does just tell the consultant that you know the patient and think it would be best if you waited outside.

After the clinic

- *Do* follow the patient journey if you encounter an interesting case. You can write up a case report from GP referral, through to investigations, diagnosis, and management. Try to watch any investigations the patient will be undergoing (e.g. spirometry, bronchoscopy, and colonoscopy). Or go with them to theatre if they are due to have any surgery.
- *Do* get in contact with the consultant if you are interested in their specialty to ask if there any audits or projects you can get involved with. Chances are they will be impressed with your enthusiasm and initiative and lead you to an interesting project. You can even participate in outpatient clinic patient satisfaction surveys.
- *Do* remember which consultants you particularly enjoyed clinic with. If you find that a consultant gave very good teaching during the clinic then do ask if you can come back and sit in another time. They will appreciate your enthusiasm and enjoy teaching you. Just make sure you do not tread on your colleagues' toes and keep things fair, as they may have plans to attend the clinic another time.

- *Do* read about anything you did not understand or know about. You will be exposed to a variety of conditions during clinic and it is quite possible to come across something you have not heard of before. A good idea is to read up on that when you get home, while the memory of the patient is still fresh in your mind. It will help you remember if you can associate a patient with it.
- *Do* attend a MDT meeting, especially if a patient you saw will be discussed. In the MDT you will get to see how different team members come together to manage difficult situations.
- *Do* reflect on how educationally beneficial you found your clinic experience. It will help you in future clinics if you know what works for you and what does not. Identify how you learn best then implement this the next time you sit in a clinic.

Overall, clinics can be a really good learning experience if you know how to utilize them. It may feel intimidating sitting in a room with just you and the consultant who is asking you questions; however, you will remember the facts having been questioned on it under a little pressure. Consultants like to see medical students who are interested in what is going on. If you show them you are keen they will in turn teach you and you will learn more.

Theatre

Before theatre

Observing surgical procedures in the operating theatre can be one of the more thrilling aspects of the medical student experience. The illustration of anatomical structures, the integration of modern imaging/viewing systems and surgical instruments/prostheses, the skill of the surgeon, and the collective functioning of an effective clinical team can illustrate modern medicine at its finest. Specialities consist of the following:

Cardio-thoracic	General (GI/vascular/ transplant/ endocrine/ breast)	Neurosurgery
Urology	Plastics (aesthetic/burns/ reconstruction)	Oral & maxillofacial
Trauma & orthopaedics	Otolaryngology (ENT)	Paediatrics
Obstetrics & gynaecology	Dentistry	Ophthalmology

Learning objectives

The complex nature of the theatre environment is such that you must set learning objectives for the session/day, perhaps based on the operating list/cases. Otherwise, you might find that you have passively seen lots of interesting things but have not learnt anything concrete or understood the significance of what you have seen. You may have to use your initiative and set these learning objectives yourself (refer to ◌ www.faculty. londondeanery.ac.uk/e-learning/explore-further/teaching_and_learning_ in_operating_theatres.pdf).

Honours

Surgery as primary management option
Acute abdomen, trauma, dislocations, fractures, skin loss, extradural haemorrhage, placenta ruptio, obstructed pyelonephritis, transplant, exsanguination, draining abscesses, tropical surgery (Buruli ulcers, obstetric fistula), debridement.

Preoperative ward round

Patients typically arrive at the hospital in good time prior to surgery to ensure that all necessary checks, investigations, and preparations can be undertaken to prepare patients for theatre in good time. You must therefore attend the preoperative ward round, if possible, on any theatre list you are attending. This is an excellent opportunity for learning to:
• identify the indication for surgery
• observe the process of informed consent (how the risks and benefits of any procedure are communicated to patients and relatives), final patient discussions, and surgical marking.

- observe communications skills on how difficult concepts are explained simply, and how surgeons respond to the patient's anxiety
- identify surgical/anaesthetic challenges, so you may understand how specific issues are addressed in theatre (a difficult airway, or a comorbidity which changes the surgical approach)
- show willingness to learn and participate. If you have seen all the patients on the preoperative ward round, you will know their medical history and aspects of their care that the consultants may not be aware of. This makes you a valuable part of the team, and they will reward this by spending extra time teaching you.

Top tips for theatre

1. Inspect the operating list in advance. This will allow you to know (excluding emergencies) the procedures to be undertaken and get a head start in reading around the relevant anatomy, pathology, and management relevant to the cases. You will seem informed to the surgeons, and they will reward this with more teaching.
2. Inspect the patient notes. This will allow you to understand the patient's presentation, results of investigations, selection for surgery, and the influence of comorbidities on surgical and anaesthetic approaches to the patient.
3. Attend the preoperative ward round to ensure you know about each patient. You must be on time as it will be difficult to get the team back on side if you are late.
4. Observe the process of informed consent. It is important to know the perioperative complications (these will be listed to the patient during this process—and are easy marks for you during the interrogation that may await in theatre) and how the risk of each complication is minimized by the surgical and anaesthetic teams.
5. Accompany the surgeons to the theatre to change—they will help you find scrubs/shoes and this way, you will not get lost! Ensure you know which colour scrub top to wear for theatre (there may be more than one colour), and check the sizes by looking at the colour-coded collar. Do not wear shoes labelled with somebody else's name—ask at the theatre reception/sister if you are struggling (you cannot wear your outdoor shoes in theatre). You must wear a hat: men generally wear tie-backs and some women prefer elastic backs. Leave valuables at home such as expensive watches/jewellery.
6. Attend the 'WHO checklist' and introduce yourself as part of the clinical team. Understand the importance of this check so that all members of the team are aware of the roles of all members of the clinical team, the needs of individual patients, and anaesthetic and surgical considerations. Note how anaesthetic technique, patient comorbidities (e.g. diabetes), and patient demographics are all taken into account in the approach to each patient, and influence the agreed order of the operating list.
7. Put your mobile phone away. Look interested and attentive.
8. Introduce yourself to the surgeons early. Let them know what preparations you have made in advance (if you have done tips 1–4); they will be more likely to provide teaching/surgical opportunities if they sense you are using your initiative, are interested, and willing.

9. Ask a member of the theatre nursing team to demonstrate how to scrub and put on gloves (including identifying your correct glove size) and gown in a sterile fashion. Remember to wash everything from your elbows down, systematically and repeatedly for at least several minutes. If assisting, remember that infection control is vital. If scrubbed, always place your hands on the patient or the sterile field, never place your hands in your lap or cross your arms (both considered dirty). If you have become desterilized, simply state so and rescrub.

10. Understand theatre etiquette. When to ask questions/when to stay quiet, where to stand (so you do not obstruct the flow of staff/ patients), respect sterile surgical fields, be professional, and try to be helpful.

11. Be well fed and rested before a theatre list. It can seem like a long day if you are not used to it. There may be lots of standing, and lots of waiting. Take this handbook to read in such quiet moments. Go to the toilet before the case starts, if you think it is likely to be a lengthy case.

12. Speak clearly and loudly to the clinical team. This is essential for communication—particularly where masks make lip reading impossible and muffle sounds. If you are asked to do something, and do not hear clearly, ask for clarification.

13. There are many things you can help out with as long as you remain supervised by the scrub team. You can help transfer the patient from bed to bed, or start writing up the discharge summary, shave the surgical area with a powered-shaver, or improve the exposure of the surgical field by holding instruments to retract and wiping blood using a surgical swab or suction.

Consent

The process of informed consent factors prominently in SJTs, interviews, and examinations. It demonstrates the essence of effective patient communication (conveying the procedure, risks/benefits, postoperative care in language patients can understand), time/consultation management, and has stark medicolegal significance. The complications explained to the patient are those that the surgeon and clinical team will aim to minimize the risk of during surgery: you can ask about such strategies during surgery (e.g. how to minimize the risk of ureteric injury during hysterectomy). You should observe this process, both in clinic or on the ward, and in the preoperative ward round, to identify effective approaches to a quality process of informed consent. You must remember to respect the confidentiality of the patient: do not take patient identifiable data (such as operating lists) home with you.

Tip

Ask the surgeon, at an opportune time, what determines which risks are discussed with a patient, and why.

WHO surgical safety checklist

The WHO devised a surgical safety checklist in 2009 in order to improve surgical safety globally. There are three phases:

1. *Sign in*: all members of the clinical team introduce themselves by name and role before the theatre list begins. Each patient on the list is discussed in the presence of all members of the team to ensure equipment is checked, surgical equipment/prostheses are present, and anaesthetic/surgical/recovery concerns are communicated effectively.

2. *Time out*: occurs before 'knife-to-skin' to ensure all members of the clinical team confirm patient identity against a wrist band, essential details of the procedure such as nature and laterality of operation, checking consent form and surgical markings, allergies, etc. Anaesthetic, surgical, and nursing staff all confirm that they feel it is safe to proceed.

3. *Sign out*: before a patient leaves theatre, the team ensures that instruments are counted, the name of the procedure is recorded, specimens are labelled, and concerns for recovery are communicated.

Observe how concerns are communicated, and how this systematic approach to confirmation of clinical details at every step decreases the likelihood of an error being made. The surgical checklist may be modified to increase its relevance to certain high-turnover procedures (such as cataract surgery).

Theatre etiquette

Theatre can be a somewhat confusing environment for a medical student at first: you may be unsure where to stand, what you are supposed to touch/not supposed to touch, when and how much you should speak, when you should ask questions, etc. Your understanding of theatre etiquette and its correct observation will endear you to all the clinical staff. Incomplete observation may frustrate them, or worse (such as violating sterility). Common sense, good manners, health and safety, and infection control are the main principles of good theatre etiquette. The following will help you to enjoy your time in theatre:

- Introduce yourself to all members of the clinical team if you were not present at the WHO check. This will mean all members of staff know you are there to learn, and will find things to teach you.

- Wear your name badge clearly: any member of staff is within their right to challenge you if it is not visible.

- Ask a theatre sister/nurse where the most appropriate place is to put your bag/valuables (you will not have a locker).

- Sense when the surgeons have time to talk (during scrubbing, while the patient is being positioned, or other delays where the surgeon is waiting), and when they do not (at a critical point in the surgery). Ask your questions at comfortable moments in the surgery if possible: you can ask as much as you want during wound closure.

- If you are feeling faint, tell a member of staff immediately so they can safely sit you down somewhere until you feel better. If you ignore the early symptoms, you will likely suffer vasovagal syncope, which can be dangerous near to a patient (and to yourself).

- Do not enter theatre through the anaesthetic room while a patient is being anaesthetized.

- Do not enter theatre through the main theatre doors while an operation is taking place. Entering theatre through the scrub room is the most appropriate route into theatre—although usually inconvenient.
- If you sustain a needle-stick injury, you must indicate this immediately. A member of staff will help you irrigate the wound, and discuss the next steps involving occupational health as per trust protocol.

Scrubbing in

Ask a theatre nurse to teach you how to scrub correctly, and in line with trust policy. There is usually a notice explaining the technique of washing your hands (more complex than you think) correctly (including use of brushes and nail picks), how to dry your hands, unfold/unravel the gown, and put on sterile gloves without touching the sterile outer surface. They may help you to identify your hand size. The average adult male hand size is 7.5 inches, and adult female is 6.5 inches (to get you started). Find your size: a glove that fits comfortably but does not restrict any manual manoeuvres. Scrubbing in will allow you a better view of the surgical field as you will be part of it. After scrubbing, stand with your hands, one over the other, on your chest. This will indicate to the team that you are sterile and you understand the sterile field (assumed to be the front of your gown above your waist). Remember that your mask is not sterile!

Tip

Remember to put your mask on before you scrub! (Masks with visors are available for procedures which risk ocular inoculation).

Observation

This is an active, rather than a passive skill. Most learning in theatre is through observation where there is plenty to see and understand. You should observe the requirements for both technical and non-technical skills. You should ask the surgeon where the most appropriate place to observe the surgery is; ask the consultant 'Where would you like me to stand?' Some procedures with viewing systems will have a monitor from which surgical anatomy can be well demonstrated. Other procedures may be viewed over a shoulder with the surgeon's permission. In general, the closer to open surgery you are, the more detailed the view, and the richer the learning experience. If this is something you might feel is appropriate, ask for the surgeon's permission. Observe how the team responds to changing circumstances: a procedure running longer than expected, complications, a change in the patient's physiology, etc.

Suturing

This is the fundamental surgical skill. It is the part of surgery, with time, you may be allowed to get most involved in assisting with during wound closure. It is a skill you can practise in the skills lab, and it is recommended that you practise beforehand if suturing is something you wish to assist with. Basic interrupted suture placement is important to learn, and will allow surgeons to build on this with suture tying techniques. Hand tying a suture is a valuable skill: ask one of the surgeons to demonstrate if there is a suitable opportunity. Be responsible with sharps in theatre since scrub nurses will become unhappy if you lose needles, as they will have to find them to balance the count. An excellent resource is available online ($\hat{\mathcal{S}}$ www.animatedknots.com).

Assisting

Being an assistant is easy. You may be asked to hold retractors, to assist the surgeons in viewing and manipulating the surgical field, cutting sutures to the correct length with scissors (if unsure, clarify how long the surgeon would like the suture ends), using suction to keep the surgical field clear, etc. If you feel you are getting tired, or cannot do something, tell the surgical team. If you are not sure of the instructions, always ask for clarification.

Other practical competencies

Urethral catheterization and gynaecological examination are competencies which may be performed under supervision in theatre while the patient is under GA. Do consent beforehand!

Logbooks

(See ➲ 'Importance of logbooks' p. 1016). It is important that you record (anonymously using hospital numbers) the procedure that you have witnessed and laterality. If you performed any part of the procedure (such as wound closure), this should be indicated on your record. This will allow you to demonstrate an objective record of your practical experience that may be important at appraisal or at interview in the future.

Reflective practice

The theatre environment offers plenty to reflect on: teamwork, patient safety, personality attributes, leadership, and managing acutely ill patients.

Surgical jargon

Suffix/prefix	Definition	Example
-ectomy	Cutting out	Appendicectomy
-otomy	Cutting open	Laparotomy
-oscopy	Looking into	Gastroscopy
-ostomy	Opening	Colostomy
-plasty	Reconstruction/repair	Rhinoplasty
Per-	Through	Percutaneous
Trans-	Across	Transoesophageal echocardiography

Useful links

- $\hat{\mathcal{S}}$ www.who.int/patientsafety/safesurgery/ss_checklist/en/
- $\hat{\mathcal{S}}$ www.faculty.londondeanery.ac.uk/e-learning/explore-further/teaching_and_learning_in_operating_theatres.pdf
- $\hat{\mathcal{S}}$ www.geekymedics.com/2015/04/06/theatre-etiquette/
- $\hat{\mathcal{S}}$ www.practicalplasticsurgery.org/docs/Practical_01.pdf

Why see patients?

Mikhail Bulgakov (see Fig. 6.1) travelled by sleigh to take up a post at a remote, snowbound hospital in rural Russia in 1916, the ink barely dry on his medical degree. The only doctor, with no telephone or electric light, wrote of his metamorphosis from bookish medical student to hands-on doctor that still rings true for new doctors a century later.

In one of his stories, a woman arrives in labour with a transverse lie. He frantically thumbs through an obstetrics textbook to try and recall how to perform a 'podalic version' but the words are a blur. Assisting him is the hospital's experienced midwife, Anna Nikolaevna. She cannot resist telling him how his predecessors carried out the procedure as he scrubs in. 'Those ten minutes told me more than everything I had read on obstetrics for my qualifying exams, in which I had actually passed the obstetrics paper with distinction.'[1]

We see patients to focus the blurred words in our imperfect lecture notes and textbooks. Good-quality YouTube videos may be an advance on written guides to practical procedures but no second-hand source can replace the experience that you build from your own histories and examinations. 'Medicine is learned by the bedside and not in the classroom' wrote Sir William Osler (1849–1919). 'Let not your conceptions of disease come from the words heard in the lecture room or read from a book. See, and then reason and compare and control. But see first.'

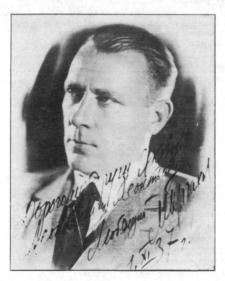

Fig. 6.1 Mikhail Bulgakov. Reproduced from https://commons.wikimedia.org. Image in public domain.

Seeing patients

What is the reality? It can be uncomfortable enough introducing yourself to the busy ward sister or to get the attention of the harassed-looking registrar on-call. But to actually go and talk to and examine the thin, yellow-looking man in bed 6 (the consultant says he will be an excellent case to see jaundice, spider naevi, and palpate a liver cirrhosed by years of alcoholism) feels plain awkward—you are not going to contribute to his care, only to your own education.

But your patient, a veteran of the medical ward, sees you looking lost, knows by your hesitant gait that you are a medical student, and beckons you over. 'The boss sent you?' he asks with a chuckle. 'Well come here and learn—and please tell the nurse that I'd like a cuppa!'

By seeing Mr Smith, you start the process of building your own, personal medical textbook, like the mental dermatology atlas the paediatrician is constantly adding to with each new rash she sees (so many do not match the colour plates of a textbook). You are also building your confidence as a communicator, able to broach difficult subjects with sensitivity, which will, in turn, inspire the confidence of your future patients. You might feel unprepared to cope with the patient who starts crying but you will learn that their tears are a sign of trust and that far from being awkward, your listening might have been therapeutic.

You will also learn a lot from the nurses and doctors around you, rejecting some bad examples but mostly absorbing fantastic ways to put patients at ease (like the registrar who asks the 5-year-old boy to flap his arms like a chicken and then hold his arms like a boxer to test power in his upper limbs).

Come your clinical exams, if you have not clerked and examined patients, it will show. Some patients will not want to see you but most will (in one study, 85.6% of women attending a gynaecology clinic were happy to have a medical student present and 63.9% said they would allow a medical student to examine them, although there was a preference for female students).[2]

And do not worry about all the things you 'missed' when the registrar or consultant goes over the history with the patient. It can often take several goes before the relevant bit of history comes out to clinch the diagnosis. Do not forget that the only difference between you and the doctor is experience and practice which cannot be rushed or bought—only earned.

Consent on the wards and in the clinic

Before seeing patients, you will have had teaching regarding consent (see ➲ pp. 141–2 and p. 861). But on a busy post-take ward round, this can sometimes be forgotten. The classic is sitting in clinic and the busy doctor forgets to explain your presence to the next patient. If you think the doctor has forgotten, you must learn how to interrupt politely and succinctly to explain who you are and if it is okay with the patient for you to be there—the consultant will thank you later for avoiding a complaint (some clinics usefully advise patients before they see the doctor that a medical student is sitting in—you could turn this into a quality improvement project).

You must gain consent for both history taking and examination. Explain to the patient not only who you are, giving your surname ('I'm Jo Bloggs, a 4th-year medical student …') but also add that it is fine for the patient *not* to see you ('It won't affect your care in any way') or to stop the interview/

examination if they are feeling tired. Giving the patient an out is far more likely to win them round.

Explain that what the patient tells you is confidential to the medical team looking after them. You will hear and be told some very private things—do not chat about their case outside the ward (what would you feel like if something you discussed with your doctor was overheard in the hospital lift or on the bus home?). Also, do not be buttonholed by friends or family to discuss the patient's case—say they must talk to the patient and the team looking after them. Ensure there are no patient identifiers if you need to write up or present cases outside the ward as part of your teaching. Be very careful about how you keep and dispose of patient lists—better not to have one. Likewise, keep your clinical life out of social media.

Get advice from the senior nursing staff or doctors on the ward when approaching patients who you think may lack capacity or when examining children (do not examine them when their parents are not there). Always consider the need for a chaperone—it is easier if you are working in pairs as then you will not have to pull a nurse or doctor away from what they are doing. However, you should be supervised for any intimate examinations (breast, genitalia, rectum, etc.) and you should have prior, written consent from the patient before any intimate examination under anaesthesia.

Medical history

It is said that 80% of the diagnosis lies within the patient's history and the rest is confirmed by investigations. Spend the first few minutes of your consult-ation listening carefully and allow the patient time to speak about their symp-toms (i.e. changes in the body) and start thinking of possible signs (i.e. clinical findings) to support your differentials. That is the mark of a good doctor!

History taking

Learning to take a history continues long after medical school. How to draw out vital symptoms from a shy patient—or how to negotiate the rapids of a patient who wants to tell you about their granddaughter's cold, her holiday in York, and the problems with her bus service—is a challenge. You will also have to learn tact, such as asking a partner to leave when taking a sexual history. The challenge is then making a coherent whole of all that you have been told so that you can communicate it succinctly to the healthcare team—not just presenting the history but giving a differential diagnosis and a management plan.

Presenting complaint (PC)

This is what brought the patient into your GP surgery/outpatient clinic. Keep the PC in the patient's own words—the differential for '*feeling tired*' is wide.

History of presenting complaint (HPC)

This is where you go over the complaint in more detail. At first, use open questions: 'What's brought you in today? How long have you had these symptoms?' The let the patient talk and simply *listen*. One study looking at history taking by optometrists showed that the median time it took for adult patients to state the reason for their attendance in their 'uninterrupted initial talking time' was 28.87 sec.[3] All your most useful information will be here and you will have gained valuable time in establishing rapport—because you listened. Once the patient has told you what the problem is, you can then start asking more closed questions: when the symptoms started, risk factors (e.g. smoking, alcohol intake, travel history), about pain and what alleviates or exacerbates this. The **SOCRATES** mnemonic is invaluable:

S: site
O: onset
C: character
R: radiation
A: associations
T: timing
E: exacerbating or relieving factors
S: severity, e.g. pain score.

Pain and past medical history (PMHx)

The patient can score their pain: 'If 1 is no pain and 10 is the worst pain ever, how would you score your pain?' Also, you can use Wong–Baker FACES® pain rating scale for children.

Each system will also have its own set of questions (e.g. asking about breathlessness on exertion for someone with chest pain or times of the day when joint stiffness is worst).

PMHx

Ask about any established medical conditions, admissions to hospital, medical conditions or previous surgery (if the patient has undergone surgery, ask about anaesthetic problems). In particular, ask about hypertension, diabetes, heart disease, stroke asthma or epilepsy. You might find important illnesses revealed from the drug history.

Medications

Important to ask about any drug allergies. If a patient has a drug allergy, ask how it affects them (e.g. anaphylaxis or a simple rash with penicillin?). Then go through all the patient's medications—you can pick up problems that a patient or parent omitted to tell you ('Oh yes, he's on folic acid and penicillin V for his sickle cell') and also alert yourself to potential problems. For instance, it is vital to know if the patient who presents with rectal bleeding is on warfarin, or to know that the normal heart rate which does not fit with the ill-looking patient in front of you because she is on a beta blocker.

Remember drugs, drug interactions (and attendant polypharmacy) can cause problems—learn to recognize drugs that will be toxic to the liver, kidneys, and hearing (e.g. the antibiotic gentamicin which can cause renal and ototoxicity).

Steroid use can have wide-ranging side effects. Remember **CUSHINGOID**:

C: cataracts
U: ulcers
S: skin—striae, thinning
H: hypertension, hirsutism, hyperglycaemia
I: infections
N: avascular necrosis of the femoral head
G: glycosuria
O: osteoporosis, obesity
I: immunosuppression
D: diabetes mellitus.

Ask about contraception, pregnancy, and breastfeeding—prescribing drugs such as certain antibiotics can reduce the combined oral contraceptive pill's efficacy while some drugs are toxic to the fetus or are present in breast milk. Start looking up medications in the *BNF* to learn how to identify common side effects, their toxicity to the liver and kidneys, especially Appendix 1, and the list of drug interactions. Ask about over-the-counter medications and alternative therapies—some of these, such as the herbal remedy St John's wort (taken for depression), interact with several medications.

Social history

The information gathered here can have big implications for managing our patients but we all too often skip over this part of the history, perhaps embarrassed to ask such personal questions. Watch in clinic or at the bedside how an experienced doctor will normalize and signpost while taking such a history. For instance, if you suspect cocaine or amphetamine use by the young patient in front of you with a tachyarrhythmia, you could say 'We need to know about any recreational drug use so we know how best to treat you'; or the child presenting with unusual bruising: 'Mrs Smith, it's a question we ask everyone who comes to the department—does Jonny have a social worker?'

Knowing who is at home is especially important for a paediatric or elderly patient, to gauge what kind of support they have. It will also be your duty as a doctor to establish any safeguarding issues to best protect your patients from any potential threat. Is the patient unemployed or receiving the benefits they need? Health follows a social gradient, whether in Angola or America.[4] Some specialties will go into much greater depth on social issues (e.g. psychiatry).

Alcohol (ETOH)

Likely to be underestimated by the patient. Ask the patient how much they drink and when they drink (e.g. binge drinking at weekends). The recommended maximum weekly alcohol intake in the UK is up to 14 units. The CAGE questionnaire remains a useful screening tool for alcoholism ('yes' to two or more suggests a problem):

C: have you felt the need to *cut* down on your alcohol intake?
A: have you felt *annoyed* by people asking about your drinking?
G: have you ever felt *guilty* about your drinking?
E: have you ever drunk an *eye-opener* in the morning?

Smoking

A major, preventable risk factor for cardiovascular disease, respiratory illness, and cancer. Smoking is measured in pack-years (i.e. 1 pack-year = smoking 20 cigarettes/day for 1 year).

Do not forget passive smoking—paediatricians see many children with their asthma and viral-induced wheeze worsened by smokers in the household. 'But I smoke outside, doc!' does not, unfortunately, lessen the harm.[5]

Systems review

This last part of the history aims to reveal important symptoms not picked up in the HPC.

- *General (constitutional symptoms)*: fever, night sweats, weight loss, fatigue (thyroid problem?), lumps/bumps, trauma, appetite.
- *Cardiorespiratory*: shortness of breath on exertion ('I run out of puff after 5 stairs'), chest pain, palpitations (thyroid problem?), orthopnoea (breathlessness when lying flat—ask how many pillows the patient sleeps on, >3 suggestive of heart failure), haemoptysis (coughing blood), wheeze.
- *Gut*: mouth ulcers, difficulty swallowing (dysphagia), acid brash, pain (SOCRATES), vomiting (haematemesis = vomiting blood, bilious = dark green), stool (blood—on surface of stool, bright red, on toilet paper; malaena = dark, tarry stool, a sign of upper GI bleeding), feeling of being unable to completely empty bowels (tenesmus, possible sign of rectal mass), testicular pain (torsion—an emergency).
- *Genitourinary*: dysuria (pain on passing urine), haematuria (blood in urine), frequency, incontinence, polyuria (passing large amounts of urine often—with polydipsia, drinking large amounts, points to a diagnosis of diabetes mellitus. Consider taking a sexual history but ensure confidentiality (rash, discharge, partners, travel, injected drug use, previous sexually transmitted diseases). Testicular pain—torsion is a surgical emergency.
- *Neurological*: headaches, dizziness, changes in vision, weakness, pins and needles (paraesthesia), speech problems, memory problems.
- *Rheumatological*: pain/stiffness/swelling of joints, when worst (diurnal variation between rheumatoid arthritis (RA) and osteoarthritis (OA)), how function affected.

Special cases

Paediatrics

Like the different array of normal values for a child's heart rate, so with how you approach the history. Along with usual schema, you will want to ask about birth history (especially in neonates—babies <28 days old) and development (a 3-year-old falling off the sofa after bouncing around and breaking their wrist is likely to be an accident, but you would be highly suspicious of the same story from a parent presenting with a 3-month-old).

Vaccination status is important not only in terms of disease prevention but a lack of immunizations can point to social problems and change your management of an 8-month-old with fever (they will not be protected against several nasty bacteria). Always take a feeding history—if a baby is not feeding, they are unwell (ask the parents how much milk she usually takes and how often and compare to how she is feeding now. Time spent on the breast is a helpful measure if the parents are not bottle-feeding the baby).

Care of the elderly (COTE)

The social history will be important (living alone/in a care home/with relatives?). Elderly patients may have non-specific presentations—a pneumonia with no cough or sputum production or a 'silent' myocardial infarction (MI; i.e. no chest pain). Elderly patients can be on several different medications—has the new antihypertensive inadvertently caused the patient to fall and fracture their hip? Ensure a thorough dug history. You will also learn how to take a collateral history from a carer or GP. Common presentations are problems with mobility and falls; dementia and confusion; infection; stroke; and incontinence (see ➔ Chapter 11).

Obstetrics and gynaecology

Be careful with confidentiality. For a gynaecological history, cover menstrual, contraceptive, and sexual history. For obstetrics, remember gravidity = the total number of pregnancies while parity is the number of pregnancies carried beyond 24 weeks (NB abortion = fetal death <24 weeks and still-birth = fetal death >24 weeks). A patient who with two children and one spontaneous abortion would be described as 2+1 (i.e. gravid 3) but less confusing simply to write '2 live children, 1 spontaneous abortion' (see ➔ Chapter 23).

Interpreters

A language barrier will greatly limit the patient's access to healthcare. In an emergency, using a family member as an interpreter might be the only option but this is the only time friends or family should be used due to issues of confidentiality etc. In the UK, you can dial Language Line, a 24/7 telephone interpreting service.

Emergency history

Take an **AMPLE** history covering the very basics for the patient arriving in the resuscitation area (see ➔ p. 262):

A: allergies
M: medications
P: past medical history
L: last time eaten
E: environment, events leading to presentation.

Presenting your findings

This takes practice and different clinicians will have their preferences (e.g. a paediatrician will always want to hear the age of the child right at the beginning as this immediately helps narrow down the differential diagnosis, an intensivist will want a systems approach). *Speak up*, and go through your history and examination findings in a systematic order (which means you are less likely to miss things). Keep the PC in the patient's own words—give your differential diagnosis at the end. Again, knowing what to leave out takes practice. Do not worry about interjections—it means the team is listening to you! Also, always give a *differential diagnosis* and have a go at making a *management plan*, both signs of a thinking doctor rather than a clerking machine. Present succinctly with positive findings before negative.

References

1. Bulgakov M (2010). *A Country Doctor's Notebook* (Tr. Michael Glenny). London: Vintage Classics.
2. Yang J, Black K (2014). Medical students in gynaecology clinics. *Clin Teach* 11(4):254–8.
3. Pointer JS (2014). The primary eye care examination: opening the case history and the patient's uninterrupted initial talking time. *J Optom* 7(2):79–85.
4. Marmot M (2015). *The Health Gap: The Challenge of an Unequal World*. London: Bloomsbury.
5. Tabuchi T, Fujiwara T, Nakayama T, et al. (2015). Maternal and paternal indoor or outdoor smoking and the risk of asthma in their children: a nationwide prospective birth cohort study. *Drug Alcohol Depend* 147:103–8.

Basic X-ray interpretation

Things to consider when requesting imaging

The key to being comfortable with radiological investigations and interpreting plain films is gaining as much exposure to imaging as possible while you are a medical student and junior doctor. There are several easy avenues to gaining exposure to imaging:

- Radiologists are all too willing to teach keen students/junior doctors and most of us enjoy it, this can be arranged by discussing with your local radiology department.
- Further exposure can be obtained by attending radiology MDTs. These occur most days within a radiology department. This will give you exposure to imaging techniques, common pathologies, and their radiological findings.
- There are also various free websites that cover imaging including ℘ www.radiopedia.org, ℘ www.radiologyassistant.nl, and ℘ www. learningradiology.com.

This section gives you the basics of how to interpret plain films but also start learning early how to orientate yourself around common CT and MRI investigations. If you have been asked by your team to request imaging, make sure there is a clear question that needs to be answered. If you or your team is unsure of the correct investigation to request, to answer your clinical question, you should discuss this with the radiology department. Most departments have a duty radiologist who will help facilitate this. Some important logistical issues to consider when requesting investigations include the following:

- Many cross-sectional techniques require the patient to remain still. If this is not possible, then the procedure may have to be performed under GA. This is more of an issue in the acutely unwell, intoxicated, and young patients.
- Many modalities require the use of contrast agents, the use of which has risks attached. CT often requires the use of IV iodinated agents which are contraindicated in those with allergies to iodine and which are nephrotoxic, and these should be used in caution in patients with renal failure. Most hospitals have guidelines relating to this.
- MRI often requires the use of gadolinium-based agents which also have relative contraindications in renal failure due to the risk of nephrogenic systemic fibrosis.
- For IV contrast to be successful, good IV access is required and the type of cannula required should be discussed with the radiology department.
- With MRI there is a relative contraindication to patients who contain metal foreign bodies (pacemakers, metal surgical clips, etc.). MRI request forms usually contain an extensive safety questionnaire relating to these issues.
- Some techniques require the use of oral contrast agents, the patient must be able to swallow these safely for the techniques to be performed.

Interpretation of a chest radiograph (chest X-ray, CXR)

- Identify the patient, their date of birth, and hospital number.
- Some pathologies are more common in certain age groups (e.g. malignancy or cardiac failure in older patients).
- Know the anatomy demonstrated on a CXR (see Fig. 6.2 and Fig. 6.3).
- Appearance of structures on the CXR are determined by their density (reflects the amount of photons that reach the X-ray plate/detector).

Bones which are dense appear white, while lungs, which essentially contain air, and bronchovascular structures are dark.

Quality of the chest X-ray

Projection

If not stated on the film, the standard projection is PA (posterior to anterior) radiograph. The heart size and mediastinal width can only be accurately assessed in a PA projection. This is because they are anterior mediastinal structures and lie closer to the X-ray plate in a PA projection.

Penetration

In a well-penetrated film, the thoracic vertebra should be visible (although now that radiographs are acquired digitally, this is less important as the image can be manipulated, or 'windowed' to see structures more clearly).

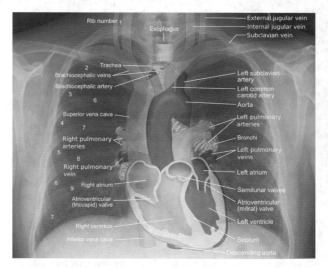

Fig. 6.2 Anatomy of anteroposterior (AP) plain chest radiograph demonstrating the mediastinal structures. Reproduced from Wikimedia Commons. Illustration by Mikael Häggström, licensed under the Creative Commons Attribution-Share Alike 3.0 Unported license.

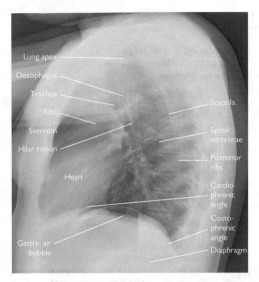

Fig. 6.3 Anatomy of the lateral chest radiograph. Reproduced from Wikimedia Commons. Illustration by Mikael Häggström, released to the public domain.

Rotation

The distances between the clavicular heads (the sternal ends) and spinous process of the thoracic vertebra should be equal. If the patient is rotated, it can make assessment of the structures difficult as they no longer lie in their correct anatomical plane.

Inspiration

To accurately assess the lungs, the radiograph should be assessed in inspiration. In a good inspiratory film there should be 8–10 posterior ribs above the diaphragm (or 6–8 anterior ribs, the ones that curve downwards and intersect the diaphragm in the mid-clavicular line). Poorly inspired films can make normal lungs look pathological by exaggerating anatomical structures.

Situs

Are the heart and gastric bubble on the left side (if not, the radiograph should clearly state which side is left)? Remember, there are patients who have dextrocardia (heart on the right side) or situs inversus (organs lie on the opposite side to normal).

Systematic approach to interpretation of the chest X-ray

When interpreting the radiographic findings on any plain film, be systematic. This results in nothing being missed, especially in stressful situations. There are many ways to interpret a CXR but a simple method to adopt is:

Lines/tubes and then the ABCDE approach

A = airways
B = breathing (lungs)
C = circulation and central structures (heart, hilum, and aorta)
D = diaphragm and review areas (apices, behind heart)
E = extras (bones and soft tissues).

Lines/tubes

These include ETTs, central lines, and enteric tubes. Ensure they are correctly located. An ETT should lie above the carina, the amount depends on the position of the neck. In a neutral position, it should lie approximately 5 cm above the carina in an adult. In a non-rotated patient, a nasogastric (NG) tube should bisect the carina and descend down the midline. The tip should lie below the level of the left hemidiaphragm.

Beware the NG tube that has entered one of the main bronchi and the associated lung (missing one of these is a 'never event' according to the National Patient Safety Agency). There are various online tools to help demonstrate the correct position. Central lines should terminate within the SVC or at the SVC/right atrial junction.

Airways

Is the trachea central? If not, is it deviated away or towards pathology? This reflects a change in lung volumes. Is the carina angle correct? This should be <90°; if ↑ this suggests left atrial enlargement as the left atrium lies directly underneath the carina. Are the major airways patent or is there an obvious obstructing mass/foreign body within them?

Breathing—lungs

Initially look at each lung individually, then compare the two. Use a systematic approach looking through all zones. This is where you are looking for pathology such as consolidation, masses, pneumothoraces, or effusions.

Circulation and central structures

Is the heart enlarged? This can only be accurately assessed on the PA projection. Heart size is assessed using the cardiothoracic ratio which is the ratio of maximal horizontal cardiac width to maximal horizontal thoracic width on a PA radiograph. The heart size should be <50%. Is the mediastinum widened (you should normally see the aortic knuckle clearly)? If the mediastinum is widened, there could be an underlying vascular (dissection) or malignant (tumour or nodes) cause.

Diaphragm and review areas

Are the diaphragms at a similar level, with the right diaphragm normally slightly higher than the left (due to the underlying liver)? The diaphragms should be clearly defined. If they are obscured, it suggests that there is something abutting the diaphragm—consolidation/mass—which obscures the air/diaphragm interface. Is there free air underneath the diaphragm? This is suggestive of an abdominal hollow viscous perforation. An erect CXR is the most sensitive plain radiograph for detecting free air (more so than an abdominal radiograph) (see Fig. 6.4). Review areas include the apices and behind the heart where pathology is not clearly visualized due to overlying structures (clavicles and heart).

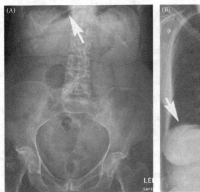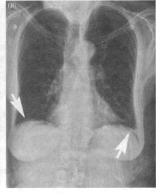

Fig. 6.4 Pneumoperitoneum on (a) supine abdominal and (b) upright chest radiographs. There is central lucency beneath the hemidiaphragm (arrow in a), representing the cupola sign. The upright chest radiograph shows free intraperitoneal air beneath the hemidiaphragms (arrows in b). Reproduced with permission from Levy, Angela, et al, *Gastrointestinal Imaging*, 2015, Oxford University Press.

Extras

It is not only the lungs and heart that are included on the chest radiograph. Often the bones and soft tissues are overlooked when looking at radiographs. Beware of pneumothoraces, fractures (ribs, clavicles), and destructive bony lesions. If significant you can also see axillary/neck adenopathy and surgical emphysema.

Tip

Since many patients will be in and out of hospital due to regular chest pathology (e.g. congenital, smokers, immunodeficient patients), make sure you go through any previous imaging to compare severity or resolution. Any prior radiological studies can usually be found in the patients electronic imaging folder with the current study. When reviewing an image, be careful to check the date of the study.

Common pathologies seen on a chest X-ray

There are numerous different pathologies that can be seen on a CXR. It is easiest to break these down into lung and cardiac pathologies.

Consolidation

Consolidation is merely fluid/tissue within the alveoli. While the term is often used in relation to infection, consolidation can be caused by pus, haemorrhage, fluid, or cells (tumour). On a CXR, consolidation appears radiopaque (white) compared to the adjacent normally aerated lung (black). When looking at consolidation you need to decide its location and distribution. Lobar pneumonia will present as a consolidated lobe. Pulmonary haemorrhage may present as diffuse, patchy consolidation throughout the affected lungs. Similarly, acute respiratory distress syndrome (ARDS) can look like diffuse patchy consolidation throughout both lungs.

> **Top tip**
> It can take up to 6 weeks before radiological resolution of consolidation can be seen. This can be ordered and followed up by the patient's GP.

Collapse

Lobar collapse has various different radiological signs depending on the lobe affected. Equally, a whole lung can collapse. Collapse causes a loss of volume within the affected hemithorax with resultant movement of structures towards the collapse (e.g. elevation of hemidiaphragm/movement of fissures and mediastinal shift towards collapse). Certain collapses have key radiological signs (see Figs 6.5–6.8).

Opacities

Similar to consolidation, an opacity refers to an area of ↑density within the normally aerated lung. Opacities can be single or multiple and the term is often used to describe malignant masses whereas consolidation is often used to describe infection. A single opacity is likely to reflect a primary lung malignancy. Multiple opacities are likely to reflect pulmonary metastases.

Cavities

Some opacities can cavitate where an air fluid level is seen within the opacity. While some malignancies can cavitate (particularly squamous cell carcinoma), cavitatory lesions are often caused by a lung abscess which can be single or multiple (*Staphylococcus* septic emboli). Some vasculitides can also cause cavitatory lesions (e.g. granulomatosis with polyangiitis (previously known as Wegener's granulomatosis)).

Effusions

A pleural effusion is fluid within the pleural space, most commonly caused by congestive cardiac failure, infection, or malignancy. Small pleural effusions cause blunting of the costophrenic angle. As they ↑ in size you get ↑density within the affected hemithorax with an associated meniscus sign.

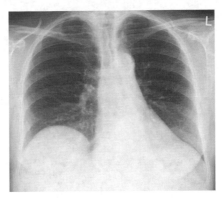

Fig. 6.5 PA CXR showing mediastinal shift to the left, depression of the left hilum, and ↑density behind the heart ('sail sign') due to left lower lobe collapse. Reproduced with permission from Darby, M. J., et al, *Oxford Handbook of Medical Imaging*, 2011, Oxford University Press.

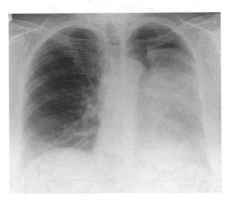

Fig. 6.6 PA CXR of left upper lobe collapse, showing 'veil like' opacification of the left chest, obliteration of the heart border, elevation of the hilum, and preservation of the arch and descending thoracic aorta. Reproduced with permission from Darby, M. J., et al, *Oxford Handbook of Medical Imaging*, 2011, Oxford University Press.

If the effusion enlarges it can cause a '*white out*' of the affected hemithorax and often causes collapse of the underlying lung which compensates for this (see Fig. 6.8). Effusions can be bilateral or unilateral. If bilateral, this usually suggests a systemic cause. Remember, if a CXR is taken with the patient lying down, then smaller effusions can be difficult to visualize as they often only cause minor ↑density within the affected hemithorax.

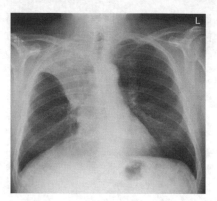

Fig. 6.7 PA CXR of patient with persistent cough, showing right upper lobe collapse. The opacity in the right upper chest has a clearly defined, curved inferior border, consisting of the elevated horizontal fissure and the inferior border of a right hilar mass (the 'golden S' sign). Note also the mediastinal shift to the right and volume loss in the right chest. Reproduced with permission from Darby, M. J., et al, *Oxford Handbook of Medical Imaging*, 2011, Oxford University Press.

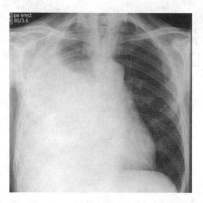

Fig. 6.8 PA CXR showing a large pleural effusion filling much of the right chest. Note the shift of the mediastinum away from the opacity and the meniscus extending up over the apex of the lung. Reproduced with permission from Darby, M. J., et al, *Oxford Handbook of Medical Imaging*, 2011, Oxford University Press.

Pneumothorax

A pneumothorax is air within the pleural space and can be spontaneous or iatrogenic. When looking for a pneumothorax, assess the lung markings and see if they extend to the thoracic wall. If they do not and there is a lung edge visualized, a pneumothorax is present. It is often easier to see pneumothoraces by inverting the image (so structures that are normally dark are white and vice versa).

If there is underlying collapse of the lung in conjunction with the pneumothorax there is often minimal mediastinal shift. If air cannot escape, the pneumothorax is at risk of tensioning (one-way valve, see Fig. 6.9). This means the pneumothorax gets progressively bigger causing mediastinal shift away from the pneumothorax. If severe, there can be cardiac compromise and a tension pneumothorax is a medical emergency. A radiograph should never be used to determine a tension pneumothorax and you should be ready to act upon this finding. A tip is to invert the CXR to make it easier to spot the pneumothorax.

Pneumomediastinum

The presence of extraluminal gas within the mediastinum. This can arise from the airways, lungs, or oesophagus and results from injury to any of these organs. There are many radiological signs but a rim of air is often seen around the mediastinal structures. If it tracks underneath the heart you get the continuous diaphragm sign. Often there is associated surgical emphysema as mediastinal air tracks into the soft tissue planes of the neck. If associated with an oesophageal perforation there will often be an associated pleural effusion which is usually left sided.

Cardiac failure

Cardiac failure can manifest in various different forms on a radiograph from an essentially normal film to having overt findings of cardiac failure. Generally speaking, the heart will be enlarged, with a cardiothoracic ratio >50%. Other radiological findings include pleural effusions, Kerley B lines (small 1–2cm horizontal lines in the periphery of the lung representing fluid within interlobular septa, typically seen at the lung bases), upper lobe pulmonary venous diversion, interstitial changes and patchy consolidation (secondary to pulmonary oedema).

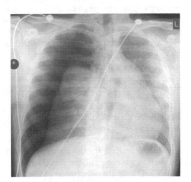

Fig. 6.9 CXR of a tension pneumothorax on the right. The collapsed lung is opacified, the mediastinum is shifted away from the affected side, and the ipsilateral diaphragm is depressed. This needs urgent decompression. Reproduced with permission from Darby, M. J., et al, *Oxford Handbook of Medical Imaging*, 2011, Oxford University Press.

Interpretation of the abdominal radiograph

There are few indications for an abdominal radiograph (AXR). These include acute abdomen (including exacerbation of IBD), bowel obstruction, renal or ureteric calculi, foreign bodies, and to assess lines/tubes. Constipation is rarely an acceptable indication, especially in children. Pregnancy is a relative contraindication.

Interpretation

An AXR is relatively more straightforward than a CXR as there is less anatomy and less pathology that can be visualized. A good AXR should include the whole abdomen (including lung bases) and pelvis. The spine should be visible. There is no set way to look at an AXR but a good approach will include looking at 'BACK the FOCK UP!':

Bones
Air (bowel gas patterns)/Aorta lining
Calcifications
Kidneys and bladder
the
Foreign bodies
Organs
Contrast
K(C)alculi
Ureters
Psoas shadow—obliteration may signify retroperitoneal pathology such as haematoma.

Bowel gas pattern

It is normal to see gas within bowel loops and you want to be able to see bowel gas down to the rectum. Small bowel is allowed to be dilated up to 3 cm, large bowel up to 6 cm, caecum up to 9 cm. Small bowel is generally central and contains *valvulae conniventes* which are thin circular folds that extend across the full width of the lumen. Large bowel contains *haustra* which are thickened folds that do not extend across the lumen. Large bowel also contains faeces. If bowel is dilated it is important to assess which parts are dilated as this will help suggest the level of possible obstruction (see Fig. 6.10–6.12)

When looking at the bowel it is also possible to assess for bowel wall thickening particularly within the colon. This may reflect colitis (infective, ischaemic, or inflammatory). In colonic wall thickening, you can get thumb printing and mucosal islands. Assess the bowel wall for evidence of intra-mural gas (*pneumatosis intestinalis*). This is concerning for ischaemic bowel (although it can be seen in benign conditions such as chronic obstructive pulmonary disease (COPD)). If there is pneumatosis intestinalis, the liver should be assessed for evidence of portal venous gas. While assessing the bowel also look for signs of perforation. The main sign in the abdomen is *Rigler's sign* which is when air is seen either side of the bowel wall. Free air can also be seen underneath the hemidiaphragm and along the falciform ligament. Remember, an erect CXR is far more sensitive for looking for bowel perforation (pneumoperitoneum).

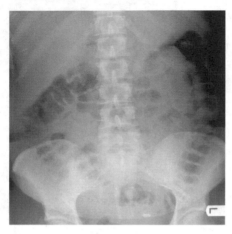

Fig. 6.10 Normal large bowel gas pattern. Reproduced from *Oxford Handbook of Clinical Medicine* 8th edition (2010), p741, courtesy of Norwich Radiology Department.

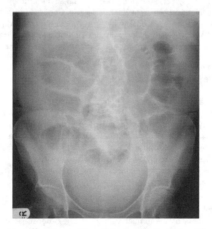

Fig. 6.11 The pattern seen in small bowel obstruction. Reproduced from *Oxford Handbook of Clinical Medicine* 8th edition (2010), p741, courtesy of Norwich Radiology Department.

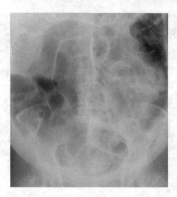

Fig. 6.12 Multiple dilated air filled loops of large and small bowel. This pattern is seen in ileus. Reproduced from *Oxford Handbook of Clinical Medicine* 8th edition (2010), p741, courtesy of Norwich Radiology Department.

Organs

Look at the outline of the upper abdominal organs, are they enlarged? While looking at the kidneys is there evidence of renal calculi (90% of renal calculi contain enough calcium to be seen on a plain film radiograph)? While looking at the liver, is there any evidence of gallstones (only 10–15% contain enough calcium to be seen on a radiograph, hence ultrasound (US) is the normal first-line investigation for gallstones)? Look for calcification within adrenal glands (past haemorrhage) and pancreas (chronic pancreatitis).

Review areas

These include bones, lung bases, hernial orifices, and abnormal areas of calcification:

- *Bones*: look at the spine, imaged pelvis, and thoracic rib cage. Look for destructive lesions and do not miss fractures (especially vertebral compression fractures and hips fractures if included).
- *Lung bases*: basal consolidation and effusions can often mimic abdominal pain and needs to be excluded.
- *Hernial orifices*: if there is bowel obstruction beware a hernia, ensure that there is no bowel gas seen below the hernial orifices.

Look for other areas of calcification—vascular calcification is common in the elderly, beware the calcified aortic aneurysm. If there is concern about ureteric calculi, trace the outline of the ureters which run parallel to the transverse process of the lumbar vertebra. They then take an arc as they descend into the pelvis where they enter the bladder. Do not forget to assess the pelvis for bladder calculi. Appendicoliths are calcifications seen in the right iliac fossa that lie within the appendix. If a patient presents with right iliac fossa pain and an appendicolith is visualized, there is a 90% certainty the patient has acute appendicitis.

Chapter 7

Anaesthetics

Anaesthetics: overview

Introduction

Anaesthesia stems from the Greek words 'an' and 'aesthesis' meaning without sensation.

General terms

- *General anaesthesia (GA)*: a complete loss of consciousness and loss of reflexes.
- *Regional anaesthesia*: analgesia, muscle relaxation, and loss of reflexes.
- *Labour analgesia*: local anaesthetic in the epidural space during labour providing sensory blockade but preserving motor function.
- *Day surgery*: a select group of patients who meet certain criteria are admitted and discharged after surgical procedures on the same day.
- *Patient-controlled analgesia (PCA)*: a drug (e.g. IV morphine or epidural) administered in a locked syringe driver with a set dose and a lock-out time, providing control to the patient and also preventing overdose.
- *Anaesthetic gases*: inhalation agents used for maintenance of GA (e.g. isoflurane, sevoflurane, desflurane).
- *IV anaesthetic agents*: IV drugs used for induction and or maintenance of anaesthesia (e.g. thiopentone, propofol, etomidate, ketamine).
- *Muscle relaxants*: drugs which cause muscle relaxation by blocking receptors at the neuromuscular junction (e.g. suxamethonium, atracurium).
- *Reversal agents*: drugs which reverse muscle relaxation (e.g. neostigmine/glycopyrrolate).

Day routine—on the seasoned anaesthetist's mind

Patient

- Preoperative assessment, examination, and type and side of surgery.
- Airway assessment and fasting history.
- Previous anaesthetic history, drug history, and allergies.
- Quantifying risk of anaesthesia and surgery.

Environment

- Familiarity with anaesthetic room and theatre.
- Anaesthetic machine check and emergency equipment.
- Drugs: pre-medication, induction/maintenance/emergence, analgesia and postoperative medications, and emergency drugs.

Team

- Surgeon, theatre team, and operating department practitioner/assistant.
- Team brief:
  - Acknowledge roles of each team member.
  - Discuss optimal running of theatre and list.
  - Any concerns regarding cases (allergies, anaesthetics).
  - Specific surgical and anaesthetic requirements.
  - WHO checklist for each case.
  - Debrief at the end.

Anaesthetics: assessments

Clinics

Usually nurse led with a named anaesthetist for advice or review.
- Checklist and proforma based.
- Assess patient suitability for the procedure and anaesthesia.
- Highlight any serious medical conditions.
- Optimize physiological variables (e.g. BP, blood glucose).
- Advice on medications (e.g. anticoagulants, antihypertensive).
- Request additional investigations.

On the day

- Corroborate the history and complete a thorough examination to elicit new changes.
- Review investigations.
- Anaesthetic plan and consent.[1]
- Emergency surgical patients require pre-optimization.

History taking and examination

A detailed history of the presenting condition and concurrent medical condition should be taken and a systematic physical examination conducted. Emphasis should be given to the cardiorespiratory system.

Drug history

- Allergies: latex, antibiotics, etc.
- Antihypertensive: risk of perioperative hypotension.
- Anticoagulants: risk of perioperative bleeding.
- Opioid analgesics: high pain scores.

Anaesthetic history

- Details of previous anaesthesia.
- Difficulties/emergencies.
- Postoperative nausea and vomiting (N&V).
- Review old anaesthetic chart for previous operations looking for issues and problems.

Things to do on your attachment

- Visit the preoperative clinic and discuss the assessment with the nurse.
- Accompany the anaesthetist on the preoperative visit round.
- Have a chat with the patients regarding any apprehensions, anxiety, and the consent process.

Airway assessment

- Mouth opening.
- Thyromental distance.
- Neck flexion/extension.
- Mallampati score.

Factors such as a class 3–4 Mallampati score (patient is asked to open the mouth with tongue protruded), thyromental distance <6 cm, restricted jaw and neck movements (e.g. arthritis), limited mouth opening, and syndromic facial presentation predict difficult intubation.

Mallampati score
See Fig 7.1.

Fasting
The Association of Anaesthetists of Great Britain and Ireland (AAGBI) recommends:
- *6 hours* for solid food, milk, and infant formula (children)
- *4 hours* for breast milk (children)
- *2 hours* for clear non-particulate and non-carbonated fluids.

Fluid balance should be assessed if the patients are elderly, have undergone bowel preparation, or have diarrhoea and vomiting (D&V). IV fluids should be prescribed.

At the end
Make sure that the following have been completed:
- Complete anaesthetic chart.
- Sign consent form.
- Mark site and side of surgery.
- Complete preoperative checklist.

Discussion with the boss
- Ask to demonstrate each airway assessment and discuss importance.
- Discuss importance of fasting and complications of full stomach.
- Read through the hospital's preoperative checklist and policies.

Scoring systems
See Tables 7.1–7.3 for different scoring systems.

POSSUM score

The POSSUM (Physiological and Operative Severity Score for the enUmeration of Mortality and morbidity) score is more commonly used for general surgical patients. The score is based on current physiological and operative parameters. It accurately predicts the 30-day mortality and morbidity scores.

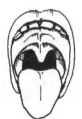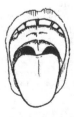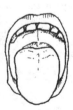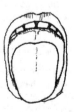

Fig. 7.1 The Mallampati score. Reproduced from Allman and Wilson, *Oxford Handbook of Anaesthesia* 4th edition, 2015 with permission from Oxford University Press.

Cardiac risk stratification based on surgical procedure

Table 7.1 Cardiac risk stratification based on surgical procedure

High risk >5%	Intermediate risk <5%	Low risk <1%
Emergency major operations	Carotid endarterectomy	Endoscopic procedures
Aortic and major vascular surgery	Head and neck surgery	Superficial procedures
Peripheral vascular surgery	Intraperitoneal and intrathoracic surgery	Cataract surgery
Surgical procedures associated with large fluid shifts and/or blood loss	Orthopaedic surgery	Breast surgery
	Prostate surgery	

Metabolic equivalents (METs)—functional levels of exercise

This score is helpful in determining the level of fitness and physiological reserve to determine the likely outcome from a general anaesthetic.

Table 7.2 MET score

METs >7	METs 5–7	METs 1–4
8. Rapidly climbing stairs, jogging slowly	5. Climbing 1 flight of stairs, dancing, cycling	1. Eating, working at computer, dressing
9. Jumping rope slowly, moderate cycling		2. Walking down stairs or at home, cooking
10. Swimming quickly, running/jogging briskly	6. Playing golf, carrying clubs	3. Walking 1–2 blocks
11. Skiing, cross country, basketball	7. Playing singles tennis	4. Raking leaves, gardening
12. Running rapidly for moderate-long distances		

1 MET = consumption of 3.5 mL O_2/min/kg of body weight. Patients with METs <4 and undergoing high-risk surgery are more likely to suffer from perioperative cardiac events.

American Society of Anaesthesiologists (ASA)

Table 7.3 ASA scoring system

ASA rating	Description	Mortality (%)
Class I	Healthy individual	0.1
Class II	Mild systemic disease	0.2
Class III	Severe systemic disease but not incapacitating	1.8
Class IV	Incapacitating systemic disease with constant threat to life	7.8
Class V	Moribund patient not expected to survive without surgery	9.4
Class VI	Brain dead patient	
Class E	Suffix added for emergency surgery	

Reference

1. Yentis SM, Hartle AJ, Barker IR, et al. AAGBI: Consent for anaesthesia 2017: Association of Anaesthetists of Great Britain and Ireland. *Anaesthesia* 72(1):93–105.

Anaesthetic equipment

Anaesthetic machine

Modern anaesthetics machines are very complex and digitalized, but the aims are the same:
1. Supply O_2 and anaesthetic gases to the patient.
2. Measure flow of gases.
3. Vaporize the anaesthetic agent.
4. Breathing system for delivering gases to the patients.
5. Provide mechanical ventilation.
6. Scavenge anaesthetic gases.
7. Monitor physiological parameters.

The anaesthetic machine is a circle system where the O_2 from the back wall is delivered into the machine. The pressure and flow of the gases are regulated by pressure regulators and flow restrictors. There is a pressure release valve, which release gases if pressure increases in the system. The patients can breathe spontaneously or can be mechanically ventilated by switching on the ventilator.

Oxygen

Facts on oxygen
- Atmospheric air consists of 21% O_2, 78% N_2, and 1% other gases.
- It is a major component of metabolism/aerobic respiration.
- Hyperbaric O_2 therapy saturates the circulatory system resulting in increased O_2 delivery to tissues.

Discussion with the boss
- Observe and perform an anaesthetic machine check.
- Learn about other methods of measuring O_2 concentrations in blood/gas mixtures.
- Ask your anaesthetist to show you the different Mapleson circuits available in your theatres and wards. Discuss the advantages and disadvantages of each.

O_2 is the most used gas in the hospital. It is supplied at the point of use by a cylinder or a piped O_2 supply. The O_2 cylinders are black with a white top (international standard for colour coding for medical gases). The piped O_2 in the hospital is either from a manifold or vacuum-insulated evaporator. The supply pressure is 4 bar. Most commonly oxygenation is measured by a pulse oximeter, which uses the principles of spectrophotometry, where the absorption of red and infrared waves is measured by application of Beer's and Lambert's laws. The ratio of absorption by oxy and de-oxy Hb is measured against a scale and O_2 saturations displayed. Breathing systems are classified into open (no rebreathing), semi-open (partial rebreathing), and closed systems (total rebreathing).

Capnography

The gases are measured by an in-stream or side-stream analyser and will give a breath-to-breath trace of CO_2 (see Fig. 7.2).

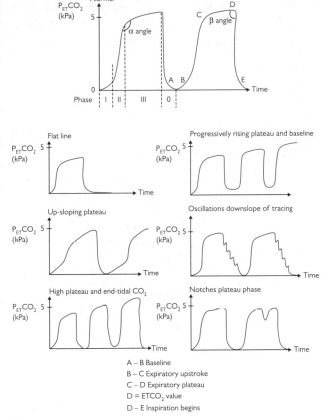

A – B Baseline
B – C Expiratory upstroke
C – D Expiratory plateau
D = ETCO$_2$ value
D – E Inspiration begins

Fig. 7.2 Capnography measurement. Reproduced from Catherine Spoors and Kevin Kiff, *Training in Anaesthesia*, 2010, Figure 4.15, Page 77, with permission from Oxford University Press.

Monitoring

The AAGBI has set minimum monitoring requirements for during and immediately after anaesthesia. This is the minimum and further monitoring such as invasive BP, urine output, arterial blood gases, cardiac output, neuromuscular blockade, temperature, and depth of anaesthesia should be considered according to the type and complexity of the surgery and anaesthesia.[1]

Discussion with the boss

Discuss monitoring options, values, ranges, parameters, and checks.

Induction and maintenance of anaesthesia

- Pulse oximeter
- Non-invasive BP monitor
- ECG
- Airway pressure
- Airway gases:
  - O_2 saturations
  - CO_2—capnography
  - Inhalation gases—infrared analyser.

Discussion with the boss

- Identify different vaporizers and their contents.
- Identify a capnography trace. Discuss different types of traces and the underlying pathology.
- Identify all the traces on your monitor and discuss the underlying physics of their measurement.
- Discuss the interference with these traces and how it is overcome in these monitors.

Reference

1. Checketts MR, Alladi R, Ferguson K, et al. (2016). Recommendations for standards of monitoring during anaesthesia and recovery 2015: Association of Anaesthetists of Great Britain and Ireland. *Anaesthesia* 71(1):85–93.

Types of anaesthesia

General anaesthesia

The principles of anaesthesia are based on a triad of hypnosis, analgesia, and muscle relaxation. The chronology of a general anaesthetic broadly involves a number of stages:

1. *Induction*: usually IV agent (e.g. propofol: white milky drug), but gaseous agent can also be used (e.g. sevoflurane—in young children or presumed difficult airway).
2. *Airway control*: starting with face mask (Hudson) and using simple adjuncts (nasopharyngeal airway, oropharyngeal airway) proceeding to laryngeal mask airway (LMA) or endotracheal tube (ETT) intubation.
3. *Intubation*: often requires a muscle relaxant. These can be divided into depolarizing agents (e.g. suxamethonium, used in rapid sequence induction) and non-depolarizing agents (e.g. atracurium, rocuronium).
4. *Maintenance* of anaesthesia with gaseous agents or propofol infusion and potent opiates (e.g. fentanyl, remifentanil).
5. *Emergence* from anaesthesia by discontinuing anaesthetic agents and leading to spontaneous ventilation and extubation.

Local anaesthesia

See Table 7.4.

- *Routes*: subcutaneous, topical cream, Instillagel® (e.g. for catheterization), IV (Bier's), intra-articular.
- *Complications*: CVS (also used as an antiarrhythmic drug) and CNS side effects avoided if not injected intravenously and if used within maximum safe dose.
- *Treatment of adverse reactions*: resuscitate, treat with Intralipid®, convulsions to be treated with IV benzodiazepine.

Regional anaesthesia

Can be provided by central neuraxial blockade (spinal/epidural anaesthesia) or by specific nerve blocks with local anaesthetic drugs (e.g. femoral nerve block for fractured hips, transversus abdominis plane block for lower abdominal surgery). IV regional anaesthesia is better known as Bier's block and uses tourniquets to exsanguinate limbs (below elbow and knee) to avoid systemic spread and toxicity. Tourniquet time should not exceed more than 2 hours. A Bier's block should not exceed more than an hour.

Table 7.4 Dosages (max.) recommended for a 70 kg adult

Anaesthetic	Dosages (max.)
Lidocaine	200 mg (3 mg/kg)
Lidocaine with adrenaline (epinephrine)	500 mg (7 mg/kg)
Prilocaine*	400 mg (6 mg/kg)
Prilocaine* with adrenaline (epinephrine)	600 mg (8 mg/kg)

* Prilocaine is not used for local infiltration but only for Bier's block.

Epidural and spinal anaesthesia

You will be asked the differences between epidurals vs spinal anaesthesia (see Fig. 7.3 and Table 7.5).

Pain management

A patient's impression of whether you are a good doctor may be based entirely on how promptly you relieve their pain. Ask the patient to score their pain intensity on a scale of 1–10. Pain is rated as:

- mild (score 1–3)
- moderate (4–6)
- severe (7–10).

Points to consider before prescribing

- Treat the cause of the pain (if possible).
- If the pain is continuous, give regular analgesia.
- Before switching analgesia, ensure a full therapeutic dose is used.
- Avoid effervescent preparations in those with hypertension (high salt content).
- Tolerance and dependence can occur with weak opioids and adverse effects are more common in the elderly, therefore start with lower doses and titrate slowly.

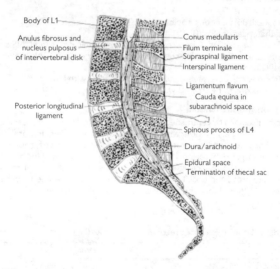

Body of L1

Anulus fibrosus and nucleus pulposus of intervertebral disk

Posterior longitudinal ligament

Conus medullaris
Filum terminale
Supraspinal ligament
Interspinal ligament

Ligamentum flavum
Cauda equina in subarachnoid space

Spinous process of L4

Dura/arachnoid

Epidural space
Termination of thecal sac

Fig. 7.3 Midsagittal section through the lumbar spinal column with spinal puncture needle in place between the spinous processes of lumbar vertebrae L3 and L4. Notice the slightly ascending direction of the needle. The needle has pierced three ligaments and the dura/arachnoid and is in the subarachnoid space. Reproduced with permission from David L. Seiden and Siobhan Corbett, *Lachman's Case Studies in Anatomy*, 2013, Oxford University Press.

Table 7.5 Epidural and spinal anaesthesia

	Epidural	Spinal
Onset	Slower: 25 min	Faster: 5 min
Site	Thoracic and lumbar spine	Below L2 to prevent spinal cord injury
Mode	Indwelling catheter	Single-shot injection, rarely indwelling catheter
Effect	Sensory loss with lower concentration and both motor and sensory with higher concentration	Sensory and motor blockade
Purpose	Postoperative pain relief, labour analgesia, and top-ups for caesarean section	Regional anaesthesia for procedures for pelvic and lower limb surgeries

WHO analgesic ladder

See Fig. 7.4.

Other treatments include neuropathic analgesia (e.g. gabapentin, amitriptyline, capsaicin) → alternative treatments (transcutaneous electrical nerve stimulation (TENS) machine, acupuncture, etc.).

Non-pharmacological

Splintage of injuries, elevation, and ice packs to reduce swelling, hot water bottle for muscle spasm pain, simple dressings for minor burns/wounds.

Psychological aspects

Fear and anxiety heighten the experience of pain. The reassurance of caring staff along with an explanation of what is happening can be very helpful, as well as the presence of family or friends.

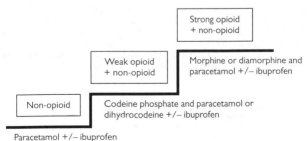

Strong opioid + non-opioid

Weak opioid + non-opioid

Non-opioid

Morphine or diamorphine and paracetamol +/− ibuprofen

Codeine phosphate and paracetamol or dihydrocodeine +/− ibuprofen

Paracetamol +/− ibuprofen

Fig. 7.4 Example of an analgesic ladder following WHO guidelines.

Critical incidents

'Can't ventilate, can't intubate'

This is an emergency scenario where the patient is asleep, not breathing, and the anaesthetist is neither able to ventilate the patient by bag mask nor intubate. The primary goal here is oxygenation. There is an algorithm produced by the Difficult Airway Society and by the end of it either the patient is woken up to breathe spontaneously or a needle cricothyroidotomy is performed. A difficult airways trolley will be around in these cases.[1]

Anaphylaxis

This is the most common critical incident during an anaesthetic, and antibiotics are the common culprits. Consider latex allergy if the presentation is slightly delayed into the surgery. The AAGBI has recommended a clear guideline and protocol to follow during an anaphylactic reaction. The main goal is initial resuscitation with oxygenation, fluids, and adrenaline (epinephrine), followed up with hydrocortisone and chlorpheniramine. Clearly document the sequence of events and take blood samples for mast cell tryptase levels at 0-, 1-, and 24-hour intervals. Follow-up and referral to the allergy clinic is very important to identify the agent causing anaphylaxis, with clear documentation in the notes and letters to the GP and patient.[2]

Local anaesthetic toxicity

This is a serious complication of using local anaesthetic agents. The risk is very high and toxicity occurs when an excess dose is administered, inadvertently administered intravascularly or the blood concentration increases when administered around highly vascular structures. The symptoms can vary from confusion, convulsions, and arrhythmias to cardiac arrest. The key to the management is early recognition, resuscitation, and administering a 20% lipid emulsion to scavenge the local anaesthetic. Adding adrenaline (epinephrine) also reduces absorption. Common ones include lidocaine (lignocaine) and bupivacaine (or Marcaine®).[3]

Malignant hyperthermia

This is a unique but very serious complication during an anaesthetic. Some patients have a genetic predisposition and are sensitive to inhalational agents and suxamethonium. When the patients are exposed to these agents there is excessive Ca^{2+} release from the sarcoplasmic reticulum due to defective receptors. The patients under anaesthetic become tachycardia, hypertensive, with raising temperature and end-tidal CO_2. The key in management is early recognition, disconnecting patients from the inhalation agent and circuit, resuscitation, temperature control, and dantrolene.[4]

References

1. Difficult Airway Society (2015). *Difficult Intubation Guidelines*. ℘ www.das.uk.com/guidelines/das_intubation_guidelines
2. Association of Anaesthetists of Great Britain and Ireland (2009). Suspected anaphylactic reactions associated with anaesthesia. *Anaesthesia* 64:199–211.
3. Association of Anaesthetists of Great Britain and Ireland (2010). *Guidelines for the Management of a Severe Local Anaesthetic Toxicity*. London: AAGBI.
4. Association of Anaesthetists of Great Britain and Ireland (2011). *Guidelines for the Management of a Malignant Hyperthermia Crisis*. London: AAGBI.

Cardiology

Cardiology: overview

Cardiology is a medical speciality dealing with disorders of the heart. It is primarily concerned with ischaemic heart disease (IHD), arrhythmias, and structural heart defects. Try to think of clinical presentations (e.g. chest pain) instead of disease processes (e.g. pericarditis). In a clinical examination, you should deploy a set approach to each possible presentation. Most patients will be actors or providing a retrospective history (see ➲ p. 875). Fortunately there are only five possible presentations: chest pain, palpitations, shortness of breath, dizziness, and incidental murmurs. Remember, as with all cardiac cases, a full cardiovascular history (see ➲ pp. 891–3) and examination (see ➲ pp. 900–4) are required.

Cases to see

Stable angina pectoris

Chest pain on activity relieved by rest. It is mostly managed in the community by GPs, although you may encounter patients with complex IHD in the clinic.

Acute coronary syndromes

An umbrella term to describe the spectrum from unstable angina, through non-ST elevation myocardial infarction (NSTEMI) to ST elevation myocardial infarction (STEMI). The former can be seen as referrals to cardiology from other inpatient teams or the ED. STEMIs are mainly seen in large teaching hospitals where the cardiac catheterization labs are situated. Only some institutions can perform percutaneous coronary intervention (PCI) which is part of the optimal early management strategy.

Aortic stenosis (AS)

These patients can be seen in the cardiology clinic referred with dyspnoea, angina, ± syncope. Those with critical AS may be referred to cardiothoracic surgeons for consideration of valve replacement.

Mitral regurgitation (MR)

This is commonly seen in the young (with mitral valve prolapse ± connective tissue disorder), and occasionally post MI (ischaemic necrosis of papillary muscle → prolapse of mitral valve leaflets). The former cohort is followed up with interval echocardiography.

Atrial fibrillation (AF)

This condition is almost ubiquitous among the geriatric population. You will see AF in all your clinical attachments but a cardiology placement is the right time to learn how it is managed. Cardiologists may also offer specialist interventions (e.g. chemical/electrical cardioversion and radiofrequency ablation).

Heart failure

Most patients with heart failure have a chronic degree of pump insufficiency. They may be followed up in the clinic for optimization of medication (e.g. diuretics). The cardiology ward will also have patients with acute heart failure and decompensated chronic heart failure.

Procedures to see

Echocardiography

This can be either transthoracic (TTE) or transoesophageal (TOE) at the ultrasound/echocardiography department. TOE is used if TTE is inconclusive and requires sedation.

Exercise stress test
Found at the cardiac investigations department.

Myocardial perfusion scan
Speak to the nuclear medicine department to find out when the next list is scheduled.

Coronary angiogram
Look for the dedicated angiography suite; if possible, look for diagnostic (angiogram) and interventional procedures (angioplasty, stent insertion).

Pacemaker insertion
This takes place in theatre or the radiology suite.

Things to do

Perform and interpret a 12-lead ECG (see ➜ p. 855). Ask a nurse to show you. You might find yourself with a sick patient without much assistance in which case you will need to know how to perform an ECG (see Fig. 8.1).

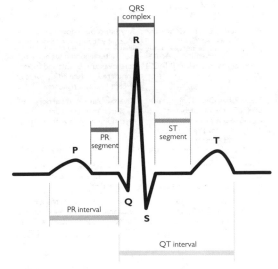

Fig. 8.1 ECG complex. Key:
- P wave—atrial depolarization.
- QRS complex—ventricular depolarization.
- Q wave—first downward wave of QRS complex (often absent).
- R wave—initial positive deflection.
- S wave—negative deflection after R wave.
- T wave—ventricular repolarization.

Reproduced from https://commons.wikimedia.org. Image in public domain.

Table 8.1 Popular recent studies

Year	Study title	Comment
2001	Randomized Evaluation of Mechanical Assistance for the Treatment of Congestive Heart Failure (REMATCH)	Left ventricular assist device reduces mortality compared to medical therapy
2001	Clopidogrel in Unstable Angina to Prevent Recurrent Events (CURE)	Clopidogrel/aspirin dual therapy reduced mortality and cardiovascular events at risk of ↑major bleeding
2003	EURopean trial On reduction of cardiac events with Perindopril in stable coronary Artery disease (EUROPA)	Perindopril reduced mortality and cardiovascular events compared to placebo in stable coronary arterial disease.
2006	Clopidogrel plus aspirin versus oral anticoagulation for atrial fibrillation in the Atrial fibrillation Clopidogrel Trial with Irbesartan for prevention of Vascular Events (ACTIVE W)	Aspirin/clopidogrel is inferior to warfarin for preventing cardiovascular events and death without improving bleeding risk
2008	Atrial Fibrillation and Congestive Heart Failure (AF-CHF)	Rhythm control does not reduce mortality (compared to rate control)
2009	Timing of Intervention in Acute Coronary Syndromes (TIMACS)	Early intervention does not ↓ risk of cardiovascular events and mortality compared to delayed intervention except high-risk patients
2011	Rivaroxaban Once Daily Oral Direct Factor Xa Inhibition Compared with Vitamin K Antagonism for Prevention of Stroke and Embolism Trial in Atrial Fibrillation (ROCKET AF)	Rivaroxaban is non-inferior to warfarin in preventing thromboembolic events in AF
2012	Early Surgery versus Conventional Treatment in Infective Endocarditis (EASE)	Surgery reduces mortality in left-sided native valve infective endocarditis
2015	Comparison of Fondaparinux and Enoxaparin in Acute Coronary Syndromes (OASIS-5)	Fondaparinux is non-inferior to enoxaparin in preventing death and cardiovascular events in NSTEMI

Cardiology: in clinic

Hypertension

Defined by BP >140/90 mmHg; optimal BP in diabetics <130/80 mmHg. 95% primary or 'essential', 5% secondary such as renal (e.g. renal artery stenosis), endocrine (e.g. Cushing's syndrome), and drugs (e.g. monoamine oxidase inhibitors). Malignant hypertension (e.g. hypertension plus end-organ damage) may necessitate acute treatment with IV antihypertensives. Treatment options consist of British Hypertensive Society guidelines (see Table 8.2).

Resistant hypertension is when a patient still has a poorly controlled BP while on three antihypertensives. Beta blockers are not first-line antihypertensives. B + D combination increases the complication of diabetes mellitus.

Stable angina pectoris

Chest discomfort due to myocardial ischaemia brought on by exertion and relieved by rest. Causes are coronary artery disease (majority) and coronary spasm (e.g. Prinzmetal's). It is distinct from unstable angina which is pain at rest. Standard cardiovascular risk factors apply. Treatment is conservative (lifestyle factors such as moderate exercise, stop smoking), medical (antiplatelet, statins, glyceryl trinitrate (GTN) spray), and revascularization (angioplasty ± stenting, coronary artery bypass graft (CABG)). Prinzmetal's coronary vasospasm is treated with calcium channel blockers.

Valvulopathy

All four valves can regurgitate or become stenosed; although one murmur may predominate, often there is mixed valvular disease on echocardiography. Some are encountered rarely (e.g. aortic regurgitation (AR), tricuspid stenosis). Murmurs can be benign (e.g. pregnancy, anaemia, hyperthyroidism) in which case they are typically soft, systolic, and positional. Focus on AS and MR.

AS is commonly due to senile calcification followed by congenital bicuspid and rheumatic heart disease. Classically, AS cardinal signs correlate with prognosis: angina → syncope → dyspnoea → worsening prognosis. If surgery is necessary, the valve is usually replaced.

Table 8.2 British Hypertensive Society guidelines for treatment

	Drug class	Examples	Combinations
A	ACEI or ARB	Ramipril or losartan	A + C in age >55 and Afro-Caribbean
B	Beta blocker	Bisoprolol	
C	Ca²⁺ channel blocker	Amlodipine	B + C in younger patients
D	Diuretics	Furosemide	

Data from *Advanced Paediatric Life Support*, 5th Edition, 2011, Wiley.

Common causes of MR are mitral valve prolapse (young females → myxomatous degeneration), left ventricular (LV) dilatation, connective tissue disorder, and acute MI (→ ischaemic papillary muscle rupture). Presentation ranges from incidental finding (medical student practising clinical examination) to infective endocarditis or acute heart failure.

Honours

Aortic sclerosis vs AS
Aortic sclerosis is a precursor state of AS. It is caused by senile calcification of the valve. Some consultants will distinguish between sclerosis and stenosis based on auscultation. Classically, AS causes an ejection systolic murmur but the murmur of aortic stenosis radiates to the carotids and is associated with a narrow pulse pressure. Pulse pressure = systolic − diastolic BP.

Atrial fibrillation

AF is an irregularly irregular atrial rhythm with intermittent atrioventricular (AV) node response and consequent irregular ventricular rhythm. The ECG appears irregularly irregular without p waves. You diagnose AF on an ECG. Slow AF must be distinguished from fast and often decompensating AF.
Causes of AF include **MITRALE**:
- **M**itral valvulopathy
- **I**nfection
- **T**hyrotoxicosis
- **R**aised BP
- **A**lcohol
- **L**one (primary)
- **E**mbolism (pulmonary embolism (PE)).

Classification

- *Recent onset/first diagnosed episode.*
- *Paroxysmal*: self-terminates, usually within 48 hours, recurrent.
- *Persistent*: lasts >7 days or cardioversion needed to restore sinus rhythm, recurrent.
- *Permanent*: rhythm control interventions abandoned.

Discussion points

Rate control versus rhythm control in AF
Management of AF can be aimed to restore sinus rhythm ('rhythm control') or permitting AF to continue but controlling the heart rate ('rate control'). Ask your consultant what factors would help determine whether to adopt a policy of rhythm or rate control for individual patients.

Management options

- *Rhythm control*: if AF present for <24 hours to restore normal sinus rhythm → cardioversion: (1) chemical: flecainide, amiodarone, vs (2) direct current (DC). If unable to cardiovert immediately, give unfractionated heparin IV and cardiovert on the next working day.
- *Rate control*: give beta blocker (atenolol, bisoprolol) and add digoxin if rate does not fall sufficiently. Factors considered when deciding between the two are age, comorbidities, structural heart disease, and prolonged AF (over 24 hours).
- *Refractory AF*: may be managed by radiofrequency ablation.
- *Thromboembolic risk reduction* since AF increases the risk of thromboembolic events (cerebrovascular accident (CVA), ischaemic bowel).

Honours

CHA_2DS_2-VASc risk scoring

Patients with AF are at ↑risk of stroke and may be treated prophylactically with anticoagulant (e.g. warfarin) or antiplatelet (e.g. aspirin) agents. This decision is informed by the CHA_2DS_2-VASc score developed from the Euro Heart Survey[1] of 5000+ patients in 35 countries. Scores of 0–9 equate to 0–15% risk respectively. Adults with non-valvular AF and a CHA_2DS_2-VASc stroke risk score of ≥2 are offered anticoagulation (warfarin, target international normalized ratio (INR) 2–3). Consider if score = 1. The factors are listed in Table 8.3.

Table 8.3 CHA_2DS_2-VASc risk factors

Risk factor	Points
Congestive heart failure	1
Hypertension	1
Age >75 years	2
Diabetes mellitus	1
Stroke/TIA/VTE	2
Vascular disease	1
Age: 65–74 years	1
Sex category	1 if female
Total	9

TIA, transient ischaemic attack; VTE, venous thromboembolism.

Lip GY et al. (2010). Refining clinical risk stratification for predicting stroke and thromboembolism in atrial fibrillation using a novel risk factor-based approach: the euro heart survey on atrial fibrillation. *Chest* 137:263–72.

Heart block

Heart block describes a failure of electrical conduction in the heart. Atrioventricular nodal block can be divided into first degree, second degree (two types: Mobitz I/Wenckebach and Mobitz II), and third degree. Mobitz II and third-degree heart blocks are associated with sudden cardiac death and may require a pacemaker. See Fig. 8.2.

First-degree AV block

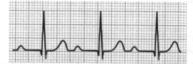

Second-degree AV block (Mobitz I or Wenckebach)

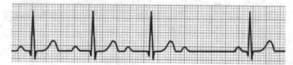

Second-degree AV block (Mobitz II)

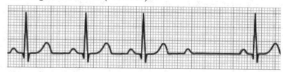

Second-degree AV block (2:1 block)

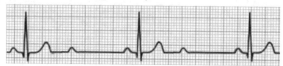

Third-degree AV block with junctional escape

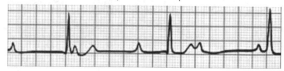

Fig. 8.2 ECG basics—heart blocks. Reproduced from https://commons.wikimedia.org/wiki/File:Heart_block.png under the Creative Commons Attribution-Share Alike 4.0 International.

Trifascicular block

A potentially fatal disease characterized by (1) prolonged PR interval (first-degree AV block), (2) right bundle branch block, and (3) left anterior or posterior fascicular block. May need pacemaker.

Chronic heart failure

Chronic heart failure is a clinical syndrome characterized by inadequate cardiac output to meet the body's metabolic needs. Essentially this means pump failure. In left heart failure, there is back pressure to the pulmonary circulation (→ haemoptysis, orthopnoea, and paroxysmal nocturnal dyspnoea), while right heart failure causes back pressure to venous return (→ peripheral oedema, ascites, and raised jugular venous pressure (JVP)). Congestive cardiac failure refers to coexisting left- and right-sided heart failure. Chronic heart failure is gradual (e.g. cardiomyopathy vs acute heart failure develops suddenly post MI). Management aims to treat the cause (e.g. valvulopathy) and optimize cardiac function (beta blocker, digoxin, diuretics, GTN), where failure → cardiothoracic intervention.

Honours

Medical treatment of heart failure

Heart failure patients often find themselves taking a concoction of different medications, some of which are at first glance surprising:

- Diuretics (e.g. furosemide) remove excess fluid through urination.
- ACE inhibitors control blood pressure and are thought to aid myocardial 'remodeling'. A number of RCTs showed that they reduce mortality in heart failure patients.
- Beta-blockers protect the heart from damaging effects of catecholamines. Some beta-blockers have been found to increase ejection fraction and reduce both hospitalisations and mortality.
- Aldosterone antagonists (e.g. spironolactone) work in a similar way to diuretics (as well as potassium-sparing) but also reduce heart failure mortality.
- Other drugs include hydralazine, nitrates and digoxin

Cardiomyopathies

These are a class of diseases of the heart muscle itself. Key types are hypertrophic (AD inheritance or sporadic) → angina, sudden death in athletes, dilated (alcohol, peripartum, congenital), and restrictive (due to infiltration (e.g. amyloidosis, haemochromatosis). Presentations vary but may show signs of heart failure.

Investigations

Troponin

Regulatory protein involved in myocyte contraction but released in infarction. Differential diagnoses for raised troponin are PE, critical illness (e.g. sepsis), heart failure, pericarditis, trauma, and renal impairment. Serial measurements are required since it can take 12 hours to peak. Troponin has replaced creatine kinase (CK) measurements.

B-type natriuretic peptide (BNP

Released upon ventricular stretch and seen in heart failure. Higher normal intervals correlate with increasing age and false positives are common.

ECG

You should be able to perform an ECG (see ➲ p. 855). Have your own method of analysing and presenting your ECG. Dedicate specific days to finding and reading ECGs on the cardiology ward, in the ED, and coronary care unit. Go with a colleague and read each ECG systematically. Present a number of interesting ECGs to a senior doctor if possible. When presenting an ECG, please adopt a system. The most common system is name, age, time, indication, rate, rhythm, axis, PR interval, QRS complexes, ST/T wave segments, QT intervals, and summary (see Fig. 8.4). For the purposes of working as a doctor, you must recognize AF and ischaemic changes (T-wave inversion, ST elevation/depression, new left bundle branch block (LBBB)). Find patients in hospital with acute coronary syndrome (ACS) and examine the ECGs that led to their diagnosis.

24-hour Holter monitor and events recorder

Intended to 'capture' arrhythmias over a longer period than a snapshot given by an ECG. One problem is that arrhythmias may not occur during the 24-hour monitored period—alternatives include a 48-hour monitor or an implantable recorder.

Echocardiography

Ultrasound of the heart to discern structure and function, performed either as TTE or TOE. A normal range of LV ejection fraction is 55–70%. Attend a clinic to understand the principles of imaging.

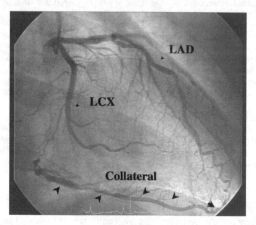

Fig. 8.3 Left coronary angiogram. LAD, left anterior descending coronary artery; LCX, left circumflex coronary artery. Reproduced with permission from Matsunaga *et al*. Angiostatin is negatively associated with coronary collateral growth in patients with coronary artery disease. *Am J Physiol Heart Circ Physiol*. 2005 May;288(5):H2042–6.

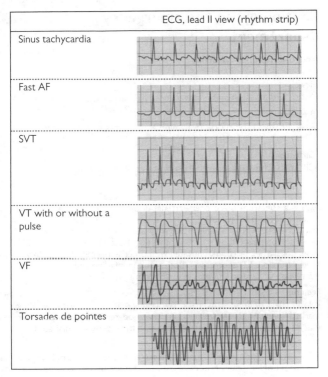

Fig. 8.4 Basic ECG rhythms. AF, atrial fibrillation; SVT, supraventricular tachycardia; VF, ventricular fibrillation; VT, ventricular tachycardia. Reproduced with permission from Tim Raine et al, *Oxford Handbook for the Foundation Programme* 4e, 2014, Oxford University Press.

Exercise ECG testing

ECG and BP assessment using a treadmill ('Bruce protocol') or by chemical stress (e.g. dobutamine) used to confirm and quantify IHD. The test might be stopped if symptomatic (e.g. chest pain) or significant ECG changes (e.g. ST elevation).

Myocardial perfusion scan

Non-invasive technetium-99 scan to assess myocardial blood flow often following exercise or chemical stress test (as previously mentioned) to determine hypoperfusion.

Cardiology: in the emergency department

Acute coronary syndrome

Airway
Assess and manage airway using manoeuvres/adjuncts.

Breathing
Assess respiratory effort, 15 L/min O_2, if no respiratory effort → call arrest team.

Circulation
CRT, pulse, heart sounds, BP, if no pulse → call arrest team.

Definition
ACS is a spectrum of coronary arterial disease from unstable angina (ischaemic chest pain at rest) to myocardial infarction (chest pain and cardiac ischaemia with elevated cardiac enzymes). MI is often classified by ST elevation (or new LBBB, STEMI, or those without ST elevation (NSTEMI, subendocardial infarction), but often with other ischaemic changes (e.g. T-wave inversion, ST depression). Both result in infarction of myocytes and the release of cardiac enzymes (e.g. troponin).

Features
Pain in chest and/or arms, back, jaw lasting >15 min, nausea, vomiting, marked sweating, breathlessness, and haemodynamic instability. Beware that MI can be 'silent' (painless), especially in the elderly and diabetics.

Risk factors
Male sex, increasing age, hypercholesterolaemia, hypertension, diabetes mellitus, smoking, family history of coronary artery disease, obesity.

STEMI
History of typical cardiac pain and:
- ≥1 mm ST elevation in at least two adjacent limb leads *or*
- ≥2 mm ST elevation in at least two contiguous precordial leads *or*
- new LBBB.

You must be able to recognize a STEMI on an ECG for your exams—this is a very common question (see ✇ http://lifeinthefastlane.com/).

NSTEMI
Raised troponin ± ischaemic ECG changes, but do not fulfil STEMI criteria.

Unstable angina
Worsening angina or a single episode of 'crescendo angina', with a high risk of impending MI. Features include angina at rest, ↑frequency, duration, and severity of pain (including ↓response to GTN).

Investigations

- ECG (within 5 min of arrival). It is helpful to review previous ECGs to look for new changes, e.g. LBBB. Repeat the ECG every 15 min to look for dynamic changes, especially if further pain.
- Full blood count (FBC), urea and electrolytes (U&E), glucose, INR, activated partial thromboplastin time (APTT), troponin T or I on arrival and at 12 hours after symptom onset (or presentation if unknown). Note, high-sensitivity troponins are being used to rule out ACS earlier.
- CXR—only if there are clinical features of LV failure and if it will not delay PCI/thrombolysis.
- The Global Registry of Acute Coronary Events (GRACE) score is used to risk stratify patients with diagnosed ACS.

Treatment

- Sit the patient up, give O_2 if hypoxic, attach cardiac monitor.
- Aspirin 300 mg PO stat (get senior advice if patient on warfarin).
- GTN spray sublingually: try one or two puffs (400 mcg per puff).
- Diamorphine or morphine IV (± metoclopramide) as required.
- Clopidogrel 300 mg PO stat if ischaemic ECG or raised troponin (600 mg or prasugrel 60 mg if going for PCI).
- IV infusion GTN if pain continues and systolic BP >90 mmHg (start at 0.6 mg/hour and ↑ as necessary).
- Atenolol IV or PO unless contraindicated.
- Glycaemic control: patients with clinical MI and diabetes mellitus or marked hyperglycaemia (>11.0 mmol/L) should have immediate blood glucose control, continued for at least 24 hours.

STEMI treatment

- Management of STEMI can be according to **MONACLES**:
  - Morphine
  - Oxygen
  - Nitrates
  - Aspirin
  - Clopidogrel
  - Low-molecular-weight heparin (LMWH), e.g. Enoxaparin
  - Stenting.
- Refer for immediate primary PCI (pPCI), ideally to be performed within 90 min of first medical contact. This is superior to thrombolysis.
- Glycoprotein IIb/IIIa inhibitor (e.g. IV abciximab) if undergoing pPCI.
- When pPCI cannot be provided within 120 min, administer immediate thrombolysis (e.g. reteplase), unless contraindicated.
- If not having pPCI, give fondaparinux 2.5 mg IV initially, then subcutaneously (SC) daily.

NSTEMI treatment

- LMWH, e.g. enoxaparin 1 mg/kg SC every 12 hours or fondaparinux 2.5 mg SC daily.
- If medium or high risk of early recurrent cardiovascular events, organize early PCI.
- Consider a glycoprotein IIb/IIIa inhibitor e.g. eptifibatide (IV) for high-risk patients, particularly if they are undergoing PCI—seek expert advice.

Unstable angina is managed according to degree of risk: antiplatelets, nitrates, beta blockers, ± angiography.

Pre-discharge
Assess LV function in all MI patients (e.g. echocardiography).
  If acute MI is confirmed, offer:
• aspirin plus a second antiplatelet agent, e.g. clopidogrel
• beta blocker, e.g. bisoprolol once stable, titrate up
• ACEI, e.g. ramipril
• statin, e.g. atorvastatin
• consider stress testing in low-risk patients with ACS.

Complications

Complication of MI are **INFARCT**:
• Inflamed pericardium (pericarditis, Dressler's syndrome weeks later).
• New murmur (e.g. papillary muscle rupture → MR, septal rupture → ventricular septal defect (VSD)).
• Failure (cardiogenic shock).
• Arrhythmia/aneurysm (LV).
• Rupture of LV → pericardial effusion/tamponade.
• Complete heart block.
• Thromboembolism (mural thrombi → systemic emboli, e.g. gut ischaemia).

Acute heart failure

This is acute onset of pump failure due to intercurrent illness (e.g. sepsis), post MI, arrhythmias, or decompensation of chronic heart failure. Patient presents with breathlessness and fatigue associated with cardiac disease. It is often accompanied by fluid retention, as indicated by an elevated JVP and oedema. Acute heart failure develops quickly, while chronic failure develops over a longer period. Causes: systolic LV dysfunction (i.e. pump failure), diastolic LV dysfunction, congenital heart disease, pericardial or endocardial disease, valvular problems, rhythm/conduction disturbance, and hypertension.

Investigations
• ECG: not often normal and may give clues to the cause (e.g. Q waves and poor R-wave progression in previous MI, LVH in hypertension/AS, low-voltage QRS in pericardial disease. Also LBBB, AF, AV block, bradyarrhythmia).
• CXR: cardiomegaly, pulmonary oedema, pleural effusion, upper lobe diversion, 'bat's wing' hilar shadows, Kerley B lines, pleural effusions, fluid in interlobar fissure (a popular exam question).
• Arterial blood gases (ABGs): if hypoxic.
• FBC, U&E, consider liver function tests (LFTs) and thyroid function tests (TFTs).
• BNP: rules out if <100 ng/L.
• Echocardiography: within 48 hours of admission for those with a new diagnosis of heart failure (raised BNP).

Treatment

Acute treatment is **LMNOP**:

- Lasix (furosemide)
- Morphine
- Nitrates
- Oxygen
- Position upright.

Treatment of the underlying cause and other steps include the following:

- Sit patient up, give O_2, and attach cardiac monitor.
- Furosemide IV 20–40 mg (more if renal impairment or already on diuretics).
- Monitor U&E, weight, and urine output while on diuretics.
- The National Institute for Health and Care Excellence (NICE) do not recommend routinely using nitrates, but consider GTN IV infusion if there is concomitant myocardial ischaemia, severe hypertension, or regurgitant aortic or mitral valve disease. Monitor BP closely (keep systolic BP >90 mmHg). New guidelines are cautious about the use of morphine but this is dependent on judicious use for the patient.
- Non-invasive ventilation (NIV) (continuous positive airway pressure (CPAP)): for cardiogenic pulmonary oedema with severe dyspnoea and acidaemia.
- Invasive ventilation indications: respiratory failure, reduced consciousness, or exhaustion despite treatment.
- Beta blocker: start when stable (i.e. not requiring diuretics) if there is LV systolic dysfunction unless HR <50, second- or third-degree heart block, or shock.
- ACEI and an aldosterone antagonist (e.g. spironolactone) if reduced LV ejection fraction.

Longer term

- Limit fluid intake to 2 L/day.
- Reduce salt intake.
- Moderate regular exercise and weight loss if overweight.
- Stop smoking and avoid alcohol.

Infective endocarditis

Infection of heart valves characterized by a new murmur and evidence of infection. Organisms include Streptococcus viridans (commonest), Staphylococcus aureus (e.g. IV drug user (IVDU), early prosthetic valve infection), and Staphylococcus epidermidis (late prosthetic valve infection). Risk factors include valvulopathy, prosthetic valve, and recurrent bacteraemia (IVDU, poor dentition). Treatment is with broad-spectrum IV antibiotics (e.g. benzylpenicillin, flucloxacillin, and gentamicin). It is possible to get through a whole cardiology attachment without seeing a patient with confirmed infective endocarditis.

Honours

Modified Duke's criteria for infective endocarditis

A confident clinical diagnosis of infective endocarditis requires two major criteria, one major and three minor criteria, or five minor criteria.

- Major criteria:
  - Two separate blood cultures growing microorganisms typical for infective endocarditis.
  - Echocardiographic evidence of endocardial infection.
  - New valvular regurgitation.
- Minor criteria:
  - Predisposing condition (e.g. valvular disease).
  - Temperature >38°C.
  - Embolic phenomenon (e.g. Janeway lesions).
  - Immunological phenomenon (e.g. Osler's nodes).
  - Microbiological evidence (e.g. single positive blood culture).

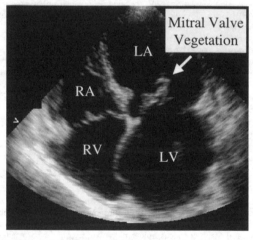

Fig. 8.5 Echocardiogram confirming infective endocarditis. LA, left atrium; LV, left ventricle; RA, right atrium; RV, right ventricle. Reproduced with permission from Cabell CH et al. Bacterial endocarditis: the disease, treatment, and prevention. *Circulation*. 2003 May 27;107(20):e185-7. http://circ.ahajournals.org/content/107/20/e185

Tachyarrhythmias

Sinus tachycardia—usually rate is <150 bpm. Can be due to fever, pain, anxiety, hypovolaemia, anaemia, heart failure, or thyrotoxicosis. The treatment approach for unstable patients is similar regardless of the specific tachyarrhythmia. Unstable patients (e.g. with shock, syncope, MI, heart failure), require DC cardioversion. Otherwise, distinguish between broad and narrow complex tachyarrhythmias. *Narrow complex* (QRS <120 ms): supraventricular tachycardia (SVT) and atrial flutter (regular), AF (irregularly irregular). *Broad complex* (QRS >120 ms): ventricular tachycardia (VT), torsades de pointes (regular), and ventricular fibrillation (VF) (irregular). Interventions vagal manoeuvers (carotid massage, Valsalva) and IV adenosine (SVT (usually >150 bpm)) and IV amiodarone (VT). With adenosine, warn the patient they will briefly feel *terrible*. You may need to spend some time in the resuscitation area, intensive therapy unit (ITU), or coronary care unit to see these unstable patients.

Bradyarrhythmias

Causes of sinus bradycardia include inferior MI, drugs (e.g. digoxin), and hypothyroidism. Unstable bradyarrhythmia (hypotension, syncope, heart failure) requires urgent pharmacological treatment (e.g. atropine 500 mcg IV) and/or transcutaneous pacing.

Pericarditis

Inflammation of the pericardium which may be idiopathic or caused by infection or post MI. It is characterized by pleuritic chest pain relieved by sitting forward and ECG might show saddle-shaped (concave-ST segment) elevation. It is typically treated with NSAIDs and these patients are not regularly admitted or followed up in clinic so the ED is your best chance of finding this condition.

Chest pain

Characterize pain, e.g. using SOCRATES: site, onset, character, radiation, associations, time course, exacerbating/relieving factors, severity. Determine whether chest pain is ischaemic. Pleurisy (sharp pain on inspiration, relieved by sitting forward) is caused by the four Ps: pericarditis, PE, pneumothorax, and pneumonia.

Features of ischaemic pain
- Central (± radiating to left arm, neck, jaw).
- Sudden onset, crushing, 'elephant sitting on chest', or heavy.
- Associated with heartburn/nausea/sweating.
- Precipitated by exercise/cold/stress.
- Relieved by rest (± GTN).

When taking a history, consider *cardiac* (ACS, pericarditis, AS, aortic dissection), *respiratory* (PE, pneumothorax, pneumonia), *GI* (GORD, oesophageal spasm, oesophagitis, cholecystitis, peptic ulcer), and *MSk* (fracture, costochondritis) causes. Ask about key features (worse on breathing/eating/moving) to satisfy examiners that you are thinking more broadly than cardiac causes alone. Stable angina is the most likely encounter in clinical examinations (see ➔ p. 181).

Honours

Brugada syndrome

A genetic cardiac disease also known as 'sudden death syndrome' due to sodium channelopathy leading to fatal VF. *ECG* shows right bundle branch block, prolonged PR and ST elevation mainly anteriorly (in V_1–V_3).

Shortness of breath

Most patients with shortness of breath have a respiratory cause. Acute heart failure is very unlikely in an examination setting, but consider chronic heart failure in any patient with a cardiovascular history (e.g. MI) or coronary risk factors. Classification for difficulty in breathing (dyspnoea) is by New York Heart Association (NYHA) classes or Medical Research Council (MRC) grades (see Table 8.4).

Table 8.4 NYHA vs modified MRC classification grades

Class	NYHA	Grade	MRC
I	Presence of cardiac disease *without* limitation to physical activity	0	No dyspnoea except with strenuous exercise
II	Presence of cardiac disease with *slight* limitation to physical activity	1	Dyspnoea when hurrying on level or walking uphill
III	Presence of cardiac disease with *marked* limitation to physical activity	2	Walks slower than contemporaries or has to stop on level ground due to dyspnoea
		3	Stops for breath after walking 100 m or after a few minutes on level ground
IV	Presence of cardiac disease resulting in the *inability* to carry on with physical activity without discomfort	4	Too breathless to leave the house or to dress/undress oneself

Palpitations

Patients experience an abnormal awareness of the heart beating. The patient will complain of 'missing a beat' or 'heart fluttering'. Adapt your standard history of presenting complaint and ask them to tap out the rhythm. Your aim is to establish whether the beat is regular or accelerated during episodes. Tachyarrhythmias cause palpitations but bradyarrhythmias do not. There are three broad causes and a good history will distinguish between these.

Causes of palpitations
- Hyperdynamic circulation: thyrotoxicosis, pyrexia, anaemia, pregnancy.
- Sympathetic overdrive: anxiety, phaeochromocytoma.
- Dysrhythmias: AF, atrial flutter, SVT, VT, VF, heart block.

It is important to ask about associated symptoms (shortness of breath, chest pain, blackouts, and feeling unwell) and family history (close relative with history of sudden cardiac death at a young age). Again, these are necessary to be considered 'safe'. Examiners' favourites include AF. Other dysrhythmias (SVT, VT, VF) are potentially unstable and unlikely to appear in clinical examinations.

Dizziness/blackouts

This is caused by cerebral hypoperfusion (e.g. hypoxia, hypotension). It is a complicated presentation, so learn the important causes. When taking a syncope history, organize your questions in terms of what was happening before, during, and after the attack.

An emotionally charged situation points to vasovagal syncope; standing up quickly or for a long time suggests orthostatic/postural hypotension. Syncope on exercise is sinister and indicates cardiac outflow obstruction (e.g. AS). Associated symptoms during (or immediately before) the attack include aura (i.e. warning of impending syncope), nausea, sweating, visual disturbance, fingertip/lip tingling, palpitations, and chest pain.

Management
Drugs commonly causing syncope include antihypertensives (e.g. diuretics, nitrates, beta blockers) and tricyclic antidepressants (e.g. amitriptyline).

Causes of dizziness/blackouts

Vasovagal
- Often during times of stress (e.g. fasting, coughing, exercise).

Cardiac
- Dysrhythmias (e.g. heart blocks, Wolff–Parkinson–White syndrome, VT).
- Obstructive lesions (e.g. AS, septal hypertrophy).
- Bradycardia (e.g. sick sinus syndrome, Stokes–Adams attacks).

Orthostatic/postural
- Standing up too quickly or for too long.
- Primary autonomic failure (e.g. Parkinson's disease).
- Secondary autonomic failure (e.g. autonomic neuropathy in diabetes).

Situational
- Cough, micturition, or hypoglycaemia.

Cardiology: in examinations

Examination

Cardiology is all about clinical signs; you are very unlikely to see a number of these throughout your entire career but that should not stop you from looking!

You need to be able to recognize important clinical signs which may be presented in photograph form or in actual patients. You may not see these in the outpatient department so visit other resources such as books and online references.

Infective endocarditis

Albeit rare signs, look for splinter haemorrhages (dark 'pen marks' under nailbed), clubbing, Janeway lesions (painless haemorrhagic macules on palms/soles, septic embolic microhaemorrhages), Osler's nodes (tender papules on pulps from immunological complex deposits), Roth spots (seen on fundoscopy), and new murmur (acutely regurgitation followed by stenosis from chronic inflammation). Other signs include splenomegaly as well as microscopic haematuria and strokes from septic emboli.

Cardiovascular risk

Obesity, tar staining, high BP, and signs of hypercholesterolaemia: corneal arcus (grey ring around iris), tendon xanthomata (small yellow papules, usually knuckles), and xanthelasma (small yellow papules on eyelids). Bear in mind that corneal arcus is pathological below the age of 50 years but geriatric patients have physiological corneal senilis.

Murmurs

Do not fear murmurs—they commonly appear in finals and are only difficult when unnecessarily complicated. It is rarely necessary to correctly diagnosis the valve lesion from auscultation alone—recognizing the existence of a murmur may be sufficient to pass. Suspect a murmur in all cardiac patients. Use the history to predict what murmur to expect. Commonly encountered cases are MR (young, endocarditis, connective tissue disorder, or post MI) and mechanical aortic valves. Diastolic murmurs (e.g. tricuspid stenosis, pulmonary regurgitation) are rarer, quieter, and less likely to appear in examinations. If you hear a murmur, state whether it is systolic or diastolic. Feel the carotid pulse while auscultating the chest. If the murmur and pulse are synchronous, it is systolic. If they are asynchronous, the murmur is diastolic. You must distinguish between these in real patients before finals—listening to recorded heart sounds is not sufficient. Do not obsess between a pansystolic (MR) vs mid-systolic ejection (AS) murmur. You can mention the difference characteristics between both murmurs but it is never that clear cut in practice.

Honours

The aortic valve replacement patient

Patients with prosthetic aortic valves (tissue or metal) often appear in examinations because they are stable, well known to the hospital, and have more obvious clinical signs. On inspecting the chest, you will see a large scar in the chest midline (median sternotomy). At this point you could divert your routine (briefly) to examine the legs for evidence of great saphenous vein harvesting. A leg scar suggests previous CABG but no scar indicates another cardiac procedure (e.g. valve replacement). Aortic valves are routinely replaced and mitral valves are usually repaired first. If there is no evidence of great saphenous vein harvesting, listen carefully and you may be rewarded by the soft 'click' of a metallic aortic valve. Report this constellation of findings out loud to the examiner—diagnosing a metallic aortic valve replacement without laying a hand (or stethoscope) on the patient has to be worth bonus points!

You are unlikely to commit the signs of each valve lesion to your long-term memory by rote learning alone. Try to think mechanically about why each sign exists. AS means blood (at high pressure being ejected from the heart) squeezing through a tight hole. The result is a loud noise on ejection (the ejection systolic murmur best heard in the aortic area at the right second intercostal space or parasternal edge) which radiates to the carotids, a slow-rising 'anacrotic' pulse (as the column of blood squeezes through the narrowed hole), and a narrow pulse pressure (systolic and diastolic pressures close together). By contrast, in AR, blood pumped from the heart falls backwards through the incompetent aortic valve leading to a 'collapsing' or 'waterhammer' pulse, wide pulse pressure, and an early diastolic murmur in the aortic area. Consider reading up on the eponymous signs associated with AR. The key feature of MR is a pansystolic murmur that radiates to the axilla. You should learn signs of other murmurs (e.g. MS, but the signs of AS, AR, and MR are particularly high yield). (See Table 8.5 for Levine's grading).

Table 8.5 Levine's grading of heart murmurs

Grade	Examination finding
I	Barely audible on auscultation
II	Faint but audible on auscultation
III	Easily heard without a thrill
IV	Loud murmur with a palpable thrill
V	Louder murmur heard over a wide area with a thrill
VI	Murmur heard without stethoscope (e.g. metallic valve)

Investigations

Almost regardless of presentation, the investigation of cardiac complaints is universal. Send routine bloods (e.g. FBC, U&E) and consider thyroid function tests (hyperthyroidism worsens angina and is a cause of AF). Most patients should have a CXR, ECG, and echocardiogram. Cardiac ischaemia may require an exercise tolerance test, and intermittent dysrhythmias should be investigated with a 24-hour Holter monitor.

Management

Depends largely on the underlying pathology but may include monitoring, medication, antibiotics for infective endocarditis, and surgery (replacement with xenograft or metal).

Honours

Eponymous signs of AR

There are many eponymous signs of AR which are unlikely to appear in formal exams but are beloved by consultants and senior trainees alike. You are unlikely to ever see them (hence their disappearance from exams) and it has been said that the last person to have seen De Musset's sign was De Musset himself! They nevertheless remain part of the rich historical tapestry of medical education:

- *Corrigan's sign*: abrupt distension and collapse of carotid arteries.
- *De Musset's sign*: rhythmic nodding of the head in synchrony with the heart beating.
- *Müller's sign*: pulsation of the uvula.
- *Quincke's sign*: capillary pulsation in the nailbeds visible on applying gentle pressure.
- *Traube's sign*: 'pistol shot' sound on auscultating femoral pulse.

Heart failure

Although it is a simple concept, heart failure is often misunderstood by students and poorly explained by their teachers. It essentially means the pump is not working effectively enough to propel blood around the body. One major consequence is that the column of blood backs up and fluid is squeezed out of the arterial circulation into inappropriate spaces. Signs of heart failure are often described as being caused by 'left-' or 'right-sided' heart failure, although these rarely present as isolated entities. Most patients will have mixed 'congestive cardiac failure'. In right ventricular failure, blood backs up along the inferior and superior vena cavae which leads to raised JVP, hepatomegaly, ascites, and peripheral oedema. In LV failure, blood backs up along the pulmonary veins. The signs (and symptoms) are therefore primarily respiratory, such as dyspnoea, respiratory distress, bibasal crepitations, pleural effusion, pleural oedema, and hypoxia.

Chapter 9

Critical care

Critical care: overview

Critical care is concerned with the diagnosis and management of serious acute conditions requiring organ support and/or invasive monitoring. The specialty consists of ITUs and high dependency units (HDUs) for both adults and children. There are also specialist ITU centres, e.g. cardiac, neurological, and liver centres. The intensive care team uses a MDT approach involving doctors, nurses, physiotherapists, dieticians, microbiologists, radiologists, and pharmacists, to name a few. There is much overlap with the specialty of anaesthesia, where intubation, ventilation, invasive monitoring, and anaesthetic, inotropic, and vasopressor drugs are commonly used. ITU doctors can be from anaesthetic, medical, surgical, or emergency medicine backgrounds. Main indications for admission are patients who have single or multiorgan failure, who require intubation and ventilation, inotropic support, and haemofiltration. The critical care team's management focuses on supporting failing organ systems, while diagnosing pathology and implementing therapy.

Cases to see
- Severe sepsis and septic shock.
- Organ dysfunction.
- Complex surgical patients.
- Pneumonia.
- Exacerbation of COPD/asthma.
- Life-threatening asthma.
- Diabetic ketoacidosis.
- Pancreatitis.
- Head injury/low Glasgow coma scale (GCS) score.
- Intracranial haemorrhage.
- Cardiac arrest.

Investigations/procedures to see
- Airway management: oro/nasopharyngeal airway devices, endotracheal intubation, tracheostomy.
- Anaesthetic and sedation techniques.
- Lines: arterial, central venous catheters (e.g. internal jugular, femoral, subclavian) using ultrasound guidance.
- ABG interpretation.
- Inotropic/vasopressor drug infusions with cardiac output monitoring.
- Haemofiltration and/or haemodialysis.
- Naso/orogastric tube.

Things to do
Attend the morning and evening ward rounds with the ITU team. This is essential to observe the systematic assessment of critically ill patients and decision-making processes. This is also a good opportunity to elicit classical signs on patient examination and hone your presentation skills. Closely shadow whoever takes ITU referrals as they will be asked to review the sickest patients in the hospital (on wards and in ED) for admission and escalation of support. Find out who carries the cardiac arrest bleep and attend arrests with them.

See Table 9.1 for common ITU drugs.

Table 9.1 Common ITU drugs

Drug examples	Class	Action	Comments
Adrenaline (predominantly β1 & β2 agonist)	Positive inotropic and chronotropic drugs	Alters the force and rate of cardiac muscle contraction, typically heart	Proarrhythmic side effects
Dobutamine (3:1 β1 to β2 agonist)			Commonly used in primary cardiac pump failure
Dopexamine (D1 and β2 agonist)			
Dopamine (D1 and D2 agonist)			
Noradrenaline (norepinephrine) (predominantly α1 agonist)	Vasopressors	Mediate systemic vasoconstriction and are often used to ↑ BP in conditions of systemic vasodilatation (distributive shock) such as sepsis	Side effects include reduced renal and splanchnic perfusion, digital ischaemia
Metaraminol (predominantly α1 agonist)			↑ SVR increases the afterload which the heart has to contract against
Vasopressin (V1 and V2 agonist)			
Suxamethonium (depolarizing)	Neuromuscular blockade	Muscle relaxation required to facilitate passage of ETT through vocal cords	Suxamethonium and rocuronium used as part of a rapid sequence induction of anaesthesia for emergency/high-risk intubations
Rocuronium (non-depolarizing)		Paralysis to improve ventilation in difficult cases	Prolonged muscle-relaxant use has been associated with intensive care unit (ICU)-acquired weakness
Atracurium (non-depolarizing)			
Propofol	Hypnotic agent	Agents can be used to induce anaesthesia and provide sedation	Can compound hypotension
Midazolam	Benzodiazepine	Hypnotic agent	Causes cardiovascular and respiratory depression
Ketamine	NMDA receptor antagonist	Hypnotic and analgesic agent	Can cause tachycardia, ↑ BP
Remifentanil	Opioid receptor agonists	Used to provide analgesia and supplement sedation. Facilitate tolerance of ETT	Bradycardia
Alfentanil			Cardiovascular and respiratory depression
Fentanyl			
Morphine			

Critical care: on the unit

Intensivists are responsible for the critical care area, supporting other teams and reviewing other critically ill patients on the wards and ED. Some patients who have return of spontaneous circulation post cardiorespiratory arrest will be admitted to the unit if they have continued severe organ dysfunction requiring support. As intensivists' interests are not confined to a specific system or set of diseases, they see a wide range of medical and surgical cases. As well as seeing a range of different diseases, your time with the intensivists can help you understand how to best to manage acutely unwell patients. This will be the part of your job as a junior doctor that most find daunting and difficult to deal with. However, with practice and more experience, you will find yourself feeling more comfortable with critically ill patients and be able to assess and initiate appropriate management faster as your insight develops.

An *Airway, Breathing, Circulation, Disability,* and *Exposure* approach represents a systematic focused assessment, where the most urgent life-threatening problems are identified and addressed first.

Organ support

Cardiovascular support: can include IV fluids (± central venous monitoring), inotropes or vasopressors (± arterial monitoring), and cardiac output monitoring. Some ITUs utilize aortic balloon pumps to improve coronary perfusion in patients with cardiogenic shock.

Respiratory support: oxygen therapy and mechanical ventilation (invasive or non-invasive). Non-invasive ventilation (NIV) may include CPAP or bilevel positive airway pressure via a tight-fitting facemask, and invasive may include intubation or tracheostomy and mechanical ventilation to provide adequate oxygenation and carbon dioxide elimination.

Renal support: involves haemofiltration and haemodialysis (see ➲ p. 211 for different renal replacement therapies). Haemofiltration is usually better tolerated in hypotensive patients (e.g. septic shock + acute kidney injury (AKI)).

GI support: patients in ITU have higher metabolic requirements and may be unable to feed themselves adequately. They may have true or pseudo-ileus as a result of surgery or systemic illness respectively. NG tubes are commonly used in ITU. This is certainly a good opportunity to learn how to insert them (under appropriate supervision). Other means of support include prokinetics (erythromycin, metoclopramide), enteral feeding (via NG, nasojejunal, or longer-term percutaneous endoscopic gastrostomy, or percutaneous endoscopic jejunostomy), and total parenteral nutrition. The ITU dietician is a valuable source of information regarding nutritional requirements of critically ill patients.

Sepsis

Overwhelming infection can have substantial systemic effects (e.g. vasodilatation → severe refractory hypotension) and → avoidable mortality, mainly due to delayed recognition and treatment. Know the difference between *SIRS, sepsis, severe sepsis,* and *septic shock.* Sepsis is managed in a similar manner almost regardless of the aetiology (e.g. UTI and LRTI): 'Sepsis Six' bundle; remember this as giving three things and taking three things ideally within 1 hour of presentation:

- *Give*:
  - High-flow oxygen.
  - IV fluids.
  - Antibiotics (after blood cultures) and source control (e.g. laparotomy for abdominal sepsis).
- *Take*:
  - Blood cultures.
  - Lactate.
  - Urine output measurement.

NB: it is worth familiarizing yourself with the Surviving Sepsis Campaign (℘ www.survivingsepsis.org/bundles/Pages/default.aspx).

Acute severe asthma or status asthmaticus

ITU may be involved in very severe or life-threatening asthma (peak expiratory flow rate (PEFR) <33%) for intubation and ventilatory support. Use this opportunity to hear widespread wheeze on auscultation.

Features

Features of life-threatening asthma include silent chest, inability to speak full sentences, reduced consciousness, exhaustion, desaturation, and rising pCO$_2$. Please read The British Thoracic Society/Scottish Intercollegiate Guidelines Network[1] guidelines on management of acute severe asthma (℘ www.brit-thoracic.org.uk/document library/clinical-information/asthma/btssign-asthma-guideline-2016/).

Management

This involves oxygen therapy, salbutamol and ipratropium bromide nebulizers, CXR, steroids, MgSO$_4$ infusion, aminophylline/salbutamol infusion, and endotracheal intubation with ventilator strategies.

Head injury

Severe head injuries are most likely to be encountered at your local MTC where neurosurgical services may be available; ask a senior doctor to point out any features visible on CT scan (e.g. concave bleed in a subdural and convex in an extradural). Try to participate in the neurological examination; familiarize yourself with the GCS (see ➜ 'Glasgow coma scale', p. 707); the most interesting signs are in the pupils (e.g. fixed unilateral/bilateral pupils indicative of coning), abnormal flexion and extension responses, and abnormal plantar responses. The primary head injury has already taken place and the focus is on preventing secondary brain injury. Management interventions are aimed at optimizing cerebral perfusion pressure and reducing intracranial pressure. Some of these interventions include:

- Surgical intervention to decompress the brain, e.g. blood clot evacuation, burr hole, or craniotomy.
- Sedate, intubate, ventilate.
- Head-up position.
- PaO$_2$ >13 kPa.

- $PaCO_2$ 4.5–5.0 kPa.
- Mean arterial pressure 80–90 mmHg.
- Avoid hypoglycaemia and hyperglycaemia.
- Avoid hyperthermia.
- Control seizure activity.

Severe intracranial haemorrhage

This may be traumatic (as previously described) or spontaneous (e.g. sub-arachnoid haemorrhage (SAH) from ruptured Berry aneurysm, or haemorrhagic stroke). Similar measures to maintain cerebral perfusion pressure are used as listed earlier.

Complex surgical patients

In complex procedures (elective or emergency) and/or in those patients with severe comorbidities, patients may be transferred pre-optimized to ITU/HDU before their surgery and returned to the unit for close monitoring, fluid and electrolyte replacement, ± vasopressors or inotropes and analgesia for a few days postoperatively.

Cardiac arrest

All calls are attended by an ITU/anaesthetist, who may decide to admit the patient in the event of successful return of spontaneous circulation (ROSC). Use this opportunity to ensure you are fully competent with basic life support (see ➲ pp. 263–265). These events can occur anywhere in the hospital, from the ward to the main entrance. You can help by carrying the transfer bag and portable suction. As a doctor you will be expected to administer advanced life support (ALS) according to the Resuscitation Council (UK) guidelines. If you can learn this algorithm (always remember *ABCDE*), it will make managing these cases easier later on. Remember to bear in mind the reversible causes: *4 Hs and 4Ts*.

Honours

Define SIRS, sepsis, severe sepsis, and septic shock (Table 9.2).

Clerking

As the patients are generally critically ill, their daily reviews are crucial in judging their progress. You will tend to find detailed proformas that need to be filled out each day for every patient. Every patient also has a parent team that reviews them daily and will determine which ward the patient is stepped down to after remaining stable. Typical contents from A to L include those in Table 9.3

Investigations/procedures to see

Airway management

A range of adjunct devices can be used in the inadequately self-ventilating patient to open their airway in the event of airway obstruction.

Manoeuvres

Simple measures of head tilt (not in cervical spine injury), chin lift, jaw thrust, and suctioning the oropharynx should be used.

Table 9.2 Definitions of SIRS, sepsis, severe sepsis, and septic shock

Definition	Explanation
SIRS (at least two criteria)	36 > Temperature (°C) <36 or >38 HR (beats/min) >90 Respiratory rate (breaths/min) >20 White cell count (WCC) ($\times 10^9$) <4 or >12
Sepsis	SIRS + infection
Severe sepsis	Sepsis + organ dysfunction/organ hypoperfusion/hypotension
Septic shock	Sepsis + intractable hypotension despite fluid resuscitation
Bacteraemia	Positive blood cultures (i.e. presence of infection in blood)

Table 9.3 Clerking

Definition	Comments
Airway	Alert, spontaneously ventilating, intubated, tracheostomy
Breathing	Chest expansion, percussion, auscultation, coughing, sputum, respiratory rate, saturation levels, ABG results, ventilation settings, CXR
Circulation	Capillary refill time, warm vs cool, JVP position, heart sounds, murmurs, HR, BP, mean arterial pressure, pitting oedema, ECG
Disability	GCS, pupil size and reflexes, blood sugar, independently moving all limbs
Electrolytes	U&E, magnesium, phosphate, calcium
Fluid balance	Total input (IV fluids, feeds, IV drugs, blood products) versus output (urine, faeces, insensible losses, NG aspirate, vomiting)
Gastrointestinal	Peripheral GI stigmata, abdomen size, palpation, percussion and auscultation
Haematology	Hb, WCC, platelets, mean cell volume
Infection	Temperature spikes, culture (blood, urine, faecal, sputum) results, duration of antibiotics
Joints	Physiotherapy, mobility, independence of feeding, washing, etc.
Kilocalories	Nutritional input: enteral vs parenteral feeding including rates of infusion
Lines	Location and type of lines (IV, per rectal, urinary catheter, drains, NG tube) and their duration

Airway adjuncts

If this has been unsuccessful, an airway adjunct such as the oropharyngeal airway (Guedel airway) and nasopharyngeal airways should be considered. Nasopharyngeal airways are often used in fitting patients with a clenched jaw and those with an active gag reflex (avoid in base of skull fracture). Learn how to size them. The correct sizing of an oropharyngeal airway is from the incisors to the angle of the jaw. Nasopharyngeal airways usually come in size 6 mm and 7 mm diameter and should fit comfortably inside the patient's nostril.

Bag valve mask

(Trade name Ambu® bag.) Bag valve mask ventilation should be used in the apnoeic patient with high-flow oxygen attached using a two-man technique. There may be an opportunity to learn this technique in simulation or in a controlled supervised environment such as theatres.

Laryngeal mask airway (LMA)

This is a supraglottic airway device which sits above the opening to the trachea and has an inflatable mask which pushes it forward to seal around the glottis. Ventilation with high-flow oxygen is achieved by attaching an Ambu® bag. This is not a secured definitive airway, but does provide some protection from aspiration. Sufficient ventilation can be achieved with a LMA so that chest compressions do not have to be stopped to deliver breaths in cardiopulmonary resuscitation.

Endotracheal tube

Intubation provides a secured definitive airway, this is achieved by:
• passing the ETT through the vocal cords into the trachea using a laryngoscope
• the cuff being inflated to seal around the trachea
• secured with a tie outside the mouth
• confirmation of ETT placement with end-tidal CO_2 monitoring
• attaches to a source of oxygen for ventilatory support.

Endotracheal intubation is the most effective at preventing aspiration and providing ventilation, even at higher inflation pressures.

Indications

• Cardiac arrest.
• Imminent respiratory failure.
• Reduced GCS.
• Unable to keep airway patent.
• High risk of gastric content aspiration.
• Transferring uncooperative patients to scans with life-threatening injuries.

Rapid sequence induction

A rapid sequence induction is used to intubate patients at high risk of aspiration of gastric contents. The patient is pre-oxygenated with high-flow oxygen. Fast-onset drugs such as thiopental and suxamethonium are used to achieve rapid intubating conditions to minimize the time between the patient being awake and being anaesthetized with an ETT *in situ*. Cricoid pressure (Sellick manoeuvre) is applied over the cricoid ring at induction of anaesthesia to prevent aspiration by temporarily compressing the oesophagus underneath.

Placement

You should know how to confirm ETT placement:
- The gold standard—capnography (for end-tidal CO_2).
- Seeing the ETT pass through the vocal cords.
- Looking for equal chest expansion.
- Auscultating both lung fields and for gastric bubbles.

Complications

Things that can go wrong include:
- intubating the oesophagus
- aspiration
- placing into a right main bronchus (unilateral chest expansion and inadequate ventilation).

If in doubt that the ETT is in the trachea – remove it and resume bag valve mask ventilation. So, 'if in doubt, take it out'.

Weaning

You may be asked when it is safe to extubate a patient in the ITU. Reasons include:
- awake, cooperative patient (off sedation)
- FiO_2 <40%
- good cough—ability to clear secretions (which should be clear, minimal, and less viscous)
- CVS stability
- near-normal physiological ABG readings
- resolution of reversible cause (e.g. pneumonia).

Tracheostomies

These are placed in patients who are slow to wean from the ventilator (e.g. COPD, ARDS, prolonged ventilation).
Advantages include:
- patient comfort
- no sedation requirements
- improved oral hygiene
- easier ongoing suctioning of secretions (toileting).

Percutaneous tracheostomies can be done on the ITU, negating transfer risks. It is associated with fewer complications than a traditional surgical tracheostomy and does not require a surgeon or theatre team.

Vascular access

Peripheral venous cannulas

These are self-explanatory and you should aim to site all of your placements confidently but firstly under supervision using aseptic technique.

Central venous catheters

These are placed in central veins including:
- internal jugular vein (risk of carotid artery puncture inferomedially)
- femoral vein (may have ↑ risk of line infection due to proximity of urethra and rectum)
- subclavian vein (risk of pneumothorax).

Central venous catheters are inserted using an aseptic technique under ultrasound guidance. This reduces the risk of complications. A vascath is a specialized central line with two lumens, for withdrawal and replacement of blood for haemofiltration/dialysis.

Indications
- Fluid administration
- Inotropic/vasopressor drug infusions
- Central venous pressure (CVP) monitoring
- Haemofiltration
- Cardiac pacing
- Parenteral administration of certain medications (e.g. amiodarone, chemotherapy, total parenteral nutrition).

Complications
- Incorrect siting
- Arrhythmias
- Infection
- Bleeding
- Thrombosis
- Pneumothorax
- Air embolus.

Other specialist lines include Hickman, peripherally inserted central catheter (PICC), Tesio®, and portacath which are used for long-term venous access.

Arterial lines
These are used as an invasive, real-time measure of BP and mean arterial pressure guiding the use of vasopressor and inotropic support. Arterial lines can be connected to cardiac output monitoring devices. Arterial lines allow for multiple ABG sampling to monitor ventilation adequacy and acid–base balance.

Ventilation
Invasive support can be given in different modes:

Intermittent positive pressure ventilation (IPPV)
This is a form of controlled ventilation, where a set volume or pressure and a set ventilation rate are given regardless of the patient's respiratory efforts (see Table 9.4).

Volume- vs pressure-controlled ventilation
Modes which give ventilator support when a patient takes a spontaneous breath can be triggered by changes in flow or negative pressure.

Synchronized intermittent mandatory ventilation (SIMV)
SIMV mode-controlled ventilations are given, but if the patient takes a spontaneous breath they can be supported with that breath. This is done using pressure support. When a spontaneous breath is detected a set '*pressure support*' is given during that spontaneous breath to give a greater tidal volume and reduce the work of spontaneous breathing for the patient. This is useful when a patient is weaning from a ventilator. The mandatory ventilation can be slowly reduced as the number of spontaneous breaths

Table 9.4 Volume- vs pressure-controlled ventilation

Volume controlled	Pressure controlled
Gives a set volume of gas (calculated by average tidal volume of 7–10 mL/kg) and a set ventilator rate	When a ventilator mode gives a controlled set inspiratory pressure (minimum required to generate an adequate tidal volume) and a set ventilator rate
Used effectively in patients with poor compliance, e.g. asthmatic patient, where a volume can be administered despite the airway pressures, hence compensating for poor respiratory compliance. However, high airway pressures cause lung trauma	Superior to volume-controlled ventilation as it reduces the risks of volutrauma, barotrauma, and biotrauma to the alveolar sacs. Generally lower peak pressures are generated in this mode

increases. As the tidal volume of the patient's breaths improves, pressure support is also reduced until the patient is breathing spontaneously without support. A disadvantage of SIMV mode is at certain points during the controlled ventilation cycle the patient's spontaneous breath is not fully supported. There is still an ↑ work of breathing as the patient's breathing may not be synchronized with the controlled ventilation cycle.

Top tip

For those who are interested, ➲ www.ccmtutorials.com/index.htm provides some interesting reading material on critical care topics.

Bilevel

This is a form of ventilator support which allows the patient to spontaneously breathe at any point during controlled pressure ventilation. The controlled breaths are achieved by cycling between two different pressures. The difference between the two pressure settings determines the tidal volume. The patient can breathe at any point during the controlled ventilation cycle and receive a set pressure support for that spontaneous breath. Each spontaneous breath is supported and controlled pressure ventilation can be reduced, as can pressure support until the patient breathes unsupported.

Non-invasive ventilation

This is the administration of positive pressure ventilatory support to a patient without an ETT or tracheostomy. This is usually achieved via a tight-fitting nasal mask, face mask, or hood. This is a short-term strategy in the acutely unwell patient and is not a substitute for endotracheal intubation if required.

Continuous positive airway pressure (CPAP)

This is the application of continuous positive airway pressure throughout the respiratory cycle in a spontaneously breathing patient. It is used in managing obstructive sleep apnoea, atelectasis and pulmonary oedema due to cardiac failure.

Positive end-expiratory pressure (PEEP)

This is the application of positive airway pressure at the end of expiration only. It is used to prevent alveolar collapse and increase respiratory compliance.

BiPAP®

This is a trade name for a portable ventilator. BiPAP® is bilevel positive pressure ventilation. This can be applied with a tight-fitting facemask. As for invasive ventilation, this mode can be used in the spontaneous breathing patient to provide pressure support, by alternating between two different positive pressures, inspiratory positive airway pressure (IPAP) and expiratory positive airway pressure (EPAP). The IPAP and EPAP are adjusted depending on the level of respiratory support required. Bilevel positive airway pressure is frequently used in patients with severe COPD and patients in type 2 respiratory failure.

Acute respiratory distress syndrome (ARDS)

ARDS is one extreme of the acute lung injury spectrum → diffuse alveolar injury. It is characterized as the following:
- Acute condition (within 1 week of insult) and potentially reversible.
- Radiographic evidence (CXR/CT) of bilateral pulmonary infiltrates (pulmonary oedema not due to cardiac failure or fluid overload).
- Respiratory failure from intrapulmonary shunting → severe hypoxaemia (measured by ratio of partial pressure of oxygen in arterial blood [(PaO_2) to fraction of oxygen in inspired air)FiO_2)). Severity of hypoxaemia correlates to mortality risk according to the Berlin criteria (see Table 9.5).
- Associated with pulmonary hypertension.
- Acute phase tends to resolve completely but residual pulmonary fibrosis occurs less commonly.

Risk factors

Pulmonary (direct) vs extrapulmonary (indirect):
- Sepsis/pneumonia
- Trauma and fractures
- Disseminated intravascular coagulation (DIC)
- Burns
- Transfusion
- Drug overdose
- Near drowning
- 20% idiopathic
- Pancreatitis
- Post-perfusion injury post CABG
- Fat embolism.

Table 9.5 Acute respiratory distress syndrome (ARDS)

ARDS severity	PaO_2/FiO_2	Mortality (%)
Mild	200–300	27
Moderate	100–200	32
Severe	100	45

Management
- 5 Ps: perfusion, positioning, protective ventilation, protocol weaning, and preventing complications.
- pH >7.2, PaO_2 >8 kPa, PaO_2:FiO_2 ≥20, PEEP ≤10 cmH_2O, FiO_2 ≤0.6.
- Recruitment manoeuvres.
- Inverse I:E ratio.
- Avoid volu-/baro-trauma.
- Prone position.
- High-frequency ventilation.
- Inhaled nitric oxide.
- Steroids.
- Surfactant replacement.
- Extracorporeal membrane oxygenation.

Renal replacement therapy
Haemofiltration and haemodialysis is used in ITU to manage:
- refractory life-threatening hyperkalaemia
- persisting fluid overload despite medical management
- resistant metabolic acidosis pH <7.1
- drug toxicity, e.g. aspirin and lithium.

ITU uses continuous haemofiltration/haemodialysis. This is a slow process, which is better tolerated in cardiovascular unstable patients.

Intermittent haemodialysis
This is used in outpatient departments where the patients are cardiovascularly stable and can tolerate large fluid shifts.
- *Principle*: haemodialysis works on the principle of diffusion of solutes and fluid across a semipermeable membrane (the haemofilter) from an area of high concentration to an area of low concentration. The rate of diffusion is dependent on the concentration gradient.

Haemofiltration
This works on the principle of convection (also known as solute drag), where a moving stream of fluid produces a positive pressure and effectively pushes solutes across the haemofilter. The rate of haemofiltration is dependent on the pressure gradient generated.
- *Anticoagulants (heparin, citrate)*: used in the haemofiltration/dialysis circuit to prolong the life of the haemofilter.
- *Complications*: associated with renal replacement therapy are those related to large-bore insertion of central venous catheters and the haemofiltration process itself (e.g. cardiovascular instability, haemorrhage, electrolyte disturbances, metabolic disturbances, and air embolism).

Dermatology

Dermatology: overview

Dermatology is a medical speciality concerned with diseases affecting skin and associated structures such as hair, nails, and oral and genital mucous membranes. There is often very little exposure to dermatology within your undergraduate medical curriculum. It is wise to plan your time carefully during your placement to ensure that you gain exposure to the common conditions that you are likely to face in your exams. If you are based in a peripheral hospital, you will spend most of your time in general clinics but larger tertiary centres will also have specialist clinics and some may even have a dermatology inpatient ward for acute cases. The significance of dermatology is that an internal disease process can initially or solely manifest as dermatological signs (e.g. autoimmune disorders). Stigma and psychological stress are also important issues to consider.

Describing lesions using dermatological terminology

- *Abscess*: localized accumulation of pus in a cavity >1 cm.
- *Atrophy*: thinning of the epidermis and/or dermis.
- *Bulla*: raised, clear fluid-filled lesion >0.5 cm in diameter.
- *Crust*: dried exudate containing sebum, blood, bacteria, and debris.
- *Erosion*: partial epidermal loss, heals without scarring.
- *Erythema*: blanching reddening of the skin due to local vasodilatation.
- *Excoriation*: scratch mark.
- *Fissure*: a linear crack in the epidermis.
- *Lichenification*: thickening of the epidermis with exaggerated skin markings due to repeated scratching or rubbing.
- *Macule*: a flat area of altered skin colour.
- *Nodule*: solid, raised lesion >0.5 cm in diameter.
- *Papule*: solid, raised lesion <0.5 cm in diameter.
- *Patch*: larger flat area of altered colour.
- *Petechiae*: pinhead-sized areas of purpura.
- *Plaque*: palpable, raised lesion >0.5cm in diameter.
- *Purpura*: (non-blanching) due to extravasation of blood into skin, ~2 mm in diameter.
- *Pustule*: raised lesion containing pus <0.5 cm in diameter.
- *Scales*: superficial flakes (stratum corneum).
- *Telangiectasia*: easily visible, blanching superficial blood vessels.
- *Ulcer*: break in the skin due to loss of the dermis and epidermis, heals with scarring.
- *Vesicle*: raised, clear fluid-filled lesion <0.5 cm in diameter.

Top tips on useful dermatology image banks

To practice your diagnostic skills in dermatology look at the following resources:
- *DermNet Nz* (⌘ www.dermnetnz.org)
- *Dermatology Image Bank* (⌘ www.library.med.utah.edu/kw/derm)
- *DermWeb Photo Atlases* (⌘ www.dermweb.com/photo_atlas).

Cases to see

The following dermatological conditions are easily seen in any general dermatology clinic.

- Eczema
- Psoriasis
- Acne vulgaris
- Solar (actinic) keratoses
- Bullous pemphigoid.

Pyoderma gangrenosum

Rare but you should be aware of this as it often comes up in written exams where you may be given a photo and a brief clinical history.

Skin cancers

There are also usually dedicated clinics for patients referred by their GP for suspected skin cancers under the 2-week referral pathway. These clinics are an excellent opportunity for you to see skin lesions at differing stages of progression.

Procedures to see

- *Ankle–brachial pressure index* (ABPI): e.g. for leg ulcers.
- *Minor procedures*: punch biopsies, excisions, curette and cauterization, cryotherapy.

Things you should practise beforehand

- *Taking a skin swab*: from lesions such as vesicles, pustules, ulcers, and mucus membranes for microbial culture/viral PCR detection.
- *Taking a skin scraping*: using a scalpel/glass slide from scaly lesions in suspected fungal infection and scabies.
- *Suturing*: practise in the clinical skills lab; there are also useful videos online demonstrating this skill.

Lesion	Definition	Morphology	Examples
Primary skin lesions			
Macule	A flat impalpable area of altered skin pigmentation		Ephelides (freckle) Lentigo ('liver spot') Café au lait macule
Papule	A palpable (raised) area under 0.5cm in diameter		Acrochordon (skin tag), viral wart, lesion of widespread eruption
Nodule	A large papule 0.5–1cm in diameter		Basal cell carcinoma
Plaque	Raised area of over 1cm diameter		Plaque of psoriasis
Vesicle	A small blister (fluid-filled lesion) >0.5cm in diameter		Herpes simplex
Bulla	A blister >0.5cm in diameter		Oedema blister, blister of bullous pemphigoid
Pustule	Pus filled papule		Acne, impetigo, folliculitis, pustular psoriasis
Secondary skin lesion			
Crust	Collection of cellular debris, dried serum and blood—a scab. Usually follows a vesicle, bulla or pustule		
Erosion	Partial focal loss of epidermis. May heal without scarring. A linear erosion produced by scratching is an excoriation.		
Ulcer	Loss of epidermis and dermis 'full-thickness' heals with scarring		Pyoderma gangrenosum
Fissure/crack	Vertical loss of epidermis +/– dermis with sharply defined walls		Complicates palmo-plantar pustulosis or hand and foot eczema
Cyst	Fluid filled nodule		Acne, epidermal cyst
Scar	A collection of new connective tissue; may be raised (hypertrophic) or indented (atrophic). Proceeded by epidermal/dermal damage		
Scale	Thick stratum corneum that results from hyperproliferation or increased cohesion of keratinocytes		Psoriasis, chronic cutaneous lupus erythematosus

Fig. 10.1 Dermatological descriptors. Reproduced with permission from Richard A. Watts et al, *Oxford Textbook of Rheumatology* 4e, 2013, Oxford University Press.

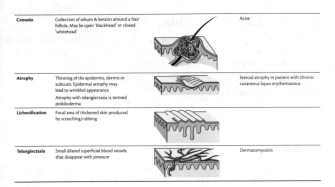

Comedo	Collection of sebum & keratin around a hair follicle. May be open 'blackhead' or closed 'whitehead'		Acne
Atrophy	Thinning of the epidermis, dermis or subcutis. Epidermal atrophy may lead to wrinkled appearance Atrophy with telangiectasia is termed poikiloderma		Steroid atrophy in patient with chronic cutaneous lupus erythematosus
Lichenification	Focal area of thickened skin produced by scratching/rubbing		
Telangiectasia	Small dilated superficial blood vessels that disappear with pressure		Dermatomyositis

Fig. 10.1 (*Contd.*)

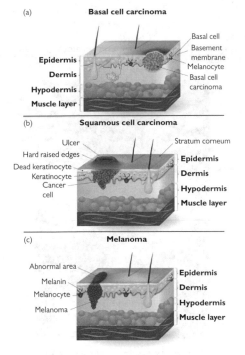

Fig. 10.2 Skin cancers. Reproduced from the U.S. National Library of Medicine (NLM). Images are in the public domain.

Dermatology: in clinic

Look out for unique features in the history and descriptions of the lesion which will allow you to diagnose the condition. Treatment often involves variations on a stepwise escalation, beginning with topical steroids eventually → systemic immunosuppression.

Eczema (dermatitis)

This is a chronic inflammatory skin condition following a relapsing and remitting course. See Fig. 10.3.

Aetiology

The commonest form is the atopic type, which predisposes individuals to other atopic conditions such as asthma, hay fever, and rhinitis and an inherited genetic defect in skin barrier function (loss-of-function variants of the protein filaggrin). Although atopic eczema can affect people of all ages, it primarily affects children and usually resolves during teenage years.

Exacerbating factors

Include infections, allergens (e.g. chemicals, food, dust, and pet fur), sweating, heat, and stress.

Presentation

Eczema commonly presents as itchy, erythematous dry scaly patches affecting the face and extensor aspects of limbs in infants, and the flexor

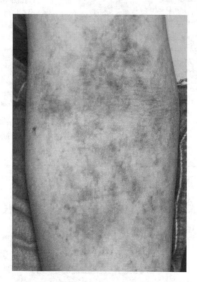

Fig. 10.3 Eczema. Reproduced with permission from Warrell, D., Cox, T., Firth, J., *Oxford Textbook of Medicine*, 2010, Oxford University Press.

aspects in children and adults. Acute lesions are erythematous, vesicular, and exudative. Excoriations and lichenification may be seen due to chronic scratching/rubbing.

Management

Avoid known exacerbating factors, use of frequent emollients, soap substitutes, antihistamines, and topical steroids for flares. Topical immunomodulators (e.g. tacrolimus, pimecrolimus) can also be used as steroid-sparing agents. Severe cases may require oral steroids or immuno-suppressants such as azathioprine or ciclosporin. Phototherapy (commonly narrow band UVB) can also be used to treat severe cases. Secondary bacterial infection is common resulting in crusted, weepy lesions requiring treatment with antibiotics (e.g. flucloxacillin).

Psoriasis

This is a chronic inflammatory skin disease due to hyperproliferation of keratinocytes in the epidermis and infiltration of inflammatory cells. It affects 2% of the population.

Aetiology

There is a genetic component to the disease, although often an environmental precipitating factor exists (e.g. trauma–known as *Koebner's phenomenon*, infection, or alcohol).

Presentation

You are most likely to see chronic symmetrical plaques like well-demarcated, erythematous, scaly, silvery white plaques on the extensor surfaces (knees, elbows, and lower back) and scalp. Gentle removal of scales causes capillary bleeding known as the *Auspitz sign*. Half of patients have associated nail changes (e.g. pitting, onycholysis) and up to 10% suffer from associated psoriatic arthropathy (see Fig. 10.4).

Management

For mild/localized diseases, topical therapies include vitamin D analogues, topical corticosteroids, coal tar preparations, dithranol, topical retinoids, keratolytics, and scalp preparations. Extensive disease may require phototherapy such as narrow band UVB or PUVA (psoralen and UVA). Systemic immunosuppressive treatments (e.g. methotrexate, mycophenolate mofetil) can also be used for severe psoriasis, or in patients with joint involvement also.

Honours

Other forms of psoriasis

Other forms of psoriasis include guttate (widespread, small plaques typically in a young patient after a streptococcal throat infection), seborrhoeic (overlap of seborrhoeic dermatitis and psoriasis, affecting scalp, face, ears, and chest), flexural (smooth, well-defined patches in body folds), palmoplantar (psoriasis affecting the palms and soles), pustular (generalized or localized to palms and soles), nail psoriasis (onycholysis, pitting, ridging, and discolouration), and erythrodermic.

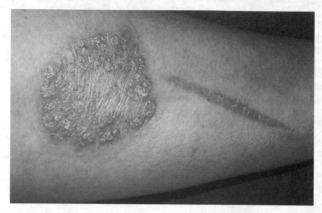

Fig. 10.4. Psoriasis (Koebner phenomenon). Reproduced with permission from Burge, S. Matin, R., and Wallis, D., *Oxford Handbook of Medical Dermatology* 2e, 2016, Oxford University Press.

Acne vulgaris

This is an inflammatory disease of the pilosebaceous follicle which commonly affects teenagers across the face, chest, and upper back.

Aetiology

Caused by a combination of factors including hormones (due to androgen), ↑sebum production, bacterial colonization by *Propionibacterium acnes*, and inflammation. Mild acne includes non-inflammatory lesions such as open and closed comedones (blackheads and whiteheads). More severe acne is associated with inflammatory lesions including papules, pustules, nodules, and cysts which → scarring.

Management

Topical treatments for mild acne includes benzoyl peroxide and topical antibiotics (due to antimicrobial properties), and topical retinoids (comedolytic and anti-inflammatory properties).

Oral therapies should be considered for moderate to severe acne such as oral antibiotics, oral contraceptive pill in females (antiandrogens), and oral retinoids (isotretinoin). Isotretinoin should be considered in patients not responding to normal treatments and where scarring is involved.

Bullous pemphigoid

This is an autoimmune, blistering skin disease usually affecting the older population. It can be localized or widespread, and crops of tense, fluid-filled, itchy blisters occur as a result of antibodies directed against components of the basement membrane (hemidesmosomes, important structural proteins between the epidermis and dermis). Some cases may be preceded by a non-specific, red, itchy rash for weeks/months prior to the blistering. (See Fig. 10.5.)

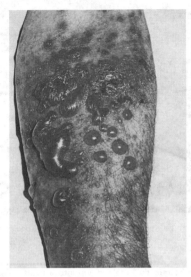

Fig. 10.5 Bullous pemphigoid. Reproduced with permission from Ramrakha, P., Moore, K., San, A., *Oxford Handbook of Acute Medicine* 3e, 2010, Oxford University Press.

Diagnosis
Is usually confirmed by skin biopsy from a blister and surrounding normal skin.

Management
If only mild and localized disease, very potent topical corticosteroids can be used to the lesions. Otherwise, most patients require immunosuppressive treatment, beginning with oral steroids or if these fail, tetracyclines (e.g. doxycycline, due to its antiinflammatory properties), azathioprine, and methotrexate.

Pyoderma gangrenosum

Although this is an uncommon cause of painful skin ulceration, pyoderma gangrenosum often comes up in written exams where you may have a clinical image to look at.

Presentation
Ulceration can occur at any site, often after minor trauma, but usually affects the lower legs and in those >50 years of age. (See Fig. 10.6.)

Aetiology
Half of cases are associated with an underlying internal disease including IBD, RA, haematological disorders, chronic active hepatitis, and vasculitis. The initial lesion may be a small pustule, a raised, red lesion, or a blood

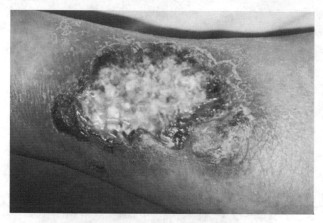

Fig. 10.6 Pyoderma gangrenosum. Reproduced with permission from Burge, S. Matin, R., and Wallis, D., *Oxford Handbook of Medical Dermatology* 2e, 2016, Oxford University Press.

blister which subsequently breaks down into a rapidly enlarging, painful ulcer. The edge of the ulcer is characteristically purplish in colour with undermined edges.

Treatment

This is by stepwise immunosuppression.

Skin cancers

Basal cell carcinoma (BCC)

This is the commonest skin tumour. Slow growing, locally invasive tumour of the epidermal keratinocytes commonly found on sites such as the head and neck. (See Fig. 10.7.)

Risk factors

Include UV exposure, fair skin type (see Table 10.1), increasing age, immunosuppression, previous history of skin cancer, and genetic predisposition.

Types

Different morphological types include nodular, superficial, cystic, morphoeic, and pigmented. The most common type of BCC you are most likely to be tested on in your exams is the nodular subtype. This typically presents as a pale papule or nodule with a pearly, rolled edge and surface telangiectasia. Sometimes these may have an ulcerated centre giving rise to the term '*rodent ulcer*'.

Management

Options include surgical excision or radiotherapy. Low-risk small lesions can be treated with cryotherapy or topical treatment (e.g. imiquimod). BCC do not tend to metastasize but may cause local tissue destruction and invasion.

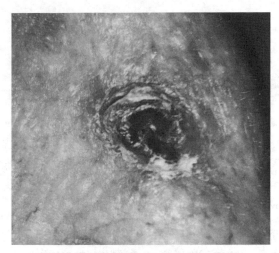

Fig. 10.7 Basal cell carcinoma. Reproduced with permission from Thomas, W.E.G. et al, *Oxford Textbook of Fundamentals of Surgery*, 2016, Oxford University Press.

Squamous cell carcinoma (SCC)

Unlike BCCs, SSCs have the potential to metastasize. SCCs are tumours arising from squamous cells within the epidermis.

Risk factors

Include those listed previously for BCCs with the addition of chronic inflammation (e.g. leg ulcers, wounds) and pre-existing areas of sun damage (solar/actinic keratoses).

Presentation

As a scaly (keratotic), ill-defined nodule which may ulcerate (see Fig. 10.8). Lesions are often tender.

Management

Surgical excision is the treatment of choice. Radiotherapy can also be used for large, non-resectable tumours. Bowen's disease is also known as SSC *in situ* (SCC confined to the epidermis) which can be treated with cryotherapy and topical treatments (e.g. Efudix®, 5-fluoruracil).

Melanoma

Invasive malignant tumour of the epidermal melanocytes which has the potential to metastasize.

Risk factors

Include excessive UV exposure, fair skin type, episodes of severe sun burn during childhood, multiple moles or atypical moles, and family history or previous history of melanoma.

Presentation

Melanomas are variable in presentation but the '**ABCDEs**' rule helps us to assess suspicious lesions. The following features are considered:

- Asymmetrical shape.
- Border irregularity.
- Colour irregularity (two or more colours within the lesion).
- Diameter >7 mm.
- Evolution of lesion (change in size, shape, colour).
- Plus symptoms (itching/bleeding).

Types

The different morphological types of melanoma includes superficial spreading melanoma, nodular, acral lentiginous melanoma (common on the palms, soles, nails beds, no clear relation to UV exposure), lentigo maligna melanoma (common on the face in the elderly population, related to long-term cumulative UV exposure).

Trivia

Sunscreens in the UK are labelled with an 'SPF' and UVA star system. 'SPF' stands for sun protection factor which indicates the level of burn protection against UVB. This usually varies between SPF 6 and 50. The UVA star system varies from 1 star to 5 stars and indicates the percentage of UVA radiation absorbed by the sunscreen compared to UVB. A sunscreen with an SPF of 30 and a UVA rating of 4 or 5 stars is recommended.

Management

Surgical excision is the definitive treatment but radiotherapy can be used in cases where excision is not appropriate.

Honours

Prognosis and risk based on Breslow tumour thickness

- Low risk = <0.76 mm Breslow thickness.
- Medium risk = 0.76–1.5 mm Breslow thickness.
- High risk = >1.5 mm Breslow thickness.

TNM (Tumour, regional Nodes, Metastases) classification system is used to predict 5-year survival rates of melanomas

- Stage 1 (T<2 mm Breslow thickness, N0, M0) = 90% 5-year survival.
- Stage 2 (T>2 mm Breslow thickness, N0, M0) = 80% 5-year survival.
- Stage 3 (N≥1, M0) = 40–50% 5-year survival.
- Stage 4 (M≥1) = 20–30% 5-year survival.

Solar (actinic) keratoses

Areas of sun-damaged skin from chronic excessive sun exposure. You will find these on sun-exposed areas (scalp, face, backs of hands, lower legs in women). Commonly seen in elderly patients and usually considered harmless with a small risk of them progressing into SCC.

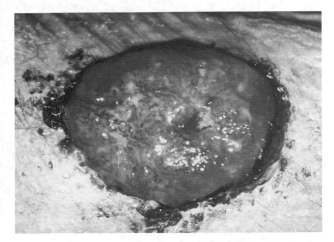

Fig. 10.8 Squamous cell carcinoma. Reproduced with permission from Thomas, W.E.G. et al, *Oxford Textbook of Fundamentals of Surgery*, 2016, Oxford University Press.

Presentation
Clinically these lesions are variable in colour but are usually scaly in appearance and rough to touch. They usually cause no symptoms.

Treatment
Options include cryotherapy, creams (e.g. diclofenac, fluorouracil, or imiquimod), surgery, and photodynamic therapy (using certain wavelengths of light to treat specific areas of damaged skin which have been treated with a photosensitizing cream beforehand).

Autoimmune disorders

Cutaneous manifestations of systemic and localized autoimmune disease are not only common but may also be the first presentation of an undiagnosed condition. Some of the common conditions you may encounter in clinic include vitiligo (loss of pigmentation), Henoch–Schönlein purpura (HSP; acute immunoglobulin (Ig)-A-mediated cutaneous vasculitis), scleroderma (e.g. CREST syndrome), and lupus.

Herpetic dermatitis
Herpes simplex (cold sores) presents with localized blistering and is often recurrent (after triggering its latent state). Triggers include trauma, upper respiratory tract infection (URTI), hormonal imbalance, and stress. Type 1 is usually associated with facial eruptions whereas type 2 results in anogenital herpes. Infectivity lasts for 1–2 weeks. Persistence should also be investigated in high-risk patients (e.g. immunodeficiency). Viral swabs from fresh vesicles can be cultured or PCR used to confirm diagnosis. Antivirals (e.g. aciclovir) may be required to treat severe eruptions.

Dermatology: in the emergency department

Urticaria, angio-oedema, and anaphylaxis

These form a spectrum of presentations. Urticaria presents as itchy wheals affecting any part of the body. Angio-oedema occurs due to oedema of the deeper structures of the skin (dermis and subcutaneous tissues).

Presentation

Whilst urticaria is normally uncomplicated, angio-oedema can be life-threatening if swelling of the tongue and lips leads to airway obstruction. Both urticaria and angio-oedema can progress to anaphylaxis which presents with hypotension, bronchospasm, facial oedema, and laryngeal oedema.

Triggers

Include food, medications, and insect bites.

Management

Antihistamines and corticosteroids can be given, while (IM) adrenaline (epinephrine) is used in cases of anaphylaxis.

Stevens–Johnson syndrome (SJS) and toxic epidermal necrolysis (TEN)

You are unlikely to see either of these two very serious conditions, and these patients are often managed in HDU or ITU due to the high risk of multisystem organ failure and death (10% and >30% respectively). SJS is characterized by mucocutaneous necrosis of at least two mucosal sites.

Presentation

Skin detachment is usually <10% of total body surface area. Drugs or combinations of infections or drugs are the main associations. SJS may have features overlapping with TEN including a prodromal illness (fever, cough, malaise). TEN is usually drug induced and patients are acutely unwell with extensive skin and mucosal necrosis accompanied by systemic toxicity. (See Fig. 10.9.)

Acute meningococcaemia

Presentation

With features of meningitis such as headache, fever, neck stiffness, along with septicaemia including hypotension, fever, myalgia, and a rash. Rash is typically a non-blanching purpuric rash on the trunk and extremities, which may be preceded by a blanching maculopapular rash. The rash can rapidly progress to ecchymoses, haemorrhagic bullae, and tissue necrosis. (See Fig. 10.10.)

Sequelae

Early recognition is important as acute meningococcaemia can lead to septicaemic shock, disseminated intravascular coagulation (DIC), multiorgan failure, and death.

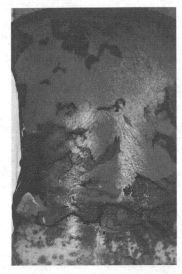

Fig. 10.9 Stevens–Johnson syndrome and toxic epidermal necrolysis. Reproduced with permission from Haddad, P., Dursun, S., Deakin, B., *Adverse Syndromes and Psychiatric Drugs: A clinical guide*, 2004, Oxford University Press.

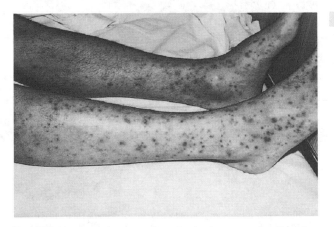

Fig. 10.10 Acute meningococcaemia. Reproduced with permission from Warrell, D., Cox, T., Firth, J., *Oxford Textbook of Medicine*, 2010, Oxford University Press.

Management

Suspected cases should be given IV antibiotics (e.g. benzylpenicillin). A LP and CT head should be performed (if signs of confusion, low GCS score, or raised intracranial pressure) but should not delay the first dose of antibiotics. Family members and close contacts should be given prophylactic antibiotics (e.g. rifampicin).

Necrotizing fasciitis

Presentation

Disproportionate limb pain following an injury should immediately bring to mind a compartment syndrome (see ➲ pp. 762–3). However, disproportionate pain without any history of an injury and in the context of skin lesions in a systemically unwell patient, should bring necrotizing fasciitis to mind. Skin changes include erythema, blisters, and necrotic skin with crepitus on palpation (subcutaneous emphysema). (See Fig. 10.11.) This may all start with an aggressive cellulitis → necrotizing cellulitis and so on.

Imaging

Plain radiography and CT may show soft tissue gas but its absence should not exclude a possible diagnosis.

Sequelae

The infection can spread rapidly through the deep fascia causing secondary tissue necrosis, and is associated with 75% mortality. Half of patients may be postoperative (e.g. abdominal surgery), have a history of poorly controlled diabetes, or malignancy.

Treatment

Requires extensive surgical debridement (see ➲ 'Debridement and reconstruction', pp. 742–3).

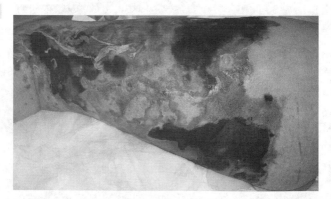

Fig. 10.11 Necrotizing fasciitis. Reproduced from Late diagnosed necrotizing fasciitis as a cause of multiorgan dysfunction syndrome: A case report. *Cases Journal* 2008, 1:125. doi:10.1186/1757-1626-1-125. Licensed under the Creative Commons Attribution 2.0 Generic license.

Dermatology: in theatre

Excisions

Are carried out under local anaesthetic (revise the maximum doses for lidocaine, bupivacaine, levobupivacaine, etc.) which can be safely administered and also sites where adrenaline (epinephrine) should be avoided (end-arterial supply as in digits and penis). Lesions are usually removed with a margin of normal skin (depending on the type of lesion). Incisions are usually elliptical and orientated in the same direction as relaxed skin tension lines for cosmesis and reducing wound tension.

Punch biopsy

Diameter varies from 3 to 8 mm. Usually used to take a small sample of skin under local anaesthetic from an area (e.g. rash).

Cryotherapy

Using liquid nitrogen to freeze localized skin → superficial destruction of the epidermis. Used to treat benign lesions such as viral warts, seborrhoeic keratoses, molluscum contagiosum, actinic keratosis, and low-risk tumours (superficial BCC and Bowen's disease).

Curette and cautery (C&C)

A curette is a sharp instrument used to scrape off skin lesions under local anaesthetic. The wound surface is then cauterized with an electrosurgical unit (diathermy) which stops bleeding and also destroys a thin layer of the epidermis (therefore useful if used to treat low-risk skin cancers). Commonly used to remove benign lesions such as seborrhoeic warts, molluscum contagiosum, viral warts, and low-risk tumours.

Honours

Sutures

Different areas of the body require different suture thicknesses and time periods for their removal (see Table 10.1).

Table 10.1 Sutures

Site	Suture	Removal of sutures
Face	4.0/5.0 Ethilon®	5–7 days
Legs and back	3.0 Ethilon®	10–14 days
Elsewhere	4.0 Ethilon®	7–10 days

Subcuticular sutures can be used in addition to interrupted surface stitches to maintain and add extra support to the wound. Useful in areas normally under tension (e.g. posterior trunk/scapula) where there is a risk of wound dehiscence. Vicryl® is commonly used and absorption is usually complete by 3 months. Methods of achieving haemostasis include applying firm pressure, chemical haemostasis (Driclor®, silver nitrate), sutures, cautery, and ligation (tie off) of vessels.

Dermatology: in exams

It is important to learn how to take a basic dermatological history. The following are important aspects to consider when taking a history from a patient with a skin-related problem. Eczema and psoriasis are the most likely conditions you will be tested on.

History station

- *Presenting complaint*: nature, site, and duration.
- *History of presenting compliant*: initial appearance, changes in appearance, symptoms such as itching and pain, aggravating and relieving factors, previous and current treatments and their effects, and potential triggers including travel, illness, stress, use of new products. History of sun burn, use of sun beds, and skin type are important for skin lesions such as moles.
- *Past medical history*: in particular, history of atopy (i.e. asthma, hay fever, and rhinitis), is important in eczema. History of skin cancer/atypical moles if a patient is presenting with a suspected skin tumour.
- *Family history*: of atopy, skin cancers, or skin disease.
- *Drug history*: enquire about any over-the-counter medications, as well as recent systemic and topical treatments.
- *Social history*: smoking, alcohol, pets, occupation (plus occupational exposure to substances if relevant), and impact on quality of life. It is important to explore patients' concerns and expectations especially in conditions such as psoriasis where the physical appearance of the condition is associated with significant psychological distress.

Examination

Practise performing a basic dermatological examination and also describing skin lesions. You are most likely to get a patient or clinical photos of a patient with chronic eczema or chronic plaque psoriasis to describe and then discuss the treatment options.

- *General inspection*: site/number of lesions and distribution of lesions.
- *Describe individual lesions*: size, shape, colour, associated secondary change, morphology, and margins. For pigmented lesions, assess according to the 'ABCD' system.
- *Palpate*: surface, consistency, mobility, and tenderness.
- *Complete systems examination*: this includes scalp, hair, mucous membranes, and nails as well as a general systems examination.
- *Eczema*: in an adult, you will generally see lichenified, dry, scaly patches of skin over flexor aspects. Practise describing the typical lesions seen in eczema including the distribution.
- *Psoriasis*: in contrast to eczema, chronic plaque psoriasis is normally seen in a symmetrical distribution over the extensor aspects of the body and scalp. Plaques are well demarcated, pink/red, with an overlying silvery scale in an asymmetrical distribution. Look for koebnerization (psoriasis at sites of scarring). Also check for nail changes—pitting/onycholysis.

Chapter 11

Elderly care

Elderly care: overview

Elderly care medicine (also known as geriatrics, care of the elderly (COTE), or ageing health) is increasingly important and relevant. Both as a student and throughout your career you will be dealing with older patients. It is one of the few specialties that incorporate every field in adult medicine. It also involves a much more holistic approach to the patient and their needs. With our ageing population, it is increasingly the specialty with the greatest demand on services.

- The fastest growing age group are people aged 65 and over.
- The proportion of people aged 65 and over will total >20% of the population by 2024.
- By 2046, one in four people will be >65 years (Office for National Statistics, 2016).
- 70% of those aged >65 have two or more long-term health conditions.

How do older patients differ from younger patients?

NAMES is a helpful mnemonic:
- Non-specific presentations.
- Atypical presentations.
- Multiple pathologies and Multimorbidity.
- Erroneous attribution to symptoms of old age.
- Single illness can have serious consequences due to underlying frailty.

Presentation

Presentation of illness is often atypical in the elderly and therefore it is important to take a thorough history and perform a detailed examination of your patients. These patients will often have multiple pathologies, which make them complicated and mean that a holistic approach to their care is essential. This means formulating a *broad differential diagnosis*, and *always* thinking about their psychological, social, and functional status.

MDT

The MDT is the backbone to providing good care to the elderly, and is essential for both initial and longer-term management. The members of the MDT include physiotherapists, occupational therapists, speech and language therapists, dietitians, pharmacists, nurses, discharge coordinators, and social workers.

Common syndromes in the elderly: the six 'I's

Geriatric giants: the so-called geriatric giants are the major categories of impairment that appear in elderly people, especially as they begin to fail. These include immobility, instability, incontinence, and impaired intellect/memory.

The following are common presentations. It is important to remember that they are often a symptom of another illness—this should always be at the back of your mind when assessing an elderly patient:

1. Instability—falls.
2. Intellectual impairment—acute confusion/delirium, dementia.
3. Immobility.
4. Incontinence and constipation.
5. Iatrogenic—always consider drug side effects and polypharmacy as a cause for presentation.
6. Infections.

The physiology of ageing

Older people are more likely to become ill than younger people, and most of the older people who are ill have more than one illness. Older adults have greater vulnerability to acute stress than younger individuals due to age-related diminution of physiologic reserves. An acute insult or stressor may push one or more organ systems 'over the brink', resulting in organ failure. When one organ system fails, others often follow. Thus, when an older adult with several chronic medical conditions develops an acute illness, those organ systems that are seemingly unrelated to the presenting problem may lack the reserve to withstand the stresses of the acute illness. (See Table 11.1.)

Ageing ('senescence') theories broadly fall into two main categories: programmed ageing and accumulation of damage. These theories may interact with each other in a complex way. The following are just two important mechanisms suggested in the ageing process:

- *Cell senescence and loss of telomeres*: telomeres determine how many times a cell can divide. Their length is a hallmark of the ageing process, and they shorten every time the cell divides. This is evidence of the cell's 'biological clock'. In addition, free radical damage acts to accelerate telomere loss.
- *Oxidative stress*: occurs when the production of reactive oxygen species (ROS)—including free radicals—outweighs the protection available from antioxidants. Interaction of ROS with DNA can result in mutations and deletions. DNA damage accumulates over time, ATP production can decline, and cells begin to die (apoptosis).

Table 11.1 Physiological changes in the elderly

CVS	Coronary artery disease Cardiac myocyte hypertrophy	↑Systolic BP ↓HR ↓Vascular elasticity
Respiratory	↓FEV₁, ↓FVC ↓Compliance	↓Surface area ↓Arterial oxygenation
Renal	↓Creatinine clearance Sclerosis of glomeruli	↓Renal plasma blood flow
CNS	Neuronal loss Neurofibrillary tangles	↓Nerve conduction ↓Auditory/visual acuity
MSk	↓Muscle mass ↓Grip strength	↓Bone mass ↓Bone mineral density
Endocrine	↓Glucose tolerance	↓Oestrogen, testosterone, and growth hormone
Skin	↓Elasticity Poor wound healing	↓Vascularity, sensation, and dermal capillarity
Oral	Loss of teeth	Altered saliva production

FEV1, forced expiratory volume in 1 second; FVC, forced vital capacity.

Frailty

Frailty is a clinical syndrome characterized by an ↑vulnerability to adverse health outcomes and is associated with ↑mortality. Frail patients accumulate physiological deficits that make them less able to adapt to stressors such as acute illness. It is also associated with an ↑rate of cognitive decline.

Care for frail older adults is frequently challenging, related to their ↑disability and multiple chronic diseases. A MDT-based approach to care is often important in meeting the needs of frail, older adults.

A person is said to be frail if they meet three or more of following five characteristics.[1]

The frailty phenotype:
1. slowness (prolonged gait speed)
2. weight loss (unintentional)
3. weakness (reduced grip strength)
4. exhaustion (self-reported)
5. low physical activity.

Finally, the Clinical Frailty Scale[2] is a rapid and easy-to-use frailty screening tool that provides a global score ranging from 1 (very fit) to 9 (terminally ill) to reflect the following domains: disability, mobility, activity, energy, and disease-related symptoms.

References

1. Fried LP, Tangen CM, Walston J, et al. (2001). Frailty in older adults: evidence for a phenotype. *J Gerontol A Biol Sci Med Sci* 56(3):M146–56.
2. Clinical Frailty Scale (K. Rockwood): ℜ http://camapcanada.ca/Frailtyscale.pdf

Elderly care: in clinic

Find out before you attend a clinic what the theme of that clinic is. Read up before you go so that you can get more out of it. Remember, elderly care is a multidisease specialty, but in general, clinics will be related to one of the following themes:

Falls clinics

'*Falls*' are one of the most common presentations in elderly care medicine.
- One-third of people aged >65 and half of those >80 fall every year.
- Falls are usually multifactorial.
- Falls can result in death and disability.
- Falls are commonly indicative of an underlying issue whether they are age-related physiological changes, such as a reduction in vision, or a specific pathology, such as an infection.
- Falls are estimated to cost the NHS >£2.3 billion/year. Therefore, falling has an impact on quality of life, health, and healthcare costs.

Commonest risk factors for falls
- Acute medical illness (virtually anything in the elderly!).
- Visual impairment.
- Polypharmacy (more than four medications is a well-recognized risk factor).
- Impairment of balance/gait—vestibular or higher-level gait disorder.
- Cognitive impairment.
- Cardiovascular—postural hypotension/arrhythmias/heart disease.
- Neurological—TIA/CVA/sensory neuropathy.
- Environmental factors (poor lighting, slippery floors, uneven surfaces).

Taking a history
- *Take a history of the fall from the patient, but if needed their friends, family, next of kin, or carers*: where, what time, how, did anyone witness the fall, does the patient recall the events?
- *Any head injury(ies)/other injuries (especially hips)*: did they lose consciousness? Any vomiting? Any pain/trauma sustained?

How many times they have fallen in last 12 months and any previous near misses?
Ask about:
- *Symptoms before and after the fall*: dizzy, palpitations, warning?
- *Cardiac symptoms*: e.g. chest pains, palpitations, (pre-)syncope.
- *Symptoms of infection*: especially urinary or chest.
- *New weakness or change*: in vision or speech.
- *Medications*: what are they on? What has been recently started?

Examination
Full examination including the following:
- Assessment for any injuries.
- *Postural BPs* (postural hypotension = >20 mmHg fall in systolic BP or >10 mmHg in diastolic BP, or if symptomatic).
- *Functional*: ask the patient to stand from a chair, walk a few steps, turn around, and sit back down ('timed up and go' (TUG) test).

- *CVS*: check pulse, assess for rhythm, and listen for murmurs (especially an ejection systolic murmur).
- *Neurological*: assess gait, identify any neurological defects, cerebellar dysfunction, visual impairment, and cognitive impairment.

Specific investigations
- *Bloods*: FBC, U&E, LFTs, TFTs, and bone profile.
- Check the *creatine kinase* if the patient has been on the floor for a significant period of time: rhabdomyolysis can cause AKI.
- *Exclude infection*: urine dipstick, midstream specimen of urine (MSU), and CXR.
- *Cardiac*: ECG, echocardiogram, postural BPs, tilt table test, 24+ hour ambulatory Holter monitor.
- *Neurological*: CT head—exclude subdural haemorrhage, look for evidence of new CVAs.

> **Honours**
> - Older patients can have a dampened white cell response or temperature so C-reactive protein (CRP) is a useful marker.
> - Patients with catheters will frequently have positive urinalysis due to colonizing bacteria so correlation with the clinical picture and blood tests/investigations are often required.

Vertigo: sensation of movement in any direction
1. *Benign paroxysmal positional vertigo (BPPV)*: extremely common. Caused by calcium debris within the posterior semicircular canal in the inner ear. Brief vertigo (<1 min) provoked by turning the head in a certain position, such as looking up, or rolling over in bed. Investigation of choice is the Dix–Hallpike manoeuvre. Treatment is a 'particle repositioning manoeuvre' such as the Epley manoeuvre which helps dislodge endolymphatic debris.
2. *Vestibular neuronitis*: acute onset lasting several days and self-limiting. Viral or post-viral inflammation affecting cranial nerve VIII.
3. *Ménière's*: recurrent vertigo lasting hours that can be associated with hearing loss and tinnitus in one or both ears.
4. *Vertebrobasilar insufficiency*: brief vertigo when looking up.
5. *Postural (orthostatic) hypotension*: can be confused with BPPV. On the whole, patients experience a presyncopal sensation rather than vertigo. Orthostatic presyncope is not usually induced by rolling over in bed or lying down.

Falls prevention: multifactoral
Address the likely medical cause (Table 11.2) and manage appropriately. Other specific interventions include:
- review of medications
- hip protectors
- Ca^{2+} and vitamin D supplementation
- exercise and balance training
- home hazard modification
- community support
- sensory evaluation (vision, hearing, neurological).

Table 11.2 Causes of falls

CNS	• Balance and gait impairment:
	• Visual impairment
	• Cranial nerve VIII problems—vestibular neuritis, BPPV
	• Neuropathy
	• Acute confusion/delirium
	• Epilepsy/fits
	• Stroke/TIA
	• Parkinson's
	• Cerebellar syndromes
CVS	• Hypotension (postural, MI, bleeding)
	• Arrhythmias (brady/tachy, broad complex/narrow) complex)
	• Valve problems—AS
	• Vasovagal
	• Carotid sinus hypersensitivity
	• Situational syncope (cough, micturition, defecation)
GI	• Diarrhoea
	• Dehydration
	• GI bleeding
MSk	• Unstable joints
	• Osteomalacia
Metabolic	• Hypo/hyperthyroidism
	• Addison's (hypotension)
	• Cushing's (myopathy, hypokalaemia)
	• Hypoglycaemia (?diabetes)
Iatrogenic/ drug causes	• Benzodiazepines (sedation)
	• Antihypertensive medications
	• Antiarrhythmics
	• Tricyclic antidepressants (TCAs), do not forget *alcohol*!

Continence clinics

- Incontinence is common among older people. It can have a major adverse impact on their quality of life. In fact, it is associated with an increase in mortality and morbidity.
- One in five women and one in ten men over the age of 65 suffer from incontinence.
- 1% of the NHS budget is spent on incontinence (£500 million).

Normal changes with ageing predispose to incontinence
- Age-related changes.
- Vaginal atrophy.
- Reduced bladder contractility.
- Weak pelvic floor musculature.
- Unable to postpone voiding.
- Prostatic hypertrophy.

Reversible causes of incontinence (Table 11.3) can be remembered with the following mnemonic (**DIAPERS**):
- Drugs/delirium
- Infection
- Atrophic urethritis
- Psychological
- Excess fluid output
- Reduced mobility
- Stool impaction.

Types of urinary incontinence
- *Stress*: involuntary urine leakage on effort or exertion or on sneezing or coughing.
- *Urgency*: involuntary urine leakage accompanied or immediately preceded by urgency (a sudden compelling desire to urinate that is difficult to delay).
- *Mixed*: involuntary urine leakage associated with both urgency and exertion, effort, sneezing, or coughing.
- *Overactive bladder syndrome*: defined as urgency that occurs ± urge urinary incontinence and usually with frequency and nocturia.

Management of incontinence
History
- What type is it?
- Any urogenital or neurological symptoms?
- Altered bowel habit?
- Mobility.
- Toilet accessibility.
- Past surgery.

Examination
As appropriate: abdominal, rectal (PR) exam including anal tone (essential), examination of perineum to assess for vaginal atrophy and prolapse.

Table 11.3 Diseases causing incontinence

Acute (often reversible)	Chronic (likely established)
Excessive diuresis (drugs, hyperglycaemia, hypercalcaemia)	Stroke
Atrophic senile vaginitis	Dementia
Mechanical (constipation)	Poor mobility
Psychological	Benign prostatic hyperplasia (BPH)
Delirium	Drugs
Iatrogenic (diuretics, oversedation, anticholinergics)	Nerve damage

Investigations

This varies but in general rule out *simple causes*:

• UTI—urine MC&S, U&E, glucose.
• Retention—perform a bladder scan initially and then kidney ultrasound scan.
• Drugs.
• Constipation.
• Voiding record.
• Urodynamic studies.
• Cystoscopy.

Management

• Pelvic floor exercises for stress incontinence.
• Timed voiding and regular toileting for dementia patients.
• Advise to avoid stimulants, e.g. tea, coffee, and soft drinks.
• Intermittent self-catheterization for overflow incontinence.
• Drug therapy: β3 adrenoceptor agonist (e.g. mirabegron), desmopressin for detrusor instability, alpha blockers for BPH, anticholinergics (but best to avoid in the elderly).
• Treat the cause.
• MDT approach.
• Surgery if required.

Memory clinics

Dementia is common in old age. The risk of developing dementia rises with increasing age: >30% of people over the age of 85. There are currently an estimated 1 million people with dementia in the UK, and it is on the increase as the population ages.

Features

• Memory loss, particularly short-term memory.
• Communication and language impairment.
• Loss of ability to focus and pay attention.
• Reasoning and judgement impaired.
• Visual perception deficits and hallucinations.

Types

• 60% Alzheimer's dementia.
• 20% vascular dementia.
• 10% dementia with Lewy bodies.
• 5% frontotemporal dementia (Pick's disease).
• 5% other dementias (e.g. vitamin B12 and thyroid deficiencies, Creutzfeldt–Jakob disease (CJD), and Huntington's disease).

Honours

Many people with Lewy body dementia are very sensitive to the older typical neuroleptic medication (e.g. haloperidol), which can lead to severe side effects and even death.

Atypical antipsychotics (e.g. risperidone and quetiapine) are better tolerated but beware of QT prolongation.

Important things to exclude in patients with memory impairment
- Systemic infection including common infections (chest and urine) and rarer causes (e.g. HIV, neurosyphilis).
- Cerebral infection/inflammation— LP to exclude infection, e.g. encephalitis/neoplasm.
- Vasculitis—suggested by elevated CRP/ESR, and antinuclear antibody (ANA).
- Alcohol-associated dementia.

Diagnosis and assessment of dementia

History
- Take as much of a history from the patient as possible, but you will also need a comprehensive collateral history from family and friends.
- Deterioration may be gradual (e.g. Alzheimer's), stepwise (e.g. vascular), or abrupt (e.g. stroke).

Features
- Unable to retain new information, and short-term memory loss.
- Unable to manage complex tasks, e.g. paying bills and shopping.
- Communication and language impairment, e.g. inability to hold conversation and word-finding difficulties.
- Behavioural changes, e.g. aggression, irritability, irrational judgement, and wandering.
- Neglect of self-care, e.g. grooming, washing, and toileting.
- Recognition, e.g. failure to recognize, friends, and family.
- Agnosia: failure to recognize familiar people, places, and objects.
- Apraxia: failure to carry out complex, coordinated movements (e.g. buttoning a shirt).

Physical examination
- Look for signs of Parkinsonism, thyroid disease, vascular disease, and neuropathy.
- AF, peripheral vascular disease (PVD; vascular dementia).
- Cognitive and mental state examination:
  - Exclude delirium (e.g. 4AT test, Confusion Assessment Method).
  - Exclude depression.
  - Measure cognitive function, e.g. Mini-Mental State Examination (MMSE), Montreal Cognitive Assessment (MoCA), Addenbrooke's Cognitive Examination (ACE).

Appropriate investigations
- Bloods to exclude infection or metabolic dysfunction.
- CT/MRI brain—excludes other cerebral pathologies, and helps detect vascular changes.
- Review of medication in order to identify and minimize use of drugs, including over-the-counter products that may adversely affect cognitive functioning (see STOPP/START Toolkit[1]).

- Electroencephalography (EEG) if concerned about seizures, and potentially a LP.
- Urinary incontinence, abnormal gait, and marked cerebral atrophy in the context of cognitive decline suggest 'normal pressure hydrocephalus', which is treatable.

Management of dementia

General approaches include:

- memory clinics
- day centres and support groups
- dementia nurse specialists
- aim to promote and aid independence
- minimize major changes such as moving home
- simplify medications and aid with a dosette box
- (lasting) power of attorneys, wills, and CPR status are all important for when the patient is unable to make decisions for themselves
- support for family and carers is very important.

Reference

1. Gallagher P, Ryan C, Byrne S, et al. (2008). STOPP (Screening Tool of Older Persons' Prescriptions) & START (Screening Tool to Alert Doctors to Right Treatment): Consensus Validation. *Int J Clin Pharmacol Ther* 46(2):72 –83.

The acute assessment of the geriatric patient: ED and on the wards

Common acute presentations in elderly patients on both the wards and in the ED are confusion and reduced mobility. Both of these two presentations are usually a sign of underlying illness and should be taken seriously.

Acute confusion and delirium

Confusion Assessment Method

1. Acute confusion and fluctuating course
Is there an acute change from the patient's baseline cognition as reported by family/carer/healthcare provider? Does this fluctuate over time?

2. Inattention
Does the patient have difficulty focusing on a topic or are they easily distracted? Can the patient count back from 10, or spell WORLD backwards?

3. Disorganized thinking
Does the patient have rambling or incoherent speech? Do they unpredictably switch from topic to topic?

4. Altered level of consciousness
Is the patient's level of consciousness hyperalert (agitated), drowsy, stuporous, or comatose?

A diagnosis of delirium requires the presence of features 1, 2, and either 3 or 4.

Delirium is a fluctuating syndrome defined by acute brain dysfunction resulting in disturbance of consciousness, change in cognition, and a reduced ability to sustain attention, precipitated by peripheral stressors/insults such as infection, hypoxia, metabolic abnormalities, stroke, and drug effects.

Delirium is common and affects 40–65% of older patients in hospital, but often goes unrecognized. It is associated with ↑mortality, ↑length of hospital stay, ↑complications, and ↑hospital costs. Delirium strongly predicts future new-onset dementia and accelerates existing dementia. (See Table 11.4 for differences between delirium and dementia.)

A common assessment of *confusion* which is used in the ED and which you will need to know for your exams and for when you start as a junior doctor is the *AMTS* score.

Common causes of delirium

Delirium can be remembered by the following mnemonic (**DELIRIUM**):
- Drugs e.g. CNS-acting drugs, anticholinergics.
- Electrolyte and metabolic disturbance.
- Lack of drugs e.g. withdrawal of alcohol.
- Infection.
- Reduced sensory input (blindness/deafness/darkness).
- Intracranial conditions e.g. stroke, meningitis, subdural.
- Urinary retention/constipation.
- Myocardial conditions e.g. MI, heart failure, arrhythmias.

Table 11.4 How to distinguish delirium from dementia

Feature	Delirium	Dementia
Timing/onset	Acute	Chronic
Precipitating illness	Common	Uncommon
Reversibility	Reversible (usually)	Irreversible
Short- and long-term memory	Poor memory	Poor short-term memory (long-term memory usually preserved until late)
Fluctuations	Hour-to hour fluctuations	Little variation/lability
Agitation and aggression	Common	Uncommon in early stages
Conscious level	Usually affected	Normally unaffected
Hallucinations	Common	Uncommon in early stages
Motor signs	Tremor, myoclonus, asterixis	Late stages only

Management of delirium
- People with delirium commonly, but not always, need to be admitted.
- Treat the underlying cause.
- Correct electrolyte disturbances and glucose levels.
- Orient patient to date and place daily, provide clocks and calendars
- Environment—low noise, low lighting at night, minimize transferring within and between wards, or changes in environment.
- Mobilize early and regularly.
- Ask family or friends to support the patient. Education of the families and carers is important.
- If a patient is confused enough to be removing cannulae or other lines, a SC needle sited in between the shoulder blades is often a good temporary measure to enable at least 2 L of hydration/day.
- Stop offending medications, e.g. discontinue benzodiazepines, anticholinergics, antihistamines, and meperidine.
- Treat any pain—start with paracetamol, use low-dose opiates → titrate up the 'pain ladder' as required.
- Check for urinary retention, which is a not uncommon cause of pain and delirium. Treat constipation. Avoid urinary catheters if possible.
- Ensure use of usual glasses, hearing aids, or other adaptive equipment. Ensure the patient can see your mouth to aid in lip reading and expressions. Optimize lighting.
- Attempt non-pharmacological strategies first.

- If sedation is required for safety: antipsychotic medications should be used with caution—start at low doses and carefully titrate up, while closely monitoring for adverse events.
  - Haloperidol 0.25–0.50 mg PO/IM.
  - Risperidone 0.25–0.50 mg PO.
  - Quetiapine 12.5 mg PO.
  - Olanzapine 2.5 mg PO/buccal.
  - Benzodiazepines are not recommended.

Mental capacity

Capacity is assumed unless proven otherwise. Assessment is based on the Mental Capacity Act (MCA) (2005).

The existence of capacity requires four criteria to be present:
- The patient can *understand* the information given to them.
- The patient can *weigh up* the information given to them.
- The patient can *retain* the information.
- The patient can *communicate* their decision.

Take all practical steps to support decision-making (e.g. hearing aids, glasses, interpreter, and family). If the patient lacks capacity, any actions must be in their best interest, and the least restrictive option. If a patient lacks capacity and is being hospitalized for a period, then a *Deprivation of Liberty Safeguarding* (DoLS) order will need to be completed as per the MCA. Contact psychiatry liaison services for support.

Mental Health Act (1983)

- *Section 5 (2):* allows detention for up to 72 hours. Completed by foundation year 2 doctor and above. Form 12 has to be completed and submitted to the duty hospital manager.
- *Section 2:* allows detention for up to 28 days and is not renewable. Completed by a social worker and two registered medical practitioners.

Patient has fallen

Much of this topic was covered in the section on falls in the clinic setting (see ➲ pp. 235–6) and is very relevant to inpatients as well as outpatients. All the same rules apply for a patient who has fallen prior to admission or who has fallen on the ward. As a junior doctor you will regularly be called to assess a person who has fallen. A thorough history and examination is required to assess for both a cause and possible consequences of the fall including injury (especially head injury and hip fractures).

In this section we will look at causes of immobility—i.e. the patient has been admitted because he/she is not able to cope at home due to sudden or insidious onset of immobility (see Table 11.5). In the elderly, once again, this is often multifactorial and a symptom of the underlying disease.

Table 11.5 Causes of immobility

Pain	Weakness	Psychological	Iatrogenic
Bone pain Fractures Osteoporosis Paget's disease Malignancy	Endocrine Hypo/hyperthyroidism Cushing's disease	Dementia + depression	Oversedation
Joint pain Arthritis: OA RA Pseudogout and gout	Metabolic Electrolyte disturbance—calcium Dehydration	Fear and anxiety of recurrent falls	Parkinsonism (drug induced)
Muscular pain PMR Polymyositis	Haematological: always think about anaemia in elderly patients		Hypotension
Soft tissue pain Pressure sores Foot problems	Neurological: stroke and Parkinson's		Bed rest

Rehabilitation

Rehabilitation is provided by the MDT, and this will be discussed at greater length later in the section on discharge planning (see ➲ pp. 250–1). It is important that the MDT, in conjunction with the patient, set goals that can be worked towards. The rehab process consists of:

- recognition of potential (rehabilitation team assessment particularly by physiotherapists and occupational therapists)
- rehabilitation goal setting
- re-ablement (interventions)
- resettlement
- readjustment.

The Barthel Index—a standardized rehabilitation measurement tool

This measures independence across ten daily living activities, including dressing, grooming, and walking, with a score ranging from 0 (dependent) to 20 (independent).[1]

Reference

1. Mahoney FI, Barthel D (1965). Functional evaluation: the Barthel Index. *Md State Med J* 14:56–61.

The holistic approach/'comprehensive geriatric assessment'

The elderly care ward round

Every elderly patient should have a 'comprehensive geriatric assessment' (CGA) during their admission. This is a multidimensional, multidisciplinary, holistic assessment of an older person that determines and addresses their medical, psychological, social, functional, and environmental needs. It encompasses joint medical, nursing, therapy, and social care services around the diagnoses and decision-making.

Randomized controlled trials show that CGA leads to better outcomes, including reduced mortality, improved function, improved quality of life, reduced hospital admission, and reduced readmission rates which is becoming even more relevant with the financial pressures placed on the NHS.

A CGA should include:
- medical diagnoses and treatment
- review of medications and concordance with drug therapy
- information about social circumstances including details of carers, social support, finances, and social services
- assessment of cognitive function and mood
- assessment of functional ability
- home environmental assessment
- formulating goals specific to the patient and agreed with the patient, their relatives, and carers.

Simplify the pill box/prescribing in the elderly

Polypharmacy

Polypharmacy and the adverse effects of drugs are common in the elderly. Up to 30% of hospital admissions are the result of adverse drug events and almost a third of inpatient complications occur due to medications.

Common adverse drug events include delirium, urinary retention, orthostatic hypotension, metabolic derangements, e.g. hyponatraemia, bleeding due to anticoagulants or antiplatelets, and hypoglycaemia related to diabetic medications. GI side effects, including nausea, anorexia, dysphagia, and constipation, are also common.

It is particularly important to ensure that a complete and accurate list of medications is obtained in older patients. Hospital pharmacists, care homes, and their GPs can be helpful sources of information.

Tips on taking a drug history in elderly patients
- Ask the patient or family to bring in all their medication.
- Include allergies and intolerances in the drug history.
- A telephone call to the GP will help confirm what medications are actually taken or prescribed.
- A discharge letter from a recent admission will often be a very useful source.

There are greater pharmacological challenges for the elderly due to:
- wasting of muscle tissue
- ↑fat accumulation
- ↓weight and ↓body water
- ↓cardiac output
- ↓intestinal motility
- impaired renal function (↓glomerular filtration rate)
- impaired homoeostasis
- ↓liver blood flow and oxidation/reduction (phase I metabolism).

Drug metabolism, absorption, and elimination all change as a patient gets older. Doses in the elderly therefore need to be carefully monitored. Doses of some commonly prescribed medications with narrow therapeutic windows (e.g. gentamicin, digoxin, and vancomycin) will need to be carefully monitored and the dose adjusted to account for reduced renal function and metabolism in older patients.

Prescribing tips for the elderly

- Is it indicated?
- Can it be stopped?
- Start low and go slow.
- Monitor renal and liver function more closely.
- Monitor therapeutic doses and serum levels (digoxin, gentamicin, lithium).
- Drugs to be regularly reviewed and discontinued if no longer indicated.
- Educate the family and patient. Use medication summaries.
- Convert to once a day or modified release if possible.
- Try to use one medication that does the same thing as two, e.g. ACEI in heart failure and hypertensive patients.
- Consider a monitored dosage system.

The following medications are potentially hazardous in the elderly and need to be prescribed with caution:

CVS

- Aspirin: high risk of GI bleed/ulcers.
- Warfarin: bleeding.
- Beta blockers in combination with verapamil or diltiazem may result in symptomatic heart block.
- Digoxin in impaired renal function: potential for digitoxicity and arrhythmias.
- Diuretics: may exacerbate gout, hyponatraemia, and hypo/hyperkalaemia.

CNS

- Benzodiazepines can worsen confusion, cause falls, and impair balance.
- Antimuscarinics and some anticonvulsants can worsen confusion.
- Avoid TCAs in dementia—risk of worsening cognitive impairment.
- TCAs exacerbate glaucoma, are proarrhythmic, and can cause constipation as well as urinary retention.
- Selective serotonin reuptake inhibitors (SSRIs) can cause hyponatraemia.
- Antimuscarinics and metoclopramide worsen Parkinsonian symptoms.

Drugs that cause falls ('BOSS VAN')

- Benzodiazepines
- Opiates, e.g. codeine and morphine
- Sedating antidepressants, e.g. TCAs
- Sleeping tablets, e.g. zopiclone
- Vasodilators, e.g. nitrates, nicorandil, calcium channel blockers
- Antihistamines (sedating), e.g. chlorphenamine
- Neuroleptics, e.g. phenytoin, carbamazepine.

GI

- Avoid NSAIDs in peptic ulcer disease or GI bleeds.
- Drugs that cause constipation: antimuscarinics, TCAs, calcium channel blockers, and opioids.

Respiratory

- Long-term steroid use can cause GI ulcers, and systemic corticosteroid/Cushingoid features.
- Nebulized ipratropium may exacerbate glaucoma.

MSk

- NSAIDS: bleeding, bruising, GI disease, exacerbate heart failure, and hypertension.

Urological

- Antimuscarinics, e.g. oxybutynin, are associated with an ↑risk of constipation, confusion, cognitive impairment, urinary retention, and glaucoma.

How to initiate warfarin

- Explain why warfarin is needed.
- Discuss risks vs benefits with patient.
- Explain about frequent blood tests and monitoring initially.
- Explain that some medications interact with warfarin, e.g. tetracyclines, more so in the elderly.
- Avoid vitamin K-rich foods, e.g. spinach.
- Inform them that alcohol will affect levels.
- Follow local hospital policy for the initial dosing of warfarin, but for most elderly patients 5 mg, 5 mg, then check INR on the third day is a safe approach.
- Initially it is important to check INR daily, then alternate days until a pattern becomes clearer.
- Give them the yellow booklet with indications for being on warfarin and their treatment schedule.

End of life and palliative care

Withholding treatment

The benefits and burdens of treatment need to be reviewed when death is imminent. It is important to recognize when the patient is in the terminal phase of their life and help make it as peaceful and dignified as possible. The palliative care team should be involved early and spiritual needs should also be addressed.

Verification of death

Check for and document the following assessments:

- Pupils fixed and dilated.
- No pulses palpable for 1 min.
- No heart sounds heard for 1 min.
- No breath sounds heard for 3 min.
- Time of death.
- Persons present.
- No response to painful stimulus/unresponsive.
- Whether next of kin/family informed or not.

Certification of death

This is an important duty and a legal requirement. A funeral cannot be arranged without it and it also provides important statistics for disease surveillance and public health. Always ask a senior before issuing a death certificate with regard to cause of death. Be as precise as possible regarding the cause, e.g. ischaemic heart disease rather than cardiac failure. Old age is an acceptable cause of death in the very elderly person who has had a non-specific decline and treatable causes have been excluded (see Fig. 11.1).

Cremation forms

You must have looked after the patient in their terminal illness to complete this form. The form asks for your details, what your role was, how long you looked after the patient, and when was the last time you cared for the patient prior to their death. It also asks for the cause of death as would be issued on the death certificate, a summary of events that led to the patient's death.

DEATH CERTIFICATE EXAMPLE GEEKYMEDICS.COM

Name of deceased..

Date of death as stated to me.................. day of .... Age as stated to me..............

Place of death..

Last seen alive by me.................. day of ....

1 The certified cause of death takes account of information obtained from post-mortem. 2 Information from post-mortem may be available later. 3 Post-mortem not being held. 4 I have reported this death to the Coroner for further action.	*Please ring appropriate digit(s) and letter*	a Seen after death by me. b Seen after death by another medical practitioner but not me. c Not seen after death by a medical practitioner.

CAUSE OF DEATH	Approximate interval between onset and death
I (a) Disease or condition directly leading to death..................	....
(b) Other disease or condition, if any, leading to I(a)..................	....
(c) Other disease or condition, if any, leading to I(b)..................	....
II Other significant conditions CONTRIBUTING TO THE DEATH but not related to the disease or condition causing it..................	....

The death might have been due to or contributed to by the employment followed at some time by the deceased ☐

I certify that this death certificate is accurate Signature.................. Qualifications..................
Residence.................. Date..................
Consultant responsible for the above-named patient..................

Fig. 11.1 Death certificate. Reproduced from Geekymedics.com

Geriatrics: in exams

Specific geriatric assessments in OSCEs

Assessment of cognition
- Introduce yourself, establish rapport/patient's name and age.
- Explain you are going to test their memory and that some of the questions you ask them may seem silly to them. Apologize for this.
- Conduct the Abbreviated Mental Test Score (maximum 10 points):
  1. How old are you?
  2. What is your date of birth?
  3. What time is it?
  4. Can you remember the following address? 42 West Street (repeat question at the end).
  5. What year is it?
  6. What place is this?
  7. What is my job? What is that person's job? (recognizing two people)
  8. Can you tell me when World War I started/finished?
  9. What is the name of the monarch?
  10. Can you count backwards from 20 to 1?

Each answer scores 1 point. A score of 8 or less is abnormal.
- Summarize and elicit any concerns from the patient.
- Present your findings and management plan to the examiner.

NB: this is a *screening tool* to establish if someone is confused; if positive, a more detailed assessment is then required—you should say this to the examiner when presenting your findings at the end of the station. You can explain that an example of this is the MMSE or the MoCA tool but you will *not* be required to do this in an examination scenario. You may be required to know what the different elements are:

The MoCA assesses several cognitive domains
- Short-term memory recall
- Visuospatial abilities
- Executive functions
- Phonemic fluency
- Verbal abstraction
- Attention, concentration, and working memory
- Language
- Orientation to time and place.

Discharge planning and functional status assessment
- Explain that you want to discuss issues surrounding their discharge home following admission (e.g. after a stroke when the patient's needs and mobility may have changed significantly).
- Establish the patients' ideas and concerns when returning home.
- Ask about the home environment (e.g. stairs, bathrooms, kitchen, etc.).

- Assessment of activities of daily living: what is the patient able to do for themselves? Ask specifically about:
  - washing
  - dressing
  - mobility and walking aids
  - transferring (e.g. bed to chair)
  - stairs
  - cooking
  - feeding
  - continence issues.
- Ask about support required on discharge:
  - Carers (for help with washing and dressing).
  - Single-level accommodation (if stairs are an issue).
  - Shopping (delivery can be arranged).
  - Cooking ('meals on wheels' are available).
  - Continence (commode in bedroom or continence pads).
- Nutrition: the Malnutrition Universal Screening Tool (MUST) is a predictor of malnutrition. There are multiple causes of weight loss due to inadequate nutrient intake. These include social (e.g. living alone, poverty, isolation), psychological (e.g. depression, dementia), medical (e.g. cancers, dysphagia), and pharmacological issues.
- Explain that there will be a MDT to help the patient prepare for discharge, which may involve social services, occupational therapists, and physiotherapists, amongst other specialist services.
- Ask the patient about any other concerns.
- Summarize.
- Present your findings and management plan to the examiner.

Formal functional scores exist that you would use to assess the patient, but you would not be expected to formally assess this in an examination. One example is the Barthel Index that focuses on reflecting the degree of independence.[1] A higher score is associated with a greater likelihood of coping and living at home with a degree of independence following hospital discharge. Ten variables are scored out of a maximum of 20.

Assessment of depression in elderly patients
- Introduce yourself.
- Ask about how the patient is feeling.
- Explain that you are going to ask some questions to assess their mood.
- *The Geriatric Depression Scale (GDS)* screening tool is used to identify depressive symptoms in the elderly.[2] It consists of 15 yes/no questions. This is a quick test which takes 5–10 min. Scoring:
  - 0–4: no depression.
  - 5–10: mild depression.
  - 11+: severe depression.
- *Ask about deliberate self-harm and suicide*: if the patient expresses any intent to harm themselves you *must* conduct a full suicide assessment.

- *Be aware of pseudo-dementia in the elderly*: the response '*I cannot remember*' may indicate some degree of cognitive impairment but also may be a symptom of depression for instance.
- Ask if the patient has any particular concerns.
- Summarize.
- Present your findings and management plan to the examiner.

References

1. Mahoney F. Barthel D (1965). Functional evaluation: the Barthel Index. *Md State Med J* 14:61–5.
2. Yesavage JA, Brink TL, Rose TL, et al. (1982). Development and validation of a geriatric depression screening scale: a preliminary report. *J Psychiatr Res* 17(1):37–49.

Emergency medicine

Emergency medicine: overview

Emergency medicine (EM) deals mostly with acute injuries and illnesses that affect patients of all age groups with a full spectrum of undifferentiated physical and behavioural disorders. During your time in this medical specialty you will gain knowledge and skills required for the prevention, diagnosis, and management of such emergent presentations along with an understanding of pre-hospital EM.

EM takes care of anyone presenting with anything at anytime

EM as it is currently known started as a specialty in the UK in 1952 and Mr Maurice Ellis at Leeds General Infirmary was the first consultant. It was initially called the Casualty Surgeons Association. Rotating through an EM placement can be a daunting task for most medical students. High patient volume, acuity, and varied pathology pose an interesting challenge during the time spent in the ED. The EM placement is unparalleled. You will gain a wide variety of medical experience and procedural skills you will not get anywhere else, from suturing to assisting in cardiac arrests. All in a day's work!

Ten ED commandments

1. *Always think ABCDE*: with every patient you see, especially in majors and the resuscitation room, think:
   • Airway: is it open? Is it maintainable?
   • Breathing: is the respiratory rate and depth normal? Is the air entry equal on both sides of the chest?
   • Circulation: are the BP and pulse normal? Is the patient adequately perfused?
   • Disability: what is the GCS score? What is the blood glucose?
   • Exposure: expose the patient for adequate examination.
2. *Know your limitations*: you will come across clinical problems and situations you have never been confronted with in the past. The sign of a safe doctor is someone who asks for help early to provide optimal patient care in a timely manner. Always do the right thing, at the right time, to the right patient, in the right place.
3. *Listen to your patient*: the majority of your diagnoses are clear from the history. If you take a good history, you will get the diagnosis. A good, relevant history is not always time-consuming.
4. *Examine the patient properly*: a good examination will give you more information about the patient's condition than state-of-the-art investigations. If a patient complains of pain in a limb, be systematic and examine the entire limb and compare it to the normal side.
5. *Anticipate the worst*: exclude the life-threatening problems first. If discharging a patient ask yourself: 'If this patient is discharged home and they die, have I thought of every potentially life-threatening problem, and have I done my best to exclude them?' If you cannot answer this question with a resounding 'yes' then ask for senior help. Examples:
   • Has a pregnancy test been done in a fertile woman with abdominal pain to exclude ectopic pregnancy?

- Has a patient with pleuritic chest pain had ABG and D-dimer tests to exclude a pulmonary embolus (PE)?
- Has a patient with a head injury who is fit for discharge gone home with an adult who can keep an eye on him/her to exclude worsening intracranial haemorrhage?

6. *Be punctual*: arrive on time for lectures and shop floor sessions. The ED runs on a shift system and the clinicians who are imparting valuable knowledge are very busy.

7. *Be courteous and professional*: to patients, colleagues, and other teams. Otherwise you will find yourself dealing with complaints from people you are working with.

8. *Keep a good clinical record*: write a clear history, important negative findings, the investigations you want to request, and your management plan. Write legibly in black ink and present succinctly. Your written record will be followed by nurses and other teams to uphold patient safety. Your record may also be used in a court of law in case patient safety has been compromised.

9. *Attend the ED teaching*: this is compulsory and subsidized. It is vital that you attend these sessions as you are taught topics which are not always covered in textbooks. You will also learn how things are done in your hospital as local policies and protocols differ.

10. *Enjoy the placement*: EM is one of the most exciting, varied, and interesting placements you will do. You will be on a steep learning curve but will be well supported if you maintain your enthusiasm and willingness to participate. If you do not take the initiative to participate and show your enthusiasm, you will quickly be ignored since it is a busy department. If you show a willingness to learn, then every member of staff will go the extra mile to make you comfortable, guide, and teach you for as long as you wish. Have the guts to do some nights and learn!

Emergency medicine: in resuscitation

Primary survey

Deals with the assessment and treatment of patients, based on the *MIST* list: Mechanism of injury, Injuries sustained or suspected, Signs (vitals), symptoms, and Treatment received. Treatment priorities of a severely injured patient must be established in a logical and sequential fashion.

Receiving and treating a severely injured patient can lead to anxiety which provokes memory loss. Therefore, one can overcome anxiety and memory loss if one develops a system for doing a rapid primary survey, resuscitation, detailed secondary survey, followed up by definitive care. This process constitutes the *ABCDEs* of trauma care and identifies life-threatening conditions according to the following sequence:

1. Airway maintenance with *cervical spine protection*.
2. Breathing and ventilation.
3. Circulation with *haemorrhage control*.
4. Disability and neurological status.
5. Exposure/Environmental control: completely undress the patient, but prevent hypothermia.

A quick (10 sec) assessment of the ABCDE in a trauma patient can be conducted by talking to the patient and asking about basic information (name and what happened). An appropriate response (ability to speak clearly) suggests that there is no major ABC issues and the brain is adequately perfused. The aim of the primary survey is to deal with the life-threatening conditions as they are identified A–E!

Airway maintenance with cervical spine (C-spine) protection

- A non-patent airway is rapidly fatal but can often be easily resolved. Think of the airway as a pipe that can be blocked (vomit/foreign body/tongue), swollen (anaphylaxis/burns), or externally compressed (haematoma/tumour/abscess).
- Ascertain patency: open, look, suck secretions, and remove visible foreign bodies. There will be no sound from a totally obstructed airway but signs of a partially obstructed airway include stridor (usually inspiratory), stertor (snoring), and gurgling (fluid). Note facial, mandibular, or tracheal/laryngeal fractures that can obstruct the airway.
- Airway opening manoeuvres: chin lift or jaw thrust (usually reserved for C-spine injury) (see Fig. 12.1 and Fig. 12.2).
- Then protect cervical spine using the trinity of devices (appropriately sized cervical collar, head blocks, and tape) if no ongoing airway concerns.
- Turning an unconscious patient on their side (into the recovery position) can help prevent aspiration of vomit or airway obstruction by the tongue (not if C-spine injury suspected—then clinical team has to log-roll vomiting patient).

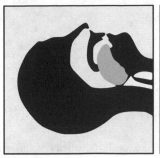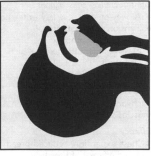

Fig. 12.1 Head tilt, chin lift. Reproduced from Wikimedia commons. Image is in public domain.

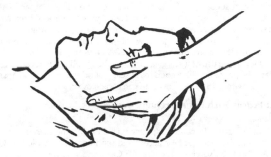

Fig. 12.2 Jaw thrust, in case C-spine injury suspected. Reproduced from Wikimedia commons. Image is in public domain.

Honours

Prior to application of a cervical collar check the following:
- *Look*: distended neck veins and neck wounds or bruising.
- *Feel*: tracheal position, laryngeal crepitus, surgical emphysema and cervical spine tenderness.
- *Listen*: hoarse voice and carotid bruits.

Breathing and ventilation

Adequately expose the patient's neck and chest. Inspect, palpate, percuss, and auscultate. The life-threatening chest injuries should be identified during the primary survey and may require immediate attention for ventilatory efforts to be effective (see Table 12.1). These can be remembered by the pneumonic '**ATOM FC**' and ensure a CXR has been requested.

Life-threatening chest injuries
- Airway obstruction/laryngotracheal injury
- Tension pneumothorax
- Open pneumothorax
- Massive haemothorax
- Flail chest
- Cardiac tamponade.

Effort
Tachypnoea, chest wall recession, stridor, grunting, and use of accessory muscles suggest ↑work of breathing.

Efficacy
↓Chest expansion, reduced breath sounds, and ↓O_2 saturations suggest reduced efficacy of breathing.

Effect
↑HR or ↓HR, cyanosis, or confusion or reduced level of consciousness would suggest secondary effects on hypoxia on the various organ systems. If there is spontaneous respiratory effort but signs of ↑work of breathing or reduced efficacy or effect, then provide high-flow O_2 via a non-rebreather mask (80% O_2 with a 15 L/min flow rate). A standard mask without the reservoir bag (Hudson's mask) provides 50% O_2 with a 15 L/min flow rate.

If trained in the use of a self-inflating Ambu® bag and mask, oxygenate and ventilate the patient. With a good mask seal around the mouth and nose, up to 95% O_2 with a 15 L/min flow rate can be achieved.

Circulation with haemorrhage control

Circulation
Check pulse rate/HR, central capillary refill time (on the sternum, normal <2 sec), and BP. Gain vascular access and send appropriate bloods. Get a venous blood gas to check for Hb, K^+, Ca^{2+}, and glucose. Get a 12-lead ECG. Prolonged capillary refill time and low BP could suggest that the patient is in shock! Shock, syncope, myocardial ischaemia on the ECG (new ST segment or T-wave changes), or heart failure (clammy skin, shortness of breath, lung crackles on auscultation, raised JVP, pitting pedal oedema) in the presence of a brady- or tachycardia suggest adverse features. Rapid and

Table 12.1 Indications for definitive airway

Airway protection	Ventilation and oxygenation
Facial injuries	Inadequate respiratory efforts: *tachycardia/hypoxia/cyanosis/hypercarbia*
Obstruction: *stridor, haematoma, laryngeal/tracheal injury*	Severe haemorrhaging and need for volume resuscitation
Aspiration risk: *bleeding, vomiting*	Closed head injury requiring hyperventilation
Unconscious or low GCS score (usually <8)	Apnoea: *paralysis, unconsciousness*

accurate assessment of an injured patient's haemodynamic status (pulse, BP, skin colour, and level of consciousness) is essential. Tachycardia is often the first sign of circulatory compromise. An injured patient who is cool and tachycardic is in shock until proven otherwise. *Shock is defined as inadequate tissue perfusion and oxygenation.* Two types include (1) haemorrhagic which is the commonest and (2) non-haemorrhagic (i.e. tension pneumothorax, cardiac tamponade, neurogenic, and septic).

There are four classes of haemorrhage, as listed in Table 12.2.

Principles of managing haemorrhagic shock

1. Identify external haemorrhage during the primary survey and control it by direct manual pressure, binders for pelvic trauma, reduction and splintage of long bone fractures, and tourniquets for extremity trauma
2. *Replace volume loss:* crystalloids = 1–2 L in adults or 10 mL/kg boluses in children and/or blood and blood products (2 units of blood in adults or 15 mL/kg of blood as 5 mL/kg boluses in children). For massive haemorrhage replace with 4 units of RBC, 4 fresh frozen plasma, 1 platelet, and 2 cryoprecipitate (if fibrinogen <1.5 g/L) aiming for:
   • Hb: 8–10 g/dL
   • Platelets: >75 × 10⁹/L
   • Prothrombin time ratio: <1.5
   • APTT ratio: <1.5
   • Fibrinogen: >1.5 g/L
   • Calcium: >1 mmol/L
   • Temperature: >36°C
   • pH: >7.35

Table 12.2 Severity of shock

Parameter	Class			
	1	2	3	4
Blood loss (mL)	<750	750–1500	1500–2000	>2000
Blood loss (%)	<15	15–30	30–40	>40
Pulse rate (bpm)	<100	100–120	120–140	>140
Systolic BP	↔	↔	↓	↓
Pulse pressure	↔	↓	↓	↓
Respiratory rate (breaths/min)	12–20	20–30	30–40	>35
Urine output (mL/hour)	>30	20–30	5–15	↓
Fluid replacement	C	C	C + B	C + B

B, blood; C, crystalloid.

3. *Vascular access—short and fat does the trick*: size 14 (orange or brown colour cap) or a 16 gauge (grey colour).
   • Consider tranexamic acid in bleeding trauma patients as soon as possible. If treatment is not given until 3 hours or later after injury, it is less effective and could even be harmful according to the CRASH-2 trial (Lancet)
   • Check acid–base balance via ABGs or Venous blood gases.
   • Monitor urinary output.
   • Base deficit and lactate are useful in determining the presence and severity of shock.
   • Hidden blood loss sites include **CRAMP**:
     — Chest
     — Retroperitoneum
     — Abdomen
     — Mediastinum
     — Pelvis.

Top tips

• *Trauma aphorism*—do not let the obvious (severed or mangled limb) distract you from the occult (tension pneumothorax/cardiac tamponade).
• If tension pneumothorax has been excluded, hypotension following trauma is secondary to hypovolaemia until proven otherwise.
• Beta-adrenergic blocking medications may dampen the shock response (i.e. patient remains bradycardic despite the blood loss).
• Bradycardia with hypotension following trauma → consider neurogenic shock.

FAST: focused assessment sonography in trauma

• Standard four views: pericardial, right upper quadrant (RUQ), left upper quadrant (LUQ), and suprapubic.
• Helpful to *rule in* haemo/haemopneumo/pneumothorax, cardiac tamponade, and haemoperitoneum *but it is not a rule out!*

Abdominal trauma

• Clinical diagnosis is difficult as clinical examination and conventional signs of peritoneal irritation are unreliable. Assume that abdominal trauma exists unless proven otherwise. Early imaging has become a standard of care.
• Management of abdominal injuries may include (1) non-operative, (2) damage control surgery, and (3) interventional radiology.

Pelvic trauma

• Largest and strongest osteoligamentous body structure and disruption usually due to high-energy (2000–10,000 N).
• Suspect in high-velocity road traffic collisions (RTCs), fall from heights, or crush injury.
• Mechanisms of injury: AP/lateral compression vs vertical shear.

- Management: *do not spring the pelvis.* Apply a pelvic binder in the primary survey. Look out for signs specific for pelvic and urethral injury including:
  - unstable or pelvic tenderness
  - blood in the urinary meatus
  - perineal bruising
  - scrotal haematoma
  - high-riding prostrate on digital rectal exam
  - request a pelvic X-ray for fractures.

Disability and neurological evaluation

Neurological dysfunction can arise out of direct cerebral injury or secondary to reduced oxygenation and/or perfusion. It is examined through:
- level of consciousness (GCS): hypoglycaemia, alcohol, narcotics, and drugs can alter GCS
- lateralizing signs
- level of spinal cord injury level if present
- pupillary size and reaction
- brain metastases.

DEFG: 'don't ever forget glucose'

Intracranial pressure (ICP)

ICP = mean arterial pressure (MAP) − cerebral perfusion pressure (CPP)
- Resting ICP is 10 mmHg. Pressures >20 mmHg sustained and refractory to treatment have poorer outcomes.
- Features of ↑ICP include headache, N&V, ↓GCS score, mydriasis, ophthalmoplegia, focal neurology, and papilloedema.

Management of raised ICP
- Elevate the head by 30°.
- Discuss with the on-call neurosurgeon and consider mannitol (osmotic diuretic) or 3% hypertonic saline and controlled hyperventilation.
- Transfer to a neurosurgical centre with neurological ITU.
- Barbiturate induced coma is also an option if the above-listed measures fail.
- Hypothermia (cooling the brain to 35°C) and decompressive craniectomies have been tried to control the ICP.

Table 12.3 Indications of CT imaging

Head	Neck
GCS score <13	
Focal neurological deficit	
Suspected open/depressed/basal skull fracture	Intubation
Post-traumatic seizure	Cervical midline tenderness
>1 episodes of vomiting	Inadequate X-rays
Risk factors: >65 years, high-energy injury (RTC)	
Risk factors: warfarin, coagulopathy, >30 min retrograde amnesia	

Exposure and environmental control

Completely undress the patient to facilitate a thorough examination and assessment following which the patient should be covered with warm blankets or an external warming device and warm IV fluids to prevent hypothermia.

> **Honours**
> Do everything you can to avoid the *triad of death in trauma*:
> 1. Acidosis
> 2. Coagulopathy
> 3. Hypothermia.

Trauma imaging

Bedside portable CXRs and pelvic X-rays can be taken at the end of the primary survey (Table 12.3). Major trauma CT examination consists of (1) head and C-spine, (2) thorax, (3) abdomen and pelvis, and (4) any other sites of injuries. The following mechanisms of injury suggest the need for a major trauma CT:

- RTC
- Fall >3 metres
- Crush injury to thorax/abdomen
- Blast injuries.

Secondary survey

The secondary survey does not begin until the primary survey is completed, resuscitative efforts are underway, and the normalization of vital functions has been demonstrated. The secondary survey constitutes a complete history and a head-to-toe physical evaluation of the trauma patient, including reassessment of all vital signs.

AMPLE history

- Allergies
- Medications currently used
- Past illnesses/Pregnancy
- Last meal
- Events/Environment related to the injury: each body region is completely examined (literally a finger/probe in every orifice).

Blood investigations

FBC, clotting screen, electrolytes, ABG (pH, PO_2, PCO_2, Hb, lactate, base excess, creatinine, glucose), group and save, and cross-match. Consider amylase/lipase in abdominal trauma, paracetamol/salicylates if history of self-harm, and troponin in chest trauma, chest pain/collapse prior to trauma, or ECG changes noted on the monitor.

Management

- IV fluid/blood
- Analgesia
- Antibiotics
- Tetanus
- Splinting.

Cardiac arrest

A sudden stop in effective blood circulation due to failure of the heart to contract effectively or at all. The patients are unconsciousness and there are no signs of life such as breathing or movement. Unless CPR is started, the person may die or suffer permanent brain and other organ damage. CPR involves chest compression (external cardiac massage) and rescue breathing. This is often termed basic life support (BLS) (Figs 12.3–12.5).

Call arrest team

Compression-only CPR for adults
1. Place the heel of one hand in the centre of the patient's chest; then place your other hand on top, interlocking your fingers.
2. Position yourself over the patient's chest, keeping your arms straight.
3. Use your body weight to compress the chest approximately one-third of the depth of the chest.
4. After each compression allow your hands to recoil.
5. Aim to deliver 100–120 compressions per minute.
6. Continue until help arrives.

Chest compression <1 year
- If alone, compress the sternum with the tips of two fingers.
- If more, use the encircling technique → place thumbs flat, side by side, on the lower sternum, with the tips pointing towards the infant's head → spread the rest of both hands, with the fingers together, to encircle the lower part of the infant's rib cage with the tips of the fingers supporting the infant's back → press down on the lower sternum with your two thumbs to depress it at least one-third of the depth of the infant's chest.

Chest compression >1 year
- Place the heel of one hand over the lower half of the sternum and give compressions and breaths at a ratio of 15:2.

The aetiology of cardiac arrest in adults can be broadly classified as *cardiac* and *non-cardiac*:

Coronary artery disease is the leading cause of cardiac arrest in adults.
Trauma is the leading cause of non-ischaemic cardiac arrests.

Types of cardiac arrest
Shockable rhythms
Ventricular fibrillation (VF): chaotic electrical activity of the heart which makes the heart quiver (fibrillate) and stops it from pumping blood. See Fig 12.6.

Ventricular tachycardia (VT): see Fig 12.7.

Non-shockable rhythms
Asystole (flatline): no cardiac electrical activity, the heart does not contract and hence there is no blood flow (i.e. cardiac output). See Fig. 12.8.

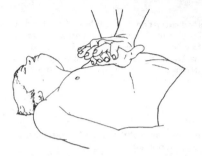

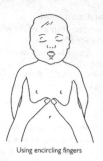

Using encircling fingers

Fig. 12.3 Chest compressions.
Reproduced from Wyatt, J. et al, *Oxford Handbook of Emergency Medicine* (4 ed.) 2012, Oxford University Press.

Fig. 12.4 Infant CPR.
Reproduced from Wyatt, J. et al, *Oxford Handbook of Emergency Medicine* (4 ed.) 2012, Oxford University Press.

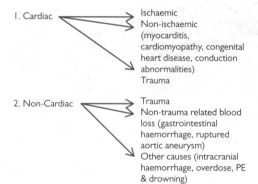

1. Cardiac → Ischaemic
Non-ischaemic (myocarditis, cardiomyopathy, congenital heart disease, conduction abnormalities)
Trauma

2. Non-Cardiac → Trauma
Non-trauma related blood loss (gastrointestinal haemorrhage, ruptured aortic aneurysm)
Other causes (intracranial haemorrhage, overdose, PE & drowning)

Fig. 12.5 Causes of cardiac arrest.

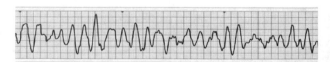

Fig 12.6 VF. Reproduced from Fiona Creed and Christine Spiers, *Care of the Acutely Ill Adult* 2010, Oxford University Press.

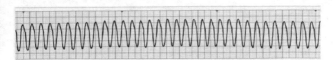

Fig 12.7 VT. Reproduced with permission from Reproduced from Fiona Creed and Christine Spiers, *Care of the Acutely Ill Adult* 2010, Oxford University Press.

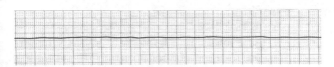

Fig. 12.8 Asystole. Reproduced from Fiona Creed and Christine Spiers, *Care of the Acutely Ill Adult* 2010, Oxford University Press

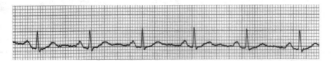

Fig. 12.9 PEA. Reproduced from Fiona Creed and Christine Spiers, *Care of the Acutely Ill Adult* 2010, Oxford University Press

Pulseless electrical activity (PEA): lack of palpable pulse in the presence of organized cardiac electrical activity. PEA has previously been referred to as electromechanical dissociation (EMD). See Fig. 12.9.

Potentially reversible and treatable causes of cardiac arrest are remembered as the 4 H's and 4 T's (Table 12.4)

When faced with an unconscious patient

- *Open* the airway.
- *Look* for chest movements.
- *Listen* at the nose and mouth for breath sounds.
- *Feel* for air movement on your cheek.
- *For* 10 sec.
- *CALL ARREST TEAM*.
- *ABCDE*.

Defibrillation

If a shockable rhythm (VF, pulseless VT, or tachycardia with adverse features) is evidence on ECG monitor, this requires a delivery of current through electrodes attached to the chest wall.

Drugs

Follow ALS and paediatric ALS algorithms for drugs used in cardiac arrest (see Fig. 12.10, Fig. 12.11, and Table 12.15).

Adults

Adrenaline

Cardiac arrest (IV)	1 mg (1:10,000)
As soon as in asystolic cardiac arrest	
After third shock in VF/VT arrest	
Anaphylaxis (IM)	0.5 mg (1:1000)

Amiodarone after third shock

Pulseless VT and VF (IV)	300 mg
Broad complex tachycardia	300 mg (10–20 min if adverse features) 300 mg (20–60 min if stable)
Bicarbonate	50 mL of 8.4% solution
Hyperkalaemia	
Tricyclic overdose	
Severe acidosis (pH <7.1 and base excess −10)	
Calcium	10 mL of 10% $CaCl_2$
Hyperkalaemia, hypocalcaemia	
Ca^{2+} channel blocker or Mg^{2+} overdose	
Magnesium	
Torsades de pointes (form of VF)	2 g

Children

Adrenaline

Cardiac arrest (IV)	0.1 mg/kg (1:10,000)
As soon as in asystolic cardiac arrest	
After third shock in VF/VT arrest	
Anaphylaxis (IM)	
>12 years of age	0.5 mg (1:1000)
6–12 years of age	0.3 mg (1:1000)
<6 years of age	0.15 mg (1:1000)
Amiodarone after third shock	
Pulseless VT & VF (IV)	5 mg/kg
Bicarbonate	1 mL/kg of 8.4% solution

Table 12.4 Reversible causes of cardiac arrest

4 Hs	4 Ts
1. Hypovolaemia	1. Toxins
2. Hypoxia	2. Tamponade (cardiac)
3. Hyperkalaemia or Hypokalaemia	3. Tension pneumothorax
4. Hypothermia	4. Thromboembolism

Calcium	0.3 mL/kg of 10% calcium gluconate
Hyperkalaemia, hypocalcaemia	
Glucose	2 mL/kg of 10% solution
Magnesium	25–50 mg/kg
in Torsades de pointes (form of VF)	

Disability

Check GCS, pupil size and reactivity, posture, tone of all four limbs, and plantar reflexes.

Exposure

Remove the patient's clothes and check for clues as to the cause of the arrest such as rashes (septicaemia, anaphylaxis), injuries, rectal/vaginal bleeding, or melaena. Measure temperature and cover the patient with a blanket to prevent hypothermia and for dignity.

Do relevant blood tests including ABGs, 12-lead ECG, CXR, and other X-rays if injury suspected.

Paediatric resuscitation

- Weight:
  - 0–12 months = 0.5 × age in months + 4.
  - 1–5 years = 2 × age in years + 8.
  - 6–12 years = 3 × age in years + 7.
- Energy: 4 J/kg
- Tracheal tube:
  - Internal diameter (mm) = (age/4) + 4.
  - Length (oral) (cm) = (age/2) + 12.
  - Length (nasal) (cm) = (age/2) + 15.
- Fluid bolus = 20 mL/kg (aliquots of 10 mL/kg in trauma).
- Lorazepam = 0.1 mg/kg (maximum of 4 mg).
- Adrenaline = 0.1 mL/kg of 1:10,000.
- Glucose = 2 mL/kg 10% glucose.

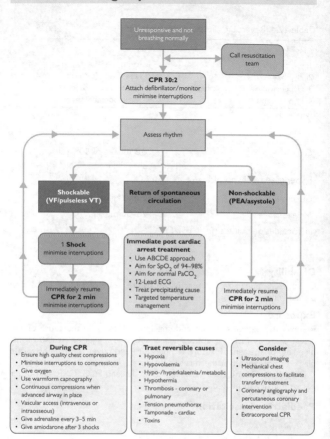

Fig. 12.10 Adult ALS. Reproduced with permission from Resuscitation Council (UK) 2015, www.resus.org.uk/resuscitation-guidelines/adult-advanced-life-support/.

Anaphylaxis

Definition

A severe systemic allergic reaction. The diagnosis is not always obvious but is highly likely if there is:
- sudden onset and rapid progression of symptoms
- life-threatening airway/breathing/circulation problems
- skin/mucosal changes (flushing, urticaria, angio-oedema).

Airway problems
- Throat and tongue swelling
- Throat 'closing up'
- Hoarse voice
- Stridor.

Breathing problems
- Shortness of breath
- Tachypnoea
- Wheeze
- Exhaustion
- Hypoxia
- Confusion
- Cyanosis
- Respiratory arrest.

Circulatory problems
- Shock (pale/clammy)
- Tachycardia
- ↓BP (late sign)
- Collapse
- ↓GCS
- Ischaemic ECG changes
- Cardiac arrest.

Common causes
- Stings, foods (nuts, shellfish)
- Antibiotics (penicillin)
- Other drugs (NSAIDs)
- IV contrast media
- Latex
- Often no cause is found.

Management

A therapeutics exam may ask you to administer adrenaline to a patient with anaphylaxis, simulated by an orange with a cannula in it. Do not be so pleased with yourself at remembering the correct dose (500 *mcg*, i.e. 0.5 mL of 1:1000 for an adult) that you forget it is an *intramuscular* and not IV injection (as in cardiac arrest situations). This is given in the mid-anterolateral thigh. (See Fig. 12.12.)

To confirm diagnosis, blood is sent for [*mast cell tryptase*]:
1. ideally at presentation
2. 1–2 hours after symptom onset
3. 24 hours or follow-up

Before discharge the patient should:
- be observed for 6–12 hours
- be advised to avoid the trigger (if known)
- be shown how to use an adrenaline auto-injector (EpiPen®)
- have prednisolone and chlorphenamine until allergic symptoms subside
- be referred to immunology clinic follow-up for further testing and prevention.

Poisoning

This is an infrequent cause of cardiac arrest, but remains a leading cause in victims <40 years old. It is also a common cause of non-traumatic coma.

Types
- *Accidental*: commonly seen in children and in the elderly population.
- *Deliberate self-poisoning*.
- *Non-accidental injury (NAI)*: fabricated illness.
- *Agents*: chemical, biological, radiological and nuclear incidents can occur secondary to industrial accidents or due to terrorism.

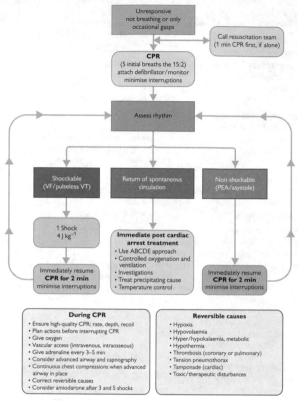

Fig. 12.11 Paediatric ALS. Reproduced with permission from Resuscitation Council (UK) 2015 www.resus.org.uk/resuscitation-guidelines/paediatric-advanced-life-support/.

Table 12.5 Normal paediatric observations (ILCOR 2010 (APLS) resuscitation guidelines)

Age (years)	Heart rate (bpm)	Respiratory rate (breaths/min)	Systolic BP 50th centile	Systolic BP 5th centile
<1	110–160	30–40	80–90	65–75
1–2	100–150	25–35	85–95	70–75
2–5	95–140	25–30	85–100	70–80
5–12	80–120	20–25	90–110	80–90
>12	60–100	15–20	100–120	90–105

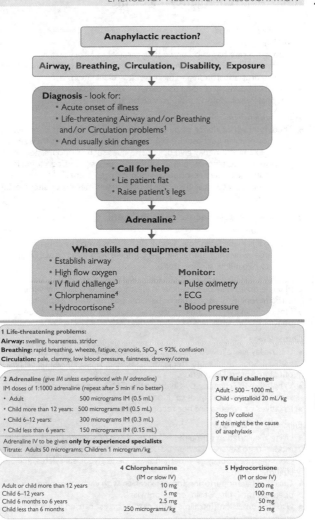

Anaphylactic reaction?

Airway, **B**reathing, **C**irculation, **D**isability, **E**xposure

Diagnosis - look for:
- Acute onset of illness
- Life-threatening Airway and/or Breathing and/or Circulation problems[1]
- And usually skin changes

- **Call for help**
- Lie patient flat
- Raise patient's legs

Adrenaline[2]

When skills and equipment available:
- Establish airway
- High flow oxygen
- IV fluid challenge[3]
- Chlorphenamine[4]
- Hydrocortisone[5]

Monitor:
- Pulse oximetry
- ECG
- Blood pressure

1 Life-threatening problems:
Airway: swelling, hoarseness, stridor
Breathing: rapid breathing, wheeze, fatigue, cyanosis, SpO_2 < 92%, confusion
Circulation: pale, clammy, low blood pressure, faintness, drowsy/coma

2 Adrenaline *(give IM unless experienced with IV adrenaline)*
IM doses of 1:1000 adrenaline (repeat after 5 min if no better)
- Adult   500 micrograms IM (0.5 mL)
- Child more than 12 years: 500 micrograms IM (0.5 mL)
- Child 6–12 years: 300 micrograms IM (0.3 mL)
- Child less than 6 years: 150 micrograms IM (0.15 mL)

Adrenaline IV to be given **only by experienced specialists**
Titrate: Adults 50 micrograms; Children 1 microgram/kg

3 IV fluid challenge:
Adult - 500 – 1000 mL
Child - crystalloid 20 mL/kg

Stop IV colloid
if this might be the cause
of anaphylaxis

	4 Chlorphenamine	5 Hydrocortisone
	(IM or slow IV)	(IM or slow IV)
Adult or child more than 12 years	10 mg	200 mg
Child 6–12 years	5 mg	100 mg
Child 6 months to 6 years	2.5 mg	50 mg
Child less than 6 months	250 micrograms/kg	25 mg

Fig. 12.12 Treating anaphylaxis. Reproduced with permission from Resuscitation Council (UK) 2015 www.resus.org.uk/anaphylaxis/emergency-treatment-of-anaphylactic-reactions/.

Principles of treatment
- ABCDE approach.
- Supportive care based on preventing cardiorespiratory arrest (correcting hypoxia, hypotension, acid/base, and electrolyte disorders).
- Limiting drug absorption and facilitate drug elimination.
- Specific antidotes according to ToxBase (www.toxbase.org) and National Poisons Information Service on +44 844 892 0111.

Watch out for these
- There is a high incidence of pulmonary aspiration of gastric contents after poisoning in unconscious patients who cannot protect their airway.
- Patient examination may give diagnostic clues such as odours, needle puncture marks, pinpoint pupils, tablet residues, signs of corrosion in the mouth, or blisters associated with prolonged coma.
- Measure temperature as hypo- or hyperthermia may occur after a drug overdose.

Substance misuse: acute management
Activated charcoal
- Charcoal is made from coal, wood, or other substances. It becomes 'activated' when high temperatures combine with a gas or activating agent to expand its surface area.
- Absorbs certain drugs but its efficacy decreases over time.
- Multiple doses may be beneficial in life-threatening poisoning with carbamazepine, dapsone, phenobarbital, quinine, and theophylline.
- Not useful in cyanide, lithium, iron, alcohol, and strong acids or alkali poisonings.

Gastric lavage
- Gastric lavage followed by activated charcoal therapy is useful only within 1 hour of ingesting the poison. Generally, this should be carried out after tracheal intubation.
- Whole-bowel irrigation by cleansing the GI tract by oral or NG tube with a polyethylene glycol solution.
- Laxatives or emetics are not recommended

Enhancing elimination
- Urine alkalinization (urine pH >7.5) by giving IV sodium bicarbonate in moderate to severe salicylate poisoning.
- Consider haemodialysis—methanol, ethylene glycol, salicylates, and lithium.
- Charcoal haemoperfusion for intoxication with carbamazepine, phenobarbital, phenytoin, or theophylline.
- Use lipid emulsion (Intralipid®) for cardiac arrest caused by local anaesthetic toxicity.

Specific antidotes
- *Benzodiazepines*: flumazenil. Caution in epileptics, in patients dependent on benzodiazepines can cause convulsions.
- *Cyanide*: amyl nitrite, sodium nitrite, sodium thiosulfate, hydroxocobalamin.

- *Digoxin*: Fab antibodies (digoxin-specific).
- *Organophosphate insecticides*: atropine (high dose).
- *Opioids*: naloxone if signs of respiratory depression/coma.
- *Paracetamol*: N-acetylcysteine (glutathione precursor) (see Fig. 12.13).
- Most common drug in overdose.
- Liver/kidney toxin.
- Just 150 mg/kg or 12 g can be fatal.
- N-acetylcysteine side effects: flushing, wheeze, hypotension, and anaphylaxis.
- Alternative to N-acetylcysteine is methionine PO (<12 hours).

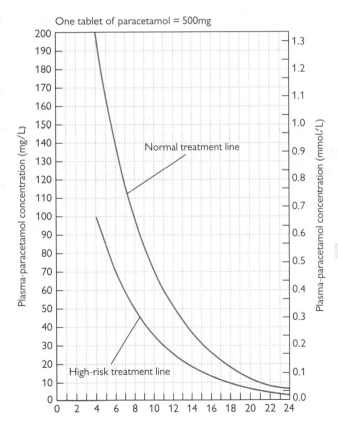

Fig. 12.13 Paracetamol poisoning nomogram. Reproduced with permission from Keith Allman, *Emergencies in Anaesthesia* (2 ed.), 2009, Oxford University Press.

Opiate
- *Classic triad*: (1) miosis, (2) hypoventilation, and (3) coma.
- May also present with bradycardia, hypotension, hypothermia, and
  ↓bowel sounds.

Withdrawal (opioid)

N&V, diarrhoea, abdominal cramps, mydriasis, tachycardia.

Withdrawal (alcohol, benzodiazepine, barbiturates)

Mydriasis, tachycardia, hypertension, hyperthermia, increased respiratory rate, diaphoresis, tremor, agitation, anxiety, hallucinations, confusion, seizures.

Emergency medicine: in majors

The chronic alcoholic

Patients with chronic alcohol problems often attend the ED. This is usually a short visit as they tend to refuse admission. Reasons for visits may be:

- fall and head injury leading to subdural haematoma
- seizures
- alcohol withdrawal
- Wernicke's encephalopathy
- hypoglycaemia.

Wernicke's encephalopathy

Occurs in around 10% of chronic alcohol misusers but fatal in up to 20% if inappropriately managed. Only 10% of patients present with a triad of (1) ataxia, (2) confusion, and (3) ophthalmoplegia. Many of these symptoms may be mistaken for alcohol intoxication so Wernicke's encephalopathy is frequently underdiagnosed. Prevented by giving IV vitamins such as Pabrinex®.

Diarrhoea and vomiting

The vast majority of patients have gastroenteritis. However, it could be the presenting complaint for many other conditions. Differential include appendicitis, femoral hernia, intestinal obstruction (initial phase), pneumonia, myocardial infarction, and ectopic pregnancy. Gastroenteritis ought to be the confirmed after excluding all other sinister differentials. Isolate patients with D&V in case of an infective cause. Admit for resuscitation if unable to tolerate oral fluids or dehydrated.

Headache

Is a common presenting symptom in the ED. It is extremely important to take a detailed history:

- A sudden onset (thunderclap) headache would suggest SAH.
- Fever with headache—consider meningitis.
- If the headache had occurred previously, it may suggest a more benign cause, but it may be a sentinel bleed (SAH).
- Aura would suggest migraine.
- Pain around the eye may be a cluster headache or in the older patient acute glaucoma.
- Painful blindness may be optic neuritis.

Sepsis

Clinical evidence of infection plus systemic response indicated by *two or more* of the following (SIRS criteria):

- Hyper- (>38°C) or hypothermia (<36°C).
- Tachycardia (HR >90/min).
- Tachypnoea (respiratory rate >20/min or PCO_2 <4.16 kPa).
- WCC >12 × 10^9 or <4 × 10^9 or 'left shift' → 10% immature band forms.

Severe sepsis

Sepsis associated with organ dysfunction:

- Hypotension
- Poor urine output
- Hypoxaemia
- Confusion
- Metabolic acidosis
- DIC.

Septic shock

Severe sepsis with hypotension (systolic BP <90 mmHg or MAP <65 mmHg) unresponsive to intravascular volume replacement (20–30 mL/kg) or lactate ≥4.

Mortality rates

- Bacteraemia: 10–20%.
- Sepsis: 20–30%.
- Severe sepsis: 30–40%.
- Septic shock: 40–60%.
- Sepsis with multiorgan failure: >80%.

Early goal-directed therapy (EGDT) in treatment of severe sepsis and septic shock

A combination of intravascular volume depletion, peripheral vasodilatation, myocardial depression, and ↑metabolism lead to an imbalance between systemic oxygen delivery and oxygen demand resulting in global tissue hypoxia or shock. Global tissue hypoxia is the key development preceding multiorgan failure and death. EGDT has been shown to significantly improve the mortality rate in patients with severe sepsis or septic shock. It reduces mortality rate from 46% to 30%, (p <0.009). Numbers needed to treat is 7 (to save one life).

1. *Select your patient.*
2. *Move patient to the resuscitation room and involve a senior.*
3. *Find focus of sepsis.* Order CXR and urinalysis. Look for other foci (e.g. meningococcal rash, necrotizing fasciitis, cellulitis, etc.).
4. *Blood tests.* FBC, U&E, LFT, bone profile, troponin, CRP, random cortisol, clotting screen, group and save/crossmatch, blood cultures (before antibiotics).
5. *Urinalysis.* If positive for a UTI, send for MC&S. If patient has pneumonia, send a urine sample to microbiology for pneumococcal and *Legionella* antigen screen.
6. *Antibiotics.* Give appropriate antibiotics within 1 hour of arrival (ideally within 30 min).
7. *Steroids.* If patient is in septic shock that is not responsive to vasopressors, give hydrocortisone 50 mg IV.
8. *Exclusion criteria.* CVA, ACS, pulmonary oedema, status asthmaticus, cardiac arrhythmia, GI bleeds, seizures, trauma.
9. *Give OXYGEN.* Insert (1) central line, (2) arterial line, (3) urinary catheter
10. *Monitor vital signs.* BP, HR, respiratory rate, temperature, GCS. Start cardiac monitor, also get an ECG and pulse oximetry.

Considerations
- *Follow protocol*: consider infusion charts for noradrenaline and dopexamine to maintain adequate perfusion.
- *Monitor glucose*: aim for glucose <8.3 mmol/L (start insulin infusion if necessary).
- *Haemoglobin*: aim for Hb >8.

Timing of antibiotics in septic shock

Timing of antibiotic treatment in septic shock is vital. A retrospective study of patients admitted to ITU with septic shock suggests that administration of antibiotics within the first 30 min of documented hypotension was associated with an 82.7% survival rate. Administration in the second 30 min was associated with 77.2% survival. The aggregate survival rate for the first hour is 79.9%. Each hour delay in the first 6 hours was associated with a 7.6% increase in mortality, resulting in a mortality rate of 42% if given at 6 hours following first drop in BP.[1]

Lactate

Lactate may be raised for several reasons. For instance, an alcoholic with liver impairment may have a high lactate due to ↓clearance. When starting EGDT based on a lactate, do so on an *arterial* lactate. A venous lactate may be raised due to a tight tourniquet.

Oxygen

It is crucial to provide optimal oxygen therapy to the acutely breathless patient. Oxygen may be delivered by well-fitted face mask with a non-rebreathing reservoir bag, Venturi mask, or nasal prongs (see Fig. 12.14).
- Oxygen is a drug and must be prescribed.
- Oxygen therapy should continue during other treatments such as nebulized therapy.
- Venturi masks should always be used in patients at risk of hypercapnia due to chronic respiratory failure.
- A well-fitted mask with a non-rebreathing reservoir bag should be used to deliver high-concentration oxygen to patients who require it.
- Patients should have continuous monitoring of pulse oximetry.
- The only role for nasal prongs in emergency treatment is to give supplementary low-flow oxygen therapy to patients with known hypercapnic COPD during bronchodilator treatment with an air-driven nebulizer.

Fixed performance masks (Venturi masks)

These masks can deliver an accurate percentage of O_2, ranging from 24% to 60% (see Table 12.6).

Nasal cannulae

These consist of a length of tubing with two prongs, which fit into the nostrils (see Table 12.7).
- Maximum 4 L/min as it can cause nasal mucosal drying and does not increase FiO_2.
- Nasal cannulae should be used to deliver O_2 to patients having nebulized medication if the driving gas is air.

Table 12.6 Venturi masks

Venturi valve	24% (blue)	28% (white)	35% (yellow)	40% (red)	60% (green)
O_2 flow (L/min)	2	4	8	10	15

Table 12.7 Nasal cannulae

L/min	% O_2
1	24%
2	28%
3	32%
4	36%

Humidification of oxygen
- Prevent the airway becoming dry and any secretions becoming tenacious and therefore difficult to clear.
- Warming inspired gases increases their ability to hold water.

Wound care

Principle
To achieve rapid and complete healing of skin and soft tissue structures producing optimal functional and cosmetic results.

Priority
Life before limb! Wound care is part of the secondary survey.

Mechanism
How the injury was caused gives clues to which structures and to what extent tissue will be injured. Then likely complications can be predicted and measures taken to avoid them.

Examples
- *Incised wounds* (glass/knife) are associated with minimal skin damage and rarely become infected or leave ugly scars. However, tissue may be divided down to bone so tendon, nerve, and vessel damage must be looked for. Exploration under anaesthesia with the use of a tourniquet is advised, particularly in children unable to cooperate with examination.
- *Crushing tissue* devitalizes it so the laceration may be stellate and some tissue may need to be excised to prevent necrosis and infection. Dirt may have been forced into tissue.
- *Shearing forces* rip skin away from blood supply, and careful examination and monitoring is required to identify ischaemic skin which initially looks viable, or compartment syndrome. This commonly happens to young pedestrians when a car tyre rolls over their limb.
- *Punch injuries* to hands need to be considered as human bites if skin is broken by a tooth/teeth. These often extend into the joint and septic arthritis can occur.

History
- How (mechanism)? When (degree of bacterial contamination/ proliferation already occurred)? Where (what kind of foreign body or pathogen to expect)? Who (in case of bite from human or animal)?
- Medical history and drug allergies (diabetes, corticosteroids, immunosuppressants).
- Vaccination (tetanus and hepatitis B status).
- Occupation, hobbies, and hand dominance.

Examination
- Pre and post anaesthesia (analgesia can be given immediately if required, but nerve function must be assessed and documented prior to local anaesthetic or sedation).
- Skin cover.
- Circulation (of the skin and distal structures).
- Nerve injury: check sensory and motor function and sweating. Remember nerves and vessels run together in bundles.
- Bone and joints (?exposed).
- Tendons, ligaments, and ducts (?any visible).

Investigation
- Plain radiograph for fracture, air, or foreign body (glass, metal, or tooth). All wounds sustained from a foreign body, especially broken glass, must have imaging since they can usually be identified.
- Bloods and cultures if septic.
- Wound swab if pus, blood, or exudate present.

Treatment
- Irrigate with copious warm saline and antiseptics.
- Debride devitalized tissue and remove dirt and foreign bodies.
- Close wound if appropriate or possible.
- Dress wound with non-adherent dressing (Mepitel® or Jelonet®) and self-adhesive dressing or gauze and crepe bandage to provide a moist, occluded healing environment and relieve pain.
- Elevate limbs, especially hands, to relieve swelling.
- Consider antibiotic use, tetanus, and boosters for blood-borne viruses.

Prophylactic antibiotic use
- Lacerations: nil.
- Heavily contaminated wounds which cannot be cleaned thoroughly: penicillin (erythromycin if allergic) and anaerobic cover depending upon contaminant as well as tetanus.
- Human/animal bites: co-amoxiclav and tetanus.
- Open fracture: IV benzylpenicillin and flucloxacillin (or cefotaxime).
- Minor (e.g. phalangeal injuries): nil but clean under local anaesthetic.
- Delay in debridement.
- Immunocompromised patients.

Refer to plastics team on-call for:
- penetrating wounds of hand or finger involving nerve, tendons, or vascular damage
- wound involving joint space
- deep facial wounds
- deep human or animal bites

Wound closure

Sutures

Use non-absorbable interrupted sutures on skin. *Absorbable* sutures are for mucosal surfaces and deep closure, but this is not required in most wounds. An approximate guide for size and time before removal:
- Face: 6/0, 3–5 days.
- Scalp: 3–4/0, 7 days.
- Trunk: 3–5/0, 7–10 days.
- Limbs: 3–5/0, 7–10 days.
- Hands: 5/0, 7 days plus.

Glue

Use on clean, uncomplicated wounds (i.e. skin only, parallel to Langer's lines) which oppose neatly with little tension. Hold wound edges together and apply the glue to the surface, do not sandwich it between tissue edges. Wait for it to dry before releasing wound. Wear gloves in case the glue trickles and sticks your finger to the patient. Be very careful in the region of the eye; position the patient so that any excess runs away from the eye.

Wound closure strips

Use on superficial wounds (skin only) in areas where the skin is not subject to much tension spreading the wound (e.g. the volar surface of the wrist as compared to the anterior thigh). Apply with no tension to prevent blisters forming. Wounds which bleed actively will probably be too wet for wound closure strips to stick, and the dressing used should be dry otherwise it will cause the strips to move. Use wide strips as the tension is more evenly distributed. Never use circumferential closure strips on digits/penis. Do not cover a flap laceration completely in closure strips as at early review they would need to be removed in order to assess viability.

Honours

The following wounds should not be sutured, closed with closure strips, or glued (i.e. where there is potential for wound infection):
- Wound older than 8 hours.
- Dehisced wounds without a senior review.
- Heavily contaminated wounds.
- Human and animal bites.

Reference

1. Kumar A, Roberts D, Wood KE, et al. (2006). Duration of hypotension before initiation of effective antimicrobial therapy is the critical determinant of survival in human septic shock. *Crit Care Med* 34(6):1589–96.

Emergency medicine: in the paediatric emergency department

Stridor

Is a harsh, vibratory sound produced by turbulent airflow through a partially obstructed airway. Stridor is a conspicuous symptom of an underlying pathology causing an airway obstruction which could be life-threatening. Stridor can be inspiratory, expiratory, or biphasic (obstruction at the level of the glottis or subglottis).

Honours

Holinger's laws of airway

1. Obstruction that is worse when the child is 'awake' suggests laryngeal, tracheal, or bronchial cause. Obstruction that is worse when the child is 'asleep' suggests a pharyngeal cause.
2. Inspiratory stridor suggests that the obstruction is 'extrathoracic' (larynx/nasopharynx). Expiratory stridor suggests that the obstruction is 'intrathoracic' (trachea and bronchus).

Causes

Age of onset

- *Birth*: choanal atresia, laryngeal web, vascular ring, vocal cord paralysis.
- *4–6 weeks*: laryngo/tracheomalacia.
- *6 months–3 years*: croup (peak incidence at 2 years of age, can occur in older children).
- *1–4 years*: foreign body aspiration (peak incidence at 1–2 years of age, can occur in older children).
- *2–16 years*: epiglottitis and retropharyngeal abscess (peak incidence at 3 years of age), bacterial tracheitis, peritonsillar abscess (peak incidence at 8 years of age).
- *Any age*: angio-oedema and laryngeal trauma.

Croup is the most common cause of acute stridor while laryngomalacia is most common cause of chronic stridor in children. Consider laryngotracheal stenosis (secondary to endotracheal intubation) in low-birth-weight infants. Stridor aggravated during feeding could suggest external compression of

Table 12.8 Signs of ineffective vs effective coughing

Ineffective coughing	Effective cough
- Unable to vocalize	- Crying or verbal response to questions
- Quiet or silent cough	- Loud cough
- Unable to breathe	- Able to take a breath before coughing
- Cyanosis	- Fully responsive
- Decreasing level of consciousness	

the trachea. If the airway is severely compromised, it has to be secured prior to any investigations. Exhaustion (quiet and shallow breathing) or silent chest on auscultation, cyanosis, saturation <85% on air, and hypotension are pre-terminal signs → call the paediatric arrest team along with the on-call ENT and paediatric anaesthetist.

All children will require high-flow oxygen but arm yourself with nebulized adrenaline, antibiotics, and steroids.

Tests

AP and lateral radiographs of the neck and chest are useful in the evaluation of a child with stridor. Flexible fibreoptic nasolaryngoscopy aids visualization of the nasal passages, naso/hypopharynx, and supraglottic larynx. It can be performed in a child who is awake. Fibreoptic and rigid bronchoscopy aids visualization below the glottis and the latter in removal of foreign bodies and with tissue diagnosis. Contrast-enhanced CT helps to identify the causes of extrinsic compression of the airway.

Choking

Is characterized by the sudden onset of respiratory distress associated with coughing, gagging, or stridor, a possible history of eating or playing with small items prior to the onset of symptoms, and in the absence of other signs of illness. When a foreign body enters a child's airway, they tend to cough with a view to expel the foreign body. A spontaneous cough is safe and much more effective than any manoeuvre (back slaps, chest thrust, or Heimlich) a rescuer performs.

Choking can lead to asphyxiation and rapid deterioration if the cough is absent or ineffective and the object obstructs the airway completely (see Table 12.8). If a child becomes unconscious and a foreign body is visible on opening the mouth, make a single attempt to remove it with a finger sweep. Beware of pushing the foreign body deeper inside.

Back blows

▶ In an infant

Deliver up to five sharp back blows with the heel of one hand in the middle of the back between the shoulder blades.

▶ In a child >1 year

Back blows are more effective if the child is positioned head down. If this is not possible, support the child in a forward-leaning position and deliver the back blows from behind.

If back blows fail to dislodge the object, and the child is still conscious, use chest thrusts for infants or abdominal thrusts for children.

Do not use abdominal thrusts (Heimlich manoeuvre) for infants.

Chest thrusts for infants

Identify the landmark for chest compression (lower sternum approximately a finger's breadth above the xiphisternum). Deliver up to five chest thrusts which are similar to chest compressions, but sharper in nature and delivered at a slower rate.

Abdominal thrusts for children >1 year

Stand or kneel behind the child. Place your arms under the child's arms and encircle their torso. Clench your fist and place it between the umbilicus and xiphisternum. Grasp this hand with your other hand and pull sharply inwards and upwards. Repeat up to four more times. Ensure that pressure is not applied to the xiphoid process or the lower rib cage as this may cause abdominal trauma.

Child abuse/NAIs

WHO definition

Child abuse is defined as any act of omission or commission by a parent or caregiver that would endanger or impair a child's or young person's physical or emotional well-being, or that which is judged by the values of the community and professionals. Younger children are at the greatest risk as they are non-verbal and defenceless.

NAI risk factors

- Poverty
- Substance abuse
- Psychiatric illness in parents
- Parent(s) victims of child abuse
- Domestic violence
- Social isolation
- Single parent
- Young parent
- Firstborn child.

Suspecting child abuse/NAI

History

Delay in seeking medical attention, vague or changing history, history or mechanism inconsistent with the degree of injury or type of injury sustained, injuries inappropriate for the developmental age, multiple ED attendances, self-inflicted injuries including repeated foreign body ingestion, alleged assault.

Observation/examination

Abnormal parental or caregiver behaviour, abnormal interaction between the caregiver/parent and the child, multiple injuries at various stages of healing, specific injuries (pattern of bruising from belts, sticks, clusters or multiple bruises of uniform shape, cigarette or rope or immersion burns, oral and genital injuries), bruising in non-ambulant children, bruising in unusual sites (medial aspect of the arms or thighs), sexual abuse.

Investigations

Unusual fracture pattern and skeletal injuries (bucket handle tear, spiral fracture in a non-ambulant child, multiple healing fractures), retinal haemorrhages on fundoscopy, subdural bleeds on CT scans.

Referral

If there are NAI concerns during the history, examination, or investigation stage, please refer to the paediatric registrar/consultant and paediatric ED sister for a more thorough, sensitive, and holistic approach to the case. They will liaise with social services, designated doctor for safe guarding, and the police as deemed necessary. It is *your* and *everyone's* responsibility to flag up vulnerable patients and cases of potential NAI. Never assume that someone else will always pick it up.[1]

Honours

If NAI is suspected, the child is likely to be admitted for further investigations including a skeletal survey. Give consideration to the siblings who may also be at risk.

Differential diagnosis of NAI

- Birth trauma
- Rickets and osteogenesis imperfecta
- Scurvy
- Copper deficiency
- Bleeding disorders
- Skin infections (e.g. scalded skin syndrome).

Reference

1. Royal College of Paediatrics and Child Health (RCPCH) *Child Protection Companion*. ℜ www. rcpch.ac.uk/resources/about-child-protection-companion

Chapter 13

Endocrinology and diabetes

Endocrinology and diabetes: overview

Endocrinology and diabetes are medical specialties related to disorders of hormone production or action. They cover the over- or underproduction of hormones from a variety of endocrine glands, notably the pancreas, thyroid, parathyroid, pituitary, adrenal glands, and gonads. Much of the work is outpatient based therefore you are likely to see the majority of cases described here in outpatient clinics.

Cases to see

Diabetes mellitus (DM)

Features of newly diagnosed diabetes covering both type 1 and type 2 diabetes. DM is caused by inadequate production and/or effectiveness of insulin, a hormone produced by the pancreas.

Thyroid and parathyroid disorders

Among endocrine disorders, thyroid problems are the commonest. Frequently encountered cases include hyperthyroidism, hypothyroidism, goitre, hyperparathyroidism, multinodular goitre, and thyroiditis.

Pituitary disease

Generally you get to see these cases in specialist clinics or patients preoperatively on neurosurgical wards.

Adrenal disorders

Try and sit in a few clinics, you might be able to catch cases of Addison's disease, endocrine hypertension, and adrenal medullary problems.

Procedures to see

Dynamic endocrine tests

Ask to see an endocrine specialist nurse or try and take time to attend the day unit and you will get to see procedures such as the short Synacthen® test, oral glucose tolerance test (OGTT), insulin tolerance test, water deprivation test, etc.

Things to do

- Meet different allied healthcare professionals such as dieticians, podiatrists, nurse practitioners, etc. and understanding their roles.
- One-to-one session with diabetes specialist nurse.
- Finger-prick capillary glucose testing.
- Dipstick urine for glucose and ketones.
- Use of glucometer.
- Treatment of hypoglycaemia.
- How to deal with a needle phobia.
- Injecting and examining injection sites.
- Measuring body mass index (BMI) and waist circumference.
- Understanding oral hypoglycaemic agents, different insulin profiles, and regimens, e.g. variable rate insulin infusion.
- Psychosocial aspects.
- Structured education programmes such as DAFNE, DESMOND, X-PERT, BERTIE, etc.

Endocrinology and diabetes: in clinic

Diabetes mellitus

Denotes a term with abnormal carbohydrate metabolism characterized by hyperglycaemia. It is associated with relative or absolute impairment of insulin secretion along with a variable degree of insulin resistance.

Honours

Diagnostic criteria

Criteria 1–3 must be repeated in the absence of unequivocal hyperglycaemia to confirm the diagnosis:

1. Glycated haemoglobin (HbA1c) ≥6.5 %. The test should be performed in a laboratory using a method that is NGSP certified and standardized to the Diabetes Control and Complications Trial assay.

Or

2. Fasting plasma glucose ≥7.0 mmol/L. Fasting is defined as no caloric intake for at least 8 hours.

Or

3. 2-hour plasma glucose of ≥11.1 mmol/L during an OGTT. The test should be performed as described by the WHO, using a glucose load containing the equivalent of 75 g anhydrous glucose dissolved in water.

Or

4. In a patient with classic symptoms of hyperglycaemia or hyperglycaemic crisis, a random plasma glucose ≥11.1 mmol/L.

Type 2 diabetes

Is by far the commonest (90%), characterized by variable insulin deficiency and resistance. Majority are asymptomatic and hyperglycaemia may be found incidentally. Clinically significant hypoglycaemia (should be in features) <3 mmol/L. Typically patients are overweight with features of insulin resistance.

Features

Sweating, pallor, tachycardia, hunger, trembling, irritability, confusion, coma, convulsion, and neurological deficit. Think of hyperosmolar hyperglycaemic state and diabetic ketoacidosis (DKA) especially in severe illness.

Type 1 diabetes

Accounts for 5–10% and is characterized by autoimmune destruction of islet cells of pancreas → absolute insulin deficiency. About 20–25% present with DKA at diagnosis. A small group of patients (2–12%) present initially with type 2 diabetes but develop autoimmune-mediated insulin deficiency later in the course and this is known as LADA (latent autoimmune disease of adult). More often than not you can differentiate between type 1 and type 2 diabetes on history and clinical grounds but occasionally it can be difficult even for an experienced diabetologist!

Gestational diabetes

Is diabetes or abnormal glucose tolerance diagnosed during pregnancy. Other rarer forms of diabetes include MODY (maturity onset diabetes of the young), secondary to exocrine pancreatic disorders, drugs, etc.

Diabetes in pregnancy

Pregnancy induces a state of insulin resistance mediated primarily by increasing levels of placental lactogen, growth hormone, progesterone, and cortisol which are all diabetogenic. These changes occur to ensure the fetus receives an ample supply of nutrients. Patients with pre-existing diabetes and those diagnosed with diabetes during pregnancy (called gestational diabetes) are at risk of maternal and fetal complications such as macrosomia, preeclampsia, and congenital malformations. Treatment usually includes dietary advice, metformin, and/or insulin therapy (basal bolus regimen). Patients have regular follow-up in joint diabetes and antenatal clinics. It is worth attending antenatal diabetes clinics.

Diabetic foot ulcers

These are complex and chronic wounds with a major impact on morbidity, mortality, and the patient's quality of life. Mostly encountered in the outpatient foot clinics or podiatry clinics but patients are admitted to hospital with severe infection. It is worth sitting in the foot MDT clinic. Successful diagnosis and treatment involves a holistic approach:
1. Optimal diabetes control.
2. Effective local wound care.
3. Infection control.
4. Pressure-relieving strategies.
5. Restoring pulsatile blood flow.

Ask the boss

Choosing insulin regimens (especially in type 2 diabetes)

Ask your senior about the facets especially in type 2 diabetes that have gone into deciding a specific patient's diabetic regimen. They are likely to discuss various factors that influence the choice include the patient's lifestyle, ability to inject or needing assistance to inject insulin, occurrence of hypoglycaemia, etc., and it is good to start to apply these risks/benefits for specific patients yourself.

Diabetes management

Evaluation

History: osmotic symptoms such as polyuria, polydipsia, nocturia, blurred vision, weight loss, etc. *Clinical examination*: BMI, CVS examination, look for any complications—neuropathy, retinopathy, and foot ulcers.

Investigations
- Bloods: FBC, U&E, LFTs, TFTs, HbA1c, fasting lipids, 12-lead ECG.
- Urine analysis.
- Insulin antibodies (anti-islet cell, anti-GAD, anti-IA-2).
- Glucose and C-peptide.

Lifestyle

Dietary advice—low-fat, low-glycaemic index diet tailored to individual. Regular exercise (30 min × five times a week), smoking cessation, reduction in alcohol consumption.

Medication
Oral hypoglycaemics: biguanides: metformin—first line in overweight patients. Sulfonylureas: e.g. gliclazide—first line in lean patients with type 2 diabetes. Other class of drugs: thiazolinediones, DDP4 inhibitors, SGLT2 inhibitors, prandial glucose regulators, and alpha-glucosidase inhibitors.

Honours
Landmark studies in diabetes mellitus
Diabetes Control and Complications Trial (DCCT)
Long-term, randomized, prospective study of patients with type 1 diabetes showed that lowering of blood glucose levels with intensive insulin therapy delayed the onset and slowed progression of microvascular complication—60% reduction in risk of retinopathy, neuropathy, and nephropathy and 41% reduction in risk of macrovascular complications.
The United Kingdom Prospective Diabetes Study (UKPDS)
This was a landmark randomized, multicentre trial of glycaemic therapies in 5102 patients with newly diagnosed type 2 diabetes. It ran for 20 years (1977–1997) in 23 clinical sites and showed conclusively that the complications of type 2 diabetes could be reduced by improving blood glucose and BP control.

Injectable therapies
Insulin
Mandatory for type 1 diabetes patients and some long-standing type 2 diabetics will need insulin to achieve better glycaemic control and prevent complications. Regimens are basal bolus regimen (type 1 diabetes) and biphasic (premixed) for type 2 diabetes.

Glucagon-like peptide-1 (GLP-1) agonists
Useful in patients who are overweight or have any occupational implications from insulin use.

Insulin pump therapy
Is usually considered in type 1 diabetes patients (not type 2) who suffer from disabling hypoglycaemia or failure to achieve optimum HbA1c despite injections and high level of care.

Key management principles in diabetes
The following are key principles in the management of patients with type 1 or type 2 diabetes:
1. Tight glycaemic control reduces microvascular complications.
2. Targets must be individualized ensuring safety.
3. *Focus on treating risk factors for cardiovascular disease*: (i) sedentary lifestyle and smoking cessation, (ii) hypertension (aim BP <130/80 mmHg), (iii) dyslipidaemia (target: LDL of <2 mmol/L; HDL >1.0 mmol/L in males, >1.3 mmol/L in women; triglycerides <1.7 mmol/L).
4. *Screen for complications*: microvascular (retinopathy—annual retinal screen; nephropathy—microalbuminuria if positive treat with ACEI/ARB; neuropathy—regular inspection of feet).

Thyroid disorders

You should have a clear picture in your mind about the classical hypo- and hyperthyroid patient. Those you encounter are likely to present with only a few of these features, but by remembering opposing characters this should serve to prompt your memory. Obviously the low and high concentrations, respectively, of TSH will usually clinch the diagnosis.

Hyperthyroidism

This patient is typically thin, sweaty, and anxious looking, and may complain of palpitations, heat intolerance, and loose stool. Elderly patients with hyperthyroidism are harder to identify. The commonest causes are autoimmune Graves' thyrotoxicosis, followed by toxic multinodular goitre, and solitary toxic nodule. Thyroiditis is common. Ask the endocrinologist to go through relevant antibodies with you, and try to find the nuclear medics who may have some old images of the now less commonly used radionuclide thyroid uptake scans.

Graves' disease signs
- Eyelid retraction
- Proptosis
- Chemosis
- Periorbital oedema.

See Fig. 13.1 and Table 13.1.

Treatment
Depends on the underlying aetiology and most common presentation you are likely to encounter is autoimmune thyrotoxicosis. Treatment is either with a dose titration regimen (carbimazole or propylthiouracil) or a block and replacement regimen. Beta blockers (propranolol) for symptom relief. In 60% of relapses, radioiodine therapy or surgery is considered.

Hypothyroidism

Insidious condition with significant morbidity but subtle and non-specific signs and symptoms. It can be easily mistaken for other illnesses and is characterized by high serum TSH and low free T4. Most common cause is autoimmune in the Western world and iodine deficiency globally. You are likely to see patients with hypothyroidism in clinic and treatment is with levothyroxine. Subclinical hypothyroidism is a biochemical entity with normal free thyroid hormone levels and ↑TSH.

Evaluation of thyroid function

The major hormone secreted by the thyroid gland is thyroxine (T4). Both T4 and triiodothyronine (T3) are bound to plasma proteins such as thyroxine-binding globulin, transthyretin, and albumin. T3 has relatively weak binding and therefore has more rapid onset and offset of action. Plasma TSH is the initial test of choice in most patients with suspected thyroid disorders. TSH alone can be misleading in non-thyroidal illness and rarer conditions such as thyroid hormone resistance and TSH-secreting pituitary adenoma. A normal TSH virtually excludes hyperthyroidism and primary hypothyroidism. Intercurrent illness can affect thyroid function and commonly TSH

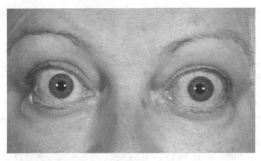

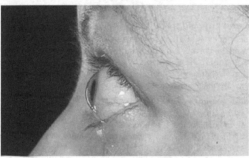

Fig. 13.1 Graves' disease. Reproduced from Jolly, E., et al, *Training in Medicine* 2016, OUP, Fig 7.16.

Table 13.1 Hyperthyroidism

Hyperthyroidism (with increased radioiodine uptake)	Hyperthyroidism (with a near absent radioiodine uptake)
Autoimmune thyroid disease:	*Thyroiditis:*
Graves' disease	Subacute granulomatous (de Quervain's) thyroiditis
Autonomous thyroid tissue:	Painless thyroiditis
Solitary toxic adenoma	Postpartum thyroiditis
Toxic multinodular goitre	*Exogenous thyroid hormone intake*
TSH-mediated hyperthyroidism:	*Ectopic hyperthyroidism, e.g. metastases*
TSH-producing pituitary adenoma	
Human chorionic gonadotropin-mediated hyperthyroidism:	
Hyperemesis gravidarum	
Trophoblastic disease	

is low normal or partially suppressed with low or normal free thyroid hormones; this is called sick euthyroidism.

Total T4 and T3

Total thyroid hormones are affected by changes in binding protein status (e.g. pregnancy/oral contraceptive pill → exogenous oestrogen increases T4 binding globulin), therefore always consider free hormone levels. An important clue is a clinically euthyroid patient with a normal TSH level.

Thyroid antibodies

Thyroid peroxidase antibodies, thyroglobulin, and TSH receptor antibodies are found in Hashimoto's thyroiditis, Graves' disease, etc.

Radioactive iodine uptake

May help in differential diagnosis of hyperthyroidism and is used to calculate dose of radioiodine therapy.

Goitre and thyroid nodules

Iodine deficiency is the commonest cause of goitre *worldwide*. In iodine sufficient areas, chronic lymphocytic thyroiditis (Hashimoto's thyroiditis) is common and this can cause hypothyroidism. Hence, TSH is measured in all goitres. Small, diffuse goitres may be asymptomatic. Large goitres → mass effect (e.g. dysphagia, dyspnoea, or dysphonia).

Multinodular goitres

Caused by nodular hyperplasia, can be euthyroid or toxic (i.e. hyperthyroid). Risk of malignancy in multinodular goitres is comparable to the frequency of incidental thyroid carcinoma. Fine-needle aspiration cytology (FNAC) evaluates thyroid nodules for malignancy; discuss with an endocrinologist the rationale for biopsy over FNAC. Single thyroid nodules are benign in 95% of patients.

Thyroid carcinoma

You need to know about four different types.
- Papillary: 80–85%
- Follicular: 7–15%
- Medullary: 3–5%
- Anaplastic: 1–2%.

Papillary thyroid carcinomas are common, slow-growing encapsulated tumours which spread via lymphatics; FNAC reveals 'orphan Annie' nuclei, and consider treatment options. These include radiotherapy, chemotherapy ± with surgical excision (thyroidectomy: lobectomy vs subtotal vs total). Total thyroidectomy involves levels of node dissection of the neck.

Honours

Multiple endocrine neoplasia (MEN) syndromes are autosomal dominant disorders. See Fig. 13.2.

Hypothalamic and pituitary disorders

Pituitary adenomas

Present with neurological symptoms, or hormonal abnormalities, or incidental masses on imaging. Classified according to size as micro- or

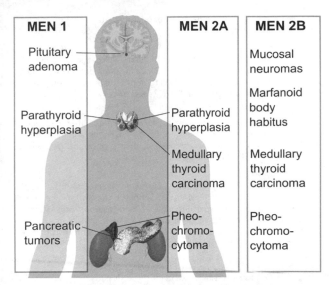

Fig. 13.2 Multiple endocrine neoplasia (MEN). Reproduced from Wikimedia.org. Image in public domain.

macroadenomas by a cut-off of 10 mm. They can be benign or malignant, non-functioning or hormone producing (e.g. acromegaly, Cushing's disease, and prolactinomas). Mostly benign but can like any malignant tumour invade adjacent structures. Perform visual acuity and visual field, to exclude bitemporal hemianopia. Functioning pituitary adenomas such as prolactinomas, acromegaly, Cushing's disease, and diabetes insipidus are encountered in the outpatient clinics. Be able to confidently describe the nature of these conditions, accounting for local mass effects (specific to location and generally raised ICP), as well as systemic hormonal manifestations.

Risk factors for carcinoma

Age <20 years, history of head and neck radiation in childhood, presence of cervical lymphadenopathy, and family history of MEN 2A or 2B or medullary thyroid carcinoma. Do not go into any medical exam without having an acronym for each MEN syndrome.

Acromegaly

Disorder caused by overproduction of growth hormone. It is a rare condition with a long lag between disease onset and diagnosis. *Clinical features*: enlarged jaw/hands/feet, ask about ↑ shoe and ring size. Can cause ↑LV mass, hypertension, impaired glucose tolerance, and ↑rate of colon cancer and premalignant polyps. *Diagnosis*: serum IGF-1 levels and OGTT.

Management: surgery, radiotherapy and/or somatostatin analogues such as octreotide and lanreotide.

Prolactinomas

Most common secretory pituitary tumours. *Clinical features*: infertility, oligomenorrhoea, and galactorrhoea. Check for bitemporal visual field defect. These tumours respond very well to dopamine agonist therapy such a bromocriptine or cabergoline and rarely need surgery.

Cushing's syndrome

Results from prolonged exposure to corticosteroids either endogenous or exogenous. Commonest cause is from exogenous administration of corticosteroids. Divided into adrenocorticotropic hormone (ACTH) dependent and ACTH independent.

Cushing's disease

ACTH-secreting pituitary adenoma. *Clinical features*: easy bruising, thin skin and violaceous abdominal striae. *Symptoms*: fatigue and centripetal obesity. *Complications*: hypertension, DM, and osteoporosis. *Screening*: overnight dexamethasone suppression test, 24-hour urinary free cortisol. Endocrinologists tend to begin with low-dose suppression tests and only use higher doses when results are equivocal.

> #### Disease vs syndrome
> Cushing's *DIS*ease describes a *DIS*tinct single diagnosis of pituitary adenoma. Syndrome is Steroids and everything else (including the Cushing's disease itself!).

Treatment

It is based on the source of hypercortisolism therefore accurate localization is very important.

- *ACTH dependent* (i.e. Cushing's disease): surgery (transsphenoidal adenomectomy) is the mainstay of treatment. In refractory cases bilateral adrenalectomy is performed rarely you encounter ectopic ACTH secreting tumours—excision of tomour is the main treatment. Adrenal enzyme inhibitors and bilateral adrenalectomy are considered in inoperable cases.
- *ACTH independent*: imaging (CT or MRI) is helpful in demonstrating unilateral or bilateral disease. If clear adrenal adenoma, unilateral adrenalectomy is performed with perioperative steroid cover until hypothalamic–pituitary–adrenal axis recovers and in patients with bilateral disease bilateral adrenalectomy is recommended. These patients require lifelong glucocorticoid and mineralocorticoid replacement.

Hypopituitarism

Congenital forms usually result in greater severity of hormone deficiencies. Patients can present with hypocortisolism, secondary hypothyroidism (TSH is not elevated and free T4 is used to guide replacement and glucocorticoids should be replaced first). Sexual dysfunction related to gonadotrophin deficiency is common. Sex hormone replacement is important to prevent osteoporosis. Growth hormone deficiency may require treatment, prolactin deficiency is rare.

Diabetes insipidus

This is a disorder of water balance caused by either defective production of antidiuretic hormone (ADH), called central diabetes insipidus (from posterior pituitary gland), or end-organ (kidneys) unresponsiveness to ADH, namely nephrogenic diabetes insipidus. Presenting symptoms include polyuria (urinary volume>3 L/day) and thirst.

Often occurs after pituitary surgery, especially if pituitary stalk is removed. Sometimes you get caught—patients are polyuric as they clear free water upon administration of hydrocortisone. In general, passing >1 L of urine in 4 hours start to get you thinking. Always rely on serum sodium (usually >145 mmol/L), urine volume, osmolality, and specific gravity.

In addition to polyuria, hypernatraemia, hyperosmolality, and low urine osmolality are present. Treatment is aimed at replacing water deficit and desmopressin for central diabetes insipidus. Nephrogenic diabetes insipidus is treated with salt restriction and thiazide diuretic.

Hyponatraemia

This is seen in 15–20% of non-selected emergency admissions. The key metrics to always think about are the severity and speed of development. Sometimes it is difficult to distinguish salt depletion and inappropriate ADH-related hyponatraemia. One way to solve this is to give a litre of normal saline slowly (water load test) and repeat the serum Na+. (See Table 13.2.)

ADH regulates water balance. SIADH causes hyponatraemia which is the commonest electrolyte abnormality frequently encountered as inpatient. However, SIADH is a diagnosis of exclusion. Low plasma osmolality together with inappropriately elevated urinary osmolality and urine sodium is consistent with SIADH: i.e. the plasma is dilute and the urine is full of salt and (therefore) inappropriately concentrated. Patients are euvolaemic with no oedema, renal failure, hypothyroidism, or adrenal insufficiency. Treatment is with fluid restriction. Very occasionally, hypertonic saline is needed in acute hyponatraemia causing neurological sequelae such as seizures. Newer agents—V$_2$ receptor antagonists (vaptans)—are available but less frequently needed.

Evaluating fluid status

You may forget everything you have learned during your endocrinology (renal or cardiac) rotation, but fail to learn to assess a patient's fluid status at your peril! Ask a friendly SHO or registrar if they can watch you examine the fluid status of a few patients on a quieter morning ward round and demonstrate the elusive JVP. Failing this, go around the patients before the ward round and use the boss's examination to confirm/refute your own assessment. You only need one word to describe your findings: hypovolaemic, euvolaemic, or hypervolaemic.

Table 13.2 Sodium and osmolality differences in serum and urine for pathologies

	Diabetes insipidus	Cerebral salt wasting	SIADH
Serum Na⁺	Up	Down	Down
Serum osmolality	>290	<290	<290
Urine osmolality	<300	>100	>100
Urinary Na⁺	Variable	>20	>20
Volume depletion	Yes	Yes	No
Treatment	desmopressin, water replacement	Yes, normal saline	No, fluid restrict

SIADH, syndrome of inappropriate ADH secretion.

Causes of SIADH
CHUMPS:
- Chest disorders: pneumonia, TB, pneumothorax
- HIV infection (uncommon)
- Unknown (idiopathic)
- Malignancies: small cell lung carcinoma
- Platinum-based and other drugs (SSRI, cyclophosphamide, carbamazepine)
- Stroke (CNS disorders).

Adrenal disorders
Cushing's syndrome
(ACTH independent.) Most common cause is adrenal adenoma.

Adrenal insufficiency
More common in females. Primary adrenal insufficiency (Addison's disease)—autoimmune destruction of adrenal gland is by far the commonest cause in the Western world. Other infectious causes included TB and HIV. Secondary adrenal insufficiency refers to loss of ACTH from the pituitary gland. Patients can present with acute adrenal crises (see ⊃ p. 300). Hyperpigmentation (only in primary as intact ACTH), hypotension (due to hypovolaemia), hypo/hyperkalaemia. Look for other autoimmune conditions: hypothyroidism, vitiligo. IV infusion and IV glucocorticoids should be given before diagnosis is established. You should be aware of how the Synacthen® test works. Hydrocortisone is necessary and all patients should have a medic alert bracelet/necklace at all times and instructed to double the dose of glucocorticoids during times of stressful illnesses.

Phaeochromocytomas and paragangliomas

You may miss seeing one of these during a short placement unless you are in a tertiary referral centre. Tumours arising from catecholamine-producing chromaffin cells in the adrenal medulla are called phaeochromocytomas and extra-adrenal tumours arising from sympathetic and parasympathetic ganglia are called paragangliomas. Usually benign and present with a classic triad: episodic headache, sweating, and palpitations. BP can be alarming high and refractory to conventional treatment. Associations are MEN, neurofibromatosis type 1 (NF1), and von Hippel–Lindau disease (hence patients may need genetic testing). Initial testing includes 24-hour urinary metanephrines (metabolites of catecholamines) or plasma metanephrines (test repeated on two occasions), imaging to guide surgery. An alpha blocker such as phenoxybenzamine is the preferred preoperative medication to control BP. Beta blockers may be required to control tachycardia but should not be started until adequate alpha blockade is achieved.

Hypercalcaemia

Symptoms

The old saying 'stones, bones, moans (psychiatric), and groans (abdominal) is useful way to remember:
- *Renal*: calculi, nephrogenic diabetes insipidus.
- *Skeletal*: osteoporosis, bony pain (malignancy).
- *Neurological*: common but subtle. Fatigue, emotionally labile, personality changes, confusion.
- *GI*: constipation.

Two commonest causes

1. Primary hyperparathyroidism: adjusted calcium usually <3.0 mol/L, chronic, seen in outpatient setting, PTH elevated or normal. Complications include osteoporosis, nephrocalcinosis.
2. Malignancy: acute hypercalcaemia frequently >3.0 mmol/L, seen in hospital setting. (See Table 13.3.)

Polycystic ovarian syndrome (PCOS)

A very common referral to the outpatient endocrinology clinic. Most common endocrine disorder in women and accounts for 75% of an-ovulatory infertility. It is characterized by polycystic ovarian morphology, hyperandrogenism, and anovulation. Treatment is aimed at presenting complaint. These patients are at ↑risk of developing type 2 diabetes, dyslipidaemia, and associated cardiovascular dysfunction.

Table 13.3 Classification of causes of hypercalcaemia

PTH dependent	PTH independent
Primary hyperparathyroidism	Hypercalcaemia of malignancy
Tertiary hyperparathyroidism	Vitamin D intoxication
Familial hypocalciuric hypercalcaemia	Granulomatous disorders
MEN syndromes	Drugs—lithium, thiazides

Dyslipidaemia

It is worth knowing when to use lipid-lowering medication: in all patients with coronary heart disease for secondary prevention and in people without diagnosed coronary heart disease or other occlusive arterial disease who have a coronary heart disease risk >20% over 10 years. You can calculate this using ✇ www.qrisk.org/lifetime.

Osteoporosis

'Porous bones' that are fragile and at greater risk of fracture. May not come to light until patient presents with a fragility fracture after minimal trauma (e.g. fall). Some go unnoticed (e.g. vertebral fractures). Always ask for smoking history and use of corticosteroids.

Endocrinology and diabetes: in the emergency department

Diabetic ketoacidosis

This is an acute medical emergency and one of the most serious complication of diabetes, particularly in type 1 DM but people with type 2 DM can also present with the same condition which is termed as ketosis-prone type 2 DM. You will come across patients with DKA on the acute admissions unit or adult diabetes ward unless they are very unwell and cared for in ITU/HDU.

DKA is characterized by the *triad* of:

1. Ketonaemia ≥3 mmol/L or ketonuria—2+ (urine dipstick).
2. Blood glucose >11 mmol/L.
3. Metabolic acidosis: HCO_3^- <15 mmol/L ± venous pH <7.3.

Management

Your hospital should have a DKA protocol which sets out the treatment algorithm; find it and prescribe a regimen for a 70 kg, 30-year-old male type 1 DM patient with normal renal function.

- IV NaCl 0.9%: give 1 L over 30 min, then 1 hour, 2 hours, and 4 hours respectively, If systolic BP <90 mmHg, give a 500 mL bolus.
- Fixed-rate insulin: 50 U soluble insulin diluted to 50 mL with sodium chloride 0.9% and infuse at 0.1 U/kg/hour (max. 15 U/hour).
- Check K^+ at 60 min, if ≥5.5 do not add K^+, if 3.5–5.4 give 40 mmol/L, if <3.5—seek help (NB the maximum rate of K^+ infusion is 10–20 mmol/hour, use a cardiac monitor). Monitor U&E.
- If taking a long-acting insulin (e.g. Lantus®), continue this.
- Prophylactic LMWH SC.
- When BM falls <14, give glucose 10% 125 mL/hour with NaCl 0.9%.
- Strict fluid balance.
- Fixed-rate insulin infusion until capillary ketones <0.6, pH >7.3, ± HCO_3^- >18.

Hyperglycaemic hyperosmolar state

A metabolic complication in patients with type 2 DM if left untreated can be fatal.

Classic triad:

- Hypovolaemia
- Marked hyperglycaemia (30 mmol/L or more) without significant hyperketonaemia (<3 mmol/L) or acidosis (pH>7.3, bicarbonate >15 mmol/L)
- Osmolality (measure osmolality 2Na + glucose+urea) usually 320 mosmol/kg or more N.B.A mixed picture of HHS and DKA may occur.

It develops over weeks precipitated by infection and dehydration → emergency admissions. It should be no surprise that treatment is robust rehydration, bringing down blood sugars slowly by IV insulin infusion, and treating the underlying precipitating factor.

- Fluid replacement is the mainstay. Typically aim for 50% of fluid replacement in the first 12 hours (3–6 litre positive balance).
- IV insulin: 50 U soluble insulin diluted to 50 mL with NaCl 0.9%. Fixed rate insulin is usually given at 0.05 units/kg/hour only if blood ketones are >1.0
- Check K^+, PO_4^{3-}, and glucose whenever a bag is replaced.
- If K >5.5—do not add K^+.
- If K 3.5–5.5—add 40 mmol KCl per 1000 mL.
- If K <3.5—seek senior input, may require central line. Prophylactic low molecular weight heparin as it is a prothrombotic state

Hypoglycaemia

This is in fact the most common diabetic emergency. Present with autonomic features (tremor, anxiety, palpitations, etc.) usually at plasma glucose levels of <3.3 mmol/L. As the blood glucose levels fall below 2.8 mmol/L, neuroglycopaenia ensues (weakness, lethargy, confusion). Treatment is with IV glucose/IM glucagon/glucogel/glucose tablets.

Endocrine emergencies

Thyroid storm/thyrotoxic crises

This acute life-threatening exacerbation of thyrotoxicosis is extremely rare, and you are extremely unlikely to encounter a case outside your exams. Presentation of high fever, >40°C (and hence sweating, tachycardia), agitation, and delirium. Supportive management which means fluids, antipyretics (paracetamol), and cooling measures (think how this can be achieved) in order to avoid cerebral complications of hyperpyrexia. Endocrinologists will prescribe propylthiouracil to block synthesis of thyroid hormones and iodides (potassium iodide) which block conversion of T4 to T3. Also useful are beta blockers, steroids, and colestyramine. Aspirin should be avoided as it exacerbates the situation.

> ### Honours
>
> The *CORTICUS* study (Corticosteroid Therapy of Septic Shock) demonstrated that hydrocortisone therapy did not improve survival or reversal of shock in patients with septic shock and at the present time the utility of steroid therapy in sepsis remains controversial.

Acute adrenal insufficiency

Usually occurs as an acute illness in a patient with chronic adrenal insufficiency precipitated by omission of steroids or concurrent severe illness. This diagnosis is hard to spot: think about the elderly patient who has been admitted for an elective knee replacement, and does not take her steroids for PMR postoperatively. A few days later, she is found to be a lethargic and unwell patient, vomiting or complaining of vague abdominal pains. She is hypotensive and not fluid responsive, and may have a low sodium on routine bloods. Treatment is with IV hydrocortisone (50–100 mg every 6 hours), IV fluids, and treating the precipitating cause. Mineralocorticoids are not necessary acutely as the receptors are saturated by glucocorticoids.

Pituitary apoplexy

Pituitary apoplexy is another rare but alarming syndrome characterized by sudden onset of headache, vomiting, visual impairment, and ↓consciousness caused by haemorrhage and/or infarction of the pituitary gland. Endocrine and neurosurgical teams will manage these patients, monitoring pituitary profile and MRI scans, and providing supportive treatment which includes (lifesaving!) rapid steroid replacement, and surgery in those with neuro-ophthalmic features.

Hyponatraemia

Acute hyponatraemia presents with headache, nausea, vomiting, lethargy, hyporeflexia, confusion, seizures, and coma. Exclude pseudohyponatraemia (caused by hypertriglyceridaemia, osmotically active solutes, e.g. glucose). A history of water consumption and different diagnostic possibilities should be worked out for cause-specific treatment. (See Fig. 13.3.)

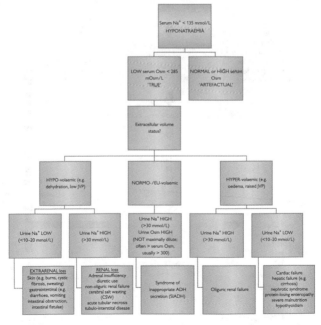

Fig. 13.3 Diagnostic approach to hyponatraemia. Reproduced with permission from Smith, Martin, *Oxford Textbook of Neurocritical Care*, 2016, Oxford University Press.

Use of hypertonic saline (3%)
- Severe symptomatic hyponatraemia requires prompt treatment.
- Institute therapy in high dependency clinical area.
- Target Na⁺ rise 2–4 mmol/L in first hour.
- Frequent measurement of serum Na⁺.
- Do not aim for a Na⁺ correction of more than 10 mmol/24 hours.

Hypercalcaemia

Hypercalcaemic crises should be considered in any patient with disseminated malignancy. Presents with polyuria, polydipsia, and altered sensorium (hypercalcaemia induces a state of nephrogenic DI by uncoupling vasopressin from its receptor in the kidney). Fluids and bisphosphonates are central to management.

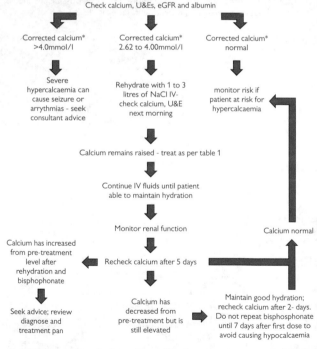

Fig. 13.4 Management of calcium abnormalities. Reproduced with permission from Scottish Palliative Care Guidelines, available at www.palliativecareguidelines.scot.nhs.uk/guidelines/palliative-emergencies/hypercalcaemia.aspx.

Hypocalcaemia

Commonly seen in postoperative setting following thyroid surgery. Typical symptoms include perioral numbness, paraesthesia, hyperreflexia, muscle cramps are quite specific for hypercalcaemia, but like most electrolyte abnormalities, at extremes seizures and coma will result. The pathognomonic signs are Chvostek's (tapping over facial nerve 2 cm anterior to ear lobe and observing for ipsilateral contract of its muscles) and Trousseau's (hand spasms by inflation of BP cuff to systolic for 3 min). Always measure total and ionized calcium (if available), magnesium, PTH, and vitamin D. ECG to look for prolonged QTc. Initial treatment is 10 mL IV calcium chloride over 3–5 min. (See Fig. 13.4.)

Top tip

Always check Mg^{2+} in patients with hypocalcaemia. Magnesium deficiency can compromise both PTH secretion and action.

Hungry bone syndrome: following removal of parathyroid gland (resulting in absence of PTH-driven bone resorption), bones serve as a sink for extracellular calcium deposition. This condition is termed hungry bone syndrome or recalcification tetany.

Endocrinology and diabetes: in exams

Unlike other specialities, most of the endocrine disorders do not present a single visible or palpable abnormality. One relies on astute observations coupled with a careful focused history to establish the diagnosis. It is therefore important that you ensure you attend as many outpatient clinics you can and perfect the art of taking a focused endocrine history, and perform a comprehensive clinical examination, e.g. foot examination. What can you look for in the hands or face that tells you a patient is hypercortisolic, hyperthyroid, or hypothyroid? (See Table 13.4.)

History station

A patient may harbour more than one endocrinopathy and usually within the first few minutes it becomes evident. Important clues include, e.g. hair growth—hypogonadism if absent; weight—loss may indicate hyperthyroidism and weight gain hypothyroidism. If you suspect diabetes, ask for onset and duration of symptoms particularly in a newly diagnosed patient, e.g. osmotic symptoms—polyuria, polydipsia, or weight loss (cardinal feature of insulin insufficiency). Are there any symptoms suggestive of microvascular (neuropathy, retinopathy) complications or the presence of macrovascular complications? Think about rarer secondary causes of diabetes, e.g. Cushing's syndrome, use of steroids, etc.

Regarding past medical history, focus on risk factors for developing complications such as hypertension, dyslipidaemia, or history of any macrovascular complications. Ask for any previous steroid use, and any drugs interfering with thyroid function. Keep an eye out for secondary prevention medications such as aspirin, statins, and ACEIs/ARBs.

Table 13.4 Summary of endocrinopathies

Hormone irregularity	Disease	Biochemical abnormality
Insulin	Diabetes mellitus	$\downarrow$Insulin
T4	Hypothyroid	$\downarrow$T4/$\uparrow$TSH
	Hyperthyroid	$\downarrow$TSH/$\uparrow$T4
GC	Cushing's	$\downarrow$GC/$\uparrow$ACTH
MC	Addison's	$\downarrow$GC/$\downarrow$Na$^+$/$\uparrow$K$^+$
	Conn's	$\uparrow$GC/$\uparrow$Na$^+$/$\downarrow$K$^+$
ADH	Diabetes insipidus	$\uparrow$Na$^+$/$\uparrow$Ca^{2+}/$\downarrow$K$^+$/ $\downarrow$urine osmolality
CC	Phaeochromocytoma	$\uparrow$Urinary/plasma metanephrines
PTH	Hyperparathyroidism	$\uparrow$PTH/$\uparrow$Ca^{2+}
	Hypoparathyroidism	$\downarrow$PTH/$\downarrow$Ca^{2+}/$\uparrow$PO$_4^{3-}$

ACTH, adrenocorticotropic hormone; ADH, antidiuretic hormone; GC, glucocorticoid, cortisol; MC, mineralocorticoid, aldosterone; PTH, parathyroid hormone; T4, thyroxine; TSH, thyroid-stimulating hormone.

A family history of diabetes or endocrinopathies (e.g. MEN, familial dyslipidaemias, etc.) is obviously relevant. The relevance of these chronic illnesses on work and social life cannot be overestimated; ask about occupation, lifestyle, and driving. Ability to comply makes a big difference (e.g. able to inject insulin and check blood glucose readings).

Examination

Cases commonly encountered in exams include the following:

Thyroid disorders (hyper/hypothyroidism, goitre)

The thyroid gland or nodule is both visible and palpable. When assessing a thyroid gland you will need to consider two separate features: the physical nodule or mass and the characteristics that go with assessing any mass along with a few nuances related to the thyroid gland—protrusion of the tongue for thyroglossal cysts, and swallowing to discriminate lesions in part of the thyroid gland that elevate (compared with skin lesions which remain static). The second part is an assessment of thyroid function which is a whole body systematic examination looking for all the features of thyroid disease.

Acromegaly

Signs can be subtle and easily missed and it is worth looking through online Google images and textbooks at a few patients with 'classic' acromegalic facies. Look for coarse facial features and soft tissue abnormalities. Presence of sweating indicates active disease. Do check visual fields even if the patient had pituitary surgery in the past. May have signs of hypopituitarism.

Diabetes complications

Examination of lower limbs for neuropathy and peripheral vascular disease.

Diabetic foot

A history would focus on a previous history of ulceration, amputation, any deformity as well as any symptoms of neuropathy (burning sensation, paraesthesia, or dead feet feeling) and vascular (rest pain, claudication), as well as renal replacement therapy and retinopathy. In addition, a smoking history is important. On examination: inspection—look for any skin changes (callus, ulceration, change in temperature, etc.) or MSk deformities such as claw toe, bunions, or rockerbottom feet. Neurological assessment should identify loss of protective sensation. Use 10 g monofilament and pinprick to assess sensory loss, and a 128 Hz tuning fork or vibration perception threshold using a biothesiometer for vibration sense and ankle reflexes.

Cushing's disease

Look for signs of cortisol excess. Easy bruising, abdominal striae, and inability to get up from the chair (proximal myopathy).

Gastroenterology

Gastroenterology: overview

Gastroenterology is the medical speciality that deals with diseases of the GI system while hepatology deals with diseases of the liver. Although these may be two separate specialties in larger (university) hospitals, liver diseases are managed by general gastroenterologists otherwise. You truly have not looked after a 'sick' patient until you have managed liver failure!

On the wards

Paracentesis is drainage of ascitic fluid (accumulation of fluid in the peritoneum due to liver failure, malignancy, and or syndromes). This is usually done when the ascitic volume is so great that it has made the abdomen tense and may lead to abdominal compartment syndrome. Patients may experience abdominal pain, shortness of breath, and difficulty mobilizing at this point. Under aseptic conditions, using local anaesthesia, a plastic drain is inserted through the abdominal wall, usually in the left/right iliac fossa (LIF/RIF) under US guidance to avoid the bowel. IV albumin is given as the ascites is drained to reduce fluid shift and support BP by increasing oncotic pressure. Volumes in excess of 10 L can be drained in one go. Drains are usually removed after 6 hours to reduce the risk of infection. Ascites is an excellent growing medium for microbes → ↑risk of spontaneous bacterial peritonitis.

Procedures to see

Gastroenterology is a very interventional medical specialty. Most of the procedures will be done in the endoscopy department. Make sure you spend several sessions there so you can see the range of diagnostic and therapeutic work performed.

Things to do

During your placement, ensure you spend time on the wards, in clinic, and in the endoscopy department. Ask about attending MDT meetings. This may include upper or lower GI oncology, nutrition support team, IBD, hepatobiliary, etc. These will give you an impression of the contribution that different professions make to the care of patients with gastroenterological conditions. You may also want to spend time with the MDT members listed in Table 14.1.

Investigations

A day spent in the radiology department seeing patients who have these investigations is a good way to understand what they involve and be able to explain them to your future patients.

Barium/Gastrografin® swallow/meal/enema

Have now largely been replaced by endoscopic investigation, but for patients not able to tolerate endoscopy or in potential oesophageal dysmotility or delayed gastric emptying it remains a useful investigation. The patient drinks

Table 14.1 MDT members in GI medicine

Dietician	IBD CNS	Stoma CNS	Nutrition CNS
Colorectal CNS	Upper GI CNS	Speech and language therapist	Alcohol support worker or CNS

a radio-opaque contrast liquid and has serial plain radiographs to show its transit through the GI tract. Distal colorectal pathology can be identified using retrograde PR contrast enema.

CT colonogram

Is an alternative to colonoscopy for some patients who may not tolerate endoscopy. Optimal images may require taking some bowel preparation and drinking an oral contrast agent (faecal tagging). Images are taken in supine and prone positions and compared allowing identification of lesions such as polyps. Biopsies for histological diagnosis or interventions (e.g. polypectomy) are not possible.

MRI

Is used as an investigation modality for complex liver lesions, accurate small bowel imaging in Crohn's disease (CD), and to assess the biliary tree in magnetic resonance cholangiopancreatography (MRCP) for instance. These procedures often require IV contrast. The presence of metallic implants, claustrophobia, noise intolerance, or inability of the patient to hold their breath for 20 sec may prevent optimal MRI.

Endoscopy

Allows internal visualization of the alimentary canal using a flexible camera. Pictures may also be taken and used for surveillance. It can be used for both diagnostic and therapeutic reasons. Capsule endoscopy has also become popular as a second-line investigation whereby >50,000 images can be recorded from mouth to anus within 8 hours. (See Fig. 14.1)

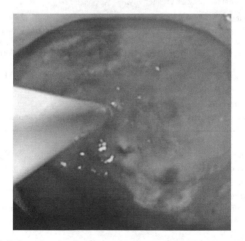

Fig. 14.1 Endoscopic view of an ulcer on the posterior wall of the first part of the duodenum. A gold probe is being used to cauterize bleeding points within the ulcer. Reproduced with permission from Matthew Gardiner and Neil Borley, *Training in Surgery: The essential curriculum for the MRCS*, 2009, Oxford University Press.

Gastroenterology: in clinic

Non-alcoholic fatty liver disease (NAFLD)/non-alcoholic steatohepatitis (NASH)

Fatty deposits within the liver that are not caused by alcohol are called NAFLD. A disease process of fatty change inducing inflammation which progresses to fibrosis then cirrhosis occurs. There is a close relation to metabolic syndrome, obesity, hypercholesterolaemia, and type 2 DM. NASH is the most severe form of NAFLD. Gradual weight loss through ↑exercise, dieting, or bariatric surgery can improve the histological findings of NAFLD. A third of cases of NASH develop into fibrosis and ~15% progress to cirrhosis over time.

Inflammatory bowel disease (IBD)

Ulcerative colitis (UC)

Affects colonic mucosa diffusely and extends from the rectum proximally in a continuous segment. Rectal disease (proctitis) is the most common form. 10% of patients with UC have total colonic involvement (pan-colitis). Associated with cryptitis and crypt abscess formation. Severe flares can cause toxic megacolon (seen on AXR) or bowel perforation.

Presentation

Presents commonly with diarrhoea, lower abdominal pain, and passing PR blood and mucus. The disease course is relapsing–remitting with acute relapses called 'flares'. Tools such as the Truelove and Witts' criteria are used to assess the severity of UC activity.

Treatment

Treatment of mild to moderate disease aims to induce then maintain remission and is with local (enema/suppositories) or oral 5-ASAs or steroids and steroid-sparing agents such as azathioprine, mercaptopurine, and ciclosporin. Biological therapies including infliximab, adalimumab, and golimumab can be used in moderately to severely active disease which does not respond to conventional treatment.

Surgical intervention

Is indicated in patients with a poor response to treatment, acute problems such as major bleeds or perforation, necrotizing fasciitis, or if colorectal cancer has developed.

Monitoring

The ↑risk of colorectal carcinoma in UC makes regular screening using colonoscopy advisable from 10 years post diagnosis of total colitis.[1]

Crohn's disease

CD can affect any part of the GI tract in a patchy or discontinuous pattern creating skip lesions.

Pathology

Transmural inflammation with epithelioid, non-caseating granulomata, fibrosis, and stricturing may occur from chronic inflammation. Fistulae (abnormal connections between two epithelial surfaces) can arise as a consequence of fissuring ('rose thorn') ulceration.

Presentation
Diarrhoea, malabsorption, weight loss, abdominal pain, and distension due to obstruction or with evidence of fistulae. A relapsing–remitting course is most common with some patients having many years between relapses.

Associations
There is an association with smoking. Genetic predispositions exist, including a link to mutations in the *NOD2/CARD15* genes which are found in ~10% of cases.

Treatment
Aims to improve symptoms by inducing and maintaining remission. Oral steroids or an elemental diet are the first-line treatments for an acute flare. Budesonide or 5-ASAs are considered if oral glucocorticosteroids cannot be used. Azathioprine, 6-mercaptopurine, or methotrexate are added in if remission is not gained or steroid dose cannot be tapered down. The biological therapies infliximab, adalimumab, ustekinumab, and vedolizumab can be used in severely active CD which has not responded to conventional treatment. Over half of patients with CD will need surgery at some point to treat obstructing strictures, fistulae, perforations, or if medical therapy fails.[2]

> ### Honours
> *Extra-intestinal manifestations of IBD*
> Include erythroderma nodosum, pyoderma gangrenosum, acute arthritis, uveitis, sacro-ileitis, and ankylosing spondylitis. UC is associated with primary sclerosing cholangitis (PSC).

Most patients with IBD are seen in the outpatient clinic although those with acute severe colitis or complications such as perforations and complex fistulae are managed as inpatients. Aim to see a range of patients with IBD—those in remission and those with active disease as well as those who are pre and post surgery—so that you can understand the spectrum of these diseases.

These are chronic conditions with potentially serious psycho-social effects and the best management is through a MDT approach. Try to understand how the different members of the MDT contribute to the care of patients with IBD. (See Table 14.2.)

Irritable bowel syndrome (IBS)

A functional disorder of the bowel present for ≥6 months with abdominal pain for ≥1 day/week on average in the last 3 months and ≥2 of the following:
- Pain related to defecation.
- Change in frequency of stool.
- Change in form/appearance of stool.[3]

Symptoms
Urgency, incomplete evacuation (tenesmus), bloating, and discharge of mucus support the diagnosis. It is important to check for other causes of similar symptoms (e.g. coeliac disease and chronic GI tract infections).

Table 14.2 Differences between ulcerative colitis and Crohn's disease

	UC	CD
Pathological features		
Tissue depth	Mucosal (shallow)	Transmural (deep)
Pattern	Continuous	Skip (patchy) lesions
Location	Colorectal	Oral → anus
Rectal involvement	Almost always	Sparing
Ileal disease	Less common (backwash ileitis)	Common
Fistulas	Rare	Common
Perianal disease	Rare	Common
Granulomas	Rare	Common
PR bleed ± mucus	+++	+
Smoking	Protective	Harmful
Colorectal cancer risk	Both increase risk (UC >CD)	
Endoscopic features		
Aphthous ulcers	Rare	Common
Mucosal friability	Common	Rare
Vascular pattern	Usually normal	Commonly distorted
Crypt abscesses	Common	Rare
Radiological features		
Strictures	Less common	More common (string sign)
Loss of haustra	Common (symmetrical)—lead pipe sign	Rare (asymmetrical)
Ulceration	Collar button	Rose thorn
Cobble stone fissuring	Rare	Common (if severe)

Management

Symptomatic relief with a combination of laxatives (macrogol), antispasmodics (peppermint oil/mebeverine), and antidiarrhoeals (loperamide). Patient education, lifestyle modification, cognitive behavioural therapy, and antidepressants may be effective in reducing symptoms.

Honours

IBS diet

The FODMAP (Fermentable, Oligo-, Di-, Mono-saccharides and Polyols) diet is an exclusion diet that aims to improve symptoms by reducing intake of foods that are poorly digested in the small bowel. Over 75% of patients report an improvement in symptoms after being on the diet.[4]

Coeliac disease

This is an autoimmune gluten enteropathy. An immunological response to the α-gliadin fraction of gluten, which is a protein found in wheat, rye, barley, and similar grains, causes a lymphocytic enteritis with villous atrophy. Clinical manifestations can include weight loss, abdominal pain, diarrhoea, iron-deficiency anaemia, and other micro-nutrient deficiencies. Diagnosis is based on serology with anti-endomysial or anti-tissue transglutaminase (anti-tTG) levels and histology of duodenal biopsies (Marsh classification) taken at oesophagogastroduodenoscopy (OGD). Treatment is with a life-long gluten-free diet with advice from a dietician.

Honours

Coeliac disease diagnosis

Most people with coeliac disease have human leucocyte antigen (HLA)-DQ2 or HLA-DQ8 serotypes. In cases of diagnostic uncertainty, HLA-DQ haplotyping can be useful. The HLA system is a gene complex encoding MHC cell surface proteins that are responsible for the regulation of the human immune system.

Nutritional deficiencies

Individual micronutrient deficiencies are relatively rare in the general population but may be more common in subgroups such as those with alcohol dependence, concurrent medical problems, hospitalization, or restrictive diets (vegans). Rates of detection of vitamin D deficiency are increasing in the UK.

Gastro-oesophageal reflux disease (GORD)

Recurrent reflux of gastric contents or secretions into the oesophagus can cause heartburn (dyspepsia), regurgitation, and dysphagia or odynophagia. An incompetent lower oesophageal sphincter is often implicated. Lifestyle and diet modifications such as attaining normal weight, eating a low-fat diet, and not eating within 2 hours of going to bed are usually tried first. PPIs such as omeprazole/lansoprazole can reduce gastric acid secretion, raise the pH of the gastric content, and reduce the irritation caused by the proximal reflux. Surgical treatment with Nissen fundoplication is usually reserved for refractory cases (proven by oesophageal pH studies) and has been largely minimized after the introduction of PPIs.

Gastritis

Inflammation of the stomach is very common and may coexist with GORD. Symptoms are those of dyspepsia and include epigastric pain and heartburn. Common causes are *Helicobacter pylori* infection (Gram-negative, flagellate bacterium), alcohol, and NSAID use. Lifestyle modification such as weight loss, stopping smoking, and moderating alcohol, spicy food, and caffeine intake may reduce symptoms. A PPI is first-line treatment. If symptoms do not improve on high dose PPIs, perform an OGD to assess for other causes.

Peptic ulceration

This term encompasses gastric and duodenal ulceration. An ulcer is the dissolution in continuity of an epithelial surface.

Aetiology

H. pylori is associated with 95% of duodenal ulcers and 70% of gastric ulcers. NSAIDs and smoking (and rarely malignancy) are common causative factors. Gastric ulceration can also be caused by corticosteroids, CD, and TB. Duodenal ulceration has been linked to stress and having blood group O although the mechanism for this is not clear.

Presentation

Epigastric pain ± signs and symptoms of anaemia such as lethargy, shortness of breath, or bleeding including haematemesis or melaena.

Treatment

This is with high-dose PPIs (IV infusion for 72 hours if an actively bleeding ulcer is seen on OGD) and eradication of *H. pylori* with a triple therapy that combines two antibiotics (clarithromycin/metronidazole/amoxicillin) and a PPI (esomeprazole/lansoprazole/omeprazole/pantoprazole) for 7 days.

Barrett's oesophagus

Is the replacement of normal squamous epithelium with metaplastic columnar epithelium in the oesophagus visible at ≥1cm from the gastro-oesophageal junction and confirmed on biopsies through OGD.

Screening and surveillance

It is most commonly an incidental finding, however screening endoscopy could be offered to patients with chronic GORD symptoms and three or more factors of age >50 years, white race, male sex, and obesity. Surveillance endoscopies and biopsies are advised (depending on the length of the Barrett's segment and histological findings) because surveillance correlates with earlier detection and improved survival from oesophageal adenocarcinoma.

Treatment

Involves optimizing antireflux medications (e.g. PPI) and surveillance. If high-grade dysplasia is detected, endoscopic resection or radiofrequency ablation can be offered. Biopsies that detect oesophageal adenocarcinoma should trigger MDT discussion at a centre where both surgical (oesophagectomy) and endoscopic treatment could be offered.

Refeeding syndrome

In patients who have been starved or had very low enteral intake for any reason for a period of time, the possibility of metabolic disturbance (especially low phosphate) known as refeeding syndrome should be considered. Daily blood tests should be done until feeding is established and deficiencies actively corrected. Look out for patients who may be at risk of refeeding on the wards and ask your team about how they are managing them.

Obesity

A BMI >30 kg/m^2 is defined as obese. Rates of obesity in the UK are growing and pose a substantial public health problem. Surgical and endoscopic interventions for obesity (bariatric surgery) including gastric banding/balloons and sleeve gastrectomy are also becoming more widespread. Dietician support in conjunction with surgery is usually offered to ensure that the more restrictive postoperative diet meets an individual's nutritional needs. You may see patients in gastroenterology clinic as part of a MDT approach to management. (See Table 14.3.)

Table 14.3 BMI = weight (kg)/height^2 (m)

BMI class	Definition
>35	Severely obese
30–34.9	Obese
25–29.9	Overweight
20–24.9	Normal
16–19.9	Underweight
<16	Severely underweight

Diarrhoea

This is a symptom, not a diagnosis. It can be defined as passing more than three unformed (Bristol Stool Chart type 5–7) bowel motions/day.

History

Duration of symptoms, number of stools/day, consistency, colour and presence of blood or mucus mixed in, with or on the paper at the end of a motion. Clues to the cause of the diarrhoea should be sought: unwell contacts, unusual foods (takeaways/buffets), travel, occupational exposure (healthcare workers, jobs with risk of sewage exposure), or recent medications including antibiotics.

Aetiology

The most common cause of acute diarrhoea is gastroenteritis: viral (e.g. norovirus) and bacterial (*Escherichia coli, Campylobacter,* and *Salmonella*) causes are common. For those with a recent travel history, parasitic infection should be suspected and stool samples sent for ova cysts and parasites. Patients who have had recent courses of (broad-spectrum) antibiotics (especially the elderly or the immunosuppressed) should be considered at risk of *Clostridium difficile* until stool samples come back negative.

Recurrent episodes of diarrhoea without a clear cause should be investigated for other differentials including IBD, irritable bowel syndrome, and colorectal cancer (especially in the elderly).

Treatment

Immunocompetent adults who are able to maintain oral fluid intake rarely need to be admitted to hospital. Admission is for supportive care with oral or IV fluids and rehydration solutions (containing Na$^+$ and K$^+$ which can both be lost), especially for those struggling with maintaining oral intake, who are severely dehydrated, or have profound electrolyte disturbances. Empirical antibiotics are not routinely used but may be considered in cases such as suspected *C. difficile*, outbreaks, IBD, or if immunocompromised.

Constipation

This is another symptom rather than a diagnosis. It should be qualified with a cause or mechanism. Constipation can be defined as passing fewer small-volume stools than the patient usually passes. An objective measure could be fewer than three stools in a week.

Table 14.4 Laxatives

Class	Example	Mechanism	Notes
Bulk-forming	Methylcellulose, ispaghula husk	Stimulate peristalsis by increasing stool bulk	Must be taken with fluids to prevent obstruction Dietary bran along with liquid such as fruit juice is an alternative
Osmotic	Macrogol Lactulose Phosphate enemas	Draw or keep water in the bowel to produce soft, large-volume motions	Must be taken with fluids to prevent obstruction Can be given in increasing amounts in a disimpaction regimen May cause bloating and abdominal pain Enemas are often used before investigations or if large, hard faecal mass is palpable on rectal exam
Faecal softeners	Arachis oil enemas Liquid paraffin Docusate sodium	Soften faecal matter—easier to pass especially if haemorrhoids or anal fissure present	Arachis oil is peanut oil—avoid in nut allergy Liquid paraffin is rarely used and only suitable for short periods of time Docusate sodium has both stimulant and non-ionic softener effects
Stimulants	Senna Docusate sodium Bisacodyl Glycerol suppositories	Increase intestinal motility	May cause abdominal pain and bloating. Avoid in intestinal obstruction Suppositories cause local irritation encouraging defaecation

Presentation

Some people with constipation may pass very small-volume, hard lumps of faeces more frequently but they will not have complete evacuation with each motion. Constipation can cause abdominal pain, perianal pain, haemorrhoids, and anal fissures if very large, hard stools are passed. Faecal impaction occurs when a build-up of solid faeces in the rectum cannot be passed, and if enemas fail, may require manual evacuation.

Investigations

These include AXR and digital rectal examination.

Aetiology

Constipation is often multifactorial. Causes consist of a diet low in fibre, dehydration, sedentary lifestyle, and anxiety.

Treatment

Chronic constipation that has not improved with lifestyle and laxative treatments may be considered for further investigations including anorectal manometry and input from colorectal or biofeedback nurse specialists. Inpatients are likely to have drug-related constipation. Co-prescription of laxatives and antiemetics with opioids is considered good practice to prevent iatrogenic side effects. Try to address hydration, diet, and mobility as well as prescribing short courses of laxatives if needed for inpatients to prevent recurrence. (See Table 14.4.)

Hepatitis B

A double-stranded DNA blood-borne virus. Spontaneous clearance is common in adults, but 5–10% of infected people will be chronic carriers. 3% will have chronic active hepatitis. Two-thirds of patients who are diagnosed with hepatitis B present with jaundice.

Vaccination

In the UK, universal vaccination for infants was introduced in August 2017. In addition, vaccination is offered to high-risk individuals including healthcare workers, injecting drug users, and sexual contacts.

Blood tests

For hepatitis B, include surface and e antigens; surface, core, and e- antibodies; and HBV DNA levels (see Table 14.5).

Treatment

For active hepatitis B (HBV DNA >2000 IU/mL and ALT >40 IU/L) is with nucleos(t)ide analogues (tenofovir/entecavir) which suppress viral replication. Treatment may be lifelong, but can sometimes be stopped if HBeAg seroconversion occurs and HBV DNA is undetectable. See European Association for the Study of the Liver guidelines for further details (ℛ www.easl.eu/medias/cpg/management-of-hepatitis-B-virus-infection/English-report.pdf).

Hepatitis C

A single-stranded enveloped RNA virus. Up to a third of patients are jaundiced at the time of identification indicating hepatic impairment. There is no effective immunization. Tests are antibody levels and viral RNA levels. Genotyping is also necessary to guide treatment. Non-invasive transient elastography (Fibroscan®) can assess the degree of fibrosis/presence of cirrhosis. Traditionally, the immuno-modulators ribavirin and interferon were used over 6–12 months but sustained virological response (SVR) or cure rates were poor. The advent of oral, directly acting antivirals (DAAs) such as Harvoni® (sofosbuvir/ledipasvir) and Zepatier® (elbasvir/grazoprevir) make almost all hepatitis C curable with a short treatment course with few side effects.

Table 14.5 Immunology of hepatitis B

Diagnosis	HBsAg	HBsAb	HBcAb	HBcIgM	HBeAg	HBeAb	HBV DNA (IU/mL)	ALT
Acute HBV	+	−	+	+	+	±	↑	↑
Resolved HBV	−	+	+	−	−	±	0	↕
HBV vaccination immunity	−	+	−	−	−	−	0	↕
HBV reactivation	+	−	+	±	±	±	≥1	↑
Immune tolerant [HBeAg+ chronic infection]	+++	−	+	−	+	−	>10⁷	↕
Immune active [HBeAg+ chronic hepatitis]	++	−	+	−	+	±	10⁴–10⁷	↑
Inactive carrier [HBeAg− chronic infection]	+	−	+	−	−	+	1–2000	↕
Immune escape [HBeAg− chronic hepatitis]	++	−	+	−	−	+	>2000	↑

ALT, alanine aminotransferase; HBcAb, hepatitis B core antibody; HBcIgM, hepatitis B core immunoglobulin M; HBeAb, hepatitis B e-antibody; HBeAg, hepatitis B e-antigen; HBsAb, hepatitis B surface antibody; HBsAg, hepatitis B surface antigen; HBV, hepatitis B virus; [new classification].

References

1. NICE (2013). *Ulcerative Colitis: Management.* Clinical Guideline 166. London: NICE. ✎ www.nice. org.uk/guidance/cg166
2. NICE (2016). *Crohn's Disease: Management.* Clinical Guideline 152. London: NICE. ✎ www.nice. org.uk/guidance/cg152
3. Rome Foundation (2016). *Rome IV Diagnostic Criteria for Functional Gastrointestinal Disorders.* Raleigh, NC: Rome Foundation. ✎ https://theromefoundation.org/
4. Staudacher HM, Whelan K, Irving PM, Lomer MC. (2011). Comparison of symptom response following advice for a diet low in fermentable carbohydrates (FODMAPs) versus standard dietary advice in patients with irritable bowel syndrome. *J Hum Nutr Diet* 24(5):487–95.

Gastroenterology: on the ward

Clostridium difficile infection

C. difficile is a spore-forming anaerobe carried in the gut of up to 3% of adults. Infection usually only follows disturbance of normal gut flora because of treatment with antibiotics. Thus *C. difficile* diarrhoeal illness is almost all iatrogenic.

Prevention

Shorter, narrow-spectrum courses of antibiotics and meticulous attention to infection control including hand washing with soap and water are effective preventative measures.

Treatment

This should be in line with local guidelines but is likely to range from oral metronidazole or vancomycin (for mild disease) to IV vancomycin, IV immunoglobulin, and oral fidaxomicin or adjunctive rifampicin for severe disease. Complications where pseudomembranous colitis develops into a toxic megacolon (colon >10 cm on AXR) is treated with surgical colectomy if the patient is deteriorating.

Liver diseases

There is a growing burden of liver disease in the UK. An estimated one in ten people in the UK have some form of liver disease. Liver disease is the only one of the five leading causes of death in the UK where mortality rates are increasing. The average age of death from cirrhosis is around 20 years lower than that of cardiovascular disease.[1]

Aetiology

The four leading causes of liver disease in the UK are NAFLD, alcohol-related liver disease, hepatitis C, and hepatitis B. Never judge when enquiring about alcohol intake, or events that may have led to blood-borne virus infection.

Transplant

Unlike in end-stage renal disease, there is no effective mechanical support for liver function in end-stage liver disease. Nearly 800 liver transplants are carried out in the UK each year. Demand for liver transplant exceeds the supply of donor organs and approximately one in ten patients on the waiting list die before they receive a liver transplant.

Treatment

You will find patients with liver disease in gastroenterology/hepatology clinics as well as on general medical and gastroenterology wards. Those with advanced or acute disease may be in HDU/ITU. If your hospital provides treatment for viral hepatitis, these patients may be seen in a dedicated clinic with MDT input. To understand the range of liver disease, try to see a variety of patients in different settings and follow them up.

Cirrhosis

Aetiology

Causes can be remembered as **HEPATIC**:
- Haemochromatosis
- ETOH

- Post hepatic (drug induced)
- Autoimmune
- alpha-1 anti-Trypsin deficiency
- Infection (hepatitis B or C virus)
- Congestive (cardiac, cancer, or cholestatic).

Pathology

Regardless of the cause of chronic liver disease, the final common pathway is fibrosis followed by cirrhosis. Cirrhosis is a diffuse process in which the normal lobular architecture of the liver is destroyed and replaced by structurally abnormal nodules of parenchyma separated by bands of fibrosis. It is irreversible and represents the end stage of liver disease.

Diagnosis

Cirrhosis is traditionally a histological diagnosis, requiring liver biopsy. However, non-invasive imaging modalities such as US, CT, MRI, and transient elastography can often permit diagnosis without risky biopsy.

Complications

Cirrhosis increases resistance in the liver causing portal hypertension which causes complications such as varices and splenomegaly. Severity can be measured by the Child–Pugh scoring system (Table 14.6).

Compensated vs decompensated

Patients with cirrhosis who are stable and have enough liver function to meet essential requirements are described as compensated. Those who have developed jaundice, hepatic encephalopathy, varices (oesophageal, umbilical, or rectal), ascites, or coagulopathy are described as decompensated.

Decompensation can be triggered by a variety of factors such as infection, development of hepatocellular carcinoma, GI tract bleeding, or exposure to toxins including alcohol. When examining patients with liver disease, it is useful to consider the following:

- Are they compensated or decompensated?
- Are there features of poor synthetic function?
  - Multiple bruises/oedema/leukonychia.

Table 14.6 Child–Pugh score

	1	2	3
Bilirubin (μmol/L)	<34	35–50	>50
Albumin (g/L)	>35	28–35	<28
INR	<1.7	1.7–2.3	>2.3
Ascites	None	Mild	Moderate–severe
Encephalopathy	None	Grade 1–2	Grade 3–4
Scores for each item are added together.			
Points	5–6	7–9	10–15
Class	A	B	C
1-year survival (%)	100	81	45

- Are there extra-abdominal stigmata of chronic liver disease?
  - Clubbing/palmar erythema/Dupuytren's contracture/leukonychia/ more than 5 spider naevi in the SVC distribution/muscle wasting/ gynaecomastia (pseudo in obesity)/excoriations from cholestatic pruritus (treated with colestyramine/rifampicin/ opioid antagonists/ ursodeoxycholic acid).

Complications of liver disease

Ascites

↑Hydrostatic pressure in the portal vein, ↑sodium and water retention, and reductions in plasma oncotic pressure because of lower levels of albumin result in ↑transduction. This results in fluid shifts into third spaces including the abdominal cavity. The fluid within the peritoneum is ascitic fluid.

Management

Ascites can be drained by paracentesis, however fluid will re-accumulate so management with a low-salt diet, fluid restriction, and diuretics is preferable to serial drainage. Spontaneous bacterial peritonitis is a risk with ascites. Any patient with ascites who also has signs of sepsis or newly decompensated liver disease, should have a sample taken for urgent MC&S.

Complication

Continuing accumulation → tense abdomen, followed by signs of abdominal compartment syndrome (i.e. intra-abdominal organ ischaemia → reduced urine output).

Peripheral oedema

Low plasma oncotic pressure also results in fluid shifts into peripheral and dependent places causing pitting oedema. Management consists of low-salt diet, fluid restriction, and diuretics.

Hepatic encephalopathy

This is a disturbance of normal cerebral function caused by ↑toxins including ammonia. Ammonia is produced as proteins are converted to carbohydrates and is usually converted to urea by the liver. In cirrhosis, ammonia levels can rise causing initially lack of attention, tremor, ataxia, and poor coordination.

At higher levels or in acute rises (seen in blood test), ammonia can cause cerebral oedema which can cause coma, decerebration, and death.

Honours

See Table 14.7.

Table 14.7 Hepatic encephalopathy grades

Grade	Symptoms	Signs	GCS score
1	Poor attention	Tremor, ataxia, poor coordination	15
2	Lethargy, disorientation, change in personality	Asterixis, ataxia, dysarthria	11–15
3	Confusion, somnolence		8–11
4	Coma	Decerebration	<8

Management

Lactulose should be prescribed to patients with cirrhosis and titrated to give at least two soft bowel motions per day to reduce GI tract protein loading and inhibit the production of ammonia by bacteria in the gut. Rifaximin is an antibiotic that is used for prevention of recurrent encephalopathy.

Oesophageal varices

Portal hypertension causes development of varicosities at the portal–systemic anastomoses (lower oesophagus, rectum, and periumbilicus). The periumbilical varices appear as caput medusae. Oesophageal and gastric varices are seen on OGD. They can obstruct the GI tract and spontaneously burst causing variceal bleeding which can be life-threatening (see ❷ pp. 328–9 for details of treatment for upper GI bleeding).

Management

Non-selective beta blockade (propranolol or carvedilol) to reduce pressure in the varices or serial endoscopies to obliterate varices by banding.

Hepatocellular carcinoma (HCC)

This is a primary liver neoplasm (also known as hepatoma). Cirrhosis predisposes to developing HCC with a risk of ~3%/year. Patients with established cirrhosis should undergo surveillance for HCC every 6 months with serial LFTs, alpha-fetoprotein (AFP), and US monitoring.

Alcohol-related liver disease

Repeated exposure to alcohol at hazardous or harmful amounts causes fatty change which can progress to steatohepatitis, then fibrosis and cirrhosis.

Recommendation

Maximum alcohol intake is 14 units per week. If drinking up to 14 units a week, it is best to spread drinking evenly over 3 or more days.

Symptoms

Symptoms of alcohol-related liver disease include fatigue, jaundice, and weight loss. Any feature of cirrhosis may occur as the disease progresses.

Abstinence

Abstinence from alcohol is a worthwhile intervention at any disease stage as there may be incremental improvement in liver function for up to 6 months after stopping alcohol exposure. All patients with cirrhosis should be advised to abstain from alcohol as liver impairment can be multifactorial. Active drinkers are excluded from transplantation waiting lists.

Management

Patients who do show dependent drinking behaviours should have supported alcohol withdrawal (with vitamins, minerals, and chlordiazepoxide or a short-acting benzodiazepine) to avoid delirium tremens which can occur if alcohol intake is rapidly stopped. Ongoing psychological and/or pharmacological (acamprosate/naltrexone/disulfiram) support can help to maintain sobriety.

Acute alcoholic hepatitis

Presents with symptoms of fatigue, weight loss, fever, RUQ pain, and jaundice. The severity of the hepatitis can be assessed using the discriminant function. Scores >32 have the worst prognosis and should be considered for treatment with steroids (if sepsis is excluded) and referral to a local or regional liver unit.

Fulminant liver failure

The time from the onset of jaundice to the development of hepatic encephalopathy is measured to allow categorization of patients (Table 14.8).

Paracetamol toxicity remains the leading cause of fulminant liver failure in the UK, despite restrictions on the number of paracetamol tablets that can be sold in a single transaction.

Management

Patients who have toxic levels of paracetamol that are above the treatment line (see ➲ *BNF*) or who have taken a staggered overdose should be treated urgently with IV N-acetylcysteine. Those with significant overdose and features of liver impairment should also receive supportive care and be discussed with a regional liver unit. Super-urgent liver transplantation is considered for those patients who may not survive more than a few days without transplantation.

Other liver diseases

You may see cases of other liver diseases including haemochromatosis, Wilson's disease, alpha-1 anti-trypsin deficiency, primary biliary cholangitis (PBC), PSC, autoimmune hepatitis, Budd–Chiari syndrome, and infiltrative diseases such as amyloidosis and sarcoidosis. Useful aspects to think about when seeing patients with these conditions would include general supportive care, specific treatments (such as venesection for haemochromatosis), indications for liver transplant assessment, and when screening of family members is advisable.

Liver function tests (LFTs)

A group of blood tests including bilirubin, albumin (Alb), alkaline phosphatase (ALP), ALT, aspartate transaminase (AST), and gamma glutamyl transpeptidase (GGT) are referred to as LFTs. Other parameters including Hb concentration, mean cell volume (MCV), platelet count, urea, creatinine (Cr), and INR are also useful to assess liver disease. Try to look at the LFTs of patients with a range of causes and stages of liver disease so that the patterns (e.g. obstructive (ALP and GGT rise >ALT and AST rise); hepatitic (AST and ALT rise >ALP or GGT rise)) become familiar. See Table 14.9 for LFT abnormalities.

Table 14.8 Duration of liver failure

Hyperacute liver failure	<7 days
Acute liver failure	8–28 days
Subacute liver failure	4–12 weeks

Table 14.9 Liver function test abnormalities

Disease	ALT	AST	GGT	ALP
Viral hepatitis	+++	+++	++	↔/+
Drug hepatitis	++	++	++	↔/+
Chronic hepatitis	++	++	++	++
Epstein–Barr virus (EBV) hepatitis	++	++	++	↔
PBC	++	++	+++	++
ETOH cirrhosis	↔	++	+++	↔/+
NAFLD/NASH	++	+	++	+
Intrahepatic cholestasis	++	++	+++	++
Extrahepatic cholestasis	++	++	+++	+++
Hepatoma	↔/+	++	++	++

Pancreatitis

This is acute or chronic inflammation of the pancreas. Damage to pancreatic cells liberates digestive enzymes which damage tissues causing local inflammation and necrosis.

Aetiology

Common causes are **GET SMASHED**:

- Gallstones
- ETOH
- Trauma
- Steroids
- Mumps
- Autoimmune
- Surgery
- Hyperlipidaemia (or hypercalcaemia or hypothermia)
- Endoscopic retrograde cholangiopancreatography (ERCP)
- Drugs (and toxins).

In most hospitals, acute pancreatitis is managed on surgical wards or in HDU/ITU if very severe. Patients with chronic pancreatitis who experience flares of upper abdominal pain are often managed by gastroenterology teams and so may be found on medical wards.

Presentation

Classically, patients present with severe upper abdominal pain that radiates through to the back. The inflammation may produce a SIRS picture. Those with chronic pancreatitis may also have weight loss, diabetes, steatorrhoea (high fat content in faeces, which may look like slimy stools which float and are difficult to flush), and malabsorption causing micronutrient deficiency (especially of the fat-soluble vitamins).

Scoring

In acute episodes, serum amylase is usually elevated to more than three times normal but is not included in the scoring. All patients who present with acute pancreatitis should have a severity score (e.g. modified Glasgow score) calculated to guide treatment and appropriate place of care (Table 14.10).

Patients with a Glasgow score of 3–4 have ~15% mortality and management in HDU for continuous monitoring is appropriate.

Management

Management of acute pancreatitis is mostly supportive with analgesia (avoid NSAIDs as these can cause pancreatitis), oxygen, IV fluids, jejunal or parenteral nutrition to rest the pancreas, and thromboprophylaxis. ERCP is considered if US and MRCP show obstructing gallstones. Surgical intervention for necrosectomy is rare, only done in severe disease, and a poor prognostic factor. The most important prognostic measurement is CRP which again is not part of the severity score.

Discussion with the boss

When to start antibiotics in pancreatitis? Since the inflammatory process is sterile from gallstones or alcohol, antibiotics are reserved after onset of opportunistic pathogens or necrosis.

Chronic disease

Amylase may be normal in chronic pancreatitis where the disease is burnt out. Faecal elastase testing is used to assess for pancreatic insufficiency. AXR or CT may show calcification of the scarred, fibrotic pancreas. Patients with chronic pancreatitis are supported with analgesia, PPIs, and pancreatic enzyme replacement (e.g. Creon®) that needs to be taken with all meals and snacks. Advice and support to avoid triggers (e.g. alcohol) should be given. Patients need to be monitored for the development of diabetes. Pain in chronic pancreatitis can be difficult to manage and early involvement of specialist chronic pain services can be beneficial.

Table 14.10 Modified Glasgow Pancreatitis Score: PANCREAS

Metric	Value
PaO_2	<8 kPa
Age	>55 years
Neutrophilia	WCC >15
Calcium	<2 mmol/L
Renal function	Urea >16 mmol/L
Enzymes	Lactate dehydrogenase (LDH) >600 IU/L or AST >200 IU/L
Albumin	<32 g/L
Sugar	>10 mmol/L

Pancreatic tumours

Investigations

They are often investigated and managed on urgent suspected cancer or 2-week wait pathways and undergo their investigations (Ca 19-9 tumour markers, CT abdomen, ERCP for histology brushings, endoscopic US) on an urgent outpatient basis. The upper GI MDT is a good opportunity to hear about patients who are being investigated or admitted for ERCP and stent placement if they have obstructive jaundice.

Symptoms

These include weight loss and jaundice ± abdominal pain.

Examination

Courvoisier's law states that a palpable gallbladder with jaundice is likely due to a pancreatic neoplasm.

Type

Most pancreatic tumours are adenocarcinoma and 80% of these are metastatic (often to the liver) at the time of first presentation.

Management

For metastatic disease, the approach is palliative with the option of chemotherapy if performance status allows. Patients with local disease and good functional status may be offered surgery at specialist centres. A Whipple's pancreatoduodenectomy is major surgery with mortality ranging from 3% to 15%. 1- and 5-year survival rates for pancreatic cancer in the UK are <20% and <4%, respectively.

Reference

1. Kaner E, Newbury-Birch D, Avery L, et al. (2007). *A Rapid Review of Liver Disease Epidemiology, Treatment and Service Provision in England*. Newcastle: Institute of Health and Society, Newcastle University.

Gastroenterology: in the emergency department

Acute upper GI bleeding

A patient with an acute upper GI bleed is a medical emergency. Large volumes of blood can be lost before the bleeding becomes apparent.

Presentation

Haematemesis (vomiting fresh or altered blood including 'coffee grounds') or melaena (passage of altered blood PR in the form of black, offensively smelling, tar-like stools). Peptic ulceration is the commonest cause.

Aetiology

Peptic ulceration, mucosal inflammation (oesophagitis, gastritis, or duodenitis), oesophageal varices, Mallory–Weiss tear, gastric carcinoma, and coagulation disorders. Ask about alcohol intake and medication history (warfarin, NSAIDs, aspirin, clopidogrel).

Investigations

FBC shows a fall in Hb and U&E may show a rise in urea (especially if melaena present). If an unstable patient has a low Hb but no overt blood loss, a PR exam to assess for occult melaena is mandatory after resuscitation. Patients with prolific haematemesis can be daunting to see but a methodical approach gives critically ill patients the best chance of survival.

Risk scores

The Rockall and Blatchford scores can be used to predict mortality and likelihood of needing blood transfusion/endoscopic intervention in the next 24 hours.

Management

- Address Airway, Breathing, and Circulation (ABC).
- High-flow O_2 and two large (14 G) IV cannulae.
- FBC, clotting, U&E, glucose, group & save/X-match (4–6 U).

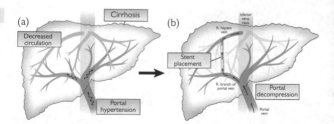

Fig. 14.2 An illustration of a TIPS placed for portal decompression. Reproduced with permission from Bhogal HK, Sanyal AJ. Using transjugular intrahepatic portosystemic shunts for complications of cirrhosis. *Clin Gastroenterol Hepatol.* 2011 Nov;9(11):936–46; quiz e123.

- If SpO$_2$ <93% check ABG. Consider CXR and ECG.
- Give IV crystalloid/blood (aim to maintain Hb at >7 g/dL).
- If unstable with low Hb, use type-specific or O-negative blood.
- Correct coagulopathy (platelets >50 and INR <1.5).
- If the patient is anticoagulated or has a clotting disorder (e.g. liver disease), discuss with a haematologist and give vitamin K/clotting factors/fresh frozen plasma accordingly.
- If varices are suspected, give terlipressin IV and prophylactic antibiotics.
- Keep fasted. Refer to specialist for admission and endoscopy.
- Urinary catheter if severe bleeding to measure urine output.
- Consider inserting a central line to guide fluid management.

Endoscopy

Patients with acute GI bleeding should undergo OGD within 24 hours or on the next working day. Those who are haemodynamically unstable should have an OGD within 2 hours of being stabilized. This requires team-working and liaison between the ED, medical, gastroenterology, endoscopy, and anaesthetics teams. Patients undergoing emergency endoscopy should be discussed with the surgical team in case endoscopic therapy fails and an open approach is needed. Emergent endoscopy is usually done under GA. Endoscopic treatment depends on the type and site of lesion but may include local injections of adrenaline (epinephrine), applying clips, or thermal coagulation. Patients with non-variceal bleeding with stigmata of recent bleeding on endoscopy should have an IV PPI infusion (pantoprazole/omeprazole).[1]

Variceal bleeding

Patients with known or suspected cirrhotic liver disease (jaundice, abdominal distension with ascites, stigmata of chronic liver disease) who present with an acute GI bleed should be treated as having variceal bleeding. Resuscitate as for acute GI bleeding and give prophylactic IV antibiotics and terlipressin. If bleeding oesophageal varices are found at endoscopy, elastic bands ('banding') can be placed to stop the blood loss. Patients with suspected variceal bleeding who, despite resuscitation, are not stable for endoscopic intervention or where endoscopic intervention does not control bleeding can have a Sengstaken–Blakemore/Minnesota tube inserted to attempt to tamponade the bleeding point. Endoscopy is then attempted 12 hours later. Transjugular intrahepatic portosystemic shunt (TIPS, Fig. 14.2) is a rescue interventional radiological procedure for intractable variceal bleeding.

Reference

1. NICE (2016). *Acute Upper gastrointestinal Bleeding in Over 16s: Management*. Clinical Guideline 161. London: NICE. ℰ www.guidance.nice.org.uk/CG141

Gastroenterology: in the endoscopy department

Endoscopy means looking at the inside. Flexible digital cameras (endoscopes) are used which allow specifically designed instruments to be passed down an internal channel in the endoscope to allow interventions such as taking biopsies and removing polyps. All endoscopies require written informed consent. It is useful to see this aspect of the procedure so you can understand the risks and benefits. Risks include infection, perforation, bleeding, failure of diagnosis and treatment, need for future endoscopies, and a small risk of mortality.

Oesophagogastroduodenoscopy (OGD)

OGD of the upper GI tract is used to investigate symptoms such as dyspepsia, dysphagia, epigastric pain, anaemia, or to treat GI tract bleeding or obstruction. Local anaesthetic to the pharynx ± conscious sedation (with e.g. midazolam) is used.

Colonoscopy

Requires patients to take bowel preparation (strong laxatives) prior to endoscopy to ensure the colon is empty and the mucosa can be clearly seen. IV analgesia ± sedation or Entonox® is given. It is used to investigate a change in bowel habit, PR bleeding, anaemia, and lower abdominal pain, as surveillance in those at high risk of colonic polyps, and as a treatment for volvulus or obstruction where palliative stenting is the only solution. The aim is to visualize the entire colon and terminal ileum. Polyps can be snared and retrieved (polypectomy) and tissue biopsies can be taken for histological diagnosis of cancer, IBD subtype, and other causes of colitis. (See Fig. 14.3.)

Flexible sigmoidoscopy

Examines the left side of the colon up to the splenic flexure, usually without sedation. Can be done after bowel preparation or in cases of possible acute colitis unprepared or after a single enema. This is the procedure used for the UK-wide bowel scope screening programme.

Percutaneous endoscopic gastrostomy (PEG)

This is the insertion of a permanent feeding tube through the abdominal wall into the stomach using PO endoscopic guidance. Sedation and local anaesthesia are used. Indications include swallowing problems after CVA, neurodegenerative diseases, or extensive head and neck carcinoma excisions.

Endoscopic retrograde cholangiopancreatography (ERCP)

ERCP is a combined endoscopic and radiological procedure treating problems of the biliary tree (e.g. gallstones) which obstruct the common bile duct or masses compressing the biliary tree → obstructive jaundice. Stenting maintains duct patency. Risk of pancreatitis is notable.

(a)

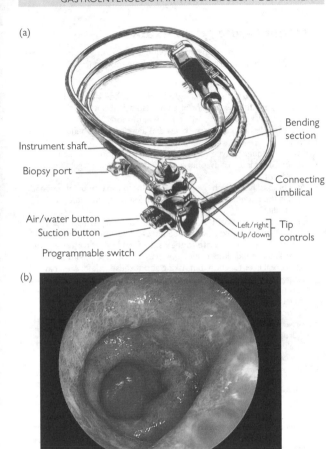

Instrument shaft

Biopsy port

Air/water button
Suction button

Programmable switch

Bending section

Connecting umbilical

Left/right
Up/down } Tip controls

(b)

Fig. 14.3 Colonoscopy. Reproduced with permission from Graham J MacKay et al, *Colorectal Surgery*, 2010, Oxford University Press, and from Daniel Marks and Marcus Harbord, *Emergencies in Gastroenterology and Hepatology*, 2013, Oxford University Press, and with kind permission from the Chelsea and Westminster Hospital.

Gastroenterology: in exams

See the full history and examination sequences for an abdominal assessment on **⮕** pp. 910–16. The following are some more detailed pointers.

History

- Abdominal pain: use a system (e.g. SOCRATES, see **⮕** pp. 148–9, p. 893) to get a full assessment of pain. Also ask about associations with meals, particular types of food, and bowel motions.
- Ensure the following areas are covered in a general gastroenterological history:
  - Bowels: frequency, type (Bristol Stool Chart), blood or mucus passed.
  - Upper GI symptoms: dysphagia, reflux, heart burn/indigestion, waterbrash.
  - Weight loss: how much over how long? Intentional or unintentional?
  - Diet: is the patient vegetarian, vegan, or following any other special diet?
  - It may also be pertinent to ask about genitourinary symptoms.
- Liver risk factors should be addressed in patients who present with liver problems. They mostly relate to the risks of viral hepatitis. Testing for viral hepatitis would almost always be part of the first-line investigations for abnormal liver function, but asking about these risk factors may help direct investigations:
  - Blood transfusions
  - Travel overseas
  - Tattoos/piercings
  - Surgery overseas
  - IV drug use
  - Family history of liver or metabolic disorders
  - Previous jaundice
  - Alcohol history
  - Drug history
  - PMHx of diabetes, hyperlipidaemia, obesity.
- Some patients may find discussing their bowel habits, genitourinary symptoms, or sexual history difficult. It is useful to give the patient a warning before asking personal questions (e.g. 'I'd like to ask you some personal questions now so I can work out what tests we need to do to find the cause of your problem. Is that OK?').

Alcohol history

Always take a full alcohol history. Patients who have a high alcohol intake should be assessed for hazardous or harmful drinking (e.g. AUDIT-C questionnaire). Maximum recommended alcohol intake is 14 units per week. Documenting that someone is a 'social drinker' is not enough as this can range from one unit twice a year (Christmas and birthday) to 10+ units in a binge every Friday night with friends. Aim to get an estimate of average weekly or daily alcohol. Also ask about duration of this pattern of drinking. Know your units!

See Fig. 14.5 for units of alcohol.

This is one unit of alcohol...

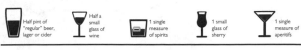

Half pint of "regular" beer, lager or cider   Half a small glass of wine   1 single measure of spirits   1 small glass of sherry   1 single measure of aperitifs

...and each of these is more than one unit

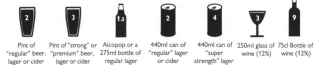

Pint of "regular" beer, lager or cider | Pint of "strong" or "premium" beer, lager or cider | Alcopop or a 275ml bottle of regular lager | 440ml can of "regular" lager or cider | 440ml can of "super strength" lager | 250ml glass of wine (12%) | 75cl Bottle of wine (12%)

Fig. 14.4 Units of alcohol. Reproduced with permission from Alcohol Learning Centre. AUDIT-C questions, available from www.alcohollearningcentre.org.uk/_library/AUDIT-C.doc

Things to practise beforehand

- Use time on clinical placements to practise taking an alcohol history, assessing for peripheral stigmata of gastroenterological disease, palpating for solid organs, and percussing for shifting dullness.
- Make sure you have talked to lots of patients about their bowels so you are comfortable discussing this with future patients.
- It is useful to have two ways of asking your patients to do any manoeuvres you may need them to do. For example, to check for asterixis ask your patient 'Please put your arms out straight in front of you and cock your wrists back'. If they do not follow you could say 'Like you're stopping traffic' and if that does not work a demonstration and request to 'Please copy me' may work.
- Present your histories and examination findings to any member of the team you are working with for practice. Aim for a coherent summary of your findings. Make eye contact with the person you are presenting to with hands behind your back.
- Be logical when answering questions, e.g. if asked for the causes of pancreatitis, although 'scorpion venom' may spring to mind, a more appropriate answer would be 'In the UK, most cases are caused by gallstones and alcohol, and rarer causes include scorpion venom, steroids, mumps, autoimmune diseases, and certain drugs'. Remember that common things are common and you are expected to identify them to demonstrate clinical competency.
- Common abdominal cases in OSCE can be IBD, stomas, hepato/splenomegaly, renal transplant, and polycystic kidney disease.

General practice

What is general practice?

Traditionally, general practice has been community family medicine. The '*Doc Martin*' model of the local GP—working in a small practice, caring for the day-to-day health issues of a known population, often a pillar of the community, mostly dealing with day-to-day minor ailments but also acting as advocate, counsellor, family therapist, and taking care of families from cradle to grave. General practice and the role of a GP have changed enormously over the last 10–20 years. Elements of this kind of practice remain but the speciality has developed rapidly and modern-day GPs deal with far more complex problems in the community than in the past.

Who are GPs and what do we do?

GPs work at the absolute coal face of medicine. We are the first port of call for everything from chest pain to cancer symptoms, from a student with suicidal feelings to a child with a snotty nose and a fever. We support individuals and families through acute illnesses, making decisions on treatment and deciding if and when a specialty opinion is needed. We look after people through chronic illness, managing symptoms when a cure is not possible, weighing up risks and benefits of different treatments, and providing palliative care to those at the end of life. We change lives through lifestyle advice as well as saving lives through identifying and providing timely treatments or referrals.

GPs have to know something about everything, but we also need to know when to ask for more help, and where to go for that help. A good GP has an enormous breadth of knowledge and skill but also has an ability to pick out the needle in the haystack—the febrile child developing meningococcal sepsis, the one person with palpitations who has a phaeochromocytoma, or the one with headaches who has a brain tumour. We have to do all this while being aware of the limitations to NHS resources, and of the harm that can occur from over-referral or over-investigation; while also keeping up to date with ever changing evidence and best practice guidelines.

Public perception, even among medical students and hospital specialists, of what a GP does every day is poor. Well people tend to only see their GP once in a blue moon, and for something fairly straightforward. The reality of a typical GP surgery is far from this. An average GP day might include some of the following examples:

- Renal colic
- Sub-fertility
- Chronic MS
- IBD
- Substance misuse
- Depression/anxiety
- Sore ear
- Breast lump
- Chest pain
- Arthritis
- Injured ankle
- Rectal bleeding.

Of about 240,000 GMC registered doctors in the UK, about 25% are GPs, 29% are hospital specialists, 25% are in training, and 20% are not in training and not on either the speciality or the GP registers. 54% of GPs are female, compared to 35% of specialists and 18% of surgeons (GMC report 2017).

The numbers of GPs per population is decreasing due to some taking early retirement and the numbers of new GPs being trained not keeping pace with population growth. The NHS needs to attract increasing numbers of newly qualified doctors into GP training if we are to retain our current model of asking people to make their GP the first port of call with any health complaint that is not an emergency. In 2012, 24.2% of doctors entering speciality training went onto a GP vocational training scheme.

What skills do you need to be a good GP?

It helps to be interested in everything! If you get bored easily, you like variety and change and enjoy being challenged academically on a daily basis then it could suit you. A bit like EM, literally any clinical presentation can walk in your door at any time. Sometimes it may not even be a clinical problem— but a question about benefits, or someone asking advice on something you never heard about at medical school, such as when to start going to the gym again after having a baby, or how to get your child to eat fish! Unlike EM, no one will ever expect you to perform an open thoracotomy.

You need to like and be interested in people and their lives. This may sound silly but do not all doctors care for their patients? In fact, there is a range in medical specialities of how much direct patient contact you will have and how much you will have to listen to people tell you about their lives and their concerns. If you do not like talking to people, then general practice probably is not for you.

GPs also develop a skill for reading between the lines of what people say and accessing the hidden agenda as to what might be really going on or causing the problems they are talking to you about. What might be underlying someone's headaches or back pain? Excellent communication skills, a good rapport, and an ongoing relationship with your patient may allow them to open up about hidden anxieties or past traumas that are causing physical manifestations that could be superficially investigated with a radiograph but will not be cured until you have addressed the underlying concerns or problems. A robust communication model includes the Calgary–Cambridge model (see Fig. 15.1).

A willingness to continue learning throughout your career is essential. Primary care research is a broad and growing specialty but you are unlikely to become the forefront expert in something niche. As most doctor–patient consultations take place in primary care, any advances in how to be effective in the consultation and in primary care treatments may have the widest impact on morbidity and mortality of all.

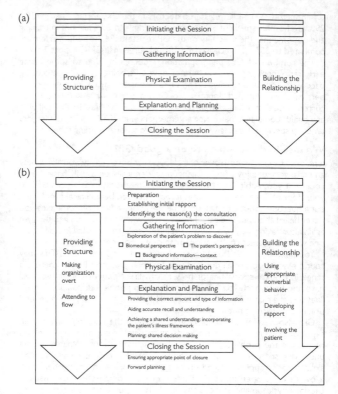

Fig. 15.1 The Calgary–Cambridge model. Reproduced with permission from Kurtz S et al. 'Marrying Content and Process in Clinical Method Teaching: Enhancing the Calgary-Cambridge Guides', *Academic Medicine*, 78:8, pp. 802–809, 2003: Wolters Kluwer Health.

How will you be assessed?

- Clinical audit or quality improvement project.
- Assessment of prescribing and delivering of urgent medications.
- OSCEs to assess communication and diagnostic skills.
- Logbook of cases, and clinical skills.

Career development

Matching the breadth of clinical acumen needed in a good GP is the breadth of potential for career development in general practice. The ways in which you might use a GP qualification are limited only by your own imagination. It is becoming increasingly popular and mainstream now to have a portfolio of different specialist interests—and these can even change over the course of your career. Many choose to train to be educators, teaching medical students or training junior doctors. Trainers get extra time when supervising students or trainees, they plan and run tutorials or may lecture at medical schools. Others have a specialist interest—many spend a day a week in a specialist hospital service, such as a cardiology clinic, conducting cardiac echocardiograms and assessing cardiac patients, or palliative care, endoscopy, dermatology, gynaecology, family planning, respiratory medicine, prison medicine, urgent care centres, or EM, etc. These skills are then brought back into the practice where they work, allowing GPs to internally refer patients with suitable issues to their own colleagues.

GPs' common-sense approach and breadth of knowledge, if supplemented with the right training, can make them useful event doctors, working on expeditions, cruise ships, or sporting events. You can travel abroad, work for international organizations, or international clinics. Some even choose to go into private practice. The growing demand for telemedicine and online app-based consultations has been largely met by GPs. Or there is also medical journalism, writing, politics, or working for the local commissioning group. It is completely up to you!

Should you choose general practice for foundation training?

- This is a chapter about general practice—of course the answer has to be YES!
- This is even more important for those of you who do not want to be GPs.

It is essential that hospital doctors have some concept of what GPs do—what the difficulties are and what the limits are. Maintaining professional and collegiate relationships between primary and secondary care avoids a lot of angst and stress for both. Medical school training entails spending a great deal of time learning about hospital medicine and very little about community medical practice. How else will you learn about what >25% of medical doctors do all day? And if you are considering a career in general practice it gives you a chance to see what it is really like. And the on-call rota is pretty good!

Getting the most out of the placement

Firstly, leave any preconceptions and prejudices at the front door and go in with a willingness to learn from the subtleties as well as maybe a new syndrome or a new clinical sign. Remember that there is no such thing as a typical GP. Your experience will vary enormously from the next student's depending on the individual trainers you are exposed to, the setting of the practice—rural or urban, wealthy or deprived, small or a large practice?

As with any medical training setting try to get as much first-hand experience and exposure to as many patients as possible. If it has not been set up for you already, ask if you can see your own patients—you will be given plenty of time for this—find out why they have come and listen to what they are telling you verbally as well as looking for the in-between information— why are they really there? What are they most worried about? Find out about their *ideas, concerns, and expectations* (ICE). Your patients will also be seen by their GP and you will have a chance to discuss each one with the trainer. Use this as an opportunity to find out what skills you can learn from your trainer, particularly in communication, as well as finding out how they approach not missing that seriously ill person.

Zola (1973)[1] suggested that patients do not seek help at their sickest point, but when they can no longer accommodate the changes they are experiencing with five 'triggers' for help-seeking:
1. *Interpersonal crisis* (e.g. death in the family), which may call attention to a person's bodily changes → prompting them to do seek help.
2. *Perceived interference with relations*: a bodily change interferes with relationships and daily life → prompting action.
3. *Sanctioning*: family, friends, or partners encourage help-seeking.
4. *Perceived interference with vocational or physical activity*: changes stop someone carrying out their job or other physical activity.
5. *Temporalizing of symptomatology*: people place a time limit on their changes, and consult if they have not resolved by that time.

Learn about risk and safety-netting. GPs are good at managing risk and at knowing how to safety-net with their patient—explaining which serious things to look out for and being clear on how they might seek further help if needed.

Go out with all the members of the GP team. Spend time with the practice nurses, the midwife, and the receptionist. Sit in on minor surgery if your practice offers it. Take any chance of doing a home visit. You learn an enormous amount about patients when you see them in a home environment. You will realize how hard it is to assess a sick, frail, elderly person who has had a collapse or a fall at home when you are not in a bright, exposed hospital setting. Think about the GP lifestyle and the practice/small business management aspects of the job. All senior jobs have admin and management responsibilities—might you like the relative freedom that comes with being contracted to the NHS?

Reference
1. Zola IK. Pathways to the doctor — from person to patient. *Soc Sci Med* 1973;7:677–89.

Genetics

Genetics: overview

Clinical genetics is the medical speciality that deals with diagnosis and genetic counselling for individuals and families with, or at risk of, conditions that may have a genetic basis. Genetic disorders can affect any body system and any age group.

Examples of genetic disorders include:

- chromosomal abnormalities, e.g. Down syndrome
- single gene disorders, e.g. cystic fibrosis (CF)
- familial cancer syndromes
- birth defects with a genetic component, e.g. cleft lip and palate.

Clinical genetics services in the UK are based at 23 regional genetics centres consisting of a clinical team of doctors and genetic counsellors and the genetics laboratories (for molecular and cytogenetic testing). Clinical genetics may be taught as part of the paediatrics rotation. Clinical geneticists usually visit district general hospitals several times a month. It should be possible to arrange to sit in on clinics. You may need to telephone the department to arrange this in advance.

Medical students can often choose to do a placement in clinical genetics such as a student selected component or special studies module. This involves a longer placement of several weeks in the department and provides an opportunity to attend a range of different clinics and clinical meetings and sometimes organize a project.

Cases to see

Clinical geneticists see a wide range of cases, some relatively common and some very rare. It will not be possible to see everything during a short attachment. Try to see a range of cases such as the following:

Prenatal genetics

Seeing pregnant couples who are concerned about a genetic disease either due to family history or abnormal results of screening tests/scans. The focus is on assessing the risk, seeing if testing is available during pregnancy, and helping couples decide whether they would like invasive testing (or non-invasive prenatal testing/diagnosis if available) and how they would use the information.

Paediatric genetics

Seeing babies and children who are suspected to have a genetic problem, e.g. due to a congenital anomaly or developmental delay. A detailed family history, pregnancy and birth history, and developmental history will be taken, and a detailed examination made. Clinical photographs are often taken to aid further discussion in the department. The focus is on trying to make a diagnosis, as this gives information about prognosis, potential complications, and recurrence risk.

Single gene disorders

E.g. CF, hereditary haemochromatosis, Marfan syndrome, NF1, and Duchenne muscular dystrophy. The focus may be on explaining the diagnosis and prognosis, implications for the wider family, or reproductive options.

Cancer genetics
Common cancer predisposition syndromes such as hereditary breast and ovarian cancer (*BRCA1* and *BRCA2* genes) or Lynch syndrome (hereditary non-polyposis colorectal cancer (HNPCC)).

Chromosomal disorders
E.g. Down syndrome, Klinefelter syndrome, Turner syndrome, chromosomal translocation (may be found during investigation of recurrent miscarriage), microdeletions, or microduplications.

Procedures to see
Clinical genetics is not a procedure-based speciality, although you may need to take blood.

Things to do
Clinical genetics is mainly led by consultants and genetic counsellors (nurses or science graduates who have had specialist training in genetic counselling usually through a master's degree). As a student, you will spend most of the time observing. You will need to practise taking family histories and drawing accurate pedigrees. You will need to be able to identify common inheritance patterns in families (e.g. autosomal dominant (AD), autosomal recessive (AD), X-linked), and explain them to patients in straightforward language. You should think about the communication skills that are very important in clinical genetics such as taking informed consent, breaking bad news, considering patient confidentiality within families, non-directional counselling (in particular about predictive testing and reproductive choices), and explaining complex information in simple language.

Common genetic conditions by specialty
- *Cardiology*: hypertrophic cardiomyopathy, Marfan's syndrome.
- *Dermatology*: NF1.
- *GI*: hereditary haemochromatosis.
- *Neurology*: Charcot–Marie–Tooth disease, Huntington disease (HD), myotonic dystrophy.
- *Oncology*: familial breast and ovarian cancer, familial adenomatous polyposis, Lynch syndrome (HNPCC).
- *Ophthalmology*: retinitis pigmentosa.
- *Paediatrics*: Down syndrome, developmental delay, dysmorphic features, fragile X syndrome, Duchenne muscular dystrophy.
- *Renal*: polycystic kidney disease (AD and AR).
- *Respiratory*: CF, alpha-1 antitrypsin deficiency.

Geneticists see a wide range of different cases and you should aim to sit in on different types of consultations as described in the overview. It will also be helpful to see families with the different inheritance patterns.

Autosomal dominant
The gene which causes the disorder is encoded on an autosome (i.e. not the X or Y chromosome) and the disorder manifests in heterozygotes, i.e. when a single copy of the gene is mutated. Examples include Marfan syndrome,

NF1, and HD. AD disorders are characterized by variability between and within families. The severity may be influenced by other modifier genes or environmental factors.

Basics
• Males and females are affected equally.
• Males and females can transmit the disorder.
• There is a one in two (50%) chance that the offspring in any pregnancy will inherit the mutation.

Penetrance
The percentage of individuals with the mutation who have clinical features of the disorder to any degree (from trivial to severe). Many AD disorders show *age-dependent penetrance*—the features of the disorder are not present at birth but become evident over time (e.g. HD). Some AD disorders show *incomplete penetrance*—meaning that not all mutation carriers develop features of the disorder over their lifetime. This can lead to a condition seeming to 'skip a generation' (e.g. Lynch syndrome).

Expressivity
Variability in the severity of the disorder in individuals with the same mutation, between and within families. Mildly affected parents should be aware of the risk of having a severely affected child.

New mutation
The rate of new mutations varies considerably between disorders, e.g. up to 50% for NF1, but low in HD.

Predictive testing

This means testing an unaffected individual who has a family history of a genetic disorder and a known mutation in the family. It is important that the individual should have genetic counselling to explain the features of the disorder, the inheritance pattern, and the pros and cons of testing. Some disorders may have screening or other treatment available (e.g. 2-yearly colonoscopy screening from age 25 in Lynch syndrome carriers, and taking aspirin decreases the risk of developing cancers), while others do not have any treatment or screening currently available (e.g. HD) so the test result would be for information only. It may affect life choices/reproductive decisions.

Autosomal recessive

The gene which causes the disorder is located on an autosome (i.e. not the X or Y chromosome) and the disorder manifests when both copies of the gene are mutated, i.e. in homozygotes (two identical mutations) and compound heterozygotes (two different mutations). They include CF, sickle cell disease, and spinal muscular atrophy. Heterozygotes (carriers) do not manifest a phenotype (e.g. CF) or if they do, it is very mild compared with the disease (e.g. sickle cell trait vs sickle cell disease).

Basics
• Disease expressed only in homozygotes and compound heterozygotes.
• Parents are obligate carriers (an exception is spinal muscular atrophy—new mutation rate ~2%).

- Risk of carrier parents having an affected child is one in four (25%).
- Healthy siblings of an affected child have a two-thirds risk of being carriers.
- Risk of carrier status diminishes by half with every degree of relationship from parents of an affected child.
- All offspring of an affected individual whose partner is not a carrier are obligate carriers.

Consanguinity

AR disorders are commoner in the offspring of consanguineous partnerships, because the parents share more of their genome than unrelated individuals. A consanguineous relationship is one between individuals who are second cousins or closer.

Carrier frequency

Population risk for carrier status can be calculated by geneticists using the Hardy–Weinberg equation. Approximate carrier frequency in the white British population = 1 in 25 for CF, and 1 in 10 for hereditary haemochromatosis.

Carrier testing

Testing relatives of an affected individual is straightforward if the mutations are known in the affected individual. Testing an unrelated partner is usually more difficult, as recessive diseases can be caused by many different mutations within the gene. Sickle cell disease is caused by one recurrent mutation, so testing is straightforward. Spinal muscular atrophy is mainly caused by a recurrent deletion, so testing of people at population risk is possible but does not give a definite answer. CF carrier testing uses a panel of common mutations which covers ~85% of mutations in the white British population, so the testing does not give a definite answer but can give a risk estimate.

Cascade testing

This means tracking a mutation through a family. This is often done for serious AR conditions (e.g. CF) to give information for reproductive choices. It is also especially important for balanced chromosomal translocations. It can be done for AD conditions, particularly if screening or treatment is available.

X-linked

Disorders are encoded on the X chromosome. Examples include Duchenne muscular dystrophy, fragile X syndrome, and haemophilia A. An X-linked recessive disorder manifests in males who have one X chromosome but generally not in females who have two X chromosomes (one normal and one mutated copy). Some disorders almost never cause symptoms in females and in some, females have symptoms infrequently (e.g. Duchenne muscular dystrophy), whereas for others (e.g. X-linked Charcot–Marie–Tooth disease, and fragile X syndrome), manifestation is fairly common but is usually less severe than in affected males. This is called X-linked semidominant inheritance.

Basics
- No male-to-male transmission.
- When an affected male fathers a pregnancy, all his daughters will be carriers and none of his sons will be affected.
- When a carrier female has a pregnancy, there are four possible outcomes, all of which are equally likely: normal daughter, carrier daughter, normal son, affected son—i.e. 50% of sons will be affected and 50% of daughters will be carriers.

Sex chromosomes

Y chromosome

The Y chromosome contains ~120 genes which mainly code for processes necessary to turn the fetus into a male.

X chromosome

The X chromosome contains >1000 genes (~1/20th of the genome), many of which are essential for normal growth and development.

X inactivation

Normal males have one X chromosome and normal females have two. In order that males and females have the same dose of the genes on the X chromosome, only one copy of the X chromosome is active in each a female cell, the other being mostly inactivated. X inactivation occurs in every cell in the female embryo 1–2 weeks after conception. X inactivation is a random process in the embryo, so there should be about 50% of cells containing the maternal X inactive and 50% containing the paternal X inactive.

Females with more severe symptoms due to a X-linked disorder may show unfavourably skewed X inactivation.

Other inheritance patterns

Mitochondrial
- Maternal inheritance: there are very few mitochondria in the sperm and many in the egg (paternal mitochondria constitute only 0.1% of the total in the fertilized egg), so the risk of paternal inheritance is essentially zero.
- Heteroplasmy: there may be two populations of mitochondria with different genotypes, and the level of mutant mitochondrial DNA has some effect on phenotype.

Multifactorial
- Some conditions tend to cluster in families more often than would be expected by chance but do not follow a Mendelian pattern.
- These probably depend on a mixture of major and minor genetic factors and environmental factors.
- E.g. cleft lip/palate, neural tube defects, schizophrenia, IBD.

Types of genetic test

Karyotype

Looks at chromosomes under light microscopy, good for detecting mosaicism and for balanced translocations.

Microarray

Detailed chromosome test (using DNA technology) for sub-microscopic deletions or duplications.

Single gene
Targeted testing of gene suspected to cause the phenotype, good if only one or two genes which cause the condition, e.g. fibrillin 1 in Marfan syndrome.

Gene panel
Testing of a specified list of genes that can cause a phenotype/condition, good if many genes can cause a similar phenotype, e.g. Charcot–Marie–Tooth disease. When a panel of genes is tested, there is a higher chance of finding variants of unknown significance.

Exome
Tests all the protein-coding genes, mainly available through research studies although starting to be used in clinical practice. This is a good approach if conventional testing has not provided an answer, but the results may be difficult to interpret, including many variants of unknown significance.

Genome
Tests nearly the whole genome, including non-coding regions. More expensive than exome sequencing and will find many more variants, but may reveal mutations in regulatory sequences which can cause disease. Currently available through research studies, e.g. 100,000 Genomes Project, although it will come into clinical practice.

Honours
Types of variant
A variant is a change from the reference human genome sequence. A pathogenic variant or mutation describes a change that is disease causing. A 'variant of unknown clinical significance' means we are not sure if it is disease causing. A benign variant is a normal (often common) finding in the population, so should not be reported.

Non-invasive prenatal testing/diagnosis
These relatively new tests are done using a sample of maternal blood to assess the genetic status of the fetus. Cell-free fetal DNA is extracted for testing. Fetal sexing looks for sequences from the Y chromosome to find out if the fetus is male or female. This is useful in X-linked recessive disorders, so that invasive testing can be offered if the fetus is male. It can also be used for sexing in disorders of sex development where ambiguous genitalia are detected on a prenatal ultrasound scan. Non-invasive prenatal testing refers to testing for common trisomies (Down syndrome, Edwards syndrome, and Patau syndrome). It can be viewed as a more accurate screening test, but is not as accurate as invasive testing. Non-invasive prenatal diagnosis can be offered for specific single gene disorders such as CF, spinal muscular atrophy, and achondroplasia. These tests mean that couples may be able to avoid an invasive procedure which causes an ↑risk of miscarriage (chorionic villus sampling or amniocentesis).

Genetics: in exams

In exams

It would be unusual to find a specific genetics station in your exams. As genetics covers all ages and systems, there are no specific genetics examination routines that you would be expected to perform. However, the skills you learn in genetics may help you in other stations, as follows.

History stations

- Taking a family history with relevant questions for the condition, e.g. heights, heart disease, sudden cardiac death, eye problems such as lens dislocation, myopia, and retinal detachment for Marfan syndrome.
- Drawing an accurate pedigree. (See Fig 16.1.)

Communication skills

Consent

Informed consent for genetic testing including benefits and harms from testing. Might include the possibility of finding a variant of unknown clinical significance, finding unexpected information, insurance implications, and implications for wider family.

Confidentiality

Be careful with sharing information with other family members (ensure that the original patient gave permission to share information with the family).

Breaking bad news

Results of predictive test that shows that someone has inherited a mutation so is likely to develop a genetic disease.

Explanation

E.g. about chromosomes and non-disjunction for Down syndrome, inheritance patterns.

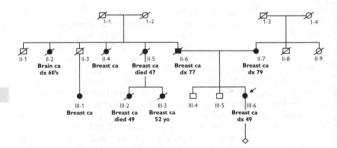

Fig. 16.1 Example of a pedigree chart. Reproduced from Kasprzak et al. Invasive breast cancer following bilateral subcutaneous mastectomy in a *BRCA2* mutation carrier: a case report and review of the literature. *World J Surg Oncol*. 2005; 3: 52, under the Creative Commons Attribution License (http://creativecommons.org/licenses/by/2.0).

Chapter 17

Genitourinary medicine

Genitourinary medicine: overview

Genitourinary medicine (GUM) involves the diagnosis and care of patients with sexually transmitted infections (STIs) and HIV. Related areas include contraceptive care, genital dermatoses, young people's clinics, sexual dysfunction and psychosexual medicine, and outreach services for sex workers and drug users. Most patients are seen as outpatients but some HIV-related cases require inpatient care. Relatively little undergraduate time is dedicated to GUM and the clinics can therefore seem like mysterious places that medical students have little understanding of. However, a huge variety of care is provided through GUM and you should aim to get as involved as possible to make the most of your very short time in this speciality.

Cases to see

Asymptomatic screen

Patients presenting without symptoms - find out what tests and vaccinations are routinely offered.

Genital ulceration/discharge/lumps

These are very common presentations to GUM clinics and you should be able to see several cases, learn the most common causes, and how to diagnose and manage them.

Pelvic pain

You should have a basic knowledge of pelvic anatomy and be able to list the most common causes of pelvic pain and how to manage them, including referral to gynaecology for ectopic pregnancies and surgeons for appendicitis. Pelvic inflammatory disease (PID) is an important and common cause of pelvic pain in GUM clinics.

Testicular pain

The most important cause of this is acute testicular torsion which is a urological emergency requiring immediate referral. Epididymo-orchitis is an important and common cause of testicular pain in SH clinics.

Contraceptive care

Consideration of contraception should form part of the consultation for all female presentations to SH clinics to identify those at risk of unwanted pregnancy, provide emergency contraception, and also information on local termination of pregnancy (TOP) services. Gain basic knowledge of the options available including mechanism of action, failure rate, and pros and cons to consider when counselling patients.

Sexual assault

Cases of sexual assault may initially present to SH clinic, or be referred from specialist services. They require specialist, experienced care. As a student it is unlikely that you will these see cases, but you should be aware of how to manage them and the referral pathways to health advisors, counsellors, and specialized sexual assault divisions of the police (e.g. The Havens in London).

Post-exposure prophylaxis (PEP)
HIV risk assessment is an important skill. Antiretrovirals can be used to reduce the risk of transmission after potential sexual exposure (PEPSE) or occupational exposure, and now also before sex (PrEP), if the risk is high enough. Occupational exposure following needle-stick injury or blood splashes is more commonly managed by occupational health. Ask someone to take you through the risk assessment table in the British Association for Sexual Health and HIV PEPSE guideline. (See British Association for Sexual Health and HIV, ℘ www.bashhguidelines.org/current-guidelines/hiv/post-exposure-prophylaxis-following-sexual-ex posure/)

HIV
This is an enormous topic and can seem daunting, but there are a few points you should focus on covering during your attachment:
• Screening programmes and opportunities for early diagnosis.
• *HIV pretest discussion and how to give the results*: spend time with the health advisors in the SH clinic who often have pretest discussions and recall those patients who test positive to give the diagnosis.
• *Partner notification*: again the health advisors do vital work in this area, and difficult cases are discussed at MDTs—you should definitely attend one of these to gain an understanding of the complex medical, social, and psychological aspects to some HIV cases.
• *Medical presentations*: of primary or established HIV infection, including the most common opportunistic infections. Spend time in HIV clinic and ask if/how HIV inpatient care is provided in your area to see if you can also spend time on the wards.
• *Basic principles of antiretroviral therapy*: Sitting in on new patient appointments in HIV clinic will be useful for this.
• *Screening programmes and opportunities for early diagnosis.*

Things to do
GUM is a fun, friendly, non-judgemental speciality so get as involved as you can. Sit in on clinics, observe the history taking, examinations, swab-taking, microscopy, and treatments such as cryotherapy. Try to follow a patient on their journey through the SH clinic to start understanding how it all works. Then aim to practise some elements yourself, in particular taking a history, examining, and taking swabs.

Examinations/procedures to see and do
In clinic
Demonstration of correct condom technique. Sit in with the health advisors when they do a 'safe sex' session with a patient.

Pregnancy tests and urinalysis
Very simple once someone has shown you how to do it.

Penile, vaginal, and rectal exam
Performed on symptomatic patients to take samples for microscopy and testing.

Microscopy
Performed in the 'GUM lab' by trained nurses; ask them to take you through the preparation of the slides and what they are looking for. Most labs will also have teaching slides they can use to show you examples.

Cryotherapy
Treatment for warts, often booked in advance for 6-week courses of weekly cryotherapy so ask if there are any patients booked in for this.

On the wards
HIV-positive patients requiring inpatient care often require procedures as part of their diagnostic workup. These can include bronchoscopy, LP, pleural aspiration/drain insertion, skin biopsy, and OGD, to name but a few. Infectious diseases wards, for example, will be more likely to have procedures such as these to see, and more regularly.

Genitourinary medicine: in clinic

General principles

- An accurate sexual history is essential in order to properly assess the risk of infection (and all potential sites) and pregnancy, and identify sexual contacts who may be at risk of infection.
- Partner notification is the process by which sexual contacts who may have been at risk of infection from an index case are traced in order to enable access to healthcare. It has huge public health implications as a core component of STI prevention—↑STI diagnosis and reduced transmission, re-infection, and complications.
- In all cases of suspected/proven STI, patients should be counselled to abstain from sex until fully treated to break the re-infection cycle.
- For HIV-positive patients, partner notification is particularly important; patients often require support from specialists to disclose their status to partners.
- Confidentiality is a core value in GUM and should be emphasized to patients to relieve any anxiety. Contacts can be traced anonymously if patients wish. In the case of HIV, patients are fully supported in the partner notification of partners at previous or ongoing risk, and any children.

Honours

Legal statement

In the UK, persons can now be prosecuted for reckless HIV transmission. In cases where disclosure is not forthcoming and identifiable partners are felt to be at ongoing risk, patients need to be aware of the legal implications of failing to disclose and failing to prevent transmission through consistent condom use and adherence to antiretrovirals.

Sexual history and examination

There is currently an aim to move away from traditional 'male' and 'female' descriptive terminology and towards 'penile' and 'vaginal', in line with increasing fluidity of gender and sexuality. See ➲ pp. 118–20.

Investigations

Microscopy

Involves sampling genital material (i.e. vaginal, cervical, urethral, and rectal swabs), placing it on slides, and viewing under the microscope in the GUM lab, allowing some diagnoses to be made in clinic. A simple Gram stain is performed and examined to identify, for example, candida, bacterial vaginosis, and gonorrhoea. 'Wet mount' is where vaginal discharge is placed onto a slide with saline on, covered with a cover slip, and examined to identify motile trichomonads in trichomoniasis. Dark-field/dark-ground microscopy is used to identify motile spirochetes in cases of syphilis.

Nucleic acid amplification tests (NAATs)

Either first-pass urine (penile) or swabs are taken and sent for testing; highly sensitive in both asymptomatic and symptomatic patients.

Polymerase chain reaction (PCR) testing

This is commonly used for herpes simplex virus, and sometimes for syphilis, on swabs taken from the ulcer.

Culture

Swabbed material is either transported in an appropriate culture medium or directly plated onto culture plates and sent to pathology; allows pathogen identification and antimicrobial sensitivities to be determined. This is important in cases of gonorrhoea as there are increasing rates of antibiotic resistance.

Serology

Blood is taken and tested for syphilis and HIV, as well as hepatitis B and C if needed.

Presenting complaints

Vaginal discharge

Bacterial vaginosis (BV)

This is the commonest cause of abnormal discharge. The vaginal pH rises above the normal 4.5 with overgrowth of anaerobic species and too few lactobacilli.

• *Presentation:* With a thin fishy-smelling discharge, but may be asymptomatic (up to 50%). Inflammation and itch are uncommon. It is not sexually transmitted; vaginal douching, use of shower gels, and antiseptic agents can precipitate the pH change. Clue cells can be seen on microscopy.
• *Treatment:* Options include metronidazole PO/gel or clindamycin gel.

Honours

Diagnosis of BV—Amsel's and Hay/Ison's criteria

Using Amsel's criteria, at least three of the four criteria need to be present to confirm the diagnosis:
• Thin, white, homogeneous discharge.
• Clue cells on microscopy of wet mount.
• pH of vaginal fluid >4.5.
• Release of fishy odour on adding alkali (rarely done now, patient report of malodour is usually seen as sufficient).
  Hay/Ison's criteria refer to Gram-stained vaginal smear appearances:
• Grade 1: lactobacilli predominate.
• Grade 2: mixed flora with some lactobacilli.
• Grade 3: mostly *Gardnerella* ± *Mobiluncus*, with few/absent lactobacilli.

Trichomonas vaginalis (TV)

This is a flagellated protozoan. In women it is found in the vagina, urethra, and paraurethral glands; transmission is almost exclusively through sexual intercourse.

• *Symptoms:* 10–50% women are asymptomatic, but symptoms include vaginal discharge (classically frothy), vulval itching, dysuria, and offensive odour. Up to 2% have the classical 'strawberry cervix' visible to the naked eye.

- *Diagnosis:* This is by detecting the motile trichomonads on light-field wet-mount microscopy, culture, or NAAT (most sensitive and specific).
- *Treatment:* This is with PO metronidazole, and PN.

Thrush (vulvovaginal candidiasis)

This is a fungal infection caused by *Candida albicans* in 90% of cases.

- *Symptoms:* Include vulval itch and soreness, vaginal discharge (typically heterogenous, but can be thin), superficial dyspareunia, and dysuria.
- *Diagnosis:* This is on microscopy and culture.
- *Treatment:* Options include topical azoles in cream or pessary form, (hydrocortisone combination if vulvitis is marked), or in PO tablet form. General measures such as use of soap substitutes and avoidance of tight-fitting synthetic clothing and perfumed substances can help prevent recurrence.

Urethritis/urethral discharge

Gonorrhoea (GC)

This is infection of the mucous membranes by Gram-negative diplococcus *Neisseria gonorrhoeae*.

- *Symptoms:* These depend on the site of infection and include penile urethral discharge, dysuria, anal discharge and perianal pain, vaginal discharge, and lower abdominal pain. Discharge is mucopurulent. Complications include epididymo-orchitis, prostatitis, PID, and disseminated gonococcal infection.
- *Diagnosis:* Gram-negative intracellular diplococci are seen within polymorphonuclear leucocytes (PMNLs) on microscopy. Specimens taken: penile—first-pass urine for NAATs and urethral swab for MC&S; vaginal—vaginal and endocervical swabs for NAATs and culture. Rectal/pharyngeal swabs are also taken if history dictates.
- *Treatment:* This is increasingly difficult due to rising antibiotic resistance. Current treatment is 500 mg ceftriaxone IM + 1g azithromycin PO but new national guidance is imminent. Visit the British Association for Sexual Health and HIV website ℘ www.bashh.org for up to date guidance.

Chlamydia trachomatis (CT)

This is the most common curable STI in the UK. It is often asymptomatic (70% women, 50% men) which leads to ongoing transmission.

- *Screening:* In 2003, the National Chlamydia Screening Programme (NCSP) was established in an effort to prevent and control chlamydia through early detection and treatment, reduce onward transmission, and prevent the consequences of untreated infection. People aged 16–25 can access free and confidential chlamydia tests as part of the NCSP at multiple sites across the UK.
- *Symptoms:* Female symptoms include postcoital or intermenstrual bleeding, lower abdominal pain, purulent vaginal discharge, cervicitis, and dysuria. In men, the main symptoms are urethral discharge and dysuria.
- *Complications:* Up to 30% of untreated women develop PID which can result in infertility, ectopic pregnancy, and chronic pelvic pain.
- *Diagnosis:* It is diagnosed on NAAT testing. All potentially exposed sites should be sampled: penile (first pass urine), vaginal (endocervical or vulvovaginal), pharynx, rectal, and conjunctival.
- *Treatment:* This is with doxycycline 100 mg twice daily for 7 days.

Non-gonococcal urethritis (or non-specific urethritis)

This refers to urethritis where GC is not identified on microscopy. It may or may not be secondary to a STI. Commonest causative organisms isolated are CT and *Mycoplasma genitalium*.

- *Symptoms:* These include urethral discharge, dysuria, and penile irritation.
- *Diagnosis:* This is made by demonstrating an excess of PMNLs in the anterior urethra on microscopy of a Gram-stained urethral smear or first pass urine in symptomatic patients.
- *Treatment:* This is doxycycline 100 mg twice daily for 7 days. All partners at risk should be identified and treated.

Genital ulceration

Genital herpes

This is caused by HSV types 1 and 2 and is transmitted through direct contact. After primary infection, the virus lays dormant in local sensory ganglia and then periodically reactivates to cause either lesions or asymptomatic virus shedding.

- *Symptoms:* These include painful ulcers, dysuria, vaginal or urethral discharge, and systemic symptoms of fever and myalgia (see Fig. 17.1).
- *Complications:* These include autonomic neuropathy causing urinary retention, and aseptic meningitis.
- *Diagnosis:* This is made clinically from the typical appearance, and detecting HSV on swabs taken from the base of the ulcer.
- *Treatment:* This includes saline baths, analgesia, topical anaesthetics (e.g. lidocaine), and oral antivirals (e.g. 400mg TDS for 5 days). Patients should abstain from sex during episodes; condom use reduces transmission but cannot completely prevent it. This condition often causes significant distress and health advisors and counsellors can be very helpful in supporting the patient.

Syphilis

This is caused by the spirochete bacterium *Treponema pallidum*. It is transmitted through direct contact (usually sexual), mother-to-child transmission, or via infected blood products. It is classified as acquired or congenital and early or late.

- *Primary syphilis:* Presents with the 'primary chancre', a classically painless, non-healing, anogenital ulcer, and regional lymphadenopathy.
- *Secondary syphilis:* Multisystem involvement with rash (often affecting palms and soles), generalized lymphadenopathy, condylomata lata (wart-like lesions), and mucocutaneous lesions.
- *Latent syphilis:* Asymptomatic infection diagnosed on serological testing, either early or late.
- *Symptomatic late syphilis:* This is very rare, but there are three types:
1. *Cardiovascular:* results in ascending aortic aneurysms and aortic regurgitation.
2. *Neurological*—three types:
   - Meningovascular (cranial nerve palsies, stroke).
   - General paresis (dementia, psychoses).

- Tabes dorsalis (dorsal column/nerve root inflammation causing sensory ataxia, paraesthesia, lightning pains, areflexia, Charcot's joints, optic atrophy, and Aryl–Robertson pupils).
3. *Gummatous*: granulomas form in the skin, mucosa, bone, joints, and rarely viscera.

● *Diagnosis:* This is made with a combination of history, examination, and investigations including dark-ground microscopy in primary syphilis, and serology.

● *Serological testing:* This can be confusing and is usually managed by senior members of the team; Table 17.1 should hopefully make interpretation easier.

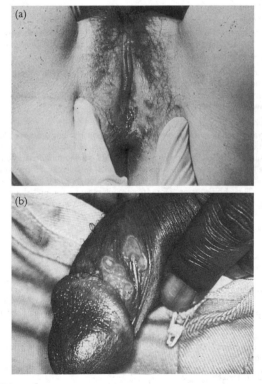

Fig. 17.1 Herpes simplex virus genital infection. (a) Female genital infection. (b) Male genital infection. Reproduced with permission from Temesgen, Zelalem, *Mayo Clinic Infectious Diseases Board Review*, 2012, Oxford University Press.

- *Treatment:* This is with either benzathine or procaine penicillin IM (or doxycycline PO if penicillin-allergic), the dosage and course length of which varies depending on whether infection is early, late-latent or late-symptomatic.
- *Follow-up:* This is necessary to monitor response to treatment and detect re-infection or treatment failure.

Tropical genital ulcer disease

A rare group of infections causing inguinal lymphadenopathy and genital ulceration from endemic areas (African-Caribbean):

1. Lymphogranuloma venereum (LGV) caused by CT serovars L1–L3.
2. Chancroid caused by *Haemophilus ducreyi*.
3. Donovanosis (granuloma inguinale) caused by *Klebsiella granulomatis*.

Genital lumps

Genital warts

These are caused by human papilloma virus (HPV) most commonly types 6 and 11. They are mostly sexually transmitted, occur at any site, and are generally asymptomatic but can cause irritation and soreness.

- *Treatment:* Depends on distribution, type, number, and patient preference and this is a point for discussion. Find out the mechanism of some topical treatment options (e.g. podophyllotoxin and imiquimod) and observe cryotherapy treatment in SH clinic.

Pelvic pain

Lower abdominal pain is a common presentation in young women. It is very important to exclude ectopic pregnancy and appendicitis. Other common causes include PID, UTI, and constipation. PID is inflammation of the upper female genital tract and supporting structures, usually caused by infection. A full STI screen is needed and pelvic examination including bimanual examination. The choice of antibiotic treatment regimen for PID depends on local antimicrobial resistance, patient preference and disease severity—consult your local guidelines.

Testicular pain

The most important causes of this are testicular torsion (emergency referral to urology (see p. 806), 6 hours to salvage the testis), strangulated hernia (emergency referral to general surgeons), epididymo-orchitis, tumour (but rarely causes pain) and trauma. Epididymo-orchitis is acute pain, swelling, and inflammation of the epididymis and/or testes. It has several causes, including GC, CT, UTI, TB (think if from an area of high prevalence or immunocompromised), and mumps. A full STI screen should be performed. To cover all potential STIs including GC, treatment is with a stat dose of ceftriaxone IM and doxycycline PO; if cover for enteric organisms is required (unprotected insertive anal sex), ofloxacin/ciprofloxacin is recommended.

PEP and PrEP

PEP is the use of emergency antiretroviral treatment to prevent transmission following exposure to HIV, either occupational or following sexual

Table 17.1 Serology testing in syphilis

Test	Examples	Notes
Treponema-specific antibody	TPHA (T. pallidum haemagglutination assay)	Positive in any stage of syphilis infection.
	EIA (enzyme immunoassay)	Used as a screening test. Also positive in non-syphilis treponemal infection (yaws, pinta).
	FTA (fluorescent treponemal antibody)	Remains positive even after effective treatment.
Cardiolipin antibody	VDRL (Venereal Disease Research Laboratory)	A high or rising titre indicates active or recent infection. Titres fall with effective treatment and become negative or serofast at a low titre (1:2)
	RPR (rapid plasma regain)	False positives seen in several other conditions (pregnancy, TB, SLE, advanced HIV).

exposure (PEPSE). The decision to use PEP involves balancing the risk of transmission (which varies according to type of exposure) against the side effects. It should be given within 72 hrs the exposure to gain maximum effectiveness (<72 hours).

PrEP is an oral tablet of antiretrovirals taken before sex by HIV negative individuals at high risk of acquiring HIV (inconsistent condom use, recent STI, recent PEP course, drug use with sex, or HIV-positive partner not taking medication appropriately) as it has been shown to significantly reduce the risk of HIV transmission (PROUD and IPERGAY studies). It is currently available from GUM clinics on the NHS in Scotland and Wales, and through the IMPACT trial in England.

Contraceptive care

A contraceptive and reproductive history forms part of the full sexual history in order to assess the risk of pregnancy and discuss emergency contraception. A basic knowledge of contraceptive methods, mechanism of action, and failure rate is required to enable patients to make informed choices. See table 17.2. All contraceptive methods are only effective if used consistently and correctly. A full medical history should be taken prior to commencing hormonal methods; the *UK Medical Eligibility Criteria for Contraceptive Use* provides guidance.[1]

Emergency contraception

This provides women with a method of preventing unwanted pregnancy following an episode of unprotected sexual intercourse (UPSI). There are three methods:

- *Copper coil* inserted up to 5 days (120 hours) after UPSI, or within 5 days from earliest estimated date of ovulation. Failure rate is <1%.

- *Ulipristal* (ellaOne®) also inhibits or delays ovulation and is licensed for up to 120 days after UPSI.
- *Levonorgestrel* (Levonelle®) primarily inhibits ovulation and is licensed for use within 72 hours after UPSI/contraceptive failure.

HIV

HIV is fairly unique in terms of the scope of conditions, infections, and malignancies that can occur as a consequence, affecting every system. It is now a treatable, manageable condition allowing HIV-positive patients to lead normal lives with normal life expectancy, including having relationships and children without transmitting the virus. However, around 1 in 4 of those infected with HIV are unaware of their infection; therefore it is important to know who to test. Testing should be offered in the presence of risk factors, HIV-associated conditions (Primary HIV infection, indicator conditions and opportunistic infections, see ➲ pp. 364–5), and to all new GP registrants and medical admissions in areas of high prevalence.

> **Trivia**
>
> Acquired immune deficiency syndrome (AIDS) began as an epidemic in 1981 with cases being reported all over the US. A retrovirus was later identified as the cause, and labelled as human immunodeficiency virus (HIV) in 1986. A similar virus was discovered that year in West Africa (HIV-2). It is believed to have originated in apes, as simian immunodeficiency virus shares many similarities with HIV, and crossed species (early 1900s).

Risk factors
Those for HIV include originating from a country of high prevalence, STI diagnosis, sexual intercourse with a known HIV-positive partner or partner from high prevalence area, men who have sex with men (MSM), IV drug use, and sex within the commercial sex trade. See Fig. 17.2 for global HIV rates.

> **Honours**
>
> *Indicator conditions for HIV testing*
> - Septicaemia, pyrexia of unknown origin, recurrent pneumonia.
> - Weight loss/diarrhoea.
> - Abnormal neurology/peripheral neuropathy/dementia/space-occupying lesions.
> - Renal failure.
> - Cancer—especially non-Hodgkin lymphoma and anal/cervical cancers.
> - Abnormal haematology—thrombocytopenia, anaemia, lymphopenia
> - Rashes—shingles, psoriasis

Table 17.2 Methods of contraception

Method	Examples	Mode of action	Failure rate
Barrier	Male condom	Physical barrier preventing sperm meeting ova	2%
	Female condom		5%
	Diaphragms		5–8%
Combined hormonal	Pill, transdermal patch, vaginal ring	Inhibit ovulation May also affect cervical/endometrial mucus	0.3%
Progestogen only	Pill	Alter cervical mucus	<1%
	Injection	Prevent ovulation Thicken cervical mucus	<4/1000 over 2 years
	Implant	Thin endometrium	<1/1000 over 3 years
Intrauterine	Copper coil	Inhibits fertilization Affects implantation Thickens cervical mucus	1–2% over 5 years
	Levonorgestrel releasing	Inhibits implantation	

Diagnosis

This is made using serum to test for HIV-1 and HIV-2 antibodies and p24 antigen. 4th generation tests can now detect HIV 2-6 weeks after exposure. A positive diagnostic test should be confirmed a second time before a formal diagnosis is made. The diagnostic 'window period' refers to the period after exposure to HIV and before seroconversion where markers of infection are absent/too low for detection and false negatives may occur (variable but roughly 4 weeks); hence, a negative test should always be followed by a confirmatory test at 3 months. A positive diagnostic test should be confirmed a second time before a formal diagnosis is made.

Point of care tests (POCT) are available in GUM clinics, antenatal units and community settings. They are finger-prick tests that take 15 minutes to give a result and are therefore useful when a result is needed urgently. They have higher false positive rates and therefore require a confirmatory serum test.

CD4 and viral load

This is a glycoprotein expressed on the surface of T-helper lymphocytes and is used as a staging marker of HIV infection, together with the HIV viral load in the blood. As time goes on post infection, the CD4 count falls and the HIV viral load increases; once the CD4 count falls <350, patients become at risk of opportunistic infections and diagnosis after this point is classified as a late diagnosis.

Honours

Consent for HIV testing

In the UK, verbal consent is required prior to testing for HIV. In some areas of high prevalence, screening programmes exist where all medical patients are tested routinely on admission and patients can 'opt out' of having an HIV test if they wish. Routine antenatal screening was also introduced in about 2000.

However, in cases where consent cannot be gained, e.g. the unconscious patient, and there is a clinical need to test for HIV, the test can be performed in the patient's best interest.

AIDS

Patients get sick if they do not know they have the disease and present late with opportunistic infections or AIDs-defining conditions, or if they do not take their medication. Late diagnosis is the most important factor in morbidity and mortality from HIV. AIDS is defined as CD4 count <200, or the presence of certain AIDS-defining conditions e.g. TB and *Pneumocystis* pneumonia.

Management

Antiretroviral therapy

The introduction of antiretroviral therapy in the 1990s revolutionized the care of patients with HIV/AIDS. There are several classes from which drugs are selected to create a combination therapy, including reverse transcriptase inhibitors (RTIs), protease inhibitors (PIs), and integrase inhibitors (IIs). Each class works differently and when used in combination forms a highly active antiretroviral therapy (HAART) which reduces the viral load and allows immune recovery. Resistance can develop if not taken at the same time every day.

Immune reconstitution inflammatory syndrome (IRIS)

Patients diagnosed at CD4 <100 are at higher risk of IRIS after commencing HAART. As the CD4 count recovers, any infection can worsen and subclinical infections can be unmasked, the symptoms and timing of which depend on the underlying infection. Examples include hepatitis C IRIS with ALT rise, herpes simplex IRIS with often very severe ulceration, and TB IRIS with fever and ↑lymphadenopathy.

Management

This can be difficult and requires specialist input; high-dose steroids may be required to manage symptoms.

Monitoring

Patients who are diagnosed and adherent to antiretroviral treatment usually remain well, but remain at risk of certain infections (encapsulated organisms), adverse effects of medications, and malignancies. They are therefore monitored closely, every 6–12 months, with both HIV and systemic monitoring bloods (renal, liver and bone) and thorough systems review. Co-morbidities are also carefully considered, and blood pressure and lipid profile are monitored due to increased risk of cardiovascular disease and diabetes.

Hepatitis B and C

It is important to perform baseline serology for infective causes of hepatitis at HIV diagnosis to identify those who are co-infected and measure their baseline hepatitis viral loads. These patients should be referred to specialist clinics for assessment of fibrosis, careful choice of HAART, initiation of hepatitis C treatment, and regular surveillance for hepatocellular carcinoma.

Reference

1. Faculty of Sexual and Reproductive Healthcare (2016). *UK Medical Eligibility Criteria for Contraceptive Use*. London: Faculty of Sexual and Reproductive Healthcare. ✆ www.fsrh.org/documents/ukmec-2016/fsrh-ukmec-full-book-2017.pdf

Genitourinary medicine: in the emergency department

GUM-related presentations

These are less common than other specialities but there are a few presentations you should be familiar with:

PID See p. 51

Epididymo-orchitis See p. 806

HSV complications

Urinary retention

This can develop due to autonomic neuropathy as a direct effect of the HSV on neurons, or secondary to severe pain preventing micturition. Patients may require catheterization; suprapubic is preferred to avoid ascending herpes infection in the urinary tract.

Aseptic meningitis

Patients present with symptoms and signs of meningeal involvement with headache, fever, meningism, and photophobia. It is different from bacterial presentations as they are less unwell, fully conscious, and CSF analysis is different (clear CSF, lymphocytosis, normal protein and glucose). Treat with aciclovir if suspected as CSF viral cultures take weeks.

Encephalitis

Presents differently with confusion, altered behaviour, and possibly drowsiness. CT/MRI, LP, and treatment with aciclovir is required, as with meningitis.

PEPSE

ED have a supply of PEPSE and are familiar with assessing risk and counselling patients.

Emergency contraception See p. 360

Disseminated gonococcal disease

This is rare but patients can present systemically unwell secondary to disseminated GC which spreads via haematogenous route causing skin lesions, arthralgia, arthritis, tenosynovitis, and sepsis.

HIV-related presentations

In general, the patients that present unwell to ED fall into one of three groups: those who do not know they have HIV, those who do not take their medication appropriately, or those who know of their status but default care completely. As mentioned before, patients with undiagnosed HIV tend to present late and sick, with either opportunistic infections or malignancies. When seeing any patients in ED with any of the indicator conditions you must test for HIV, particularly in areas of the UK with high prevalence and if the patient originates from a high-prevalence country.

Primary HIV infection

Primary HIV infection and acute seroconversion illness symptoms happen in 80% of newly infected patients, at around 4–6 weeks post infection, with non-specific symptoms of fever, rash, pharyngitis, and myalgia. It is a golden time to test as it may be the only time that patient presents to healthcare services until their disease is much more advanced as HIV infection is so often asymptomatic.

Pyrexia of unknown origin (PUO)

HIV-related disease is an important cause of this and must be tested for. It mostly occurs when CD4 count falls to <100 and is less common in patients established on HAART. Infectious causes are by far the most common, followed by neoplasia and drug reactions.

Candidiasis

Oral/pharyngeal/oesophageal candidiasis is associated with advanced HIV infection. It presents as white plaques and dysphagia/odynophagia. Easily spotted but also easily missed if you do not look. It usually responds well to azoles, e.g. fluconazole.

Pneumocystis pneumonia (PCP)

This is caused by the fungus Pneumocystis jirovecii. Most cases occur in patients with CD4 counts <200. It typically presents with progressive exertional dyspnoea over weeks with dry cough. The CXR is deceptively normal but CT thorax classically reveals perihilar ground-glass opacification. It is diagnosed on silver staining or immunofluorescence of bronchoalveolar lavage (BAL) samples. First-line treatments are co-trimoxazole and HAART.

Tuberculosis

HIV/TB co-infection can be very difficult to manage due to diagnostic challenges in immunosuppression, drug toxicities/interactions, and IRIS with HAART—flare of TB symptoms with fever and malaise as the immune system recovers and directs action at the mycobacteria. TB can occur at any CD4 count and can be pulmonary or extrapulmonary. Pulmonary disease is suspected in the presence of fevers, night sweats, weight loss, respiratory symptoms, and abnormal CXR findings with lymphadenopathy. Send sputum for acid-fast bacilli staining, BAL if sputum is smear negative and tissue cultures if extrapulmonary disease is suspected. Anti-TB treatment should be commenced before HIV treatment due to the effects of immune recovery in the context of untreated TB.

Toxoplasmosis

This is infection with Toxoplasma gondii, an obligate intracellular pathogen transmitted from cats, which most commonly causes cerebral abscess mass lesions. It presents with focal neurological signs and symptoms, raised intracranial pressure (headache and vomiting), and sometimes seizures. It is diagnosed by finding multiple ring-enhancing lesions on CT brain and treated with sulfadiazine and pyrimethamine. Primary CNS lymphoma is the main differential.

Cryptococcosis

This is the commonest systemic fungal infection associated with HIV, caused by the encapsulated yeast Cryptococcus, but is now very rare since the advent of HAART. It can present as cryptococcal meningitis (headache, fever, and meningism), with serum/CSF positive for cryptococcal antigen. Treatment is with amphotericin B.

Genitourinary medicine: in exams

History station

Taking a sexual history is less likely to come up in exams but is something that every medical student should be able to do; you will at some point in your career (especially in gynaecology, urology, and general practice) come across a case where knowing the sexual history is crucial to treat the patient correctly. It involves eliciting details which enable accurate assessment of the risk of STI, site, type, risk of pregnancy, and dictates all further investigations:

Symptoms
Discharge, soreness, bleeding, pain.

Sexual contacts
In the last 3 months.

For each contact
- Date of last sexual intercourse.
- Type of relationship (casual or regular) and duration.
- Sex.
- Condom use (always, occasional, mostly, never).
- Route of sex:
  - Vaginal.
  - Oral—giving/receiving and condom use.
  - Anal—insertive/receptive and condom use.
  - Country of origin of partner.

Risk of blood-borne viruses
- Previous STIs.
- History of IV drug use.
- Previous homosexual sex.
- Commercial sex.

Other relevant background information
- Present/past medical history
- Contraceptive/obstetrics and gynaecology (O&G) history
- Drug history/allergies
- Drug/alcohol use.

Start by introducing yourself, be aware of body language and consider acknowledging any distress the patient may be feeling. A good way to begin is with an open question such as '*How can I help you today?*' This enables the patient to say why they have come and perhaps what they are worried about. You can then move on to ask about any symptoms they might have at the moment. To lead on to obtaining details of their recent sexual activity, you could ask the question, '*When did you last have sex?*' and proceed to ask all the above-listed questions regarding this sexual encounter, and then ask about any previous encounters moving chronologically back through the last 3 months. When it comes to asking details about route of sex, this will be awkward if you are feeling awkward and embarrassed—a way to dispel this is by practising with a fellow student, working out what phrases feel natural to you to use when asking about whether sex was vaginal, oral or anal, receptive/insertive, active/passive, etc. Explaining to patients that the information is needed in order to direct investigations can help if they are feeling the questions are too intrusive.

Communication skills station

Scenarios that could come up in communication stations include pre-test discussion for HIV, delivering a positive result, or issues regarding confidentiality.

Pretest discussion

This should begin with the rationale for testing. Patients are often anxious for many possible reasons including lack of understanding, stigma, and perceived effects on employment, immigration status, and relationships. The positive message as outlined earlier regarding diagnosis and treatments and the advantages of testing should be made clear. Details should be given of how the patient will get the results and when, and the patient's contact details should be checked for accuracy. Treatment for HIV-positive patients is free on the NHS regardless of immigration status.

Giving the test result

Negative results

Patients should understand the significance of the window period in the context of a negative result, and that a repeat confirmatory test may be required.

Positive results

The result is best given by the person who performed the test, in a private environment. Beware the pitfall of patients misunderstanding the word 'positive' and believing this to mean good news. It may be better to say something like 'the blood test shows you have HIV' rather than 'you are HIV-positive' to avoid misinterpretation. Consider avoiding phrases like 'I'm afraid to say...' or 'I'm very sorry but...' as this re-enforces the negative connotations of an HIV diagnosis. Emphasize the positive message, and that the patient is far better off *knowing* they have it than *not knowing*. Explain that their care will be managed by a specialist HIV team and make arrangements for the patient to see them. Stress the importance of confidentiality, but that it is standard practice to inform the GP for managing future care.

Examination

As with history taking, you will at some point in your career have to examine genitalia; misdiagnoses are frequently made because doctors do not examine 'down below'. Therefore, use your placement to improve these skills and overcome any reluctance to perform the examinations. Practise asking questions about sexual practices so you can do this without getting embarrassed and in a non-judgemental way.

Male (penile)

Good lighting is required, the patient should be comfortable, and a chaperone present.

1. General inspection: skin lesions, rashes, generalized lymphadenopathy, oral lesions, hair loss, joints (extragenital manifestations of STIs/ systemic diseases).
2. Inspect the pubic area and palpate for inguinal lymphadenopathy.
3. Penis: examine the prepuce, glans, urethral meatus, and foreskin, looking for ulcers, lumps, rashes, and urethral discharge. Swabs depend on symptoms:
   • Symptomatic → urethral swab (microscopy) & GC culture.
4. Scrotum: inspect scrotal skin then palpate the testes which should be equal in size, non-tender, and smooth. Look for any swelling and if present, evaluate further:
   • Can you get above it? If not, it may be an inguinal hernia so proceed to examine for this.
   • Is it solid or cystic? Use a torch to differentiate; cystic swellings will transilluminate.
   • Is it attached to the testis or separate?
5. Urine for CT/GC NAATs, and urinalysis if symptomatic of UTI.

Female (vaginal)

Preparation is key: with the help of a chaperone, position the patient on the couch, supine, with feet together/in stirrups, knees bent and legs relaxed out to the sides, and buttocks in line with the edge of the couch. Place a sheet over the abdomen and ensure illuminating light is available. Then with disposable gloves on, proceed, explaining to the patient what you are doing:

1. General inspection as for males.
2. Inspect the pubic area and palpate the inguinal nodes.
3. Examine the vulva: labia majora, labia minora, introitus, urethra, clitoris; examine for any ulceration, lumps, lesions, rashes, swelling, irritation, etc. A methodical approach means you will not miss important yet potentially subtle changes such as those caused by female genital mutilation and vulval dermatoses.
4. Insert the speculum, lubricated with gel/water:
   • *Vagina*: look for irritation, ulcers/lesions, atypical discharge.
   • *Cervix*: again looking for atypical discharge, pain, and any abnormality of the cervical epithelium.
   • *Swabs*: vaginal wall for microscopy for BV/candida, posterior fornix wet mount for microscopy for TV, and endocervical swabs for CT/ GC NAATs, Gram stain microscopy, and GC culture.
5. *Bimanual*: perform if any history of pelvic/abdominal pain. Insert two fingers into the vagina to reach the cervix while palpating per abdomen with the other hand to assess for cervical excitation and adnexal tenderness (e.g. infection), and any adnexal or pelvic masses (do not forget possible pregnancy!).
6. Pregnancy test and urine dip/MSU if needed.

Haematology

Haematology: overview

Haematology is a unique speciality that combines both medicine and pathology. Haematologists manage patients with diseases affecting the bone marrow, blood, and lymphatic system. As well as treating patients with primary haematological disease, haematologists are essential to ensure the safe and effective running of hospitals by managing anticoagulation and transfusion services.

Cases to see

Leukaemia, lymphoma, and multiple myeloma

With most haematological malignancies, the diagnosis and initial assessment can be made either as an inpatient or outpatient. In the presence of certain complications, these patients will need to be treated as inpatients, as well as with some more intensive regimens of chemotherapy.

Idiopathic thrombocytopenia

Patients often present to hospital with signs and symptoms of bleeding although investigations and treatment can often occur as an outpatient.

Thrombotic thrombocytopenic purpura

Is a rare but fatal disorder of haemostasis that presents acutely to hospitals and requires urgent treatment.

Sickle cell disease

Patients attend clinic regularly and are admitted for management of complications such as a sickle cell chest crisis or strokes.

Therapeutic anticoagulation

Patients with a variety of medical problems require anticoagulation. Understanding the rationale and duration of anticoagulation, as well as the recommended agent and reversal of anticoagulation, is important.

Transfusion reaction

Blood transfusions are commonly administered on surgical wards, ICUs, and medical units. Understanding the theory behind transfusions, the indications for transfusions, and the recognition and management of complications is vital.

Procedures to see

Examination of a blood film

Is an essential diagnostic tool in medicine and haematology and provides important qualitative and quantitative information.

Bone marrow aspirate and trephine

Is a liquid sample of bone marrow taken and smeared on a slide and stained to primarily observe the morphology of the bone marrow cells.

A bone marrow biopsy (or trephine) is a core of bone tissue which allows the observation of the architecture of the tissue as well as morphology.

Things to do

Laboratories

Are an important place to learn about haematology. Most hospitals will have a laboratory and blood bank and the scientists there will be happy to teach you about the laboratory and techniques used. Understanding how a test works and why it is used is an excellent way to gain a deeper knowledge of medicine and haematology.

Day unit

Most haematology departments have a day unit where patients attend for chemotherapy, blood products, and other treatments. Attending the day unit will give you an opportunity to speak to and examine more physiologically stable patients.

MDT meetings

As with all specialities, attending a MDT meeting will allow you to see a breadth of cases and to observe the diverse expertise required to care for patients with haematological disease. Get a list of cases beforehand to familiarize yourself with the cases using the patient's notes.

General principles

Blood films examination of a peripheral blood film is an essential part of a haematologist's work. Take time to read the following terms, see examples and to think about why the abnormalities occur, what the abnormalities mean, and in which diseases the abnormalities are detected. Morphological abnormalities occur in primary haematological disorders as well as disorders of other systems. The following are examples of morphological terms that are of importance and terms you need to be familiar with.

- *Anisocytosis*: variation in RBC size—iron deficiency, thalassaemia, vitamin B12/folate deficiency.
- *Blasts*: refers to immature blood precursor cells not normally present in the blood: leukaemia, myelofibrosis.
- *Fragmented RBC*: irregular, broken RBC—microangiopathic haemolysis.
- *Haematopoiesis*: the process of haematopoiesis is an important concept in haematology.
- *Howell–Jolly bodies*: DNA inclusions in the RBCs—hyposplenism.
- *Hypochromia*: pale RBCs due to reduced haemoglobinization—iron deficiency, thalassaemia.
- *Left shifted*: immature neutrophils present in the peripheral blood—sepsis.
- *Leucoerythroblastic*: early immature white and red blood cells present in the peripheral blood—marrow infiltration, e.g. cancer.
- *Macrocytic RBCs*: large RBCs—vitamin B12/folate deficiency, myelodysplastic syndromes (MDS), alcohol/liver disease, haemolysis (increase in reticulocytes).
- *Microcytic RBCs*: small RBCs—iron deficiency, thalassaemia, anaemia of chronic disease.
- *Pencil cells*: elongated RBCs—iron-deficiency anaemia, thalassaemia.
- *Poikilocytosis*: variation in RBC shape, e.g. sickle cell disease, iron deficiency anaemia.

- *Polychromatic RBC*: immature RBCs (blue tinge)—haemorrhage, haemolysis, bone marrow infiltration.
- *Rouleaux*: stacking of RBCs—chronic inflammation, paraproteinaemias (e.g. multiple myeloma).
- *Sickle cells*: sickle-shaped RBCs—sickle cell disease.
- *Spherocytes*: round RBCs—hereditary spherocytosis, haemolysis, post-splenectomy.
- *Target cells*: RBCs with area of central staining—liver disease, hyposplenism.
- *Teardrop RBC*: teardrop-shaped RBCs—myelofibrosis, marrow infiltration by malignancy.

Each cell lineage has a complex maturation process which is assisted by growth factors as seen in Fig. 18.1. In haematological malignancy, disruption of this process results in excess proliferation without maturation. Identifying the lineage from which this occurs is essential in understanding haematological malignancy and its treatment.

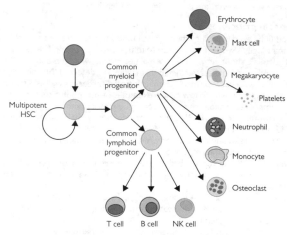

Fig. 18.1 Haematopoiesis. Reproduced from Qasim et al. Normal haematopoiesis and the concept of stem cell transplantation. *Expert Reviews in Molecular Medicine.* Vol. 6; Issue 13; 2 July 2004.

Haematology: in clinic

A patient can present with symptoms due to bone marrow dysfunction. Think about the three main types of cells the bone marrow produces (Fig 18.1) and you can extrapolate these symptoms: (1) anaemia—fatigue/shortness of breath or polycythaemia—headaches/blurred vision, (2) thrombocytopenia—bruising/bleeding or thrombocytosis—thrombosis, and (3) leucopaenia—infection; or leucocytosis—headaches) and infiltration of any organs (e.g. hepatomegaly, lymphadenopathy), ± adjacent tissue compression (e.g. spinal cord compression → leg weakness).

Laboratory tests in malignant haematology

There are several important diagnostic methods utilized in malignant haematology. No one technique is used in isolation: multiple techniques are used to accurately identify the malignancy and provide information which influences treatment decisions.

- *Morphology*: characterizing the appearance of cells in the blood or bone marrow.
- *Immunohistocytochemistry*: detecting a protein in a tissue section.
- *Cytogenetic analysis and fluorescent in situ hybridization (FISH)*: detecting the karyotype and chromosomal abnormalities (e.g. translocations).
- *Flow cytometry*: detecting antigen expression on or in cells ('the immunophenotype').
- *Molecular studies*: detecting DNA sequences or expression of genes in malignant cells.

Honours

WHO classification of tumours of haemopoietic and lymphoid tissue
This was developed to ascertain a consensus on the diagnosis of malignancy in the haemopoietic and lymphoid tissues. The classification stratifies neoplasms based on their cell lineage of origin (e.g. myeloid, lymphoid, or histiocytic). Within each category, diseases are further classified based on their morphology, immunophenotype and genetic abnormalities.

Leukaemia

The leukaemias are a group of highly heterogeneous diseases characterized by the accumulation of a clonal population of white blood cells in the bone marrow and/or lymph nodes and can spill into the blood. They are classified according to the cell of origin (myeloid vs lymphoid (i.e. T or B cells)), and as usual the diagnosis is established on bone marrow aspiration and biopsy.

Acute myeloid leukaemia (AML)

Commonest <u>acute</u> leukaemia in adults with increasing incidence with age; presents with acute signs/symptoms of bone marrow failure (although WCC can be high due to the malignany myeloid cells spilling into the blood). Chemotherapy is used to produce remission, followed by further of chemotherapy cycles as consolidation. You may see patients receiving an allogenic stem cell transplant (SCT) which is reserved for patients who have aggressive disease (see Honours: *Haemopoietic stem cell transplantation (HSCT)* p. 376).

Acute lymphoblastic leukaemia (ALL)

Commonest cancer in children. These malignant cells are lymphoid (unlike AML) and can be either B or T cells. Similar presentation with bone marrow failure, but high WCC or lymphadenopathy may be seen. Treatment is as for AML, with allogenic SCT or maintenance chemotherapy offered for high-risk disease.

Chronic lymphocytic leukaemia (CLL)

The malignant cells are mature B cells, and this is the most common adult leukaemia in the West. While they may present with bone marrow failure symptoms, these patients are often asymptomatic and diagnosis is made after a blood test which shows lymphocytosis. These patients are treated with chemotherapy although newer 'targeted' treatments are now being used.

Lymphoma

The lymphomas are a heterogeneous group of disorders characterized by accumulation of malignant *lymphocytes* in the lymph nodes and/or extranodal sites including the CNS. They are broadly classified into Hodgkin lymphoma (HL; characterized by the presence of Reed–Sternberg cells) and non-Hodgkin lymphoma (NHL).

Hodgkin lymphoma

HL occurs in a bimodal age distribution and is associated with EBV infection. The malignant cell is derived from the *B-cell* lineage. Classical HL is characterized by the multinucleated Reed–Sternberg cell. Nodular lymphocyte-predominant HL is characterized by the lymphocytic and histiocytic cells.

Presentation

Patients typically present with painless lymphadenopathy and may have 'B' symptoms such as weight loss and high temperatures, and are diagnosed by core biopsy or lymph node excision. Try to see a CT or positron emission tomography (PET)-CT which is used to stage the disease and ask the radiologist to talk you through his/her assessment of the size and location of lymphadenopathy (they may discuss the Ann Arbor Classification with Cotswold modification).

Treatment

Chemotherapy ± radiotherapy. When this fails or in relapse, haemopoietic SCT is offered. Find out about the short- and long-term complications associated with these treatments such as second cancers and heart failure.

Non-Hodgkin lymphoma

Are a very diverse group of clonal disorders of *B- and T-cell* lymphoid cells (if you think it includes every lymphoma other than the relatively rarer Hodgkin). You should be able to name a few common types: diffuse large B-cell lymphoma, follicular lymphoma, and Burkitt's lymphoma.

Presentation

Irrespective of the type, the presentation is largely dependent on the grade of disease. 'Low-grade' lymphoma typically presents with widespread disease with an indolent course, whereas 'high-grade' lymphoma typically presents with a rapidly enlarging lymph node, organ infiltration, and 'B' symptoms.

Treatment
Treatment is dependent on the type and distribution of NHL. Broadly speaking, chemotherapy and radiotherapy are used to induce disease control or remission. However, monoclonal antibodies and 'targeted therapies' are being employed in isolation or in combination with traditional treatment modalities.

Honours

Monoclonal antibodies
Monoclonal antibodies are monospecific antibodies. Monoclonal antibodies are designed to target a specific protein and are used therapeutically. For example, rituximab specifically targets CD20, a protein found on B cells. This contrasts with chemotherapeutic agents which have the potential to destroy all dividing cells as defined by their mechanism of action. Monoclonal antibodies are in widespread use in haematology and in other medical specialities.

Multiple myeloma (MM)

In healthy individuals, *plasma cells* are responsible for producing antibodies and are derived from the *B cells*. MM is a haematological malignancy characterized by clonal proliferation of plasma cells, usually in the bone marrow, the presence of a monoclonal protein in the serum/urine, and tissue damage (**CRAB**: **C**alcium (elevation), **R**enal Impairment, **A**naemia, **B**one disease—often resulting in lytic lesions and fractures). Multiple cycles of combination chemotherapy and an autologous stem cell transplant are used to prolong remission but there is no cure. Find radiographs of patients who have these typically appearing lytic lesions and fractures. Bisphosphonates are used to prevent the progression of bone disease.

Myeloproliferative neoplasms (MPNs)

The MPNs are a group of disorders characterized by clonal proliferation of haemopoietic cells with preserved maturation (lots of 'normal looking' cells) resulting in an increase in the number of cells of a particular lineage. This can affect the erythroid, granulocytic, or megakaryocytic lineage. Gene mutations in the *JAK2* and CALR genes are common in MPNs. Patients with an MPN are at increased of developing an acute myeloid leukaemia ('transformed disease').

Chronic myeloid leukaemia (CML)
CML is a clonal disorder of the *myeloid* progenitor cell. It is characterized by the Philadelphia chromosome t(9; 22) (q34;q11) abnormality resulting in an abnormal fusion protein, BCR-ABL. Clinical features are high WCC and splenomegaly. Tyrosine kinase inhibitors (e.g. imatinib), are used to inhibit the the activity of the BCR-ABL fusion protein.

Polycythaemia rubra vera (PRV)
This is the commonest MPN and is characterized by an erythrocytosis. Do not forget to think about differential diagnoses of a secondary polycythaemia (e.g. secondary to chronic hypoxia in COPD) as well as a relative erythrocytosis secondary to reduced plasma volume (e.g. dehydration).

Thrombosis or transformation to myelofibrosis or AML are significant complications. Venesection is the main treatment along with cytoreductive therapy, aspirin, and a JAK2 inhibitor.

Primary myelofibrosis (PMF)

PMF is a clonal proliferation of *megakaryocytes* and *monocytes*, which results in activation of fibroblasts initiating a fibrotic response within the bone marrow. Clinical features include splenomegaly and bone marrow failure, and is treated with cytoreductive therapy, or an allogenic SCT.

Essential thrombocytosis (ET)

ET is characterized by an elevation in platelet count in the absence of a secondary cause. Patients are often asymptomatic or present with vasomotor symptoms such as headaches, thrombosis, or paradoxical bleeding; treated with aspirin and cytoreductive medication.

Myelodysplasia

The myelodysplastic syndromes are a group of clonal disorders of the bone marrow characterized by ineffective haematopoiesis and cytopenias, classified by clinical features, morphology (from blood film/bone marrow aspirate), karyotype, and molecular tests. There may also be a relative excess of myeloblasts (immature myeloid cells, although still <20% of all nucleated cells on a bone marrow aspirate), and MDS can progress to AML. Previous chemotherapy family history and age are risk factors, and presentations vary between bone marrow failure and being asymptomatic.

Treatment

Options are tailored to each individual, but can be categorized as follows:
• Supportive: blood product support, iron chelation therapy.
• Low intensity: demethylating agents such as azacitidine (epigenetic modification).
• High intensity: chemotherapy and/or an allogenic SCT.

Honours

Haemopoietic stem cell transplantation (HSCT)

The aim of haemopoietic stem cell transplantation is to achieve reconstitution of haemopoiesis by the transfer of haemopoietic stem cells. Broadly speaking, this has two sources: autologous—from oneself; allogeneic—from another (sibling, unrelated). Stem cells can be harvested from the umbilical cord, bone marrow, or peripheral blood (after the administration of G-CSF) and can be stored frozen or given fresh.

HSCT can be used in the following circumstances:
• Following high (myeloablative) doses of chemotherapy in the treatment of malignant disease.
• Less commonly to replace abnormal bone marrow/immune system/ inherited errors in metabolism (e.g. thalassaemia, lysosomal storage disorders).

Allogenic SCT has an additional therapeutic benefit not restricted to high-dose chemotherapy: i.e. graft vs disease effect. However, this is associated with a major short- and long-term toxicity: i.e. graft vs host effect. This effect can be modulated post transplant by adjusting immunosuppression.

Attending the MDT

Cases are discussed at regional MDT meetings and this is an opportunity for doctors to review clinical details and investigations and agree a management plan.

Infection

Patients with haematological malignancy are at risk of infection due to the disease and the treatment administered. These infections are often not seen in immunocompetent people. Haematologists work closely with microbiologists to treat infection.

Vascular access

Central venous access ('line') is often required to ensure safe administration of chemotherapeutic agents, blood products, and antibiotics.

Blood requirements

Patients often require transfusion support as part of their management due to the myelosuppressive nature of their disease and the treatment administered.

Tumour lysis

The initiation of treatment can result in rapid destruction of tumour cells which release metabolites into the bloodstream, which can be fatal. Fluid hydration as well as specific agents such as allopurinol and rasburicase can prevent the sequelae of tumour destruction.

Psychological and social support

Psychological and social support is required to minimise the impact of a diagnosis of haematological disease, as well as treatment, on a patient's life.

Reproduction

Cytotoxic treatment is associated with infertility. Patients should be counselled about this and be offered reproductive conservation.

CNS disease

Malignancy can affect the CNS and specific treatment is required to prevent and treat this (e.g. intrathecal methotrexate).

Haemostasis and thrombosis

The haemostatic system is tightly regulated to ensure an appropriate cessation of bleeding in haemorrhage with appropriate clot dissolution. Clotting should not occur in the absence of haemorrhage. When a blood vessel is damaged, there are three distinct phases:

1. *Vascular phase*: vascular spasm reduces blood loss.
2. *Platelet phase*: platelet aggregation acts as a plug as well as releasing platelet factor 3, which acts to promote the coagulation cascade.
3. *Coagulation cascade*: biological amplification process acts to create fibrin which stabilizes the platelet plug. Diseases can be thought of as thrombophilic (increased propensity to clot) or haemophilic (increased propensity to bleed). These can be inherited or acquired.

Laboratory tests in haemostasis and thrombosis

Coagulation screening tests are designed to identify which part of the clotting cascade is dysfunctional (Fig 46.2, although it is important to remember, these tests are performed on blood that has been removed from the body and are therefore surrogate tests for the haemostatic performance in a human body):

- *Activated partial thromboplastin time (APTT)*: the time taken in seconds for a citrated blood sample to clot after calcium and contact factor are added. The APTT is a functional determination of the intrinsic and common pathways. Prolonged by unfractionated heparin, DIC, dilutional coagulopathy, factor VIII, IX, XI deficiencies, antiphospholipid antibodies (although *in vivo* is procoagulant).
- *Prothrombin time (PT)*: time taken in seconds for blood to clot after calcium and thromboplastin (a preparation of tissue factor) is added. The PT is a functional determination of the 'extrinsic pathway'. Prolonged by warfarin, vitamin K deficiency, and liver disease.
- *INR*: the thromboplastin used in the PT is not the same in different laboratories and this alters the result of the PT, making results incomparable. The INR is calculated as a ratio of the patient's PT and a standard and thus permits comparison.
- *Thrombin time*: time in seconds for a citrated blood sample to clot after thrombin is added. Prolonged in unfractionated heparin and hypofibrinogenaemia.
- *Mixing studies*: a patient's plasma (with APTT prolongation) is mixed with normal plasma (usually a 1:1 ratio). If the mixture fails to correct, this suggests a coagulation factor inhibitor is present in the patient's serum (as a factor deficiency would correct with replacement via the normal plasma).
- *Fibrinogen*: levels are low in DIC (consumption) and dilutional coagulopathy.

Venous thromboembolic disease (VTE)

Deep vein thrombosis (DVT) of the lower limb and PE are the most common sites of venous thrombosis encountered in clinical practice. Referring to Virchow's triad is a sensible way to classify the risk factors associated with thrombosis:

- *Hypercoagulability*: malignancy, oral contraceptive pill, hyperviscosity.
- *Stasis of blood*: prolonged immobility, AF, varicose veins.
- *Vessel wall injury*: trauma, infection/inflammation, catheters.

Thromboprophylaxis

VTE is a preventable cause of hospital death. Patients are assessed based on their risk of developing thrombosis and bleeding. Interventions include thromboembolic deterrent stockings, heparin injections, and mechanical compression devices. It is important to note that the approach in medical, surgical, and obstetric patients is different.

DVT

- *Symptoms*: pain, swelling, and discolouration of the leg.
- *Investigations*: the Wells score is used to provide a 'pretest probability' of DVT. The D-dimer test is a measure of fibrin degradation products and is positive in thrombosis as well as malignancy, infection, and pregnancy—it is therefore not specific for thrombosis.

- In patients with a low pretest probability and a negative D-dimer—a DVT may be excluded. Compression ultrasonography should be carried out on patients with a low pretest probability with a positive D-dimer or those with a moderate/high pretest probability.
- If a negative initial ultrasound result is obtained in selected patients, a repeat ultrasound in 1 week may be required to exclude a DVT.
- *Differential diagnosis*: muscle strain, cellulitis, ruptured Baker's cyst.

PE
- *Symptoms*: shortness of breath, chest pain, haemoptysis.
- *Investigations*: Wells score is used to provide a 'pretest probability' of PE.
- In patients with a low pretest probability and a negative D-dimer—a PE may be excluded. CT pulmonary angiography should be carried out on patients with a low pretest probability with a positive D-dimer or those with a high pretest probability. If a negative CT pulmonary angiogram is obtained, PE is excluded.
- *Differential diagnosis*: acute coronary syndrome, costochondritis, pneumonia, aortic aneurysm.

Treatment of DVT and PE: anticoagulation initially with LMWH (or unfractionated heparin if significant renal dysfunction) and then with orally administered anticoagulation for 3–6 months (duration variable and dependent on bleeding risk) for first thrombosis and for longer if a subsequent thrombosis. Consideration must be given for any patient with VTE as to whether a secondary reversible cause exists, e.g. malignancy or inherited thrombophilia.

Honours
Thrombophilia testing
Selected patients should be investigated for inherited thrombophilia, e.g.:
- First thrombosis <40 years without a major provoking factor.
- Individuals from apparent thrombosis-prone families (more than two other symptomatic family members).
- Multiple unexplained miscarriages before 12 weeks of gestation.

Thrombophilia screen
- Consists of antithrombin, protein C and protein S, factor V Leiden and activated protein C ratio, prothrombin gene mutation, lupus anticoagulant, and anticardiolipin antibodies.
- Heritable thrombophilias include factor V Leiden, prothrombin gene mutation, protein C or protein S deficiency, antithrombin deficiency.
- Thrombophilia testing should not be carried out in the acute episode and should ideally be deferred till 8 weeks after pregnancy or 4 weeks after cessation of anticoagulation.

Antiplatelet therapy
Aspirin
Mechanism: inhibits the COX enzyme, irreversibly reducing platelet thromboxane A2. *Indications*: ischaemic stroke, acute coronary syndrome.

Clopidogrel
Mechanism: ADP receptor antagonist. *Indications*: ischaemic stroke, acute coronary syndrome.

Anticoagulant therapy

Heparin
Indications: therapeutic anticoagulation in patients with significant renal impairment, anticoagulation perioperatively. *Mechanism*: potentiates the activity of antithrombin III. *Pharmacokinetics*: quick onset of action and has a short half-life. Renally eliminated. Given as a bolus and infusion. Patients commenced on a heparin infusion are closely monitored and the infusion is titrated to APTT results. *Reversal agent*: protamine

Low-molecular-weight heparin
E.g. enoxaparin. *Indications*: therapeutic anticoagulation in VTE, thromboprophylaxis. *Mechanism*: potentiates the effect of antithrombin III. Renally eliminated. Given as a SC injection once a day. *Reversal agent*: protamine, recombinant factor VIIa.

Vitamin K antagonist
E.g. warfarin. *Indications*: therapeutic anticoagulation in VTE, AF, anticoagulation for metallic heart valves. *Pharmacokinetics*: inter-patient variable dose determined (dose adjusted as per INR). Patients are required to attend an anticoagulant clinic where the INR is measured and appropriate dose of warfarin prescribed.

New oral anticoagulants
E.g. rivaroxaban. *Indications*: stroke prevention in non-valvular AF. *Mechanism of action*: dependent on specific agent. *Pharmacokinetics*: dependent on specific agent. Oral tablet once/twice per day. *Reversal agent*: are currently under development and are specific to each agent.

Reversal of anticoagulation therapy
Reversal of anticoagulation is considered in patients who present with haemorrhage or require an urgent procedure. This requires a balance of risks and benefits and is a frequent topic of discussion for the on-call haematologist.

Acquired thrombotic disorders

Thrombotic thrombocytopenic purpura (TTP)
This is a rare but often fatal disease characterized by: (1) thrombocytopenia, (2) microangiopathic haemolytic anaemia (physical destruction of RBCs by fibrin mesh on small blood vessels), (3) fluctuating neurological signs, (4) renal impairment, and (5) fever. Antibodies are found to ADAMTS13 (which breaks down large von Willebrand factor (vWF) multimers) in adults with idiopathic TTP. Untreated TTP has a high mortality rate and the treatment is with urgent plasma exchange.

Haemolytic uraemic syndrome (HUS)
This has features in common with TTP although with predominant renal dysfunction and diarrhoea. Many cases are associated with *Escherichia coli* and other organisms such as *Shigella*. Treatment is with BP control and supportive therapy.

Inherited bleeding disorders

A specialist haemophilia centre should manage patients with inherited bleeding disorders.

Von Willebrand disease (vWD)

This is one of the most common heritable bleeding disorder characterized by reduced vWF levels and/or dysfunction in vWF due to a genetic mutation (inheritance often autosomal dominant). vWF is produced by endothelial cells and megakaryocytes and is responsible for promoting platelet adhesion and for preventing factor VIII destruction. vWF is classified as follows:

- Type I: quantitative deficiency in vWF (accounts for 75% of cases).
- Type II: qualitative dysfunction of VWF (further subclassified).
- Type III: absence of vWF (rare).

Clinical features: variable depending on the type and the causative mutation. Mucocutaneous bleeding and excessive bleeding following cuts and surgery. Haemarthrosis occurs in type III vWD. *Treatment*: mild bleeding—antifibrinolytics (e.g. tranexamic acid). Moderate disease and minor surgery—desmopressin (DDAVP®, releases vWF from endothelial cells). Major surgery—significant bleeding, severe disease (vWF concentrate).

Haemophilia A and B

X-linked bleeding disorders that are distinguishable on specific clotting factor assays. The genetic defect results in a low level of plasma factor VIII and factor IX respectively. *Clinical features*: soft tissue bleeding is noted which may lead to compartment syndrome. Recurrent joint bleeding causes chronic arthropathy secondary to haemarthroses and large encapsulated haematomas. *Investigations*: see Table 18.1 for a comparison of the inherited bleeding disorders.

Treatment

Desmopressin and tranexamic acid for minor surgery. Recombinant factor concentrates are recommended (donor-derived products have a risk of virus transmission) but are not accessible worldwide.

Table 18.1 Comparison of haemophilia types

Laboratory test	Haemophilia A	Haemophilia B	von Willebrand disease
Platelet count	↔	↔	↔ (reduced in a subtype)
PFA-100 (platelet function test)	↔	↔	Prolonged
PT	↔	↔	↔
APTT	Prolonged	Prolonged	Prolonged/↔
Factor VIII	Low	↔	↔/↓
Factor IX	↔	Low	↔
vWF	↔	↔	Low/abnormal function

Honours

Inhibitors

A complication of haemophilia treatment is the development of anti-bodies (inhibitors) to infused factor concentrates, rendering the patient refractory to additional replacement therapy. Factor VIII bypassing agents can be used in those with inhibitors who are bleeding.

Acquired bleeding disorders

Disseminated intravascular coagulation (DIC)

DIC is a medical emergency and is characterized by systemic activation of coagulation resulting in consumption of platelets and coagulation factors which leads to excessive bleeding. Causes include sepsis, trauma, organ necrosis, malignancy. *Investigations*: ↑PT, ↑APTT, ↑fibrin degradation products, ↓fibrinogen, thrombocytopenia. *Treatment*: treatment of the underlying cause with blood product support.

Idiopathic thrombocytopenia purpura (ITP)

ITP is a disorder characterized by peripheral platelet destruction with a reduction in platelet production by megakaryocytes (immune mediated). *Clinical features*: patients typically present with non-palpable purpura (in contrast to vasculitis) and is located in dependent areas of the body. *Investigations*: exclude other causes of thrombocytopenia—causative drugs, autoimmune screen, viral screen, thyroid screen, infection screen. A blood film should demonstrate true thrombocytopenia (with no platelet clumping). There must be an absence of a secondary condition associated with destruction of platelets (e.g. SLE) and no other unexplained cytopenias must be present. Bone marrow tests are performed in those >60 years of age or to exclude another cause. *Differential diagnosis*: DIC, TTP/HUS, myelodysplasia, splenic sequestration. *Treatment*: adults with a platelet count of <30 are treated due to a risk of bleeding whereas children often require no treatment as the majority undergo spontaneous remission. IV immunoglobulin, steroids, and anti-rhesus (Rh)-D have all been used.

Red cell disorders

Laboratory tests

- Haemoglobin (Hb): measures blood concentration of Hb (g/L).
- Haematocrit (Hct): proportion of blood occupied by RBC (%).
- Mean corpuscular volume (MCV): average volume of RBC (fL).
- Mean cell haemoglobin: average mass of Hb in the average RBC (pg).
- Mean cell haemoglobin concentration: average concentration of Hb in the average RBC (g/L).
- Red cell distribution width: variation in the size of RBCs (%).
- Reticulocyte count: measure of immature red cells (% or $\times 10^9$/L).

Anaemia

In adults is defined by WHO as Hb <12 in women or Hb <13 in men. It can be classified as per the MCV as microcytic (iron deficiency anaemia, anaemia of chronic disease, thalassaemia), normocytic (recent bleeding, anaemia of chronic disease, combined iron and folate/vitamin B12 deficiency, leukaemia, aplastic anaemia), and macrocytic (vitamin B12/folate deficiency, alcohol abuse, hypothyroidism, liver disease, myelodysplasia).

Anaemia of chronic disease (ACD)

The recent discovery of the protein hepcidin and its elevation in inflammatory disorders is thought to be crucial in the pathogenesis of ACD. However, the pathogenesis of ACD is complex and involves the dysregulation of iron absorption, transport, and storage. *Diagnosis*: microcytic anaemia with an elevated ferritin.

Iron deficiency anaemia (IDA)

The most common cause of a microcytic anaemia is IDA—although this is not a diagnosis and a cause must be established. Causes include hookworm infestation, chronic blood loss (e.g. bleeding from the GI tract secondary to cancer, menorrhagia), malabsorption, and dietary deficiency. *Diagnosis*: microcytic anaemia with a low serum ferritin level. Serum ferritin is also elevated in inflammatory states and in patients with coexisting IDA and systemic inflammation (common), iron indices are useful. *Treatment*: iron can be replaced through oral iron salts although unwanted side effects are common. Reducing the dose or liquid iron salts can be helpful. IV iron is an alternative. Iron indices are useful in establishing ACD vs IDA. (See Table 18.2.)

Vitamin B12 deficiency

Vitamin B12 is required for DNA synthesis and is important in haematopoiesis and neurological function. Vitamin B12 deficiency presents with symptoms of anaemia (which is macrocytic) and neurological symptoms (peripheral neuropathy affecting proprioception and vibration sense). Vitamin B12 is absorbed at the terminal ileum following binding to intrinsic factor (produced by gastric parietal cells). Causes include malabsorption (pernicious anaemia, gastrectomy, ileal disease, coeliac disease) and dietary deficiency. Treatment: vitamin B12 replacement can be given IM and orally (although less well absorbed).

Folate deficiency

Causes a derangement in haematological parameters indistinguishable from vitamin B12 deficiency. Folate absorption occurs in the proximal jejunum and is required for DNA synthesis. Causes include malabsorption (coeliac disease, Crohn's disease), dietary deficiency, ↑requirements (pregnancy, haemolysis), and drugs (methotrexate, barbiturates).

Table 18.2 Comparing anaemia subtypes

	IDA	ACD
Iron	↓	↓
Transferrin	↑/↔	↓
Transferrin saturation	↓	↓
Hepcidin	↓	↑

Honours

Subacute combined degeneration of the spinal cord

In patients with folate deficiency, vitamin B12 deficiency should be excluded prior to administering folate replacement therapy. This is because isolated folate replacement in patients with a combined folate and vitamin B12 deficiency can result in subacute combined degeneration of the spinal cord.

Haemoglobinopathy

The haemoglobinopathies are a group of conditions characterized by mutations in the genes which are responsible for the synthesis of Hb. This can result in either a qualitative change in Hb function (e.g. sickle cell disease) or a quantitative change (e.g. thalassaemia). There are areas of ↑prevalence of haemoglobinopathies due to selection pressures (e.g. malaria infection). Hb electrophoresis is used in the diagnosis of haemoglobinopathies. The Hb is separated across a gel based on electrical charge and size.

Sickle cell disease

Is prevalent in West Africa, Middle East, and parts of India. The mutation is a single base change in the beta globin gene resulting in the amino acid at position 6, glutamine, being substituted for valine. The resulting haemoglobin polymerizes in hypoxic environments resulting in sickling of the RBCs. Heterozygotes tend to be asymptomatic. Despite a specific genetic mutation, there is a broad phenotype associated with homozygosity for the sickle cell mutation.

Painful vaso-occlusive crisis

Sickle cells cause blockage of blood vessels resulting in tissue ischaemia. This can affect any tissue (e.g. skin—ulcers, brain—stoke, chest—embolism, bone—avascular necrosis of the hip, renal—papillary necrosis, spleen—hyposplenism).

Aplastic crisis

Sudden drop in Hb production by the bone marrow due to nutritional deficiency or infection with parvovirus.

Haemolytic crisis

Sudden drop in Hb due to ↑breakdown of RBCs. Long-term haemolysis predisposes to gallstone formation.

Sequestration crisis

Mainly occurs in children and can be precipitated by a viral infection. Pooling of blood occurs in the liver and spleen resulting in hypotension and profound anaemia.

Diagnosis

Sickledex®, haemoglobin electrophoresis, sickle cells demonstrated on blood film.

Management

Of an acute sickle cell crisis is a medical emergency. Oxygen, fluids, analgesia, and antibiotics if infection is suspected. Transfusions are recommended for red cell aplasia secondary to parvovirus infection, sequestration crisis, and chest crisis. Repeated transfusions are associated with antibody formation making subsequent transfusions complex. Exchange transfusion is reserved for patients with a chest crisis or for patients with a CVA. Hydroxycarbamide can be used long term and works via multiple mechanisms including increasing fetal Hb levels. Phenoxymethylpenicillin is given (long term) as patients are hyposplenic.

Thalassaemia

The thalassaemias are prevalent in the Mediterranean, Middle East, and Indian subcontinent. Adult haemoglobin is formed from two α-globin chains and two β-globin chains. Diminished or absent production of these chains result in thalassaemia. The globin chains in excess form tetramers and precipitate within RBS → chronic haemolysis.

α-Thalassaemia

Two α-globin genes are present on each chromosome 16 resulting in a total of four α-globin genes per cell ($-\alpha/\alpha\alpha$).
- *Silent α-thalassaemia* ($-\alpha/\alpha\alpha$): one gene is deleted. Asymptomatic.
- *α-Thalassaemia trait* ($--/\alpha\alpha$) or ($-\alpha/-\alpha$): two genes deleted. ↓Hb and ↓MCH. Requires no treatment.
- *Haemoglobin H (HbH) disease* ($--/-\alpha$): three genes deleted. Moderate anaemia with ↓Hb, ↓mean corpuscular Hb (MCH), and ↓MCV. Blood film shows reticulocytes, hypochromia, target cells. Brilliant cresyl blue stain on peripheral blood shows HbH inclusions (tetramers of β-globin). Clinical features: hepatosplenomegaly (extramedullary haematopoiesis) and jaundice (haemolysis). Treatment: folic acid supplementation and prompt treatment of infection.
- *Haemoglobin Bart's* ($--/--$): four genes deleted. γ-globin chains form tetrameters which have a high affinity for oxygen resulting in tissue hypoxia. The result is a stillborn fetus or one that dies soon after birth. Intrauterine transfusions have been used.

β-Thalassaemia

One β-globin gene is present on each chromosome 11 resulting in a total of two β-globin genes per cell.
- *β-Thalassaemia trait*: heterozygous for a β-globin gene mutation. Mild anaemia (microcytic). Blood film: microcytic, hypochromic RBCs with target cells. Clinical features: asymptomatic. No treatment required.
- *β-Thalassaemia intermedia*: arises through a variety of different genetic mutations: by definition these patients do not require regular transfusions. Clinical features: moderate anaemia with hepatosplenomegaly, iron overload. Some patients demonstrate skeletal abnormalities, chronic leg ulceration, and impaired growth. Treatment: iron chelation, folic acid supplementation, and prompt management of infection

- β-*Thalassaemia major*: abnormality of both β-globin genes. Clinical features: severe anaemia with ↓MCV, ↓MCH, reticulocytosis. Extramedullary haematopoiesis, hepatosplenomegaly, and skeletal abnormalities. Blood film: anisopoikilocytosis, target cells, nucleated RBCs. Methyl blue stain demonstrates α-tetramer inclusions within the RBC. Treatment: regular lifelong blood transfusions every 2–4 weeks. Iron chelation. Splenectomy may reduce transfusion requirements. HSCT has been used.

Haemolytic anaemia

Haemolysis is the premature destruction of RBCs (normal life span ~120 days). This can be classified as hereditary vs acquired, extravascular vs intravascular, or immune vs non-immune.

Hereditary
- Red cell membrane disorders (e.g. hereditary spherocytosis).
- Red cell enzyme disorders (e.g. glucose-6-phosphotase deficiency).
- Abnormal haemoglobin e.g. (sickle cell disease, thalassaemia).

Acquired and immune
- *Alloimmune*: e.g. haemolytic disease of the newborn—anti Rh antibodies from a Rh-negative mother crossing the placenta and causing haemolysis of the fetus
- *Autoimmune*: e.g. warm autoimmune haemolytic anaemia in SLE, cold haemagglutinin disease, *Mycoplasma* infection.

Acquired and non-immune

E.g. microangiopathic haemolytic anaemia (MAHA), TTP/HUS, prosthetic heart valves, malaria, paroxysmal nocturnal haemoglobinuria.

Investigations

Confirm whether haemolysis is occurring: ↓Hb, ↑reticulocyte count, ↑serum bilirubin, ↑lactate dehydrogenase (released from RBC), ↓haptoglobin (binds free Hb). Blood film: polychromasia, spherocytes, fragmentation, helmet cells, echinocytes. Is the haemolysis immune mediated? Direct antiglobulin test (DAT): a positive test indicates the red cells are coated with antibodies and the haemolysis is immune mediated.

Treatment

Treat underlying cause. Give folic acid and iron supplementation.

Transfusion medicine

A transfusion involves the safe transfer of blood products from a donor to a recipient. Blood product transfusion should only be administered when the benefit outweighs the risk and there are no other options (such as cell salvage, haematinics replacement). The benefits and risks of transfusion should be discussed with the patient and the indication for transfusion documented in the notes. The decision to transfuse is based on clinical assessment of the patient and the application of evidence, not the results of a laboratory test in isolation. Errors related to blood product transfusions are associated with significant morbidity and mortality.

Honours

Haemovigilance

This is the 'systematic surveillance of adverse reactions and adverse events related to transfusion' with the overall aim of reducing the risk associated with transfusion. Transfusion reactions and adverse events should be investigated by the hospital as well as reported to the Serious Hazards of Transfusion (SHOT) scheme.

Blood group and antibodies

Blood group antigens

These are proteins present on the surface of RBCs and some are present on platelets as well as other tissues in the body. There are >300 human blood groups described. In clinical practice, the ABO and Rh systems are of most importance.

Blood group antibodies

These are produced when an individual is exposed to blood of a different group or during pregnancy. Antibodies to AB antigens are naturally occurring and are found in all adults.

The ABO system

There are four main blood groups: A, B, AB, O. An individual will have antibodies to the A or B antigens that are not present on their own red cells (see Table 18.3).

The Rh system

Consists of five main Rh antigens, the most clinically important is RhD. Unlike the ABO system, anti-RhD antibodies are only present in RhD-negative individuals who have been exposed to RhD-positive blood (transfusions or fetomaternal haemorrhage).

Compatibility testing in hospitals

Transfusion of an incompatible blood group to a patient can be fatal by causing activation of the immune system and intravascular haemolysis. It is therefore important to accurately determine the recipient's blood group. Hospitals have a strict policy as to how this is done, how samples are taken and processed, and when the samples are taken with respect to when the blood is transfused.

Table 18.3 Comparing ABO subtypes

Blood group	Antigens on red cells	Antibodies in plasma	Compatible red cell product
O	None	Anti-A and anti-B	O
A	A	Anti-B	A, O
B	B	Anti-A	B, O
AB	A and B	None	AB, A, B, O

Group and screen
The recipient's blood group is established and their plasma tested for antibodies.

Cross-matching
The recipients plasma is mixed with a panel of red cells to ensure no significant antibodies are present. In certain circumstances, this process is now being replaced with a computer cross-matching system, which is quicker.

Blood products
Processing whole blood into different components allows the transfusion of specific components to patients. Whole blood is filtered to remove white blood cells and was introduced in 1998 to reduce the risk of variant CJD, febrile transfusion reactions, and alloimmunization. Here are the most commonly used products:

Packed red cells
Are used to restore the oxygen carrying capacity of the blood in patients with blood loss or anaemia where alternative interventions are not appropriate. They are stored at 4°C for 35 days.

Platelets
Are used to prevent or stop bleeding in patients who are thrombocytopenic (one pool is often sufficient). They should be matched for ABO groups as they have reduced survival if incompatible. A pool of platelets consists of platelets from four donations. If a patient's platelet count fails to increment with a transfusion of a pool of platelets, a single donor (apheresis) unit or HLA-matched units can be used. Platelets are stored at room temperature on an agitator. The introduction of bacterial screening can increase the shelf life from 5 days to 7 days.

Fresh frozen plasma (FFP)
Is used to replace clotting factors in patients who are actively bleeding with a derangement in their clotting factors (e.g. in DIC). The recommended dose is 12–15 mL/kg. FFP can be stored up to 36 months at <−25°C but once thawed to 4°C, it must be used within 24 hours.

Cryoprecipitate
Is a fibrinogen-rich product derived from FFP. It is used as a concentrated method to replace fibrinogen.

Acute transfusion reactions
If a transfusion reaction is suspected, the patient should be reviewed and action taken quickly with frequent clinical assessment. Ensure the laboratory is aware as additional investigations and specific action will need to be taken. Seek help early.

Honours

Special requirements

There are a number of blood product special requirements and anyone that can prescribe products should be aware of these. Here are some examples:

Irradiated products

Are used for patients at risk of transfusion-associated graft vs host diseases. This includes patients who are undergoing haemopoietic stem cell transplantation, patients with HL, and patients treated with purine analogues.

Cytomegalovirus (CMV)

Negative products should be provided for intrauterine transfusions and neonates as well as pregnant women (unless in an emergency).

Urticaria

Symptoms: an isolated urticarial skin rash. Management: chlorphenamine and reducing the rate of transfusion.

Febrile non-haemolytic transfusion reaction

Symptoms: a temperature rise of <1.5°C. Management: paracetamol and reducing the rate of transfusion.

Severe allergic reaction

Symptoms: angio-oedema, pain, hypotension, bronchospasm. Management: stop the transfusion and return the bag and set to the blood bank. Administer oxygen, salbutamol nebulizer, adrenaline (epinephrine), chlorphenamine.

Haemolytic reaction/bacterial infection

Symptoms: pyrexia, shortness of breath, pain. Management: stop the transfusion and return the bag and set to the blood bank. Give oxygen, antibiotics, fluid support, and maintain satisfactory urine output.

Fluid overload

Symptoms: shortness of breath, hypoxia, elevated JVP, fluid overload. Management: administer oxygen and diuretics.

Transfusion-related acute lung injury

Symptoms: shortness of breath, hypoxia, pyrexia, JVP not elevated. Management: stop the transfusion and return the bag and set to the laboratory. Administer oxygen and contact ITU.

Major haemorrhage

Each hospital has a major haemorrhage protocol, which consists of quick and safe access to compatible (O RhD-negative) blood products in the absence of a cross-match.

Haematology: in the emergency department

Neutropenic sepsis

This is defined as the presence of signs and symptoms of infection in a patient with an absolute neutrophil count of <0.5 × 10⁹/L. This is one of the most common emergencies in haematology and in 2012 accounted for two deaths per day in England and Wales. Patients who are neutropenic are susceptible to invasive infection and can deteriorate rapidly. Many patients do not exhibit classic features of sepsis (e.g. pyrexia), often due to concomitant chemotherapy and steroid therapy.

Conduct a primary survey: ABCDE

Investigations: FBC, U&E, LFTs, CRP, bone profile, coagulation studies, blood cultures (peripherally and from any lumens of the line), ABG (beware patients with low platelets—ensure pressure applied after), urine dipstick and culture, CXR.

If possible, take a brief history from the patient ascertaining the chronicity of symptoms, whether the patient has had previous infections and source, history of malignancy (if so, which type, treatment stage, last dose of chemotherapy, physician they are under the care of), and allergies.

Cultures should ideally be taken prior to the administration of antibiotics but cultures should not delay the administration of antibiotics. Antibiotics administered should provide an anti-microbial effect against a large number of bacteria (so called 'broad spectrum'). Individual hospitals have local policies but a suggestion for empirical antibiotic therapy is piperacillin/tazobactam and amikacin (beware aminoglycosides and renal impairment). Previous cultures if available are informative (e.g. previous MRSA) and may alter antibiotic therapy and for patients who have a prolongued history of neutropaenia, other opportunisitic infections should be considered (e.g. infection with pneumocystis jiroveci). Consider removing the line if this is the source of sepsis and discussing the patient with the intensive care unit if the patient is significantly unwell or at risk of further clinical deterioration.

Honours

Granulocyte-Colony Stimulating Factor

G-CSF is a growth factor which stimulates the bone marrow to produce and release neutrophils into the blood stream. A significant side effect ties bone pain/discomfort. Different preparations are available but are given subcutaneously. Consider giving G-CSF in patients with neutropenic sepsis providing the patient does not have active leukaemia. G-CSF is however not recommended for prophylaxis.

Haematology: in exams

As haematological disease can affect the whole body, it is important that you can demonstrate the ability to perform an accurate and systematic history and clinical examination of a patient. One must be able to identify the signs associated with other diseases and be able to perform an examination of the reticuloendothelial system.

History station

- *Symptoms related to anaemia and chronicity*: tiredness, shortness of breath, reduced functional ability, peripheral oedema, angina.
- *Symptoms related to immunocompromise*: pyrexia, specific sites of infection, sore throat.
- *Symptoms related to haemostatic dysfunction*: e.g. bruising, bleeding, joint swelling, leg swelling. Assess for haemostatic function when the patient has been 'challenged', e.g. surgery, trauma.
- *Symptoms related to organ infiltration*: CNS (headache, leg weakness), lymphadenopathy (abdominal pain/swelling), chronicity.
- *Past medical history*: other diseases are associated with haematological conditions (e.g. autoimmune disorders) or may have a relation to their presenting complaint (e.g. anaemia secondary to chronic blood loss).
- *Past surgical history*: surgical procedures may be related to haematological disease (e.g. gastrectomy and vitamin B12 deficiency) and represent an event where the body is challenged. Identifying complications such as bleeding and thrombosis during these periods is useful.
- *Past obstetric history*: number of pregnancies, complications, and relationship to symptoms.
- *Past transfusion history*: have they received blood products? If so, when, where, which products, and for what reason?
- *Drug history and allergies*: prescribed and non-prescribed medications can cause haematological abnormalities.
- *Social history*: haematological diseases can interfere with daily functioning. This interference can provide considerable insight into the severity of disease. Management of haematological disease is often long term and the impact on patients' lives can be profound. Haematological disease can be associated with particular jobs. Lifestyle factors can predispose patients to certain infections.
- *Tobacco and alcohol*: consumption can affect the haematological system.
- *Travel history*: important when considering infections.
- *Family history*: many haematological diseases are inherited or demonstrate familial susceptibility.

Clinical examination

- *General examination*: vital signs, pallor, jaundice, weight, skin rashes, pigmentation.
- *Mouth*: dentition, gingival hypertrophy, ulcers, bleeding.
- *Hands*: koilonychias.
- *Abdomen*: abdominal scars (splenectomy), assess for hepatomegaly and splenomegaly.
- *Lymphadenopathy*: examine the cervical, axillary, and inguinal nodes. Quantify the location, the number, and size of the lymph nodes. Note the consistency and whether tender.
- *Bones and joints*: joint swelling and range of movement (important in haemophilia) and bony tenderness (malignancy).
- *Optic fundi*: examine for signs of hyperviscosity (e.g. hyperleucocytosis in leukaemia with a high WCC, paraproteinaemias).
- *Neurological exam*: peripheral neuropathy in vitamin B12 deficiency.

Things to do beforehand

There are clinical scenarios which frequently present to haematology clinics, one of which is anaemia. The second is lymphadenopathy. Understanding the differential diagnosis will assist in planning the necessary investigations.

Clinical scenarios

Lymphadenopathy

Lymphadenopathy can be caused by a wide range of different pathological processes.

Causes

- Infection:
  - Bacterial, e.g. tonsillitis, cellulitis, TB, syphilis.
  - Viral, e.g. CMV, EBV, HIV, hepatitis B and C, rubella.
  - Other, e.g. toxoplasmosis, histoplasmosis.
- Neoplastic:
  - Haematological:
    — Lymphoma (HL and NHL).
    — Leukaemia (CLL and ALL, rarely AML).
  - Non-haematological:
    — Systemic disorders, e.g. RA.
    — FBC and peripheral blood film examination.
    — U&E, LFTs, CRP, bone profile.
    — ESR.

Viral screen

- Imaging: consider CT of the chest abdomen and pelvis to assess extent of lymphadenopathy (lymphadenopathy may be deep, e.g. para-aortic and therefore not palpable).
- Lymph node biopsy (core or excision): to achieve a definitive diagnosis.
- Microbiology: blood and urine cultures, serology, consider sending tissue samples, TB testing.
- Bone marrow examination: not necessary unless staging as part of haematological malignancy.

Interpreting laboratory results

The key to being successful when interpreting laboratory results is to develop a systematic method. Clinical correlation is important as well as thinking about further informative tests to help achieve a diagnosis.

Anaemia

- Microcytic : low Fe, thalassaemia, chronic disease, sideroblastic.
- Normocytic: leukaemia, aplastic anaemia, haemolysis, acute blood loss, pregnancy.
- Macrocytic: vitamin B12/folate deficiency, myelodysplasia, reticulocytosis, cytotoxic, hypothyroidism, liver disease.

Neutrophilia

- Primary: myeloproliferative neoplasms.
- Secondary: bacterial infection, inflammation, e.g. MI, trauma, surgery, burns.

Neutropenia

- Reduced production: viral infection, sepsis, bone marrow failure (e.g. leukaemia), cytotoxic drugs.
- ↑Destruction: viral infection, sepsis, antineutrophil antibodies, splenic sequestration.

Lymphocytosis

- Primary: leukaemia and lymphomas, e.g. CLL.
- Secondary : acute viral infections, chronic infections, e.g. TB.

Lymphopenia

- Reduced production : HIV, uraemia, bone marrow failure (e.g. leukaemia), cytotoxic drugs.
- ↑Destruction: HIV, steroid therapy, SLE.

Thrombocytopenia

- ↓Production: vitamin B12/folate deficiency, leukaemia or myelodysplastic syndromes, reduced production of thrombopoietin in liver failure, sepsis, hereditary syndromes, e.g. congenital amegakaryocytic thrombocytopenia.
- ↑Destruction: ITP, TTP/HUS, DIC, SLE, post-transfusion purpura, neonatal alloimmune thrombocytopenia, splenic sequestration, dengue fever, HIV.

Eosinophilia

- Primary: leukaemia and lymphomas, hypereosinophilic syndrome.
- Secondary: allergy, drug reaction, GvHD.

Immunology and allergies

Immunology and allergies: overview

Clinical immunology and allergy explores defects of the immune system. It combines both clinical and laboratory principles in the context of clinical medicine. You will have exposure to a vast array of interesting and complex medical conditions, some of which you may have heard of, some which you did not even know existed! This discipline truly combines basic sciences with clinical medicine, making the field both exciting and challenging. Cases seen can vary from simple food allergies to rare inherited diseases. Often diagnostic workup is complex, and the laboratory aspect introduces you to novel diagnostic approaches and procedures. In view of this, both management and treatment approach can be innovative and complex.

Cases

The majority of immunology-based diagnoses can be multifaceted and difficult to diagnose. Patients can present with a constellation of symptoms which require good history taking, careful clinical consideration, and specialist diagnostic work (see Table 19.1). Reasons for referral can include recurrent infections despite multiple and frequent antibiotic usage, syndromic features, recurrent swellings and rashes, and symptoms which do not seem to fit other diagnoses. Cases may overlap with other specialities including dermatology, haematology, and respiratory medicine to name a few, which makes it an interesting platform for MDT-based management.

Table 19.1 Examples of patients seen in clinical immunology

Type of cases	Examples of diseases seen
Primary immunodeficiency	• X-linked agammaglobulinaemia • Combined immune deficiency • Common variable immunodeficiency disorders • Complement deficiencies • Hyper IgE syndrome • Hereditary angio-oedema
Secondary immunodeficiency	Secondary to: • Chemotherapy • Steroid therapy • Infections • Immunosuppressant therapy • Antiepileptic drugs
Allergy	• Food allergy • Drug allergy • Chronic spontaneous urticaria

Immunology and allergies: in clinic and exams

What do we do?

The majority of clinical work is outpatient based under allergy and immunodeficiency. Referrals can be GP sourced, or from other specialities seeking a secondary opinion on complicated cases. The increase in cases of patients with secondary immunodeficiency across disciplines has seen the emergence of combined clinics with other specialities to deliver optimum care. Although inpatient lead care is seldom found, advice with regard to management of patients with primary immunodeficiency, anaphylaxis, immunoglobulin therapy, and allergy testing is common. There may be a day unit offering immunoglobulin infusions.

Laboratory

(See → 'Pathology: in the pathology laboratory' pp. 563–4.) The laboratory aspect of immunology and allergy training is just as significant as the clinical aspect. Clinicians are taught about the principles of laboratory organization and management, through dedicated laboratory time during training. Clinicians are expected to learn about:

- laboratory organization and management
- laboratory quality management
- principles of immunoassays including assays such as immunofluorescence and flow cytometry
- analytical techniques and instrumentation
- interpretation of specific immunology assays.

Procedures

The majority of procedures fall under the remit of allergy medicine. Procedures include the following:

- *Skin prick testing*: to multiple allergens—performed in allergy clinics.
- *Challenge testing*: this can be skin prick, intradermal, or oral challenges to a wide variety of allergens including (mainly) drug and food-related allergies.
- *Inpatient desensitization*: e.g. to antibiotics in complicated CF cases.
- *Immunotherapy*: delivering small quantities of allergen to patients to invoke desensitization—often outpatient based.

Exam questions

It is likely that the majority of questions based on immunology will be under the pathology section or integrated within exams of other specialities. You may be asked about laboratory investigations, serology, clinical features, and diagnostic testing. It is unlikely that you will see patients with primary immunodeficiency in the practical exams but it is important to consider some of the conditions as important differential diagnoses, e.g.: hereditary angio-oedema in the context of recurrent swelling and anaphylaxis. Exam questions could be MCQs, an essay, photos, and a viva.

Infectious diseases and tropical medicine

Infectious diseases and tropical medicine: overview

The infectious diseases/tropical medicine placement is an excellent opportunity to see a wide variety of presentations and exotic diseases; patients will have various stories and different systemic involvement. Your overall medical skills such as history taking (especially the travel history), clinical examination, and diagnostic skills will be vital throughout this placement and will be developed further.

On the wards

You could see anything from skin and soft tissue infections such as cellulitis, and necrotizing fasciitis to more deep-seated infections such as septic arthritis, osteomyelitis, meningitis, encephalitis, and infective endocarditis (covered elsewhere in the book).

In clinic

You will get the opportunity to meet patients from various ethnicities and social backgrounds, each with a different story and illness. Patients that come to mind include the migrant labourer with reactivation of TB, the keen hiker who caught Lyme disease from trekking in the New Forest, and the farmer who developed Q-fever during the lambing season.

In the ED

You will meet others with exciting travel histories, some will present with a simple diarrhoeal illness, others with potentially life-threatening infections such as malaria.

Overall, in infectious diseases you will see very ill people improve dramatically following your intervention. Your expertise will not be limited to one system or organ, which keeps things fresh. You will also work closely with various specialties, as well as public health agencies and community teams to improve patient outcomes and prevent outbreaks.

Infectious diseases and tropical medicine: cases to see

Malaria

In the UK, malaria is a serious imported infection caused by single-celled parasites from the *Plasmodium* species. Transmitted by the female *Anopheles* mosquito, it is a medical emergency and prompt diagnosis and management is vital. Globally, malaria continues to be a major issue. Figures released by the WHO estimate the burden was over 200 million cases worldwide, with nearly half a million deaths in 2015. Most of these cases were in sub-Saharan Africa and South-East Asia. In 2016, there were 1618 reported malaria cases in the UK (real numbers are probably double that) with six deaths/year over the past decade. There are five *Plasmodium* species where 80% of infections in the UK are due to *P. falciparum*. Species include:

- *P. falciparum*
- *P. vivax*
- *P. ovale*
- *P. malariae*
- *P. knowlesi*.

Factoid

Documented as an illness for >4000 years; the name probably originates from the Italian word *Mal'aria* meaning '*bad air*'. It was not until 1880 that the malaria parasites were discovered and since have been studied extensively and treated. (See Fig. 20.1.)

History

Patients are returning travellers from endemic areas who often present with fever, rigors, sweats, and malaise; but it could also present with non-specific symptoms such as headaches, myalgia, diarrhoea, and cough. The symptoms can occur anywhere from 6 days to 3 months following exposure in cases of *P. falciparum*. However, *P. ovale* and *P. vivax* can present months or (rarely) years later, especially if treated in the past, as these two can present following auto-infection with the dormant liver stage of the parasite (hypnozoite). You will need to take a thorough travel history, noting country and area of travel, including stop-overs, and date of return to the UK. Do not forget to ask about malaria prophylaxis, i.e. the name of drug, dosage, and adherence.

Diagnosis

Once malaria is suspected, *thick and thin blood films* for microscopy should be sent to the haematology lab urgently. This is in addition to a FBC, U&E, LFTs, clotting, and blood gas analysis including lactate and glucose. If the first sample is negative but the clinical suspicion remains, further samples should be sent 12–24 hours later. If three films are negative, malaria is unlikely. Clinical assessment and systemic examination will exclude severe malaria or concurrent infections.

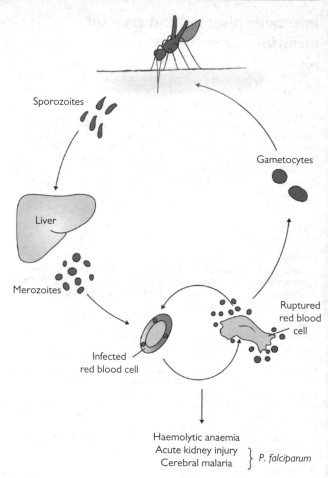

Fig. 20.1 Malaria life cycle. An infected mosquito injects sporozoites into blood which home to the liver and multiply in hepatocytes, forming merozoites. Merozoites released into blood infect red blood cells and multiply again, rupturing the red cells and infecting more red cells. Some merozoites mature into gametocytes which newly infect a mosquito, completing the life cycle. Reproduced with permission from *Clinical Pathology* (Oxford Core Texts), Carton, James, Daly, Richard, and Ramani, Pramila, Oxford University Press (2006), p. 26, Figure 3.5.

Major features of severe or complicated falciparum malaria in adults

- Impaired consciousness or seizures.
- Renal impairment (*oliguria <0.4 mL/kg/hour or creatinine >265 mmol/L*).
- Acidosis (pH <7.3).
- Hypoglycaemia (<2.2 mmol/L).
- Pulmonary oedema or ARDS.
- Hb ≤8 g/dL.
- Spontaneous bleeding/DIC
- Shock (algid malaria—BP <90/60 mmHg).
- Haemoglobinuria (without G6PD deficiency).
- Parasitaemia >10%.

Treatment

Uncomplicated falciparum malaria

There are three therapeutic options for the treatment of uncomplicated falciparum malaria. *Artemisinin combination therapy* (ACT, e.g. Riamet® or Eurartesim®) is the preferred option as they are more effective against the parasite throughout its life cycle. However, if ACT is not available, *atovaquone–proguanil* (Malarone®), and *oral quinine sulfate + doxycycline* are other available options.

Complicated falciparum malaria

Parenteral therapy is the mainstay treatment of complicated falciparum malaria. Parenteral therapy should also be considered in cases of parasitaemia >2% and pregnant women with artesunate (IV for 1–5 days followed by a full course of an oral ACT) or quinine dihydrochloride (IV followed by a course of quinine + doxycycline/clindamycin).

Non-falciparum malaria

Either an oral ACT or chloroquine can be used to treat the blood forms of all non-falciparum species. In cases of *P. vivax* and *P. ovale*, the treatment regimen should include primaquine to eliminate the dormant liver stage (hypnozoite) to prevent relapse. Test patients for G6PD deficiency before treatment with primaquine.

Viral haemorrhagic fevers

You have probably heard of the recent devastating outbreak of Ebola in West Africa. Patients are returning travellers from endemic areas who present with non-specific symptoms such as fever, malaise, vomiting and diarrhoea. Patients could present with bruising or active bleeding (hence the haemorrhagic in viral haemorrhagic fevers). It is important to be aware of current outbreaks which you could find on Public Health England's website (⌘ www.gov.uk/guidance/viral-haemorrhagic-fevers-origins-reservoirs-transmission-and-guidelines). Patients present within 3 weeks of returning from an endemic area but malaria needs to be excluded first! Patients will require specific infection control precautions including patient isolation according to local policies as well as special sample handling by the lab. Treatment for viral haemorrhagic fevers is supportive, focusing on correcting metabolic and electrolyte abnormalities, as well as treating potential concurrent infections and organ support if needed. Viral families include Arenaviridae, Flaviviridae, Bunyaviridae, Filoviridae.

Amoebiasis

Caused by the single-celled (protozoan) parasite *Entamoeba histolytica* in ~10 % of the world population. It is transmitted via the faeco-oral route so ask about eating habits, as well as water sources for drinking, ice, cooking, and brushing teeth! *Symptoms*: vary from asymptomatic to the commoner diarrhoeal illness; however, amoebiasis could cause dysentery and colitis in severe cases. Extraintestinal amoebiasis can occur if the parasite spreads beyond the intestine, and causes an amoebic liver abscess → RUQ pain and fever. *Diagnosis* requires imaging of the abdomen (e.g. US scan), stool MC&S, or aspiration (dark red-brown colour described as '*anchovy paste*'). *Treatment*: pharmacotherapy and an interventional assessment in cases of severe colitis and liver abscess. Paromomycin, iodoquinol, and diloxanide furoate are luminal agents (minimal GI absorption) that can be used for asymptomatic or mild infections. Metronidazole is reserved for severe disease.

Soil-transmitted helminth infections

Affects ~1.5 billion people worldwide, mostly children. The infection is prevalent in areas of poor sanitation. Transmitted via the faeco-oral route by the ingestion of eggs present in contaminated soil, water, and vegetation. There are three main species that infect humans:
- Roundworm (*Ascaris lumbricoides*).
- Whipworm (*Trichuris trichiura*).
- Hookworms (*Necator americanus* and *Ancylostoma duodenale*) could also be transmitted by walking barefoot on contaminated soil, as larvae can penetrate the skin.

Mostly asymptomatic but could cause abdominal pain and diarrhoea. Chronic infection could → nutritional deficiencies and anaemia. Diagnosed by microscopy of stool samples. Treatment is with albendazole or mebendazole.

Schistosomiasis

Is a parasitic worm infection of the blood trematode (fluke) class. It is estimated that 200 million people worldwide are infected. The infection is transmitted through swimming in contaminated water in endemic areas. Free swimming larvae (cercariae) are released by the intermediate host (fresh water snails) and penetrate the human skin. This causes a pruritic rash, known otherwise as the 'swimmer's' itch'. The larvae then migrate through the lungs or the liver to their final organ. Depending on species, the adult worm could settle in either the venous plexus of the urinary bladder (*Schistosoma haematobium*) or the portal venous system (*S. japonicum, S. mansoni*), and lay their eggs which in turn are released through urine and faeces. The eggs hatch in fresh water and penetrate the snail, continuing the infection cycle. In the travel history, it is important to ask about leisure activities especially swimming and rafting in fresh water. The stereotypical location to contract the infection is Lake Malawi in Africa (prime destination for medical students on electives). Schistosomiasis can cause a myriad of systemic syndromes including acute schistosomiasis (Katayama fever), intestinal, urinary, hepatic, CNS, and chronic schistosomiasis:

• Acute schistosomiasis (Katayama fever) presents within 2 months of infection with fever, headache, hepatosplenomegaly, lymphadenopathy, and peripheral eosinophilia.
• Urinary schistosomiasis (*S. haematobium*) presents with terminal haematuria, if untreated → urinary obstruction or in some cases bladder cancer due to chronic granulomatous inflammation.

The diagnosis is confirmed by detection of eggs in urine or faeces, serological tests are also helpful. Treatment is with praziquantel.

Traveller's diarrhoea

Is the commonest travel-related illness worldwide. ~90% of cases are caused by bacteria; enterotoxigenic *Escherichia coli* is commonest, followed by *Campylobacter, Shigella*, and *Salmonella* species. Viruses such as norovirus, rotavirus, and astrovirus cause ~5–8% of cases. Rarely, traveller's diarrhoea is caused by parasites such as *Giardia* and *Entamoeba* species. Spread is via the faeco-oral route, and depending on the organism, symptoms could start hours to days after ingestion of contaminated food or drink. Symptoms range from mild abdominal discomfort and nausea to vomiting and frequent diarrhoea which could contain blood and mucous (*dysentery*). Diagnosis is often presumptive if mild, but could be made by microscopy and culture of stool samples if moderate or severe. Treatment is mostly supportive for mild cases, using oral rehydration solutions and antimotility agents (not to be used in bloody diarrhoea or patients presenting with fever). Antibiotics (e.g. azithromycin or fluoroquinolones) are reserved for moderate to severe cases.

Dengue fever

Is caused by a flavivirus, endemic in the tropics, and transmitted by the *Aedes* mosquito. Symptoms start within 2 weeks of infection and include fever, headache, retro-orbital pain, myalgia, and a maculopapular rash. In cases of repeated infection, patients can present with confusion, petechiae, bruising, and signs of shock due to hypovolaemia and coagulopathy (Dengue shock syndrome). Diagnosis is often made by serology (raised Dengue IgM in acute infection) or detection by PCR. Treatment is supportive with antipyretics, rehydration, and circulatory support in severe cases. The Chikungunya virus is an *alphavirus*, also transmitted by the *Aedes* mosquito, and therefore endemic in the same areas as Dengue with similar management.

Extrapulmonary tuberculosis

TB most commonly presents as a primary lung infection. However, following the initial infection which could be asymptomatic, *Mycobacterium tuberculosis* can lie dormant for years to reactivate later in the form of extrapulmonary TB. Profound immunosuppression due to frailty, biologic agent use, cancer chemotherapy, or HIV infection are known risk factors; however, reasons for reactivation in apparently immune competent individuals are poorly understood. The mainstay of diagnosis is biopsy and culturing the organism from tissue or bodily fluid samples, this is often difficult due to the low yield from culturing bodily fluids such as CSF. Detection by

PCR could also be used, especially in determining resistance to rifampicin. Interferon-gamma release assays (QuantiFERON-TB Gold®, T-SPOT®.TB) are helpful in determining prior exposure to TB, but their sensitivity is reduced in profound immunosuppression. Systemic manifestations include the following:

- *TB meningitis (e.g. bacterial meningitis)*: presents with fever, meningism (headache, neck stiffness, and photophobia), reduced consciousness, and coma. The CSF shows a lymphocytic predominant pleocytosis, with a very high protein level but very low glucose.
- *CNS tuberculoma*: presents as a space-occupying lesion, symptoms depend on the area of the CNS affected. It is typically formed of a caseating granuloma. Diagnosis is with biopsy and culture.
- *TB osteomyelitis*: confirmed by culture.
- *TB adenopathy*: presents with fever, night sweats, and lymphadenopathy. Diagnosis is confirmed by culture/PCR from biopsied lymph node.
- *Intraocular TB*: rare and presents with reduced vision or pain in cases of TB uveitis. Diagnosis is often presumptive; but the organism can be detected by PCR/culture from aqueous/vitreous samples.

Treatment is similar to pulmonary TB initially, with a 2-month induction phase with quadruple therapy (rifampicin, isoniazid, ethambutol, and pyrazinamide + pyridoxine to prevent isoniazid-induced peripheral neuropathy). This is followed by a consolidation phase with rifampicin, isoniazid, and pyridoxine for the remainder of the course. The total duration depends on the location. CNS involvement requires a total of 9–12 months of treatment, others usually require at least 6 months. Investigation of the immune status is vital (i.e. HIV testing).

Epstein–Barr virus

Is a widely-disseminated herpes virus that spreads by intimate contact with body fluids, primarily saliva, from asymptomatic carriers or infected patients. The virus remains latent in most infected cells and can be reactivated after the acute phase. Most of the EBV infections are subclinical. *Infectious mononucleosis/glandular fever/kissing disease* is common in adolescence and consists of fever, tonsillitis ± pharyngitis and cervical lymph node enlargement with atypical lymphocytosis preceded by 1–2-week prodromal phase of anorexia and malaise. Lymph node enlargement could be out of proportion producing upper airway obstruction. Pharyngitis (with palatal petechiae in 25–60%), hepatomegaly, splenomegaly, periorbital oedema, and lymphadenopathy are common on examination. Some complications include mild hepatitis (95%), cytopaenias (usually self-limited), splenic rupture, and neurological complications of meningitis, encephalitis, and seizures. *Morbilliform rash following the administration of penicillin (possibly immune-mediated) is also a common complication.* EBV is associated with a variety of lymphoproliferative disorders and some malignancies such as African Burkitt lymphoma and nasopharyngeal carcinoma. EBV-infected B cells produce monoclonal IgM antibodies (heterophile antibodies) that are measured using various agglutination tests (Paul–Bunnel/monospot test). 90% have developed these antibodies by week 3 and they usually disappear within the first 3 months. EBV-specific antibodies (viral capsid antigen and

Epstein–Barr nuclear antigen) confirm acute, late, or past infection. Most cases are self-limited and do not require specific therapy. Steroids may be indicated in cases of severe thrombocytopenia, haemolytic anaemia, impending airway obstruction, and for CNS or cardiac involvement.

Typhoid

Salmonella enterica serotypes Typhi and Paratyphi (A, B, and C) can cause a potentially severe bacteraemic illness referred to as typhoid and para-typhoid fever, respectively. It is acquired by consumption of water or food contaminated by faeces of an acutely infected, convalescent person, or a chronic asymptomatic carrier. Endemic areas include southern Asia (India, Pakistan, Bangladesh), south-east Asia, and Africa. Incubation period 6–30 days. Insidious onset with increasing fatigue and high fever (with rela-tive bradycardia) followed by headache, malaise, anorexia, abdominal pain, and diarrhoea or constipation. Complications include cholecystitis, intes-tinal haemorrhage, and perforation. Diagnosis with blood cultures (+ve in 50% of patients) or bone marrow (highest yield). Urine and stool sam-ples are positive at a late stage. Quinolones are the drug of choice, but if there is suspicion of resistance (i.e. >80% in most of Asia), ceftriaxone or azithromycin are alternatives. 1% of patients become chronic carriers (will need treatment if at risk of spreading disease, e.g. food handlers). Typhoid vaccine exists just for typhoid fever and is recommended for all travellers to endemic areas. Immunization is not 100% effective

Influenza ('flu')

Is caused by influenza viruses type A, B, and C spread from person to person through respiratory droplets. Subtypes of influenza A are clas-sified based on surface proteins: haemagglutinin and neuraminidase. Distribution of influenza varies every year between geographic areas and time of year. Avian and swine influenza viruses can occasionally infect and cause disease in humans, associated with close exposure to infected ani-mals. Incubation period is 1–4 days. Uncomplicated influenza symptoms in-clude fever, muscle aches, headache, malaise, non-productive cough, sore throat, vomiting, and rhinitis. Complications include primary influenza viral pneumonia, secondary bacterial pneumonia, myocarditis, myositis, and encephalopathy. Adults >65 years, children <2 years, and patients with comorbidities are at higher risk of complications. Diagnostic tests include viral culture, rapid influenza diagnostic tests, immunofluorescence and re-verse transcription PCR. The cornerstone of management is an effective vaccination strategy recommended in 'at-risk' groups included all patients >65 years, those with diabetes, immunosuppression, and/or with cardiac, lung, or renal disease, and health workers. Early antiviral treatment (<48 hours after onset of symptoms) can shorten the duration of illness and reduce the risk of complications. Oseltamivir (neuraminidase inhibitor) is the preferred agent, recommended in hospitalized patients and patients at higher risk of complications.

Chickenpox

Is caused by varicella zoster virus (VZV). Common in childhood and highly contagious (85% secondary attack rates). After primary infection, the virus remains dormant in the sensory nerve ganglia and can reactivate at a later time causing herpes zoster (shingles in 20% of population). Transmission occurs from person to person by inhalation of aerosols from vesicular fluid of skin lesions and infected respiratory tract secretions. The period of transmission begins 1–2 days before the onset of rash and ends when all lesions are crusted. Incubation period 10–21 days. 1–2 days of pro- dromal symptoms (fever, malaise) usually precedes a pruritic rash con- sisting of crops of macules, papules, and vesicles that resolve by crusting. The presence of lesions in different stages of development at the same time is characteristic of varicella. Complications are more frequent in in- fants, adults >65 years, and immunocompromised people and include bac- terial skin infection, pneumonia, cerebellar ataxia, meningitis, encephalitis, and haemorrhagic conditions, rarely resulting in death (1/40,000 for chil- dren, ↑15-fold for adults). Diagnosis is usually clinical. Vesicular swabs or scrapings from crusted lesions can be used to identify VZV DNA by PCR (preferred method) or direct fluorescent antibody. Serologic tests are less reliable. Oral/IV aciclovir should be considered in high-risk populations (>65 years, chronic cutaneous or pulmonary disorders, and immunocom- promised patients) and in serious complications. Live, attenuated vaccine is recommended in non-immune healthcare workers and close contacts of immunocompromised patients. Its effectiveness is 80% after one dose, 95% after two doses.

Measles (rubeola)

Caused by a virus from the genus *Morbillivirus* and transmitted from person to person by aerosolized droplets. It is highly contagious with an incubation period of 7–21 days. Symptoms include fever, conjunctivitis, rhinitis, and cough followed by small blue-grey spots on an erythematous base on the buccal mucosa (Koplik spots) and a maculopapular rash that usually begins on the face. Infected people are usually contagious from 4 days before until 4 days after rash onset. Common complications include diarrhoea, middle ear infection, and pneumonia. Risk of encephalitis is higher in children <5 years and adults >20 years and in malnourished population. *Subacute sclerosis panencephalitis* is a chronic, degenerative, neurological complication occurring years after infection. Positive serology test confirms the diagnosis. Treatment is supportive. Vitamin A is recommended for all children with acute measles to reduce the risk of complications. It is preventable with a live, attenuated vaccine given at 1 year and in preschool.

Poliomyelitis

Is produced by poliovirus (genus *Enterovirus*) which is highly contagious via faecal–oral or oral transmission. Incubation period is 10 days. Most in- fected patients are asymptomatic and just a minority develop acute flaccid paralysis of a single limb or quadriplegia. Respiratory failure and death are rare. There may be delayed progression or paralysis (*post-polio syndrome*). Diagnosis requires identifying poliovirus by cell culture or PCR in clinical specimens (usually stools) obtained from an acutely ill patient. Only sup- portive treatment is available. Prevention includes routine infant immun- ization by inactivated poliovirus vaccine (IPV) at ages 2, 4, 6–18 months, and 4–6 years. Vaccine confers lifelong immunity. Poliovirus disease is now confined to only two countries: Pakistan and Afghanistan. Adults travelling to these areas who are unvaccinated or whose vaccination status is unknown should receive a series of three doses of IPV.

Rabies

Is a neurotropic virus from the family *Rhabdoviridae* transmitted by inoculation of saliva from a bite of a rabid animal (e.g. bats, dogs, cats, and foxes). Symptoms can develop 9–90 days after exposure. Pain and paraesthesia at the site of exposure are often the first symptoms followed by fever, headache, malaise, and rapidly progressing into a fatal, acute encephalitis. It causes 50,000 deaths/year worldwide and is often fatal. Advise travellers to avoid animal contact. If bitten, clean bite wound with soapy water. Pre-exposure prophylaxis is recommended to travellers highly exposed to rabies (e.g. vets, zookeepers, and bat handlers). Treatment if bitten (and previously vaccinated) consists of rabies vaccine on days 0 and 3 after exposure. Post-exposure prophylaxis for an unvaccinated patient consists of rabies immunoglobulin ± vaccine on days 0, 3, 7, and 14. Rabies is a notifiable disease.

Creutzfeldt–Jakob disease (CJD)

Is a human prion disease, classified as a transmissible spongiform encephalopathy (TSE). It is a rapidly progressive, invariably fatal neurodegenerative disorder caused by an abnormal isoform of a cellular glycoprotein known as the prion protein. It occurs in 85% of cases as a sporadic disease. 5–15% develop CJD because of inherited mutations. It presents as a rapidly progressive dementia with myoclonus → eventually developing extrapyramidal signs and visual symptoms. Infection usually → death within first year of onset of illness. Diagnosis relies on presence of 14-3-3 protein in the CSF and/or a typical EEG pattern (periodic sharp wave complexes). Confirmatory diagnosis requires neuropathological and/or immunodiagnostic testing of brain tissue. No therapy has been shown to stop the progression of this disease and treatment is supportive.

Tetanus

Is produced by tetanospasmin, the exotoxin of *Clostridium tetani*, transmitted by contact of non-intact skin with contaminated objects. Susceptible wounds include those contaminated with dirt, human or animal excreta or saliva, burns, punctures, or crush injuries. 20% of patients have no evidence of recent wounds. Produces 50 deaths/year in the UK with 40% mortality (80% in neonates). Incubation period 3–10 days. Prodrome of fever, malaise, and headache before classical acute symptoms of muscle rigidity and spasms, often in the jaw (*trismus*), facial muscles (*risus sardonicus*), and neck. Progression to generalized tetanus (*opisthotonus*) may occur → respiratory failure and death. There are no confirmatory diagnostic tests available. Treatment includes human tetanus immune globulin (hTIG) to neutralize toxin, agents to control muscle spasm (e.g. diazepam), antimicrobials (first choice metronidazole 500 mg/6 hours), and aggressive wound care included debridement and excision if possible. Prevention includes routine tetanus vaccine: three doses during first year of life and a booster dose during adolescence and early adulthood.

Lyme disease

Is caused by the bacteria *Borrelia burgdorferi* transmitted to humans through the bite of infected blacklegged ticks (*Ixodes scapularis*). Incubation period 3–30 days. Typical symptoms include fever, headache, fatigue, joint and muscle pains, and a characteristic, painless, annular skin lesion centred on the bite called erythema migrans. 60% of patients do not recall a tick bite. Later features of Lyme disease (weeks to months after the tick bite) can include mono- or polyarthritis (often knee), Bell's palsy, meningitis, carditis, and severe fatigue. A positive serology test for *Borrelia burgdorferi* antibodies confirms the diagnosis if added to a suggestive clinical history, they could develop late (90% +ve at 4–6 weeks). CSF serology should be obtained in patients with neurological symptoms. Early-stage manifestations are treated with a course of oral doxycycline or amoxicillin for up to 28 days. If symptoms persist or neurologic symptoms appear, IV ceftriaxone should be considered for 14–30 days.

Infectious diseases and tropical medicine: in exams

The returning traveller from the tropics

The most common presenting complaint you will find in your exam is a patient presenting with fever.

History
- It is important to clarify the onset, duration, and progression. Think about incubation periods (see Table 20.1). The pattern of fever is classically described by textbooks for various tropical infections but unlikely to be diagnostically reliable. However, persistent fever at night for months may point towards TB. Is the fever accompanied by drenching sweats?
- Associated symptoms are vital to fish out, especially rigors, described as uncontrolled teeth clattering and shaking, as opposed to goosebumps, chills, or simply feeling hot and cold.
- Go through the systematic review as you would normally. In addition to taking a history of GI, respiratory, and genitourinary symptoms, do not forget to ask about sore throat symptoms, lymphadenopathy, myalgia, arthralgia, and rashes.

Travel history
First, you would want to put on your travel agent cap here; you will need to find out the full travel itinerary, including dates of travel, stopovers, locations, and purpose of travel.

Ask about the following:
- Accommodation for the whole trip (hotels vs huts, urban vs rural), food and water sources, do not forget about water used for ice and brushing teeth (food- and water-borne illnesses, e.g. amoebiasis and traveller's diarrhoea).
- All outdoor activities, especially fresh water activities such as swimming or rafting (schistosomiasis), caving (viral haemorrhagic fevers), and interaction with the locals and animals, if any.

Table 20.1 Importance of incubation periods

Short <10 days	Medium 10–21 days	Long >21 days
Malaria	Malaria	Malaria
Arbovirus (dengue)	Typhoid	Viral hepatitis
Enteric bacterial	Rickettsial	TB
Haemorrhagic fevers	Haemorrhagic fevers	Acute HIV
Plague	Leptospirosis	Amoebic liver abscess
	African trypanosomiasis	Katayama fever

- *Bites and injuries*: mosquito bites? Tick bites? Is there an eschar? Animal or human bites? Cuts or needle-stick injuries?
- How good a prevention strategy did they have? Vaccinations, insect repellents, bed nets, and malaria prophylaxis. Ask about drug name, dosage, and compliance. Note that full compliance does not rule out malaria!
- Is anyone else in the group affected?
- Any hospitalizations abroad?

Sexual history

(See ➜ Chapter 17.) Taking a comprehensive sexual history is vital in returning travellers—you do not want to miss HIV seroconversion! Ask about the number of partners if any, gender, type of sex, protection, and prophylaxis (pre- or post-exposure prophylaxis).

Examination

- *General examination*: rule out sepsis (capillary refill time, BP, HR, and temperature), look for rashes, bruises, petechiae, and lymphadenopathy.
- *Systemic examination*: looking for respiratory signs and hepatosplenomegaly; do not forget to examine the throat!

Investigations

- You will find that the central dogma in infectious diseases is nailing a microbiological diagnosis by sending samples for microscopy, culture, serology, and PCR (choose wisely).
- However, in cases of returning travellers from the tropics with fever:
  1. Rule out malaria.
  2. Rule out malaria.
  3. Rule out malaria.
- In addition to regular blood tests as mentioned in the malaria section (see ➜ p. 401).

Management

- Once you form a differential diagnosis, management should be specific to each condition.
- In cases of sepsis or systemic compromise, does the patient need assessment by your seniors or an intensivist?
- Does the patient need any special infection control precautions?

Chapter 21

Nephrology

Nephrology: overview

Nephrology is the medical specialty that manages diseases of the kidney and renal replacement therapy (RRT; e.g. dialysis and transplant). While only larger hospitals will have a renal unit, most will have a visiting nephrologist, and *all* hospitals will have inpatients with renal impairment. The principles of fluid balance and managing a patient with renal failure are vital skills for every clinician.

Cases to see

- *Acute kidney injury (AKI)*: a common reason for emergency admission and it also frequently develops in hospital. The commonest cause is 'pre-renal' haemodynamic disturbance such as dehydration, sepsis, or hypotension combined with drugs including NSAIDs, ACEIs, and diuretics. It is often multifactorial.
- *Nephrotic syndrome*: caused by a number of glomerular diseases and is generally managed in the outpatient clinic. However, some are admitted for renal biopsy/fluid management.
- *Chronic kidney disease (CKD)*: managed in the community and clinic. However, patients admitted for unrelated problems are at risk of further renal deterioration (acute-on-chronic failure).
- *Haemodialysis*: patients attend the hospital three times weekly for life-sustaining treatment. Hospital admissions are common, e.g. with complications of dialysis access or comorbidity such as ischaemic heart disease.
- *Renal transplant*: a subspecialty field encompassing both surgery and medicine that you will only find at larger teaching hospitals. Most renal units will care for transplant patients after the first few months.

Procedures to see

Renal biopsy

Usually done as a day-case procedure under US guidance.

Dialysis access

Either an emergency/temporary dialysis line (vascath or tunnelled catheter) or for patients nearing end-stage renal failure elective arteriovenous fistula.

Nephrostomy

Usually done by an interventional radiologist to relieve upper urinary tract obstruction, especially where there is intercurrent infection.

Surgery

Renal transplant or donor nephrectomy if based in specialist/teaching hospital.

Things to do

Practise fluid balance assessments, learn about intrinsic renal disease, and speak to a dialysis patient to understand the restrictions they face (e.g. dietary, fluid, lifestyle, and psychosocial). See Table 21.1 for recent studies.

Causes of renal failure

Pre-renal

Occurs in response to renal hypoperfusion, e.g. in dehydration, hypotension, and sepsis (or more rarely in heart failure or renal artery stenosis). Urine is appropriately concentrated to retain water and salt. Serum urea is often elevated proportionately more than creatinine. Usually responds to treatment of underlying cause. Uncorrected pre-renal failure → acute tubular necrosis (ATN).

Renal

Usually ATN following pre-renal insults. Often results in established renal failure despite fluid replacement and BP support. May require temporary haemodialysis. Also includes intrinsic renal disease such as glomerulonephritis and interstitial nephritis.

Post-renal

Secondary to blocked urinary drainage. Lower urinary tract obstruction often due to prostate disease → urinary retention. Upper tract obstruction may be caused by stones, intrinsic (e.g. urothelial tumour) or extrinsic (metastases) compression.

Vital components of a renal assessment

Fluid assessment

To diagnose dehydration as cause of renal failure or fluid overload due to reduced urine output. Cannot be done over the phone! Aim for euvolaemia rather than a given urine output in patients with established renal impairment.

Urinalysis

Blood or protein in the urine is suggestive of glomerular disease. Leucocytes (pyuria) and nitrites are seen on a urine dipstick in UTI which is confirmed by MC&S.

Renal tract imaging

US to exclude urinary tract obstruction and assess size of kidneys and cortical thickness. Also diagnoses structural kidney disease (e.g. autosomal dominant polycystic kidney disease (ADPKD)). CT of kidneys/ureters/bladder gives more detailed information about entire urinary tract and identifies renal calculi.

Medication review

Often forgotten but it is vital to identify agents that may have contributed to or compounded renal failure (ACEI, NSAIDs, diuretics). Drugs that are renally excreted must be given in reduced doses in renal failure to prevent accumulation toxicity (e.g. some opiates and antibiotics).

Renal haemodynamics: the key to understanding most cases of AKI

The kidney filters about 200 L of blood per day. This function is expressed as the glomerular filtration rate (GFR; mL/min/1.73 m²). This can be measured indirectly by nuclear medicine renography or can be estimated based on serum creatinine/cystatin C and sex/age/weight.

GFR is maintained across a wide range of systemic blood pressure and changes in circulating volume by renal autoregulation; vasoconstriction of the efferent arteriole maintains hydrostatic pressure within the glomerulus at times of low blood pressure. Afferent arteriolar tone protects the glomerular vessels from high systemic blood pressure.

Sepsis and drugs (e.g. ACE inhibitors and NSAIDs) interfere with these mechanisms and cause renal failure especially in the context of dehydration or hypotension. Initially this will cause prerenal failure but it will progress to ATN if not corrected in time.

Table 21.1 Recent studies in nephrology

Details	Trial	Comments
2002 JAMA N = 1094	African American Study of Kidney Disease and Hypertension (AASK)	No difference in CKD progression among African American patients with either intensive vs conservative BP control
2006 NEJM N = 1432	Correction of Hb and Outcomes in Renal Insufficiency (CHOIR)	Erythropoietin therapy targeting a higher Hb level of 13.5 g/dL (vs 11.3), → higher mortality risk + hospitalizations for congestive heart failure in patients with non-dialysis CKD + anaemia
2007 NEJM N = 1645	Efficacy Limiting Toxicity Elimination-Symphony trial (ELITE-Symphony)	Immunosuppression with tacrolimus in renal transplantation → higher estimated glomerular filtration rate, graft survival, and lower rates of rejection at 12 months (compared to 3 other regimens)
2010 NEJM N = 828	The Initiating Dialysis Early and Late (IDEAL)	No difference in survival/clinical outcomes between early vs late initiation of dialysis in CKD (stage V)
2016 NEJM N = 620	Artificial Kidney Initiation in Kidney Injury (AKIKI)	No mortality difference between early or delayed RRT in ICU patients with AKI

Nephrology: in the emergency department

You should be aware of the life-threatening complications of renal failure requiring emergency haemodialysis.

Pulmonary oedema

Patients with reduced or no urine output will become fluid overloaded. A trial of high-dose diuretic is reasonable if the patient has some residual renal function but if they are anuric or a chronic haemodialysis patient they need immediate dialysis to remove excess fluid.

Symptoms/signs

Dyspnoea, hypoxia, fine bibasal crackles, and CXR showing 'bat's wing' appearance, alveolar shadowing.

Hyperkalaemia

Mild (5.5–6.0), moderate (6.1–6.9), severe (>7.0 mmol/L). Serum K^+ >6.5 requires immediate attention. *Features*: weakness/cramps, paraesthesiae, hypotonia, focal neurological deficits and cardiac arrest.

ECG changes (a common exam question):
- Peaked T waves.
- Small/broad/absent P waves.
- Widening QRS complex.
- Sinusoidal ('sine wave' pattern) QRST.
- Atrioventricular dissociation.
- VT/VF.

Management
- 12-lead ECG (can be normal) and cardiac monitor.
- 10 mL of 10% calcium chloride IV (stabilizes the myocardium).
- Insulin (10 units soluble insulin)/glucose (50 mL of 50%) infusion (drives K^+ into the cells).
- Nebulized salbutamol 10–20 mg.
- Enteral calcium polystyrene sulfonate can be given but takes hours to take effect.
- Consider dialysis if severe or refractory.

Uraemia

Systemic complications from accumulation of uraemic compounds (not urea per se). Neurological features include myoclonus and fluctuating GCS score. Can also cause haemorrhagic pericarditis. Initial dialysis should be short and slow to avoid disequilibrium syndrome. Gastric protection (e.g. PPI) may reduce risk of GI bleeds. *Symptoms/signs*: twitching, drowsiness, pericarditic chest pain with widespread ST changes on ECG and effusion on echocardiography.

Metabolic acidosis

Usually normal anion gap. Exclude other causes (e.g. DKA and lactic acidosis). Difficult to correct high K^+ in presence of acidosis.

Symptoms/signs

Kussmaul breathing, low pH, low HCO_3^-.

Poisoning

Uncommonly, dialysis is used to remove poisons/toxins (e.g. ethylene glycol and salicylates) even in patients with normal renal function.

Discussion with the boss

Intermittent haemodialysis vs continuous renal replacement therapy?

Haemodialysis

Typically 3–4-hour sessions, quickly corrects high K^+ or high urea, can ultrafiltrate about >1 L fluid/hour using dialysis line or arteriovenous fistula. Not suitable for haemodynamically unstable patients or those with multiorgan failure.

Continuous RRT

(E.g. haemofiltration): lower efficiency but causes less haemodynamic instability. Takes place continually over 24–48 hours. Used in critical care setting and where patient requires inotrope/vasopressor support. May improve inflammatory milieu in sepsis.

There is no clear survival benefit of either technique. Consider on an individual patient basis (vital signs, comorbidities, other organ involvement, vascular access, availability of resources, etc.).

Approach to the patient with renal failure

Deal with any life-threatening complication (high K^+, pulmonary oedema, etc.).

History
- Baseline renal function if known (acute vs chronic).
- Previous renal failure or relevant renal history.
- Recent dehydrating illness or symptoms of fluid overload.
- Urinary problems such as prostatism, reduced output or UTI.
- Symptoms in keeping with multisystem disorder (e.g. weight loss, fever, joint pain, rash, ear or nose discharge, haemoptysis).
- Cardiovascular comorbidities especially PVD, hypertension, or heart failure.
- Diabetes (micro- or macrovascular complications?).
- Medications, especially ACEIs, ARB, diuretics, antibiotics, PPIs. Over-the-counter drugs including NSAIDs or herbal remedies.
- Family history (e.g. ADPKD, Alport's syndrome).

Examination
- Fluid assessment:
  - Intravascular: HR, BP (postural), capillary refill, JVP, urine output (NB urine output is not a useful indicator of fluid status in established renal failure).
  - Extravascular: peripheral/pulmonary oedema, ascites, weight.
- Stigmata of systemic disease (joints/lungs/skin/chest/eyes).
- Exclude urinary retention/BPH.
- Exclude uraemic complications (e.g. pericarditis/encephalopathy).
- Palpable kidneys in ADPKD.

- Peripheral pulses (PVD and renal artery stenosis coexist) and arterial bruits.
- Urinalysis for protein/blood.

Imaging: to exclude urinary tract obstruction and to assess renal symmetry (renal artery stenosis or congenital shrunken kidney), cortical thickness (reduced in CKD) and scarring (e.g. in reflux nephropathy).

Correct fluid imbalance: IV fluids where dehydrated, diuretics/fluid restriction/ultrafiltration where overloaded.

Medication review: stop any drugs which may contribute to renal failure or cause toxicity.

Dietary advice: low K^+ or PO_4^{3-} diet may be appropriate. Variable fluid restriction where oliguric/anuric.

Further investigations
- Urine albumin:creatinine ratio (ACR) to quantify proteinuria.
- Autoimmune panel to exclude vasculitis.
- Myeloma screen (serum and urine electrophoresis, immunoglobulins).
- Renal biopsy if suspicion of intrinsic renal disease (other than ATN) or diagnosis/prognosis unclear.
- Septic screen where appropriate.
- Bone profile, PTH, and haematinics (iron studies, vitamin B12, and folate) to manage complications of renal failure.
- Call GP or other hospital to establish baseline renal function.
- Other renal imaging (e.g. CT kidneys, ureters, and bladder (KUB) for stones, renal angiogram for renal artery stenosis).

Discussion of management options: such as modes of RRT, or conservative management if patient unlikely to benefit from RRT. Immunosuppression if immune-mediated renal disease.

Vascular access: avoid cannulae and phlebotomy in forearm veins, which may later be needed for arteriovenous fistula!

Renal syndromes

Acute kidney injury

See Table 21.2 for definition.

Epidemiology

- 2% of all hospital inpatients, 40% on admission to critical care.
- Community AKI particularly in elderly, ACEIs/ARBs, prostate disease.
- Assume all renal failure is acute until proven otherwise (historical bloods, shrunken kidneys).

Pathophysiology

Commonly ATN in response to ischaemic insult. Mechanisms include acute inflammation in response to sterile tubular cell injury and intrarenal vasoconstriction. AKI has deleterious effects on other organ systems (organ 'cross-talk').

Risk factors and causes (pre-renal, renal, post-renal)

See Fig. 21.1.

Pre-existing

- DM
- CVD
- CKD
- Liver disease
- Vasculitis/VTE
- Obstruction (stones, BPH, catheter).

Admission related

- Major surgery
- Sepsis
- Dehydration
- Rhabdomyolysis
- Urinary tract obstruction.

Table 21.2 AKI defined using RIFLE criteria

	GFR	U/O
Risk	1.5 × Cr 25% ↓GFR	<0.5 mL/kg/hour (6 hours)
Injury	2 × Cr 50% ↓GFR	<0.5 mL/kg/hour (12 hours)
Failure	3 × Cr 75% ↓GFR	<0.3 mL/kg/hour (2 hours) Anuria (12 hours)
Loss	No renal recovery after 4 weeks	
End-stage failure	No renal recovery after 12 weeks	

Cr, creatinine; GFR, glomerular filtration rate; RIFLE, Risk, Injury, Failure, Loss of kidney function, and End-stage kidney disease; U/O, urine output.

Drugs
- ACEIs, ARBs
- Diuretics
- NSAIDs
- Radiocontrast agents
- Antibiotics (e.g. gentamicin, penicillins).

Intrinsic renal disease
- Glomerulonephritis
- Interstitial nephritis
- Tubular (ischaemia, myeloma, rhabdomyolysis, contrast).

Management
- Assess volume status (pulse, BP, peripheral perfusion, JVP).
- Check urine dipstick for evidence of renal damage (blood + protein).
- Treat the cause:
  - PO/IV rehydration if hypovolaemic.
  - Relieve any obstruction (US scan renal tract can help diagnosis).
  - Stop nephrotoxic drugs.
  - Treat sepsis.
- Treat any associated hyperkalaemia.
- Adjust doses of other medication in relation to renal function.
- Monitor creatinine regularly.

A *renal biopsy* indicated where a specific treatment (e.g. immunosuppression) is available or where renal prognosis is important to guide further management.

Prognosis
- 40–50% mortality in critical care patient requiring RRT.
- 5% mortality if single organ failure.
- 70–80% renal recovery (age and comorbidities as determinants).
- Worse outcomes in oliguric/fluid overloaded patients.
- ↑risk subsequent CKD.

Honours

'Adding insult to injury': National Confidential Enquiry into Patient Outcome and Death (NCEPOD) report into AKI deaths 2009

Recommendations:
- Earlier recognition of AKI that develops in hospital.
- Involvement of senior and specialist staff early on.
- 24-hour access to renal US and nephrostomy service.
- Prompt recognition of the sick patient and critical care referral.
- Renal biochemistry and urinalysis for all emergency admissions.

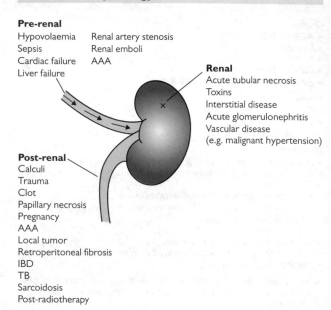

Pre-renal
Hypovolaemia   Renal artery stenosis
Sepsis   Renal emboli
Cardiac failure AAA
Liver failure

Renal
Acute tubular necrosis
Toxins
Interstitial disease
Acute glomerulonephritis
Vascular disease
(e.g. malignant hypertension)

Post-renal
Calculi
Trauma
Clot
Papillary necrosis
Pregnancy
AAA
Local tumor
Retroperitoneal fibrosis
IBD
TB
Sarcoidosis
Post-radiotherapy

Fig. 21.1 Causes of reduced urine output. AAA, abdominal aortic aneurysm; IBD, inflammatory bowel disease; TB, tuberculosis. Reproduced with permission from Piers Page and Greg Skinner, *Emergencies in Clinical Medicine*, 2008, Oxford University Press.

Rapidly progressive glomerulonephritis (RPGN)

This renal emergency is caused by immunologically mediated disease → the following:
- Rapid deterioration in renal function.
- 'Crescents': inflammatory infiltrate within Bowman's capsule which can compress and destroy glomerulus.
- Hypertension is common.
- Blood/protein in urine (beware anuria).
- Often extrarenal features (e.g. pulmonary haemorrhage, rash, and joint pain).
- Pulmonary haemorrhage is life-threatening and requires aggressive management.

May respond to immunotherapy so early recognition, biopsy, and treatment are a priority.

Causes of RPGN

Pauci-immune (60%): usually antineutrophil cytoplasmic antibody-associated small vessel vasculitis; microscopic polyangiitis (MPA) or granulomatosis with polyangiitis (GPA, previously known as Wegener's granulomatosis).

Immune-complex mediated (20%): Worldwide post-infectious glomerulonephritis is a common cause but lupus nephritis and Henoch–Schönlein purpura/IgA nephropathy are more common in the West.

Anti-GBM disease (Goodpasture's disease) (15%): caused by IgG autoantibodies to alpha-3 (IV) chain of collagen found in glomerular (and alveolar) basement membrane.

Specific treatments:
- Pulsed methylprednisolone and high-dose oral steroids.
- Alkylating agent such as cyclophosphamide followed by azathioprine or mycophenolate mofetil.
- Plasma exchange (where severe renal failure at presentation or pulmonary haemorrhage).

Investigations

Urine and blood test abnormalities (haematology, biochemistry, and immunology) in renal failure are highlighted in Table 21.3.

Nephrotic syndrome

A triad of:
1. Peripheral oedema.
2. Proteinuria >3 g/24 hour (equivalent to urine ACR >210 mg/mmol).
3. Hypoalbuminaemia.
4. (Hypercholesterolaemia is usually present as well.)

Patients may notice swollen ankles or frothy urine.

Causes (can only be distinguished on renal biopsy)
- Focal segmental glomerulosclerosis (FSGS)
- Minimal change disease (MCD)
- Membranous nephropathy (MN)
- Amyloid
- Diabetes mellitus
- Rarely SLE, IgA.

FSGS, MCD, and MN can be primary/'idiopathic' or secondary (drugs, infection).

Complications
- Postural hypotension.
- AKI.
- Hypertension.
- High cholesterol.
- Immobility/debility from oedema and skin breakdown.
- Infection (immunoglobulins lost in urine, complication of treatment).
- Thromboses (usually venous, arterial seen in antiphospholipid syndrome).

Table 21.3 Abnormalities in renal failure

Parameter	Normal range	Renal failure
Biochemistry		
Urea (U)	3–7	↑ (esp. pre-renal)
Creatinine (Cr)	80–120	↑ (esp. rhabdomyolysis)
Sodium (Na^+)	135–145	↑ (dehydration) ↓ dilution/urinary loss
Potassium (K^+)	3.5–5	↑ in impaired excretion
Bicarbonate (HCO_3^-)	18–25	↓ in renal wasting/↓H+ excretion
Calcium (Ca^{2+})	Corr 2.1–2.3	↓ in impaired absorption/↓ vitamin D
Phosphate (PO_4^{3-})	0.8–1.2	↑ in reduced urinary excretion
Parathyroid hormone (PTH)	25–75	↑ in renal failure
Serum electrophoresis		Monoclonal band in myeloma
Immunoglobulins (Ig)		Immunoparesis in myeloma ↑ Ig M/G in infection ↑ Ig A in IgA nephropathy
Creatine kinase (CK)	25–200	↑ in rhabdomyolysis
Haematology		
Haemoglobin (Hb)	11.5–15	Renal anaemia (↓ EPO secretion)
Platelets (Pl)	150–400	↓ in thrombotic microangiopathy
Ferritin	>20	↓ in iron deficiency
Transferrin saturation	20%	Functional iron deficiency
Vitamin B12/ folate		Exclude other causes of anaemia
Immunology		
ANCA		Autoimmune vasculitis
ANA/anti dsDNA		SLE
C3/C4		↓ in lupus, SBE, cholesterol emboli
Anti-GBM		Goodpasture's disease
Urine		
Albumin:creatinine	>2.5	Quantify proteinuria
Microscopy		Crystals, red cell casts
Bence Jones protein		Immunoglobulin light chain
24-hour collection		Investigate stone

Treatment depends on cause

General

- Stop smoking.
- Optimize BP, cholesterol, and proteinuria (ACEI).
- Infection prophylaxis (vaccines, co-trimoxazole, etc.).
- Anticoagulation if serum albumin <20.
- Primary FSGS/MCD: steroids and/or calcineurin inhibitor (e.g. tacrolimus).
- Idiopathic MN: one-third remit spontaneously but one-third progressive. 6 months of conservative management followed by high-dose steroids/alkylating agent if evidence of progression. Recently found to be caused by anti-PLA2R antibodies.
- Amyloid: cytotoxic myeloablative therapy to deplete pathogenic plasma cells.
- Diabetes: optimize HbA1c, BP, and ACEI.

> **Proteinuria: why all the fuss?**
> - Albuminuria is a sensitive sign of renal disease.
> - Proteinuria in itself is a risk factor for progression of CKD, hence indications for ACEI/strict BP control.
> - Microalbuminuria in the general population is predictive of cardiovascular morbidity and mortality.
>
> Most labs now do ACR on a spot urine sample. 24-hour collections are inconvenient and rarely required.

Chronic kidney disease

Important information for investigations and diagnostics
See Table 21.4.

Causes

- Diabetes mellitus.
- Glomerulonephritis.
- Hypertension.
- ADPKD.
- CAKUT (congenital abnormalities of kidney and urinary tract).
- Inherited disorders, e.g. Alport's syndrome, cystinosis.
- Other (e.g. tubulointerstitial nephritis).
- Often unknown ('small kidneys').

Presenting symptoms: usually discovered incidentally or on screening.

Things to address in clinic
Cause of CKD
Often deduced from comorbidities such as diabetes with microvascular complications, cardiovascular disease, smoking, or known urological disease. Biopsy indicated where diagnosis unclear and result will change management.

Table 21.4 Classification and biochemical findings in CKD (according to NICE CKD guidelines 2014)

GFR and ACR categories and risk of adverse outcomes			Urine ACR (mg/mmol)		
			<3	3–30	>30
			A1	A2	A3
GFR categories (mL/min/ 1.73 m²), description and range	≥90 Normal and high	G1	No CKD unless other markers of kidney damage	Moderately ↑risk	High risk
	60–89 Mild reduction	G2		Moderately ↑risk	High risk
	45–59 Mild–moderate reduction	G3a	Moderately ↑risk	High risk	Very high risk
	30–44 Moderate reduction	G3b	High risk	Very high risk	Very high risk
	15–29 Severe reduction	G4	Very high risk	Very high risk	Very high risk
	<15 Kidney failure	G5	Very high risk	Very high risk	Very high risk

Blood pressure
NICE guidelines <140/90 or <130/80 mmHg if diabetic or urine ACR >70.

Proteinuria reduction
With ACEI/ARB if ACR >3 and diabetic, or >30 and hypertension, >70 with neither.

Prevention of cardiovascular disease
Statin and antiplatelet.

Secondary hyperparathyroidism
Occurs in response to phosphate retention and impaired hydroxylation of cholecalciferol. Treat with vitamin D analogue (alfacalcidol or calcitriol).

Phosphate
Dietary advice or phosphate binders for PO_4^{3-}<1.5 mmol/L.

Renal anaemia
Consider iron supplements and erythropoietin aiming for Hb 10–12 g/dL.

Fluid management
Diuretics or fluid restriction if overloaded, encourage fluid intake if myeloma or polyuria (e.g. lithium).

Renal replacement therapy
Education, counselling and provision of arteriovenous fistula or peritoneal dialysis catheter where required.

Transplantation

Evaluate for renal transplantation (live donor where appropriate) in those likely to benefit.

ACEIs: hero or villain? Hero—where used appropriately!

- ACEIs preserve remaining GFR and reduce proteinuria through physiological fall in GFR via efferent arteriolar vasodilatation. Hence <25% fall in GFR or <30% rise in creatinine acceptable/expected.
- If greater change than this, consider renal artery stenosis/dehydration and stop/reduce.
- Stop in event of dehydrating illness.
- Do not give to any woman likely to conceive/pregnant.

Important conditions causing renal failure

Multiple myeloma

Is caused by a malignant clone of plasma cells, which produce either immunoglobulins (usually IgG) or light chains. These infiltrate bone marrow (causing bone marrow failure) and cause lytic bone lesions throughout the skeleton.

Renal failure at presentation is common and affects up to one-half of all patients during the course of the disease. Renal function is an important prognostic factor in myeloma.

Causes of renal failure in myeloma

- Cast nephropathy or 'myeloma kidney': light chains which are filtered at the glomerulus bind to Tamm–Horsfall proteins in the tubular lumen forming casts. These obstruct urinary flow and cause ATN. A reactive tubulointerstitial infiltrate is also seen. Myeloma kidney is diagnosed on renal biopsy (check for normal platelets first).
- Hypercalcaemia from skeletal involvement causes polyuria and dehydration. Remember that serum calcium is usually low in AKI so the combination of AKI and hypercalcaemia should prompt myeloma investigations. All patients with myeloma (except those who are anuric) should be encouraged to drink at least 3 L/day.
- Infections: myeloma patients often have *immunoparesis* with low immunoglobulin levels predisposing them to infections. Sepsis with a disproportionate degree of AKI is commonly seen in myeloma and all such patients should have a complete septic screen.
- Treatment: most myeloma treatments are not nephrotoxic. However, patients may use over-the-counter NSAIDs, especially to treat bone pain.
- Less common: AL amyloidosis or light chain deposition disease.

Management of renal failure in myeloma

Investigations: bone profile, immunoglobulins, serum and urine electrophoresis, serum free light chains for disease monitoring, renal biopsy where indicated.

1. Aggressive rehydration, particularly where hypercalcaemia present.
2. IV bisphosphonate if hypercalcaemia persists despite rehydration.
3. Prompt treatment of infections.
4. Treat anaemia (transfusion or erythropoietin).
5. Renal biopsy usually undertaken at presentation.
6. Definitive myeloma treatment regimens such as cyclophosphamide/ dexamethasone/thalidomide or newer agents such as the proteasome inhibitor bortezomib will reduce the production of paraprotein/ light chain.
7. Light chain removal treatment: there is evidence that extended dialysis sessions using high cut-off membranes (which remove higher-molecular-weight molecules than conventional ones) can reverse AKI in myeloma kidney. This should be done in conjunction with definitive therapy as listed above.

Rhabdomyolysis (crush injury)

Is caused by skeletal muscle breakdown in response to physical trauma or biochemical disturbance. Necrotic myocytes release myoglobin, a metabolite of which is directly toxic to renal tubules causing ATN. Additionally, ischaemic or necrotic muscle can sequester very large quantities of fluid causing severe dehydration. Significant muscle cell death also releases potassium, phosphate, CK, and urate, which are disproportionately high in rhabdomyolysis. Hyperkalaemia can develop rapidly and is a medical emergency.

Urine is typically 'Coca-Cola' coloured due to the presence of myoglobin. Urine dipsticks cannot distinguish this from haemoglobin but the biochemistry lab can.

You should suspect rhabdomyolysis in patients with compartment syndrome or significant limb injuries, anyone who has been on the floor for a long time (frail elderly, alcohol-dependent patients), and following recreational drug use.

Management
Investigations
CK (often >100,000 U/L), K^+, PO_4^{3-}, urate, urine dip, and urine myoglobin.

Renal failure from rhabdomyolysis can be prevented by *early and aggressive* fluid regimens driving large-volume diuresis to 'flush out' myoglobin and to replace fluid losses in injured muscle. This may require >10 L/day and should only be done in HDU setting. There is limited evidence for urinary alkalinization with sodium bicarbonate to reduce the formation of toxic myoglobin metabolites.

In practice, most patients with rhabdomyolysis have established renal impairment at the time of presentation. In these cases, aggressive fluid resuscitation may still be beneficial but should be done with extreme care due to the risk of fluid overload in the face of falling urine output. Oliguria and hyperkalaemia mandate immediate haemodialysis treatment. Patients usually recover renal function but may remain dialysis dependent for weeks.

Beware that calcium may precipitate with extracellular phosphate causing severe hypocalcaemia. This should be treated only if the patient has symptoms (e.g. tetany or cardiac arrhythmia) due to the risk of further calcium deposition.

Tumour lysis syndrome (acute uric acid nephropathy)

Occurs in patients with very cellular/proliferative malignancies such as leukaemias and lymphomas, usually at the initiation of treatment but sometimes spontaneously. Sudden lysis of metabolically active and purine-rich tumour cells → massive release of intracellular uric acid (and $K^+/PO_4^{3-}/$ LDH as in rhabdomyolysis) which crystallizes in the renal tubules → AKI.

Preventative measures before cancer therapy is started include allopurinol (xanthine oxidase inhibitor) and IV fluids. Rasburicase is a new recombinant urase oxidase which rapidly oxidizes uric acid. This is increasingly used prophylactically.

As in rhabdomyolysis, the combination of falling urine output and hyperkalaemia would prompt emergency haemodialysis. Renal function usually recovers with appropriate management.

Renal failure in liver disease

Patients with advanced liver disease have a number of problems predisposing them to AKI: ascites and hypoalbuminaemia, spontaneous bacterial peritonitis, shock from oesophageal varices, and drugs such as spironolactone.

A particular condition called hepatorenal syndrome occurs due to renal vasoconstriction in response to a fall in useful circulating volume. It is diagnosed only where no other cause of ATN or kidney disease is identified, and generally confers a poor prognosis.

Management

Optimize fluid balance (CVP monitoring, 20% human albumin solution), treat infections, and stop nephrotoxic drugs. The use of the IV vasopressin analogue terlipressin causes redistribution of circulation via splanchnic vasoconstriction and may reverse renal vasoconstriction. It should not be used in ischaemic heart disease.

Renal replacement therapy

If the patient is a candidate for liver transplant then RRT is appropriate. Renal function in hepatorenal syndrome should improve with the restoration of normal liver function but where a patient is established on RRT, combined liver–kidney transplant may be undertaken.

Renal replacement therapy

1. Haemodialysis
2. Peritoneal dialysis
3. Renal transplantation
4. Conservative management.

Haemodialysis

Solutes such as urea and K^+ are removed by diffusion across a dialysis membrane, and H_2O by osmosis. Ultrafiltration removes additional fluid. Look out for 'crash landers' who present at end-stage renal failure without having any pre-dialysis work-up.

Pros

- Fast and efficient compared to continuous techniques.
- Does not require active patient involvement.
- Can be done through temporary line.

Cons

- Haemodynamic instability.
- In-hospital or satellite units.
- Line infections and other complications of vascular access.

Peritoneal dialysis

Uses peritoneum as dialysis membrane.

Pros

- Gradual/continuous so well tolerated haemodynamically.
- Better fluid and K^+ control.
- Home therapy and 'normal routine' allows patient empowerment.
- May preserve residual renal function more than haemodialysis.

Cons
- Peritoneal dialysis peritonitis.
- Planning/access required with Tenckhoff catheter.
- Technique failure.
- Encapsulating peritoneal sclerosis.

Renal transplantation
Kidney transplanted from deceased or living donor usually into iliac fossa.

Pros
- Provides more renal function than any form of dialysis.
- Better quality and quantity of life with improved cardiovascular health.
- Relative independence from medical interventions (dialysis, fluid restriction, etc.).

Cons
- Surgical/anaesthetic risk.
- Complications of immunosuppression (infections, haematological, diabetes, malignancy).
- Paucity of donor organs.

Conservative management
Is appropriate where dialysis is unlikely to improve quality or quantity of life.

Pros
- Symptom-based care.
- Fewer hospital visits and admissions.
- Preferred place of death.
- Patient choice.

Cons
- Ultimately patient will die from renal failure.
- May experience uraemic symptoms and fluid overload.

Procedures in nephrology

Dialysis line insertion

Ideally this is an elective procedure in a patient with a planned dialysis start, in which case a semi-permanent tunnelled line is inserted. Sometimes, however, a breathless or hyperkalaemic patient requires a temporary vascath for emergency dialysis.

The catheter

Dual lumen although both are contained within a single tube in the vein and only split after exiting the skin. Both sit in a central vein but one lumen is called 'arterial' as it removes blood from the body. Usually about 24 cm long and 12 French gauge.

Preferred sites

- Right internal jugular vein (RIJV): follows a shorter straight line to the junction between SVC and right atrium. Cleaner than femoral.
- Left internal jugular vein (LIJV): longer more tortuous course hence higher resistance to flow (Poiseuille's law) and more opportunity for wire to take a wrong turn.
- Femoral: often easiest in an emergency and compressible if patient is anticoagulated/coagulopathic. Less clean and may restrict mobility and predispose to DVT.
- Subclavian: avoided by nephrologists where possible due to risk of causing central venous stenosis.

Procedure

- Consent patient for risk of bleeding/infection/pneumothorax (if jugular or subclavian) and misplaced line.
- Strict adherence to aseptic technique is critical for central venous lines especially semi-permanent tunnelled lines. Vancomycin frequently given post procedure.
- US guidance is recommended by NICE for central venous cannulation. It is particularly valuable in chronic renal patients with previous lines/ thrombosed veins.
- Local anaesthetic to skin. Aspirate before injection to avoid bolus of IV lignocaine.
- Prepare the line by flushing lumens with normal saline to avoid air embolism.
- Seldinger technique: the vein is cannulated under US guidance with a wide-bore needle until venous blood is aspirated. A guide wire is inserted through the introducer needle which is then removed. Skin and soft tissue are then dilated using sheaths inserted over the guide wire. Dilators are removed and the vascath inserted over the guide wire, which must then itself be withdrawn. Venous blood should be aspirated freely through both lumens which are then flushed with saline and locked with heparin to reduce clot formation. Non-absorbable sutures are used to anchor the line to skin.
- CXR to confirm position at SVC/right atrial junction and exclude pneumothorax before using the line. Femoral line does not require imaging and can be used immediately.

Complications
- Carotid/femoral arterial cannulation: withdraw immediately and compress for several minutes to avoid haematoma and to achieve haemostasis.
- Pneumothorax: seek expert help.

Native renal biopsy

Usually an elective procedure in patients with nephrotic syndrome or AKI/CKD, of unknown cause. Patient should be sufficiently mobile/fit to lie on their front for up to 30 min and be able to cooperate with instructions such as breath holding.

Pre-procedure preparation
- Control BP to reduce bleeding risk (usually <160/100 mmHg).
- US to exclude obstruction/tumour or single kidney.
- Normal platelets and clotting. Ask about warfarin/antiplatelet drugs.

Procedure
- Consent patient for risk of visible haematuria (<5%; see Fig. 21.2), urinary clot retention (<2%), bleeding requiring blood transfusion (<1%), further intervention (e.g. embolization/nephrectomy (<0.5%)).
- Patient lies in supine position often with pillow beneath abdomen to encourage kyphosis.
- Skin cleaned and local anaesthetic infiltrated to level of kidney under US guidance.
- Biopsy needle advanced to kidney (with US). Ask patient to hold breath to reduce movement of kidney. Biopsy gun will retrieve sliver of renal tissue ~1 × 10 mm. Usually two cores taken.
- Bed rest for 4–6 hours after with frequent BP/HR monitoring and visual inspection of urine.

Complications
- Bleeding: interventions as listed previously.
- Upper or lower tract obstruction due to clot and need for nephrostomy/stent or bladder irrigation/catheter respectively.
- Arteriovenous fistula formation at biopsy site; usually only a problem in transplanted (i.e. single) kidney where significant shunt may require embolization.

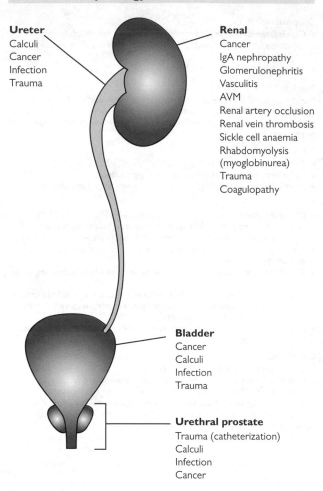

Ureter
Calculi
Cancer
Infection
Trauma

Renal
Cancer
IgA nephropathy
Glomerulonephritis
Vasculitis
AVM
Renal artery occlusion
Renal vein thrombosis
Sickle cell anaemia
Rhabdomyolysis
(myoglobinurea)
Trauma
Coagulopathy

Bladder
Cancer
Calculi
Infection
Trauma

Urethral prostate
Trauma (catheterization)
Calculi
Infection
Cancer

Fig. 21.2 Causes of frank haematuria. AVM, arteriovenous malformation.
Reproduced with permission from Piers Page and Greg Skinner, *Emergencies in Clinical Medicine*, 2008, Oxford University Press.

Nephrology: in exams

Renal patients are frequently asked to help with clinical exams; they have chronic conditions, stable clinical signs, and regular hospital visits. The examination routines are covered elsewhere, but here are a few things to look out for:

Is there any clue to the cause of renal failure?

- *ADPKD*: large, bilateral, ballotable masses in the flanks. Often associated with polycystic liver too.
- *DM*: finger pricks from BM testing, insulin injection marks on abdomen, visual impairment/guide dog, sugar-free drink on table, Medic Alert bracelet.
- *Alport's syndrome*: hearing aid.
- *Nephrectomy scars*: flanks, often well healed and concealed by skin folds.

Is there evidence of renal replacement therapy?

- *Haemodialysis*: arteriovenous fistula especially at wrist or elbow. Is there a thrill? Has it been needled recently (plaster/scab)? Defunct fistula elsewhere? Haemodialysis catheters, usually tunnelled over chest wall inserted into jugular vein. Look for scars near clavicle. Some haemodialysis patients have central vein obstruction causing signs of SVC obstruction or dilated collateral veins over chest wall.
- *Peritoneal dialysis*: Tenckhoff catheter exiting few cm lateral to umbilicus, tunnelled to midline, and small midline scar. Offer to check exit site but do not remove dressing without instruction due to infection risk. Catheters are removed at transplant, so look for scars.
- *Renal transplant*: smooth palpable mass beneath 'hockey stick' scar in iliac fossa. There may be a failed graft on other side. Listen for bruit.

Are there any complications of renal failure?

- *Fluid overload*: look for peripheral oedema (including ankles and sacrum), and raised JVP.
- *Anaemia*: pale conjunctivae.
- *Hyperparathyroidism*: parathyroidectomy scar (identical to thyroidectomy).
- *Pruritus*: look for linear scratch marks (excoriations) especially limbs/torso.

Are there any drug side effects? (Immunosuppression for transplant or immunological renal disease)

- *Steroids*: bruising/moon face/buffalo hump/diabetes mellitus/acne.
- *Tacrolimus*: fine, resting tremor.
- *Ciclosporin*: hirsutism, gum hypertrophy.

Fluid balance

As many as one in five patients on IV fluids and electrolytes suffer complications or morbidity due to their inappropriate administration.

However, here are some general tips from the NICE IV fluid therapy guidelines:

- If the gut works—use it! Consider using oral or nasogastric rehydration before IV. Stop IV fluids as soon as they are no longer needed.
- Prescriptions should include the type, rate, and volume of the fluid to be given (e.g. '500 mL 0.9% sodium chloride IV over an hour').
- Remember the 5 Rs:
  1. *Resuscitation* (500 mL boluses of crystalloid).
  2. *Routine maintenance*.
  3. *Replacement*.
  4. *Redistribution* (is fluid leaking into their gut/interstitium?).
  5. *Reassessment* (pulse, BP, mucous membranes, skin turgor, capillary refill time, mental status. Keep urine output >0.5 mL/kg/hour (only if renal failure not present)).
- Do not forget to consider all other sources of fluid and electrolyte intake (IV or enteral), including drugs, IV nutrition, blood, and blood products.
- All patients on IV fluids must have a fluid balance chart and daily review including body weight and U&E.

When on the wards, take time to look at the bags of fluid and what they contain. Fluids are treated as a prescribed drug so it is important you know what is in them (see comparison table of different IV fluids at ℘ www.frca. co.uk/article.aspx?articleid=295).

Clinical notes
- HR increases will be masked in the elderly and by beta blockers.
- Interpret BP in the light of any history of hypertension.
- Oliguria may be masked by diuretics.
- Capillary refill time is also ↑ by a cold environment, hypothermia, pain, and anxiety.
- Never infuse fluids containing >5 mmol/L potassium rapidly (can cause arrhythmias).

Neurology

Neurology: overview

Neurology is a fascinating specialty with increasingly sophisticated tools of diagnosis and a range of therapies for diseases affecting the brain and nerves. It is clinically wide ranging, from acute inpatient stroke services to outpatient clinics managing chronic degenerative conditions such as Alzheimer's and Parkinson's diseases.

Cases to see

Headache

Attend headache clinics to differentiate between primary headache syndromes and headaches secondary to alternative diagnoses and note the subtle differences between numerous primary headache syndromes.

Epilepsy

Common outpatient referrals for 'fits' and 'funny turns', observe how important history is in diagnosing epilepsy or, frequently, its many mimics. Observe how choosing treatment options is a fine balance between benefits in reducing seizures while minimizing side effects; be aware of how a diagnosis of epilepsy can change a patient's life, e.g. ability to drive.

Parkinson's disease and movement disorders

Frequently encountered among older inpatients as a comorbidity, managed in outpatients either by geriatricians or neurologists. Try to see complex patients with limitations of maximal treatments, treatment complications, significant non-motor symptoms, and assessments of neurosurgical treatment options such as deep brain stimulation.

Dementia and memory

Cognitive impairment secondary to Alzheimer's disease, vascular causes, or Lewy body disease is commonly encountered among older inpatients and outpatient memory clinics. Attend tertiary centre dementia clinics for typically younger and atypical patients with more unusual causes of cognitive impairment, such as frontotemporal dementia, CJD, and corticobasal degeneration.

Motor neuron disease

Typically encountered in specialist outpatient clinics. Try to obtain a grasp of neurophysiological testing in diagnosis. Be aware of the multidisciplinary input required including palliative care physicians, dieticians, and potentially respiratory and gastroenterological inputs as this degenerative condition progresses.

Emergency cases

Stroke

Shadow the stroke registrar on call to attend thrombolysis calls for patients presenting within 4.5 hours of symptoms starting and watch a National Institutes of Health Stroke Scale (NIHSS) international) examination, then follow the patient through their hyperacute neuroimaging.

On acute wards, the emphasis changes to finding the underlying cause of stroke and preventing further events while a MDT begins intensive rehabilitation.

Guillain–Barré syndrome

Potentially rapidly progressive, frequently encountered as an emergency on the acute medical take; urgent cardiac monitoring, spirometry, and swallowing assessments are required. Relatively stable patients can be found receiving IV immunoglobulin on the neurology ward while more unwell patients may require intubation on the ICU.

Meningitis

Frequently a differential diagnosis on the acute medical take; good opportunity to watch a lumbar puncture and familiarize yourself with local hospital policies on CNS infections

Myasthenia gravis

Familiarize yourself with the emergency investigations when encountering a patient with fatiguable muscle weakness: is their respiratory function compromised? Can they swallow? If the diagnosis was previously known, are there metabolic or infectious causes for this patient's decompensation?

Idiopathic intracranial hypertension

A good opportunity to practise fundoscopy and see swollen optic discs; often another good opportunity to observe a LP.

Procedures to see

Lumbar puncture

Performed on either the ward or outpatient day-case unit, LPs are performed aseptically using local anaesthetic. The needle passes between the spinous processes at L3/L4, anatomically defined as the intersection of two iliac crests. The opening pressure is measured and samples collected for cell count, protein, glucose, and other specialized tests such oligoclonal bands helpful in the diagnosis of MS. Before the back is cleaned, make sure you ask the doctor and patient to feel the anatomical landmarks.

Nerve conduction studies

Neurophysiologists test peripheral nerve conduction by passing electricity via needle electrodes through two points of a nerve, calculating conduction velocity and signal amplitude, the pattern of which helps to determine the underlying cause of a neuropathy. Loss of the myelin coating causes a reduction in conduction velocity; axonal loss reduces amplitude in the presence of conduction block across a defined segment.

Electroencephalography (EEG)

Scalp electrodes can be used to record brain electrical activity. One of the main uses is to find seizure activity suggestive of epilepsy.

Abnormalities may be found in between seizures ('interictal abnormalities'). Activation procedures such as hyperventilation, photic stimulation (strobe lighting), or sleep deprivation may be used to enhance subtle abnormalities. Patients may be admitted for a prolonged period of EEG recording while under close observation (video telemetry), allowing observed attacks to be correlated with the EEG. This is helpful in identifying a focus that may be triggering seizures, which can be a target for surgical resection, or for diagnosing non-epileptic attacks. Find your nearest neurophysiology department and arrange to attend for a couple of hours to see some of these procedures being performed.

Things to do

The majority of learning comes from taking as many focused histories and examining as many neurological patients as possible. Most departments have regular neuroradiology MDT meetings (see Fig. 22.1), where radiologists point out significant and interesting features on CT and MRI scans. Neurosurgical MDTs can be useful to see the overlap between medical and surgical treatments in difficult to manage patients with epilepsy and Parkinson's disease. Shadow the stroke registrar to encounter how speed can make all the difference in a thrombolysis call and attend the stroke MDT to experience how a multidisciplinary setting helps patients with neurological deficits improve their mobility and cope at home.

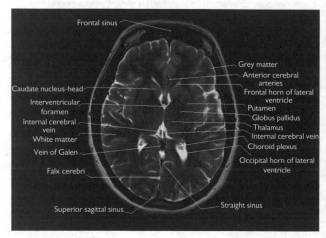

Fig. 22.1 Axial MRI of brain. Reproduced from ✍ www.mrimaster.com.

Neurology: in clinic

Idiopathic intracranial hypertension

A condition of uncertain aetiology in which intracranial pressure is raised (>25 cm water), not secondary to a space-occupying lesion or other 'physical' causes such as venous sinus thrombosis.

Presentation

It is most common in young, overweight women, and the main symptom is headache, typically worse on lying flat, coughing, or straining. Visual symptoms include blurring, field loss, and fleeting blackouts of vision, and if untreated, the major risk is visual loss.

Diagnosis

Patients may be admitted for lumbar puncture, which measures the pressure and provides temporary relief as CSF is removed. Perform fundoscopy as many will have papilloedema, and examine eye movements as sixth nerve palsies can occur as a false sign of raised pressure.

Treatment

Is with weight loss, and acetazolamide to reduce CSF production. If vision is threatened, surgery (LP CSF shunting) is required.

Parkinson's disease

'Parkinsonism' describes the combination of bradykinesia, rigidity, resting tremor, and postural instability, of which the most common cause is idiopathic Parkinson's disease, caused primarily by degeneration of nigrostriatal dopaminergic neurons in the basal ganglia. Idiopathic Parkinson's disease can also present with non-motor features such as postural instability, bladder and bowel dysfunction, and cognitive impairment, ranging from mild to dementia.

Differentials

Conditions mimicking idiopathic Parkinson's disease include vascular disease, encephalitis, and drug-induced Parkinsonism, classically by MPTP (1-methyl-4-phenyl-1,2,3,6-tetrahydropyridine), used by 1980s Californian meperidine addicts.

Parkinson's plus syndromes

Display atypical Parkinsonism features such as lack of asymmetry, anosmia, and poor response to levodopa, as well as their individual characteristic symptoms, and you should learn one or two distinct features of multisystem atrophy, progressive supranuclear palsies, and corticobasal degeneration. It is a safe bet to be asked about dopamine metabolism, levodopa precursors, and monoamine oxidases in clinic when you are discussing drug treatments which target this pathway.

Prognosis

As affected dopaminergic neurons continue to degenerate, patients often become resistant to therapy after 5 years, and develop new involuntary movements: levodopa induced dyskinesias and increasing psychiatric features.

Management
See Fig. 22.2.

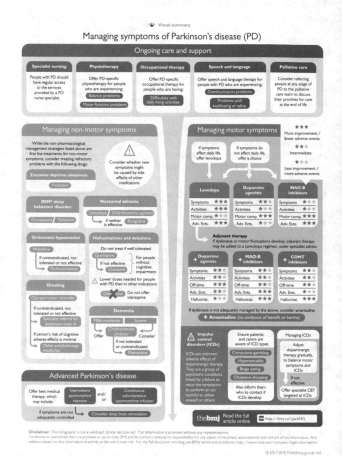

Fig. 22.2 Parkinson's medical treatment. Reproduced from Rogers et al. Parkinson's disease: summary of updated NICE guidance. *BMJ* 2017;358:j1951.

Headaches

It is important to distinguish between primary headache (no underlying pathology, e.g. migraine, tension and cluster headaches) and headaches secondary to other conditions (underlying pathology, e.g. infectious, neoplastic, vascular or drug induced. 10–15% of ED attendances with headache have a serious underlying cause). See Table 22.1 for subtypes and features.

Red flags

For secondary headaches: new/change in headache in patients >50 years; sudden-onset 'thunderclap' headache; neurological symptoms; headache that changes with posture, wakes the patient, or is precipitated by physical exertion; jaw claudication; visual disturbance; neck stiffness; fever; and history of cancer/HIV.

Investigations

All patients should have their BP checked and a neurological exam including fundoscopy. Investigation is rarely needed for primary headaches. Perform CT on those with a first presentation of thunderclap headache (98% sensitive for SAH at 12 hours, dropping to 93% sensitive at 24 hours). Consider LP looking for xanthochromia at 12 hours post onset if CT negative. This can be positive for up to 2 weeks. Perform ESR and CRP if giant cell arteritis (GCA) is suspected.

Treatment

* Try simple analgesia first: paracetamol and NSAIDS (aspirin/ibuprofen/naproxen). Avoid opioids.
* Antiemetics (prochlorperazine/domperidone/metoclopramide) and 5HT1 receptor antagonist (e.g. sumatriptan) for migraines.
* Beta blockers (propranolol) or TCA (amitriptyline) can be used for migraine prophylaxis.
* Give high-flow oxygen for cluster headache.
* Provide high-dose prednisolone for GCA.
* Advise stress management, adequate hydration, good sleep hygiene, minimal TV/PC screen time, and review by the optician.

Migraines

Are by far the most common primary headache, classically unilateral, pulsating headaches lasting between 4–72 hours, exacerbated by movement, and associated with nausea, photophobia, and phonophobia, and needing to lie in a dark room. Family history of migraines is common. Patients are asked about preceding symptoms such as flickering lights in the hour before the headache (the aura).

Management

Acute attacks are treated with NSAIDs and antiemetics, before escalation to specific antimigraine drugs such as triptans. Frequency of migrainous attacks are reduced with beta blockers (e.g. propranolol) and anticonvulsants (e.g. sodium valproate).

Multiple sclerosis

MS is an autoimmune disease resulting in the inflammation and damage of myelin sheaths around the white matter of the CNS.

Table 22.1 Subtypes of headache

Type	Age	Location	Duration	Timing	Severity	Quality	Features
Migraine	5–40	Unilateral around temple	Hours–3 days	Varies	++/ ++++	Throbbing/ pulsating	Photophobia, N&V, visual disturbance
Tension	10–50	Whole head	30 min–1 week	Varies	+/++	Tight pressure around head	Sore shoulders
Cluster	15–40	Unilateral/ retro-bulbar	30 min–2 hours	1–8 times/ day/at night	++++	Stabbing/piercing	Unilateral tearing, nasal congestion
Cervicogenic	Varies	Neck base	1–6 hours	Daily	++/+++	Dull to severe	Neck pain, nausea

Presentation

It classically affects women in their 30s and can present with a variety of symptoms depending on the area affected: weakness, loss of sensation, paraesthesia, and visual disturbances can all present.

Diagnosis

Read about the McDonald diagnostic criteria, which aim to establish two or more episodes of CNS inflammation separated in time and location. MRI brain and spine can be helpful in detecting small areas of inflammation or old plaques; detection of oligoclonal bands in CSF but not in serum is suggestive of CNS inflammation and supportive of MS as a diagnosis.

Progression

Of MS is highly variable between patients and you will better understand this after spending half a day in an MS clinic, where you will also learn about MDT management which also seeks to better address the patient's symptoms. The disease can continue to deteriorate (primary progressive) or progress in relapsing/remitting pattern with episodes of recovery.

Management

Steroids are used to reduce the length of symptoms in acute relapses but only DMARDs affect progression (e.g. interferon beta).

Honours

Internuclear ophthalmoplegia

Beloved sign of neurologists and examiners, internuclear ophthalmoplegia describes impaired oculomotor circuitry at the medial longitudinal fasciculus (MLF) at the pons. On eye abduction, the sixth cranial nerve innervates the lateral rectus muscle of the ipsilateral eye and also gives off a branch via the MLF to the contralateral third nerve nucleus, which subsequent adducts the contralateral eye to produce conjugate horizontal eye movements. Disruption of this circuitry is classically caused by demyelination such as MS or pontine strokes, resulting in diplopia on horizontal gaze only.

Motor neuron disease

A progressive degenerative disease of upper and lower motor neurons, frequently presenting as asymmetric bilateral limb weakness, dysphagia, dysarthria, and dyspnoea (eventually → possible respiratory failure). See Table 22.2 for subtypes.

Clinical examination

Typically demonstrate a combination of lower motor neuron signs such as muscle wasting and muscle and tongue fasciculations; and upper motor neuron signs such as brisk reflexes and upgoing plantars. There is no single diagnostic test and treatment is symptom control. Disease subtypes are shown in Table 22.2.

Table 22.2 Motor neuron disease subtypes

Type	Upper motor neuron degeneration	Lower motor neuron degeneration
Progressive muscular atrophy (PMA)	No	Yes
Progressive bulbar palsy (PBP)	No	Yes (bulbar region)
Primary lateral sclerosis (PLS)	Yes	No
Amyotrophic lateral sclerosis (ALS)	Yes	Yes

Myasthenia gravis

An autoimmune disorder in which antibodies attack nicotinic acetylcholine receptors of the neuromuscular junction.

Presentation

The hallmark is muscle weakness with fatiguability on exertion which makes for some interesting examination techniques to elicit this feature. Muscles commonly affected are those of the eyes, speech and swallowing, neck, proximal limbs, and respiration (most dangerous).

History

In the history ask in particular about fatiguability or fluctuation of symptoms (e.g. may be worse in the evening).

Examination

You should examine these patients for ptosis, which may be brought out with sustained upgaze, complex ophthalmoplegia which does not fit the pattern of a particular cranial nerve, and fatiguable weakness of the neck and limbs.

Diagnosis

Is by identification of the antibodies and by neurophysiological studies.

Management

During acute episodes, patients may receive IV immunoglobulin or plasma exchange. Symptomatic treatment is with pyridostigmine, a cholinesterase inhibitor, with the mainstay of treatment by immunosuppression. Some patients have an abnormality of the thymus and may respond to thymectomy.

Peripheral neuropathy

To understand peripheral nerve disorders it is important to have a good knowledge of anatomy. Make sure you know which nerves and nerve roots supply the major muscles, and the sensory coverage of the dermatomes and major peripheral nerves (median, radial, ulnar, and common peroneal).

Mononeuropathy

Means dysfunction of a single peripheral nerve, and is usually due to compression, e.g. carpal tunnel syndrome affecting the median nerve.

Mononeuritis multiplex

Means dysfunction of multiple named peripheral nerves (e.g. median and common peroneal), and can result from multiple sites of compression or systemic vasculitis. Generally, however, the term peripheral neuropathy is taken to mean a condition of damage to all peripheral nerves (polyneuropathy). Usually the longest nerve fibres are worst affected, giving a characteristic pattern of distal weakness and 'glove and stocking' sensory loss. There is a long list of causes including diabetes, alcohol, vitamin B12 deficiency, and certain drugs. Inflammatory causes such as Guillain–Barré syndrome (and its chronic counterpart, chronic inflammatory demyelinating polyradiculoneuropathy) are important causes as they can be treated with immune-modulating drugs. Patients with peripheral neuropathy are often admitted for investigations such as LP and nerve conduction studies, or for treatments such as IV immunoglobulin—so use the chance to take a careful history and perform a full examination. Expect to find all lower motor neuron signs, and look closely for wasting and fasciculations which can easily be missed. Try to determine the pattern of nerve damage. Is it motor, sensory, or both?

Does the sensory component involve small fibres (pain and temperature), large fibres (proprioception and vibration), or both? Are autonomic nerves involved (check postural BP)?

Confusion: delirium and dementia

You should know the difference between delirium and dementia.

Delirium

A form of organic brain syndrome characterized by:

• disturbed conscious level (overactivity, excitement, drowsiness, stupor)
• global disturbance of cognition (memory, orientation, attention, speech, motor function)
• rapid onset with fluctuating course (often worse at night) and brief duration.

Delirium can occur at any age, but is more common in the elderly.

Aetiology

Infections (UTI, pneumonia), medications (digoxin, steroids, diuretics), withdrawal (alcohol, opioids), metabolic (hypoxia, hypercapnia, hypoglycaemia, hyponatraemia), cardiac (acute MI, cardiac failure), neurological (head injury, chronic subdural, post-ictal), organ failure (respiratory, renal, hepatic), endocrine (DM, thyrotoxicosis).

Dementia

Definition

An acquired, progressive decline in intellect, behaviour, and personality. It is irreversible and typically occurs with a normal level of consciousness. Note that patients with dementia are at risk of delirium resulting from an acute infective or metabolic origin.

Diagnosis

Patients with progressive deficits in two or more cognitive domains affecting the patient's daily life. See Table 22.3 for subtypes.

Aetiology

The most common causes are Alzheimer's disease, Lewy body dementia, vascular dementia, and frontotemporal dementia. It is worth being aware of the existence of some of the rarer types, but more detailed knowledge of these four should suffice.

Reversible causes

Where dementias are by definition progressive and irreversible, it is essential to exclude a number of reversible mimics resulting in cognitive deficits: depression, vitamin B12 deficiency, normal pressure hydrocephalus, intracranial haematomas and masses, HIV, neurosyphilis, and hypothyroidism are importantly all reversible or treatable.

Other types include mixed dementia, CJD, Huntington's disease, and Wernicke–Korsakoff syndrome.

Table 22.3 Types of dementia

Dementia	Prevalence	History	Signs/symptoms	Pathology/imaging
Alzheimer	50–80%	Gradually progressive	• Rapid amnesia • Language deficits • Early *normal* neuro and gait exam • Affective/behavioural symptoms	• Brain atrophy • Beta amyloid plaques
Vascular	20–30%	Abrupt with stepwise decline	• Focal neuro signs • Associated vascular disease	• CVA • Lacunar infarcts • Brain atrophy • Ischaemic changes
Lewy body	10–25%	Insidious onset	• Visual hallucinations • Shuffling gait • Parkinsonism • Neuroleptic sensitivity	• Generalized brain atrophy • Lewy body in cortex and midbrain
Fronto-temporal	10–15%	Insidious onset but rapid progression	• Disinhibition • Socially inappropriate • Apathy • Poor executive function	• Frontal and temporal atrophy • Pick cells/bodies in cortex

Alzheimer's disease

Accounts for 70% of dementias affecting nearly half a million people in the UK, characterized by the formation of amyloid proteins and neurofibrillary tangles in the cerebral hemispheres.

Clinical features

Are characterized by the 6 A's:

- *Amnesia* (impaired formation of short-term memory).
- *Apraxia* (impaired ability to perform tasks).
- *Agnosia* (impaired recognition).
- *Alexia* (inability to read).
- *Acalculia* (inability to perform simple arithmetic).
- *Aphasia* (impaired understanding and word production).
- Visuospatial deficits can also become prominent in later disease.

Vascular dementia

Is the second commonest type and affects patients differently depending on the site of brain ischaemia. Yet it often progresses in a step-like fashion whereby symptoms may remain at a constant level for some time and the illness progresses in obvious steps rather than a gradual reduction in skills/abilities as with Alzheimer's disease. Life span is also shorter most likely due to CVS risk factors.

Frontotemporal dementia/frontal lobe dementia

Is a neurodegenerative disease, with an insidious onset and slow (usually years) progression.

Presentation

person may behave very differently as a result of their illness. For instance, someone who was previously very quiet and unassuming might become loud and aggressive and use offensive language. Some people become withdrawn, while others may become disinhibited or even sexually inappropriate by exhibiting sexual behaviour in public.

Family history

Is positive in 50%.

Dementia with Lewy bodies (DLB)

Takes its name from abnormal collections of protein within nerve cells, known as Lewy bodies.

Presentation

In addition to symptoms of Alzheimer's disease, people with DLB are likely to experience *hallucinations* (particularly visual ones) and delusions. The condition tends to have an insidious onset, fluctuates, and parkinsonism is common. DLB is also associated with Parkinson's disease (however it can occur without this). Many features are similar to those seen in delirium (e.g. fluctuations, effect of drugs, psychosis—hallucinations and delusions). DLB often progresses more rapidly than Alzheimer's disease.

Diagnosis

Is frequently clinical after excluding the aforementioned reversible causes with neuroimaging and graded by cognitive screens such as the MMSE, and Addenbrooke's Cognitive Examination-Revised (ACE-R).

MMSE

This is a screening tool to assess cognitive function. The maximum score is 30. A score of ≤23 is the cut-off point for significant impairment.

Management

The unfamiliar surroundings of the hospital environment are likely to make confusion worse. It can be very disorienting having lights on all the time. These patients are best nursed by the same people in a calm environment, with large wall clocks to help them orientate to time. Be patient. It may be impossible to get a reliable history from the patient so seek other sources of information, including relatives, carers, GP, and previous medical records. Pharmacological treatment for Alzheimer's disease is with acetylcholine esterase inhibitors such as galantamine and the NMDA receptor antagonist memantine. MDT discussions involving specialist nurses, therapists, psychiatrists, and counsellors with the patient and their families are critical at diagnosis.

Neurology: in the emergency department

Status epilepticus

Definition

Prolonged seizure or series of seizures lasting ≥5 min (newly defined as when anticonvulsants are started), or when a second seizure occurs without recovering consciousness from the first during the same time period. This could lead to incomplete recovery often defined after 30 min duration but emergency treatment begins much earlier.

Management

You will see doctors following the 'ABC Don't Ever Forget Glucose' approach:

- **A**: airway, recovery position in case airway is compromised from low GCS score and obstructive vomitus/tongue.
- **B**: high-flow oxygen.
- **C**: venous access, bloods (FBC, U&E, CRP, LFT, Ca^{2+}, Mg^{2+}, antiepileptic drug concentration), venous/arterial blood gases.
- **D**: hypoglycaemia is quickly corrected with IV 50% glucose.
- Check blood glucose and serum electrolytes from a quick venous blood gas test.

Many seizures will self-terminate after a 5 min, but if not, initial treatment is with a benzodiazepine such as IV lorazepam or diazepam; buccal midazolam or PR diazepam in the community. Repeat this dose 10 min later if still fitting, but if not subsiding escalate to IV anticonvulsant loading (over 20 min), usually phenytoin, before escalation to intubation and general anaesthesia (IV propofol, midazolam, or thiopental) in an intensive care setting. EEG may be used to monitor termination of seizure activity. True status epilepticus is a medical emergency with a 20% mortality rate, causing irreversible brain damage in survivors.

Investigations

5 mL of serum and 50 mL of urine samples should be saved for future analysis, including toxicology, especially if the cause of the convulsive status epilepticus is uncertain. CXR if there is concern about aspiration. Consider CT head and LP if an intracranial lesion or meningitis is suspected.

Clinical tips

Check for head injuries (can be cause or consequence of seizure). If alcohol abuse is suspected, give IV thiamine (Pabrinex®). Be aware of pseudo-seizures (often in psychiatric patients). Advise the patient not to drive if discharged (see Driver and Vehicle Licensing Agency (DVLA) guidance).

Seizure and epilepsy

Patients with 'fits, faints, and funny turns' commonly present to neurologists. The diagnosis usually lies in the history of the attack, which is best supplemented by a collateral history from a witness.

History

Ask about the temporal pattern of attacks, and symptoms between attacks. Are the attacks stereotyped? Talk through a typical attack and identify the timings and what happens before, during, and after.

In attacks with loss of consciousness, identify the first clear memory on regaining consciousness. It is important to elicit the *before* (aura, triggers, prodromes, *warning signs*), *during* (loss of consciousness, head injury, eye-witness account for duration of seizure, foaming at mouth, tongue biting, limb jerking, urinary/faecal incontinence) and *after* (feeling weak/tired, memory of event, aftermath symptoms) the event.

Seizure

Is an episode of abnormal synchronous brain electrical activity.

Epilepsy

Is the tendency to have recurrent unprovoked seizures.

Generalized seizures

Originate with discharges in both hemispheres, so consciousness is always affected. The classic form we tend to think about is the tonic–clonic seizure, where usually without warning the patient becomes rigid and unresponsive, associated with tongue biting and incontinence. Synchronous jerking of all four limbs typically lasts for a few minutes, reducing in frequency until stopping. Afterwards, the patient is drowsy and confused ('post-ictal') for minutes to hours, and once fully recovered will have no recollection of events during the attack and poor recollection of events during the post-ictal state.

Partial (focal) seizures

Originate from a localized area, the clinical manifestations of which depend on the parts of the brain involved. They may be 'simple' or 'complex', depending on whether awareness is preserved or altered respectively. There may be secondary generalization, where the abnormal discharges spread into a generalized seizure. After a partial seizure in the motor cortex, the affected limb may be weak in the post-ictal state (Todd's paresis). The most common site of onset for partial seizures is the temporal lobe, causing odd symptoms such as olfactory hallucinations, déjà vu, and motor automatisms.

Aetiology

Seizures may be caused by an idiopathic epilepsy syndromes or be secondary to an underlying brain disorder such as hypoxia, head injury, infection, or metabolic derangement; or a focal lesion such as a tumour, stroke, or vascular malformation.

Investigation

Since epilepsy is a condition of attacks, examination and investigation in between attacks may be normal. EEG can be helpful and brain imaging can look for an underlying cause, especially in focal seizures.

Treatment

Is primarily with anticonvulsant drugs, such as lamotrigine or carbamazepine for focal, and sodium valproate for generalized seizures—the choice of which frequently depends on their side effect profiles. Surgery may be an option if there is an underlying resectable structural lesion which is proven to be the epileptic focus.

Differentials

Not all episodes of collapse and shaking are seizures, and not all seizures cause *collapse and shaking*. A common mimic is syncope, a transient loss of consciousness due to cerebral hypoperfusion; this is common and results from vasovagal, postural hypotension, cardiac, or carotid sinus disease.

Thunderclap headache

Sudden severe headache which reaches peak severity within 60 sec is termed 'thunderclap', which when occurring spontaneously (e.g. non-traumatic) is frequently associated with SAH following rupture of an intra-cranial berry aneurysm.

Clinical manifestations

Vary: there may be neck stiffness and photophobia due to meningeal irritation; a pupil-involving third nerve palsy may be present due to compression by an underlying posterior communicating artery aneurysm; while focal signs such as hemiparesis can occur due to vasospasm and infarction. Reduced conscious level can occur due to hydrocephalus (non-obstructing CSF accumulation due to impaired resorption).

Investigations

CT is first performed, which if negative is followed by LP performed 12 hours after headache onset to analyse for xanthochromia, a haemoglobin degradation product.

> **To ask the boss**
>
> *'Does the timing of CT scan after the thunderclap headache affect its sensitivity in detecting subarachnoid haemorrhage?'*
>
> The combined sensitivity of a CT scan and xanthochromia in picking up a SAH varies depends on the time of the scan from headache onset, resolution of the scanner, and the radiologist. Ask the consultant about their threshold for CT or formal angiography in patients who present late with negative investigations but strong clinical features of a SAH.

Management

Confirmed SAH requires angiography to find the culprit aneurysm and secure it by surgical clipping or endovascular coiling.

Stroke and transient ischaemic attack

Definition

Any acute neurological deficit with a cerebrovascular cause, strokes and TIAs are rather arbitrarily differentiated by neurological deficits lasting for longer (stroke) or less (TIA) than 24 hours.

Aetiology

Strokes can be caused by ischaemic arterial occlusion (80%) or intracranial haemorrhage (20%); it is important to differentiate on initial diagnosis with imaging because the treatment is obviously distinct.

Screening

The Recognition Of Stroke In the Emergency Room (ROSIER) scale is designed to aid diagnosis:

New acute onset (or on awakening from sleep):
- Asymmetric facial weakness   +1
- Asymmetric arm weakness   +1
- Asymmetric leg weakness   +1
- Speech disturbance   +1
- Visual field defect   +1
- Seizure activity   −1
- LOC/syncope   −1

Scores can range from −2 to +5. Stroke is likely if total score is >0 and unlikely if ≤0.

Investigations

Aim to find the underlying cause of the stroke: carotid Doppler US for carotid artery stenosis, 24-hour ECG for tachyarrhythmias, echocardiograms for cardiac regional wall and valvular abnormalities, in addition to blood tests for DM and lipid disorders. The aim on discharge is optimization of vascular risk factors to prevent further strokes (so-called secondary prevention).

The NIHSS (National Institutes of Health Stroke Scale) is a tool used to quantify the impairment from a stroke (www.mdcalc.com/nih-stroke-scale-score-nihss).
- Bloods (beta-2 microglobulin, FBC, U&E, ESR, blood glucose), ECG (AF is a risk factor), CXR.
- CT head immediately if any of the following apply:
  - Indications for thrombolysis or anticoagulation.
  - On anticoagulant.
  - A known bleeding tendency.
  - GCS score <13.
  - Unexplained progressive/fluctuating symptoms.
  - Papilloedema, neck stiffness, fever, headache.

Imaging

When the time of onset is unclear, such as patients who present with deficits on waking, CT perfusion determines whether an ischaemic penumbra exists, where an area of salvageable brain tissue exists around an infarct and hence could make thrombolysis potentially therapeutic. MRI is increasingly available for acute infarcts when ischaemic strokes are difficult to distinguish from mimics such as seizures, migrainous syndromes, intracranial tumours, and demyelinating disease. Know the mechanism of drug action of some of the common thrombolytics prior to shadowing the stroke registrar.

Management

Ischaemic stroke

Typically treated with 300 mg aspirin (exclude haemorrhagic stroke first and supplement with PPI if history of dyspepsia) for 2 weeks followed by 75 mg clopidogrel.

Honours

Antiplatelets and anticoagulation

Two large randomized controlled trials, the IST and CAST, demonstrated early high-dose aspirin significantly reduced stroke recurrence and mortality after ischaemic stroke. Evidence for combination antiplatelets with adjunctive clopidogrel + dipyridamole is inconsistent, with different trials recruiting different stroke and TIA cohorts of varying ethnicities: one of the largest trials, MATCH, demonstrated no benefits but significantly ↑risk of intracerebral haemorrhage with aspirin + clopidogrel. Evidence from IST found no benefit of anticoagulation with heparin over antiplatelet therapy.

Haemorrhagic stroke

If the patient is anticoagulated, normalize INR using prothrombin complex concentrate and IV vitamin K. Patients are admitted onto a hyperacute stroke unit with specialist stroke physicians, therapists, and dieticians, an arrangement proven to improve survival. Maintain blood glucose level between 4 and 11 mmol/L. Only control BP if there is a hypertensive emergency or for thrombolysis candidates with BP >185/110 mmHg. Swallow screen on admission.

To ask the boss

'Beyond thrombolysis in acute stroke'—endovascular clot retrieval

Treatments other than IV thrombolysis are currently being investigated for patients presenting with acute ischaemic strokes, including intra-arterial thrombolysis and mechanical clot retrieval. With the appearance of a new generation of thrombectomy devices, current trials are investigating whether improved re-canalization rates transfer to improved patient outcomes. Ask the consultant about the technical difficulties and potential complications of mechanical clot retrieval.

Thrombolysis

Ischaemic strokes presenting within 4.5 hours of onset may be eligible for thrombolysis treatment, intended to break up the offending arterial blood clot (but with a significant risk of intracranial haemorrhage). Thrombolysis with alteplase (tissue plasminogen activator) if <4.5 hours from onset (current NICE guidance although controversial—direct comparisons of alteplase with no alteplase at 3–4.5 hours after stroke suggest an absolute ↑ in mortality of 2% and no clear benefit).

TIA: ABCD² system

The **ABCD²** scoring system helps identify those at high early risk of stroke as follows.

Criteria

(Points allocated.)
- Age (≥60 years = 1).
- BP (systolic >140 mmHg and/or diastolic ≥90 mmHg = 1).

- Clinical features (unilateral weakness = 2, speech disturbance without weakness = 1, other = 0).
- Duration of symptoms in minutes (≥60 = 2, 10–59 = 1, <10 = 0).
- Diabetes (present = 1).

Risk of stroke in next 2 days based on total score: score of 0–3, risk = 1%; score of 4–5, risk = 4%; score of 6–7, risk = 8%.

Honours
Thrombolysis
It is useful to know the evidence behind the rationale for management of acute ischaemic stroke during your neurology firm. The NINDS trial demonstrated thrombolysis administered within 3 hours of symptom onset resulted in improved rates of near full recovery at 3 months (38% vs 21%) associated with an ↑ in intracerebral haemorrhage complications (6.4 vs 0.6%) but with no difference in 3-month mortality. The ECASS 3 trial demonstrated a significant albeit smaller benefit when the therapeutic window was extended to 4.5 hours, again associated with a higher risk of intracerebral haemorrhage but no difference in 3-month mortality. Evidence for thrombolysis up to 6 hours from symptom onset is controversial: only the open-label IST-3 trial recruited patients up to 6 hours with evidence neither concluding or excluding thrombolysis benefits at this extended therapeutic window.

Management
Admit high-risk patients: ABCD^2 score of ≥4 or those with crescendo TIA (two or more TIAs in a week). Aspirin (300 mg daily) started immediately. Specialist assessment and investigation within 24 hours of onset if high risk, and 7 days if low risk (ABCD^2 ≤3). Measures for secondary prevention (e.g. BP and cholesterol control, smoking cessation). If carotid artery imaging (Doppler) shows significant stenosis, carotid endarterectomy should be performed within 2 weeks of the TIA.

Guillain–Barré syndrome
An autoimmune-mediated peripheral neuropathy triggered by GI or lower respiratory infections, classically includes mycoplasma pneumoniae, CMV, and EBV.

Presentation
Progressive ascending weakness with absent reflexes, and sometimes sensory loss or back pain.

Diagnosis
Is based on clinical suspicion and may be supported by block of peripheral nerve conduction on electrophysiological testing and ↑protein on CSF. Autonomic nerves can also be involved and you should be able to thereby explain some of the other wider manifestations of Guillain–Barré syndrome.

Honours

Autoantibodies against peripheral nerves (anti-GM1) may be positive in Guillain–Barré syndrome while anti-GQ1b may be present in Miller–Fisher syndrome, a similar autoimmune condition resulting in ophthalmoplegia, areflexia, and ataxia.

Treatment

May involve IV immunoglobulin or plasma exchange.

CNS infections

Organisms may enter the CNS through the blood, via nerves, or via direct spread from adjacent structures. Infections generally take the form of either meningitis, encephalitis, or a space-occupying lesion. Fever is a common feature to all. Immunosuppression may predispose and a HIV test should be done in all patients with CNS infection.

Bacterial meningitis

Presentation

Acute neck stiffness, photophobia, headache, and fever. Beware of additional features such as seizures, cranial neuropathies, and systemic features if the patient becomes septic.

Risk groups

Meningitis should be particularly suspected in high-risk groups, such as patients with skull trauma, CSF shunts, and systemic immunosuppression who may present with more uncommon organisms (e.g. TB).

Diagnosis

Is made via a combination of clinical features, blood tests, and CSF examination unless contraindicated. CSF in meningitis typically demonstrate raised white blood cells, predominantly neutrophils in bacterial meningitis and lymphocytes in TB, raised proteins, and CSF glucose below 40% of serum levels.

Trivia

- Worldwide, neurocysticercosis from the pork tapeworm is the most common cause of epilepsy.
- TB causes meningitis and space-occupying lesions ('tuberculomas').
- Cerebral malaria is a highly dangerous complication of falciparum malaria.
- HIV causes a wide range of neurological problems due to opportunistic infections such as cryptococcal meningitis, toxoplasma encephalitis and abscesses, and CMV encephalitis.

Treatment

Is with prompt initiation of third-generation IV cephalosporins until the organism is isolated and particular attention paid to complications such as features of raised ICP and seizures. The European Dexamethasone Study[1] demonstrated that the use of steroid reduced morbidity and mortality in *Streptococcus pneumonia* type.

Viral encephalitis

Types

The majority of viral infection of the brain parenchyma results from HSV, EBV, CMV, VZV, and enteroviruses.

Presentation

Like all infections of the brain, it can involve headache, confusion, seizures, or focal neurology, and can be complicated by combination with meningitis (meningoencephalitis).

Diagnosis

Is made clinically, supported by raised serum inflammatory markers and positive viral serology in blood, lymphocytosis, raised protein, and viral serology in CSF; neuroimaging may demonstrate non-specific areas of oedema or haemorrhage.

Treatment

Patients should be promptly treated with IV aciclovir.

Reference

1. de Gans J, van de Beek D, European Dexamethasone in Adulthood Bacterial Meningitis Study Investigators. Dexamethasone in adults with bacterial meningitis. *N Engl J Med* 2002;347(20):1549–56.

Neurology: in exams

During your neurology placement, ensure that you can perform and elicit the symptoms and signs described in this section.

History station

Cover all the usual areas including family and social history. Ask in detail about function and any practical limitations, e.g. with walking or writing. Ask about driving, which may be limited by law in many neurological diseases. Neurological problems can be very difficult to describe, so be ready to ask discriminating questions that will narrow the differential. For example, if faced with weakness, always ask if there is associated sensory disturbance, and vice versa. If dealing with visual loss, work out if the problem is in one eye or in one visual field—what happens when the patient closes each eye in turn? If a patient uses the word 'numb', ask what they mean—insensitive, painful, clumsy, or weak?

Always ask: what is the time course? A *sudden onset and slow recovery* is typical of vascular events such as stroke. A *relapsing–remitting* course where symptoms come on over hours or days, reach a peak, and then gradually fade away, with multiple attacks, perhaps with incomplete recovery in between, is typical of inflammatory diseases such as MS. A *progressive* course is typical of neurodegenerative conditions such as Parkinson's disease and expanding structural lesions such as tumours. Finally, *paroxysmal* disorders are characterized by stereotyped attacks, with relatively symptom-free periods in between attacks. Examples of paroxysmal disorders are epilepsy, migraine, and TIAs. Are the symptoms positive or negative? Examples of positive symptoms would be abnormal movement of a limb, or flashing lights in the vision, whereas the converse negative symptoms would be paralysis or loss of vision. Are the symptoms stereotyped—exactly the same with each attack? Are the attacks provoked or unprovoked? Epilepsy tends to cause unprovoked, stereotyped attacks, lasting less than a few minutes, and which may feature positive symptoms and/or altered consciousness. Migraine aura causes positive symptoms which evolve over minutes. TIAs tend to cause negative symptoms which are maximal at onset, and rarely affect consciousness.

When taking a history of loss of consciousness, a collateral history from a witness is essential. Ask the patient exactly what they remember leading up to the attack, and the first thing they remember afterwards. If the patient collapsed, ask if they remember hitting the floor. Ask the witness what they observed before, during, and after the attack, including any abnormal movements or colour change. Finally, ensure that your history has covered the major elements of the nervous system: limbs, eyes, face, swallowing, speech, bladder/bowel, and cognition.

Things to do

Lumbar puncture

You need to be competent to perform this on clinical models. See Table 22.4 for CSF analysis. Be prepared to answer:

- What structures does the needle pass through?
  - Skin, subcutaneous fat, supraspinous and interspinous ligaments, ligamentum flavum, epidural space, dura, subarachnoid space, CSF.
- Where does the spinal cord end?
  - Between L1 and L2; below this level the nerve roots float in the subarachnoid space as the cauda equine and safe space for LP.
- What is the normal CSF pressure?
  - Vary between 8–16 cm water but >20 cm water is abnormal.
- What is the CSF volume and how quickly is it made?
  - Volume is ~120 mL, and 500 mL are made (and reabsorbed)/day.

Neurology examination

Holding the arm flexed and leg extended is common in hemiparesis. Look for movement disorders, which broadly speaking feature either too little movement (akinetic-rigid syndromes including Parkinson's disease), too much movement (hyperkinetic disorders including chorea), or abnormal postures (dystonia). Also look around the patient, for functional aids or signs of treatment before inspecting the gait. Ask the patient to get out of the chair or bed without using their arms—a good test for proximal weakness. Test for *Romberg's sign*—ask the patient to stand with their feet together and arms by their side, then to close their eyes. The sign is positive if the patient is steady with eyes open but unsteady with eyes closed, and implies sensory ataxia (loss of joint position sense). Then assess gait, walking normally, and then heel–toe to bring out the unsteadiness of cerebellar ataxia.

Table 22.4 CSF analysis

	Normal	Bacterial	Viral	Fungal
Pressure (cmH$_2$O)	5–20	>30	Normal	Normal
Appearance	Normal	Turbid	Clear	Turbid
Protein (g/L)	0.18–0.45	>1	<1	0.1–0.5
Glucose (4.4 mmol/L)	2.5–3.5	<2.2	Normal	1.6–2.5
Gram stain	Normal	Positive >60%	Normal	Normal
Glucose CSF:serum	0.6	<0.4	>0.6	<0.4
WCC (/mm³)	<3	>500 (90% PMN)	<1000 (monocytes with some PMN)	100–500

Obstetrics and gynaecology

Obstetrics and gynaecology: overview

Obstetrics and gynaecology (O&G) is a surgical specialty that deals with pregnancy, childbirth, and diseases of the female reproductive tract including infertility and cancer. Most hospitals provide both O&G services, with some tertiary units acting as stand-alone trusts, with a link to a local ED. If you are placed at a peripheral hospital, you are likely to see both O&G services that are required for your training. However, those of you placed at tertiary centres may also get the opportunity to see subspecialist clinics or services (e.g. fertility, fetal medicine, and advanced laparoscopic surgery).

Antenatal care

Antenatal care is the complex of interventions that a pregnant woman receives from organized healthcare services. This includes planning for pregnancy and continues into the early neonatal and postpartum period. The objectives are to:
- promote and maintain physical, mental, and social health of mother and baby through:
  - education
  - detecting and managing complications
  - a birth plan
  - preparing the mother to experience normal puerperium.

Pre-pregnancy counselling

This is essential for women with pre-existing diseases such as diabetes or epilepsy, or those with a drug or alcohol abuse concern. Both pre-pregnancy and antenatal visits are used to reinforce positive health messages including:
- good diet
- smoking cessation
- alcohol
- recreational drugs
- folic acid—400 mcg or 5 mg depending on whether they are higher risk.

Counselling for a woman with type 1 diabetes

Women who have diabetes are at a higher risk of miscarriages, fetal cardiac anomalies, small babies, and still births. It is important to optimize their glycaemic control and ensure they have appropriate check-ups throughout their pregnancy including ophthalmology and renal review. You will see these women in diabetic antenatal clinics where they will come for their pre-pregnancy counselling, monitoring of their ideal HbA1c before they conceive, and a plan for a future pregnancy.

Pregnancy test

A urine pregnancy test can be performed at any time from the first day of a missed period, where a woman can be pregnant around 2 weeks after conception. The test measures the beta subunit of human chorionic gonadotropin (hCG) (in urine or blood), which is produced by trophoblasts on day 6 after fertilization. The first antenatal visit (before the 12th week) includes:
- detailed history
- physical examination
- making a risk assessment
- estimating the due date
- support services.

Calculating the 'due date'

The average pregnancy "gestation" is 40 weeks or 280 days from the first day of the last menstrual period (LMP). You can also use Naegele's rule:
• Subtract 3 months from the first day of the LMP.
• Add 7 days.
• Correct the year if necessary.

Booking visit

Observe a newly pregnant woman have her booking visit with the antenatal department around 10–12 weeks of her pregnancy. You will see this in antenatal clinic with the midwives for low-risk pregnancies, and with the doctors for high-risk pregnancies.

Honours

Customized growth chart

During their booking, women will have a due date provided according to their dating scan (first scan). This EDD (estimated date of delivery) can be used to create a customized growth chart specific to the woman bearing in mind her height, weight, ethnicity and previous babies. Learn about why this is important especially with monitoring fetal growth (symphysiofundal height measurements).

Normal delivery (stages of labour)

• First stage: from the onset of labour until full dilatation of cervix.
• Second stage: from full dilation of the cervix until delivery of the baby.
• Third stage: from the delivery of the baby until complete delivery of placenta and membranes.

Normal vaginal delivery

Observe the care of a woman during normal delivery. Differentiate the different stages of labour, and either observe or actively participate in the delivery of the baby.

Preterm delivery

A delivery that occurs after 24 weeks and before 37 weeks of gestation. Most babies born closer to 37 weeks do very well, with minimal intervention from the neonatal unit, or without requiring intensive care or resuscitation. Babies born earlier, or those where the pregnancy has an underlying pathology (e.g. severe pre-eclampsia) with growth restriction, require liaison with an appropriate neonatal unit for a suitable level of care for the neonate. IM steroids need to be administered to the mother to improve fetal lung maturity, which in turn improves neonatal outcome.

Retained placenta

All or part of the placenta is left behind in the uterus during delivery beyond 30 min with an active third stage and beyond 60 min with a passive third stage. This can be due to some adherence or invasion of the placenta into the myometrium. The latter tends to occur where there have been scars on the uterus, e.g. a previous caesarean section (CS) or myomectomy. A retained placenta can → haemorrhage, and infection of the retained tissue. There are various methods of dealing with this at delivery, or if patients present back to the delivery suite with some pieces retained.

Twin pregnancy and delivery

Twin pregnancies, although a source of much joy to the parents, have a high-risk start during pregnancy. Multiple pregnancies are known to have a higher risk of congenital anomalies, cerebral palsy, twin-to-twin transfusion syndrome, growth restriction, preterm labour, pre-eclampsia, still birth, maternal anaemia, morbidity, and mortality. There are different types of twins. During a booking scan of a twin pregnancy, the state of the amniotic sac determines whether the pregnancy is dichorionic (i.e. two placentas) or monochorionic (i.e. one placenta). Look for the 'lambda (λ) sign' for the dichorionic twin pregnancies.

Twin-to-twin transfusion syndrome

This occurs in monochorionic pregnancies, where the fetuses share a placenta. As a result of this shared blood flow, anastomoses that develop can result in ↑blood supply to one of the twins, with conversely reduced blood supply in the other. The syndrome starts off with an imbalance in liquor in the amniotic sacs, resulting eventually in fetal mortality if untreated. *Laser ablation*: stopping the blood flow through these anastomoses is necessary to avoid unequal distribution of blood between the fetuses.

Miscarriage

~20% of pregnancies miscarry. There are different types of miscarriage:
• *Threatened*: admitted with pain and/or bleeding, cervical os closed.
• *Inevitable*: admitted with pain and/or bleeding, cervical os open.
• *Incomplete*: admitted with pain and/or bleeding, cervical os open, passed some products of conception.
• *Complete*: admitted with pain and/or bleeding that are resolving, cervical os closed, passed all products of conception.
• *Missed*: asymptomatic or pain and/or bleeding, cervical os closed, scan shows no fetal HR.
• *With sepsis*: admitted with pain and/or bleeding, signs of infection.
• *Recurrent*: more than three recurrent consecutive miscarriages.

Management

Options must involve psychological evaluation with access to formal counselling if required, and information on support groups.
• Conservative: watch and wait with follow-up appointment.
• Medical: mifepristone for cervical priming followed by misoprostol for uterine contractions.
• Surgical: evacuation of retained products of conception (ERPC/ERPOC/EVAC).

A woman with early pregnancy (up to 12 weeks) bleeding and/or pain: if she has a little bleeding with no pain, she may be followed up in the early pregnancy assessment unit with a scan. If she has heavy bleeding, she will be admitted and if haemodynamically unstable, may require an ERPC in theatre. If she presents only with RIF or LIF pain and/or minimal bleeding, an ectopic pregnancy will need to be ruled out with an US scan. Learn to take a history and perform an examination of a woman who comes into hospital in early pregnancy (up to 12 weeks) with bleeding and/or pain. Consider how to differentiate between miscarriage and ectopic pregnancies.

Gestational trophoblastic disease

These are a group of disorders including complete and partial molar pregnancies, invasive mole, choriocarcinoma, and the very rare placental site trophoblastic tumour.

Complete molar pregnancies (75–80%)

Are diploid and only contain genetic material from one sperm. This usually arises due to a duplication of a single sperm following fertilization of an 'empty' ovum. There is no evidence of any fetal tissue. Some complete moles (20–25%) can arise after dispermic fertilization of an 'empty' ovum.

Partial molar pregnancies

Usually have two sets of paternal haploid genes and one set of maternal haploid genes, making it triploid. This occurs after dispermic fertilization of an ovum. In this, there is usually evidence of a fetus or fetal RBCs.

Presentation

Some women may remain asymptomatic, and others commonly present with irregular vaginal bleeding, hyperemesis, excessive uterine enlargement, and an early failed pregnancy on US scan.

Diagnosis

US is easier with a complete molar pregnancy which can have a 'snowstorm appearance'. However, a final diagnosis is only made on histological examination of the products of conception.

Management

Involves removal of the products of conception by suction curettage or evacuation, ± chemotherapy depending on their level of hCG which needs to be monitored.

Down's syndrome screening and counselling

All women, regardless of age, are offered screening for Down's syndrome. The risk of Down's syndrome rises with maternal age. The aim of this screening programme is to identify those at higher risk of having a baby with Down's syndrome and offer diagnostic testing using either chorionic villus sampling or amniocentesis. Women found to be carrying a baby with Down's syndrome will be offered expert counselling and support; they may be offered a termination of pregnancy or they may choose to continue with the affected pregnancy with support. The challenge of a prenatal screening programme is to identify women in whom a risk of Down's syndrome is sufficiently high to justify such an invasive test and to minimize the risk of miscarrying a healthy baby.

Chorionic villus sampling

This procedure takes between 11 and 13 weeks of gestation and involves transabdominal or transcervical sampling of the placental/chorionic tissue. There is a 1–2% risk of miscarriage and it offers a diagnostic answer of chromosomal anomalies with the fetus.

Amniocentesis

This procedure takes place after 15 weeks of gestation. A spinal needle is inserted through the maternal abdominal and uterine walls into the pocket of amniotic fluid within the amniotic sac. 10–20 mL of fluid is aspirated. There is a 0.5–1% risk of miscarriage.

Obstetrics and gynaecology: cancer

Endometrium

Endometrial cancer is the most common gynaecological malignancy in developed countries.

Risk factors

Include ↑oestrogen exposure (early menarche, late menopause, nulliparity, unopposed oestrogen use in HRT), tamoxifen use, increasing age, PCOS, HNPCC, obesity combined with diabetes, and hypertension.

Presentation

Women usually present with postmenopausal bleeding, where vaginal bleeding occurs after 12 months of amenorrhoea.

Investigations

Include performing a transabdominal/transvaginal US scan where an endometrial thickness <4 mm is considered low risk. Other tests include an endometrial biopsy (Pipelle®/curettage) as well as hysteroscopy. The majority of endometrial cancer is histologically adenocarcinoma, and rarely sarcoma. CT scans stage the disease.

Treatment

The mainstay of management is surgical ± radiotherapy, and possibly chemotherapy.

Postmenopausal bleeding

Women present with postmenopausal bleeding and are investigated in rapid access gynaecology clinics to rule out endometrial cancer. They will have a pelvic US with endometrial Pipelle® biopsy and may proceed to have a hysteroscopy.

Hysteroscopy

This is an investigation where a camera is inserted through the vagina and cervix into the uterus to examine the endometrial cavity and look for abnormalities including polyps, fibroids, or abnormalities in the endometrial lining. Advances in this area mean this can be done as an outpatient procedure with some local anaesthetic, or can be offered traditionally under GA.

Ovary

Ovarian cancer is the fourth most common malignancy in women. Unfortunately, due to non-specific symptoms, a majority present with advanced disease with poor survival. This usually occurs in postmenopausal women with a 1:80 lifetime risk.

Predisposing factors

Include unopposed oestrogen production (nulliparity, early menarche, late menopause), familial (*BRCA1*, *BRCA2*, HNPCC), and iatrogenic (*in vitro* fertilization (IVF), clomifene).

Protective factors

Include pregnancy, breastfeeding, and the use of the combined oral contraceptive pill.

Types and markers

Ovarian cancer can be of epithelial, germ cell, or metastatic origin. Epithelial cell tumours include cystadenocarcinomas, which comprise 90% of cancer: serous cell (cancer antigen (CA)-125), mucinous (CA19-9), endometrial (CA125), and clear cell carcinoma. Germ cell tumours occur in 10% of women who are younger, e.g. dysgerminomas (LDH) and yolk sac tumours (alpha fetoprotein). Metastatic tumours can be of endometrial, breast, stomach, or colorectal origin.

Presentation

Women usually present with abdominal pain and swelling, anorexia, and bladder and bowel symptoms due to pressure effects.

Investigations

Include US scan, CT, and bloods, following which staging is performed surgically. Multidisciplinary assistance is sought to decide between debulking surgery versus chemotherapy.

> **Honours**
>
> *Risk Malignancy Index (RMI)*
> - A RMI helps differentiate benign from malignant ovarian masses.
> - RMI >200 increases risk of malignancy.
> - *RMI − CA125 × menopausal status × US features.*
> - US (1 point for each): multilocular cysts, solid area, metastases, ascites, bilateral lesions (U = 1 if 1 point, U = 3 if 2–5 points).
> - Menopausal status: M = 1 if premenopausal, M = 3 if postmenopausal.
> - CA125 level in IU/mL.

Cervix

Cervical cancer is the third commonest gynaecological malignancy, with a peak incidence at 45–50 years of age.

Aetiology

99.7% is due to HPV, and other causes include smoking, HIV, and the combined oral contraceptive pill.

Histology

80% squamous cell carcinoma, and 20% adenocarcinoma.

Presentation

Postcoital/intermenstrual or postmenopausal bleeding. Women can have persistent vaginal discharge, and only in late stages present with pain or thrombosis.

Examination

The cervix usually has an exophytic lesion and looks friable.

Investigations

Include colposcopy, biopsy ± MRI or CT scans.

Management
The case is usually discussed at an MDT meeting with surgery and chemoradiotherapy depending on the staging (see Table 23.1 for action plans).

Intermenstrual/postcoital bleeding
Women present with intermenstrual and/or postcoital bleeding and are examined to find cervical abnormalities (i.e. ulceration or a nodular cervix on palpation). Their smear history is taken and investigations include colposcopy ± hysteroscopy.

Smears
Women aged >25 years are routinely invited every 3 years to attend for a cervical smear. About 1 in 20 women will have an abnormal smear that requires further testing or treatment. The screening programme runs as follows:
• 25 years: first invitation to cervical screening in England and Northern Ireland (age 20 in Scotland and Wales).
• 25–49 years: cervical screening tests are every 3 years.
• 50–64 years: cervical screening tests are every 5 years.
• 65 years: routine cervical screening ceases.

Women >65 years of age should be screened if:
• they have not had a cervical screening test since the age of 50
• a recent cervical screening test has been abnormal.

Colposcopy
(See Fig 23.1 for cervical intraepithelial neoplasia.) This is where the woman is placed in the lithotomy position and her cervix is examined using a speculum and microscope. Cervical biopsy or treatments such as excision can be performed under local anaesthetic.

Table 23.1 Smear test action plans

Result	Means	Action
Normal (90%)	Normal	Routine recall
Inadequate (2%)	Not enough cervical cells picked up	3 consecutive—colposcopy
Borderline changes squamous cells (3–4%)	Cells are not quite normal	3 consecutive—colposcopy
Borderline changes endocervical cells (3–4%)	Cells are not quite normal	Colposcopy
Mild dyskaryosis (2%)	Mild changes in the cells	Colposcopy
Moderate/severe dyskaryosis (0.6–0.7%)	Moderate/severe changes in the cells	Colposcopy
Invasive/glandular neoplasia (<0.1%)	New growth of cells suggesting cancer	Urgent colposcopy within 2 weeks

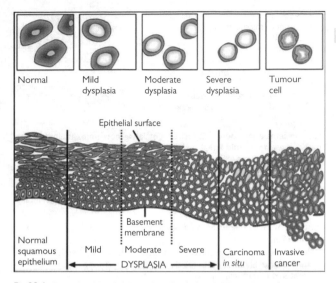

Fig 23.1 Cervical intraepithelial neoplasia. Reproduced with permission from Graham H Barker, www.colposcopy.org.uk.

Infertility

Is the inability to conceive after 1–2 years of regular unprotected intercourse in the absence of pathology. The cumulative pregnancy rate after 1 year is 85%, and after 2 years is 92%. Infertility affects 15% of couples and can be divided into primary (70%) and secondary (30%).

Aetiology

Causes of infertility and treatments:

Female
- Anovulatory (hypothalamic–pituitary–ovarian axis):
  - Ovarian dysfunction (PCOS) → weight loss, clomiphene, ovarian drilling.
  - Hypergonadotropic hypogonadism (premature ovarian failure) → ovum donation.
  - Hypogonadotropic hypogonadism (stress, weight loss, hyperprolactinaemia) → weight gain.
- Tubal (pelvic inflammatory disease, endometriosis) → surgery, IVF.
- Uterine (fibroids/Asherman's syndrome) → myomectomy, adhesiolysis.

Male
- Primary testicular
  - Trauma (torsion)
  - Infection (mumps)

- Neoplastic (chemo/radiotherapy)
- Genetic (microdeletions)
- Steroids
- Obstructive:
  - Congenital (vas deferens)
  - Iatrogenic (vasectomy)
  - Cystic fibrosis
- Endocrine: hyperprolactinaemia
- Drugs and environment: smoking, alcohol.

Investigations

For the female include day 2 follicle-stimulating hormone/luteinizing hormone; oestradiol; mid-luteal progesterone; hysterosalpingography/laparoscopy and dye; and US scan pelvis. For the male, the most important test is the semen analysis.

Management

Includes correcting lifestyle factors e.g. stop smoking; reduce alcohol intake; diet and exercise.

Polycystic ovarian syndrome-related infertility

Presentation

Women with PCOS present with oligomenorrhoea, biochemical features (raised luteinizing hormone to follicle-stimulating hormone ratio), and physical features (hirsutism).

Management

Includes stimulating regular ovulation, metformin, or operating for ovarian drilling to stimulate normal ovulation.

Chronic pelvic inflammatory disease-related infertility

Women with pelvic inflammatory disease present with chronic pelvic pain and inability to conceive due to hydrosalpinx (swollen fallopian tubes filled with fluid) or pyosalpinx (filled with pus). Damage to the cilia in the fallopian tubes as well as adhesions result in inability to conceive.

Treatment

Options include Filshie clip sterilization and IVF. By mechanically blocking the tubes, it protects implanted embryos from adverse effects of fluid collected in the fallopian tubes.

Incontinence

There are two main causes of incontinence:

Stress incontinence

Involuntary urine loss associated with stress due to ↑intra-abdominal pressure (while coughing, exercising, etc.), but in the absence of bladder muscle (detrusor) contractions.

Causative factors

Include raised BMI, multiparous, high birth weight or medical conditions predisposing to chronic cough (COPD/asthma).

Overactive bladder/urge incontinence

Involuntary loss of urine associated with frequency and urgency with or without urge incontinence. The diagnosis is based on symptoms alone, and assumes there is no underlying organic pathology.

- Frequency: voiding more than eight times a day or more than 2-hourly
- Nocturia: interruption of sleep due to more than one micturition every night. Voiding twice at night over the age of 70 years and three times over the age of 80 years is within normal limits
- Urgency: feeling of a sudden, compelling desire to pass urine, which is difficult to defer

Aetiology

Include urological (UTI/bladder masses); gynaecological (cystocele/pelvic masses e.g. fibroids/previous pelvic surgery); genital (urethral caruncle/atrophy); medical (upper motor neuron lesion/impaired renal function/congestive heart failure/diabetes); or general (excessive fluid intake/anxiety/habit/pregnancy). Rare causes include fistulae, congenital abnormality, and urethral diverticula.

Treatment

Is usually surgical.

Urodynamics

This is a procedure to assess the function of the bladder in response to filling, ↑intra-abdominal (coughing), and emptying. The volume of urine and the rate at which the bladder empties are measured. A catheter is inserted into the bladder to measure internal pressure. This is to determine whether the woman has stress incontinence, an overactive bladder, or mixed incontinence.

Prolapse

Is descent of the pelvic genital organs towards or through the vaginal introitus. There are different types and degrees of prolapse:

- *First degree*: descent of the cervix and uterus but not up to introitus.
- *Second degree*: descent of the cervix up to the introitus.
- *Third degree*: descent of the cervix and whole uterus through introitus.
- *Procidentia*: whole of the uterus out of the introitus.

Causative factors

Include childbirth, increasing age, connective tissue disorder (collagen defects), chronic cough, chronic constipation, intra-abdominal masses or ascites, obesity, or pelvic surgery.

Types

- Urethrocoele
- Cystocoele
- Uterine/vault
- Enterocoele
- Rectocoele
- (Cystourethrocoele is the commonest.)

Cystourethrocoele/prolapse

Women usually present with a dragging sensation of 'something coming down' and a lump/fullness in the vagina, which is worse at the end of the day and relieved with lying down. They may also present with difficulties in passing urine or stools, and/or dyspareunia.

Treatment

Is either conservative or surgical. These include physiotherapy (pelvic floor exercises) ± electrical stimulation, intravaginal ring or shelf pessary, or surgery.

Honours

Surgical correction for prolapse

- Anterior/posterior vaginal wall repair.
- Uterine descent:
  - Vaginal hysterectomy
  - Laparoscopic sacrohysteropexy.
- Total vault prolapse:
  - *Sacrocolpopexy*: abdominal or laparoscopic suturing of vault to the body of the sacrum directly or via graft (e.g. Prolene® mesh).
  - *Sacrospinous fixation*: vaginal fixing of vault to the sacrospinous ligament. Complications: damage to sciatic nerve and pudendal vessels; buttock pain; recurrent anterior compartment prolapse.

Obstetrics and gynaecology: emergencies

The following are all O&G emergencies, which you will either have a chance to observe, participate in, or at least read about and discuss at tutorials. *The mother's life always takes priority.*

Ectopic pregnancies

Occur in ~11:1000 pregnancies.

Risk factors

There is an ↑incidence in women who have had previous ectopics, undergone IVF, tubal surgery, or diagnosed with pelvic inflammatory disease. It is a preventable cause of maternal mortality (0.2:1000 ectopic pregnancies).

Presentation

Women present with a history of amenorrhoea, bleeding, and uni/bilateral pelvic pain. They can also present with diarrhoea, shoulder tip pain relating to the side of the ectopic, as well as symptoms of shock.

Investigations

Include blood hCG and US scans.

Management

The cornerstone of diagnosis is laparoscopy, where simultaneous management involving removing the ectopic (salpingotomy) or removal of the tube and ectopic (salpingectomy) can be performed. Methotrexate can be used for smaller ectopics with a lower hCG level and follow-up monitoring.

Antepartum haemorrhage

Differential diagnoses

For bleeding in pregnancy include placental abruption (most common pathology), placenta praevia (second commonest pathology), and others including vasa praevia, cervical polyp, erosion, carcinoma, and uterine rupture.

Placental abruption

Presentation

Painful bleeding where there are tetanic contractions of uterus.

Cardiotocography (CTG)

Demonstrates fetal distress and is pathological, denoting a lack of blood (and oxygen) supply to the fetus. US scanning is of no relevance as this is a purely clinical diagnosis.

Risks

Abruption are ↑ by a previous abruption (×10), maternal diseases (hypertension/thrombophilia), abnormal placentation (praevia), smoking, cocaine and amphetamines, or abdominal trauma.

Placenta praevia

The placenta covers or is within 2 cm of the internal cervical os. It occurs in 0.5–1% of pregnancies.

Risks

Are ↑ by previous CS (×6), multiparity (×2.6), previous dilation and curettage, and smoking.

Presentation

This usually presents with painless bleeding and is diagnosed by clinical acumen and/or US.

Complications

Can include placental abruption, intrauterine growth restriction, fetal malpresentation, or postpartum haemorrhage.

Pre-eclampsia

It is a multisystem disease of pregnancy with pregnancy-induced hypertension (>140/90 mmHg) and proteinuria (0.3 g/24 hours) after 20 weeks of gestation. Pre-eclampsia is the second highest cause of maternal death (source: CEMACH). This occurs in 2–3% of all pregnancies, of which 2% develop eclampsia.

Risks

Women who suffer with essential hypertension have a 15% risk of developing pre-eclampsia. Organs affected can include the heart, kidneys (ATN), liver (subcapsular haemorrhage), blood (DIC), lungs (pulmonary oedema), and brain (CVA).

Spectrum

There is a spectrum of hypertensive disorders of pregnancy ranging from pregnancy-induced hypertension → pre-eclamptic toxaemia → HELLP → eclampsia, with a gradual ↑ in fetal/maternal morbidity and mortality. Eclampsia is the occurrence of a tonic–clonic seizure with incidences of 38% antenatal, 18% intrapartum, and 44% postnatal.

Pathology

Although the pathophysiology is not confirmed, it is understood to be related to poor trophoblastic invasion into the maternal myometrial spiral arterioles. This results in uteroplacental underperfusion and placental hypoxia → the release of antiangiogenic factors causing endothelial damage.

Symptoms

Include headache (frontal), blurred vision/flashing lights, nausea, vomiting, epigastric pain, and peripheral oedema.

Signs

Include pedal/hands/facial oedema, RUQ tenderness, hyper-reflexia, clonus, and tonic–clonic seizures.

Investigations

Include urine for proteinuria >0.3 g/24 hours urine protein (protein:creatinine ratio). Blood tests to check for FBC (thrombocytopenia), LFT (elevated transaminases), U&E, clotting (DIC), and elevated uric acid. USS is performed to identify *in utero* fetal growth restriction, liquor volume, and umbilical artery Doppler.

Management

Is multidisciplinary and can require HDU admission. The main aim is to control BP and control or prevent seizures.

Drugs

Drugs that can be used to control hypertension include labetalol, nifedipine, hydralazine, and methyldopa. $MgSO_4$ is used for seizure prevention. Fluid management is important to avoid overload. Fetal monitoring, and planning the time and mode of delivery are essential.

Honours

$MgSO_4$ for seizure prevention in pre-eclampsia

$MgSO_4$ is recommended by the MAGPIE trial that demonstrated 58% risk reduction in seizure occurrence. It needs to be continued 24 hours from the last fit or from the time of delivery, whichever is most recent. Clinical monitoring is essential, i.e. respiratory rate, urine output, reflexes, ECG, SaO_2 Mg^{2+} level monitoring can be conducted if signs of toxicity. Fluid management is important to avoid pulmonary oedema, which is a major cause of mortality. Fluid intake should be restricted to 85 mL/hour with monitoring on an input–output chart, with the assistance of CVP monitoring if necessary.

Uterine inversion

This is a rare complication occurring in 0.05–0.5% of pregnancies. It is a result of excessive traction on the placenta to deliver it during the third stage. The woman suffers vasovagal shock and resulting massive bleeding.

Management

Involves manual repositioning of the uterus.

Amniotic fluid embolus

This is a rare emergency occurring in 2:100,000 pregnancies. However, there is a very high mortality rate of 80%.

Pathology

An anaphylactic reaction to fetal antigens or due to severe sepsis. It occurs at delivery and results in pulmonary hypertension, left ventricular dysfunction or failure, coagulopathy, and a massive postpartum haemorrhage.

Presentation

It can present with rigors, perspiration, restlessness, coughing, cyanosis, hypotension, tachycardia, arrhythmia, convulsions, or with a cardiac arrest and DIC.

Diagnosis

Is clinical and CXR, ABG, and ECG can be performed.

Management

Is purely supportive with an aggressive treatment of coagulopathy with fresh frozen plasma.

Risk factors
Include multiparity, placental abruption, abdominal trauma, external cephalic version, fetal death, and amniocentesis.

Prolapsed umbilical cord

This is a rare complication occurring in 0.2–0.6% of pregnancies.

Risk factors
Include long umbilical cord, breech/transverse, small fetus, multiparity, twins, and artificial rupture of membranes.

Diagnosis
By inspection of the vulva ± vaginal examination.

Management
Involves elevating the presenting part of the fetus to relieve pressure off the umbilical cord. If the fetal head is low and cervix is fully dilated, an instrumental delivery can be performed. If not, a CS is advised.

Shoulder dystocia

After the delivery of the fetal head, the anterior shoulder of the fetus is 'stuck' behind the mother's symphysis pubis. The midwife or doctor will diagnose this once there is difficulty in delivering the body of the baby with gentle traction. The incidence is <1%, but has implications for fetal and maternal morbidity and mortality. Mothers can suffer from postpartum haemorrhage, third- and fourth-degree tears, and psychological sequelae. Brachial plexus injury is the most important complication that can affect babies, where they end up with Erb's or Klumpke's palsy.

Risk factors
Include macrosomia, previous dystocia, obesity, multiparity, and diabetes mellitus.

Sepsis

Is currently the leading cause of direct maternal deaths; with group A streptococcal infection one of the main culprits. Other organisms include *Streptococcus* groups B and D, pneumococcus, and *Escherichia coli*. Severe sepsis with acute organ dysfunction has a mortality rate of 20–40%, which ↑ to 60% if septic shock develops.

- *Sepsis:* infection + systemic manifestations of infection.
- *Severe sepsis:* sepsis + organ dysfunction or tissue hypoperfusion.
- *Septic shock:* persistence of hypoperfusion (i.e. refractory) despite adequate fluid replacement therapy.

Risk factors
For maternal sepsis have been identified as obesity, impaired glucose tolerance/diabetes, impaired immunity/immunosuppressant medication, anaemia, vaginal discharge, history of pelvic infection, history of group B *Streptococcus* infection, amniocentesis and other invasive procedures, cervical cerclage, prolonged spontaneous rupture of membranes, group

A *Streptococcus* infection in close contacts/family members, and women from minority ethnic groups.

Symptoms

Include fever or rigors, D&V, rash, abdominal/pelvic pain and tenderness, offensive vaginal discharge, productive cough, or irritative urinary symptoms.

Signs

Include pyrexia, hypothermia, tachycardia, tachypnoea, hypoxia, hypotension, oliguria, impaired consciousness, and failure to respond to treatment. An Early Warning Score should be utilized to highlight patients that require urgent review, or those that require transfer to ITU.

> ### Honours
>
> *Surviving Sepsis Campaign Resuscitation Bundle*
> - Serum lactate.
> - Obtain blood cultures/swabs prior to antibiotics.
> - Broad-spectrum antibiotic within the first hour.
> - Hypotension/lactate >4 mmol/L:
>   - 20 mL/kg crystalloid/colloid.
> - Hypotension despite fluid resuscitation (septic shock)/lactate >4 mmol/L:
>   - CVP >8 mmHg.
>   - Steroids.
> - Maintain O_2 saturations, transfuse if Hb <7 g/dL.

Breech

In ~3–4% of pregnancies at term, the bottom of the fetus is the presenting part towards the pelvis. Antenatal diagnosis through clinical examination or US should have a further US scan. If no contraindicating factors, an external cephalic version should be arranged around 37 weeks' gestation, where an attempt is made to 'turn' the baby into a cephalic position with pressure placed on the abdomen.

Management

If a woman presents in the early stages of labour with a previously undiagnosed breech presentation, she should be informed that a planned CS carries a reduced perinatal mortality and early neonatal morbidity for the baby at term compared with planned vaginal birth. There is no evidence that the long-term health of babies with a breech presentation delivered at term is influenced by how the baby is born. A breech delivery is more complicated due to the delivery of the after-coming head once the body is delivered. A CS should be considered if there is a delay in the first or second stage of labour, or there is suspected fetal distress. A fetal blood sample from the buttocks of the baby should be avoided. Breech extraction should be performed by a skilled practitioner.

Venous thromboembolic events (VTE), see ⭕ p. 378

This is the third commonest cause of direct maternal death. The risk of VTE/PE is ↑sixfold in pregnancy.

Aetiology

This occurs because of Virchow's triad where there is a change in the composition of blood (↑clotting factors), venous stasis (uterine pressure), and damage to endothelium (operative delivery). Other risk factors are similar to any VTE scoring, i.e. obesity, thrombophilia.

DVT

Presents with calf pain ± oedema with signs of tenderness and increasing swelling.

Investigations

Include USS leg Doppler ± venogram.

PE

Presents with pleuritic chest pain, haemoptysis, dyspnoea, tachypnoea, pyrexia ± collapse.

Investigations

Include ABG, CXR, leg venous Doppler, V/Q scans ± CT pulmonary angiogram.

Management

For both DVT and PE includes LMWH and warfarin.

Prophylaxis

Women need to be risk assessed at booking during pregnancy for appropriate prophylaxis in the antenatal and postnatal period.

Gynaecology: in theatre

Abdominal hysterectomy: total/subtotal ± ovarian conservation

A hysterectomy is surgery to remove the womb, tubes, and ovaries. This can be performed via different routes, e.g. abdominal incision, vaginal, or laparoscopic. The hysterectomy can be *total* (removal of womb, tubes, ovaries, and cervix) or *subtotal* (womb, tubes, and ovaries). Women who have a subtotal hysterectomy require ongoing cervical smears. In younger women requiring a hysterectomy, the ovaries can be conserved to avoid early menopausal symptoms. Although laparoscopic hysterectomy requires greater skill, it results in reduced hospital stay, ↓infection rates, and ↑mobility.

Incision and drainage of Bartholin's abscess

The Bartholin glands are pea-sized mucous secreting glands occurring at 4 and 8 o'clock on the labia minora. When the gland duct is blocked, fluid collects within the gland resulting in a cyst. If the contents of the cyst get infected, an abscess forms which may respond to oral ± IV antibiotics, or require surgery: incision and draining; or marsupialization to avoid recurrence.

Evacuation of retained products of conception

This is a procedure to remove any products of pregnancy that may still be *in situ* within the uterus, either as a missed miscarriage requiring surgical management, or an incomplete miscarriage requiring removal of remaining tissue products. Otherwise, it may → bleeding or sepsis. This procedure also takes place during the postnatal period if there are symptoms/signs of retained placental tissue. Cervical priming with prostaglandin preoperatively is followed by cervical dilatation, and the use of suction catheter to extract pregnancy/placental tissue.

Diagnostic laparoscopy

This procedure is done now most commonly as a day case, where women can go home the same evening, unless they have underlying medical problems. A small, vertical incision is made within the umbilicus (intra-umbilical) to allow the Veress needle to be inserted. Two clicks should be audible: one for piercing the rectus sheath, and one for piercing the parietal peritoneum. CO_2 gas insufflation is used to distend the abdomen. A trocar and port are inserted carefully into the intra-umbilical port. Once within the abdominal cavity, the trocar is removed and the port allows for a laparoscope to be inserted. Multiple small incisions in the suprapubic and iliac fossa can be created for initial diagnosis, followed by treatments such as tubal sterilization, oophorectomy, excision, or ablation of endometriosis. Once the procedure is completed, the peripheral ports are removed under direct vision to ensure no ongoing bleeding, followed by expulsion of the gas and removal of the main intra-umbilical port. The incisions can be closed using sutures, wound closure strips, or special glue.

Diagnostic hysteroscopy

Is commonly performed to evaluate the uterine cavity. This can be performed without anaesthetic, or with regional or general anaesthetic. Other procedures can be conducted at the same time (e.g. removal of polyp, excision of fibroid, endometrial ablation). Saline solution is used to distend the uterine cavity and the hysteroscope is usually inserted with hydrostatic pressure.

> *One-stop clinics/'see and treat'*
> One-stop hysteroscopy clinics are being set up, where patients are having a vaginoscopy and hysteroscopy without anaesthetic, and having other procedures such as polypectomy, resection of fibroids, or insertion of Mirena® intrauterine device.

Anterior/posterior vaginal wall repair

Relieves the symptoms/signs of prolapse. This could be related to the anterior vaginal wall where the urethra ± bladder can be affected, or posteriorly where the rectum can be affected. An incision is made in the vaginal wall and the excess vaginal tissue is dissected. Caution is exerted to avoid excising too much tissue and narrowing the vagina. Underlying defective fascia is repaired with sutures ± placement of a mesh. Anterior/posterior vaginal walls are sutured, and a vaginal pack inserted with urinary catheter *in situ*.

Tension-free vaginal tape (TVT)

Is a procedure that helps women suffering from stress incontinence. The bladder is catheterized to allow urine to empty, and also to provide a guide for urethral positioning later on. The anterior vaginal wall in opened in a vertical incision and the underlying tissue is dissected. Two small cuts are made in the suprapubic region. The TVT is passed from the anterior vagina to the suprapubic area using metal trocars on either side of the urethra, using a metal guide within the urethra to deflect it away from each side as the mesh is inserted. A cystoscope is inserted to ensure no bladder perforation before adjusting the sling (mesh) to stabilize the urethra.

Colposcopy procedures (biopsy/LLETZ)

This is a procedure where the cervix is examined closely using magnification. The indications are abnormal smears requiring further investigation. It is performed after a vaginal speculum is inserted to visualize the cervix, where a colposcope is used with a light and magnifying lens to visualize cervical abnormalities. The use of acetic acid on the cervix stains abnormal areas white. Cervical biopsies ± large loop excision of the transformation zone (LLETZ) can also be performed at the same time.

Myomectomy

This is a procedure that can be performed laparoscopically or via an abdominal incision (vertical/transverse) to remove subserosal or intramural fibroids, or also hysteroscopically to remove submucosal fibroids. If performed laparoscopically, morcellators are used to shred the fibroid tissue so it can be removed via the small incisions.

Obstetrics: in theatre/procedures

Caesarean section

CS is one of the commonest obstetric procedures to witness in the delivery suite, and students can get involved either during emergency or elective CSs. Once the woman has appropriate analgesia, regional or general, she is catheterized aseptically to empty the bladder. An incision is made transversely in the suprapubic region where layers of subcutaneous tissue, muscle, and peritoneum are opened and the bladder is deflected downwards to protect it from injury. The lower segment of the uterus is incised transversely to allow delivery of the fetal head with concurrent pressure by the assistant on the uterine fundus to deliver the fetus. The cord is clamped and cut and the placenta is removed by controlled cord traction. Once the uterus is checked to be clean with no placental tissue remaining, it is sutured most commonly in two layers. The parietal peritoneum is opposed only and rectus sheath is sutured to prevent hernias. The skin can be sutured with either dissolvable or other sutures to be removed within 5 days.

Honours

Surgical skills

Scrub up for a CS and identify the anatomy of the abdominal wall, i.e. layers incised in order from skin to uterine lower segment. Learn how to suture the skin with different methods: subcuticular, interrupted, and mattress sutures.

Fetal blood sampling

This is a procedure where a small volume of blood is obtained from the fetal scalp to determine fetal distress via analysis of pH values. It can usually be performed after cervical dilatation of 4 cm and provides an indication whether the fetus requires delivery or labour can be continued.

Honours

See Table 23.2.

Table 23.2 Fetal blood sample results: pH

7.25 or more	Normal result
7.21–7.24	Borderline result—repeat 30 min
7.20 or less	Abnormal result—deliver

Ventouse delivery

A vacuum extractor, which is either soft or hard plastic or a metal cup, is attached to the baby's head by suction. This cup fits firmly onto the fetus. During a contraction, with the mother pushing, the operator pulls to allow delivery of the fetus. It can leave a small swelling on the fetal head called a chignon. The risks of a vacuum extractor are a resulting cephalohaematoma.

Trivia

Categories of CS

- Category 1: immediate threat to life of the mother or fetus (decision–delivery time = 30 min)
- Category 2: no immediate threat to life of the mother or fetus (decision–delivery time = 60 min).
- Category 3: requires early delivery.
- Category 4: at a time to suit the woman and maternity services.

Forceps delivery

These are metal instruments that curve around the head of the fetus to allow for delivery when the mother pushes and the operator pulls. They can leave marks around the fetus, which take a few days to settle. These are more likely to result in maternal perineal tears and may require creating an episiotomy.

To ask the boss

Operative delivery

- Indications for operative delivery: CS, ventouse, forceps.
- Consent process for operative delivery: CS, ventouse, forceps.

Episiotomy

Around one in seven deliveries involves an episiotomy. NICE recommends that an episiotomy should be considered if the baby is in distress and needs to be born quickly, or if there is a clinical need, such as a delivery that needs forceps or ventouse. An episiotomy is usually made in a right mediolateral incision to avoid tearing down towards the anus.

Obstetrics and gynaecology: in exams

Exams in medical schools vary, with some testing for competence during the O&G block, with others testing for competence during the OSCE.

Need to know how to take a ...

Gynaecology history
- Name.
- Age.
- Gravidity and parity: miscarriages/terminations/stillbirths/other losses.
- PC.
- HPC.
- Duration of symptoms: days, weeks, months, years.
- Progression of symptoms: worsening, improving, stable, fluctuating.
- Cyclical: do symptoms have any relationship to the menstrual cycle?
- Pain: SOCRATES (see ➌ pp. 148–9).

Menstrual history
- Age of menarche.
- LMP (first day of last menstrual period).
- Duration and regularity (X/28 days).
- Flow: heavy/light—number of sanitary towels/tampons useful to estimate loss.
- Menstrual pain.

Other symptoms
- Irregular bleeding.
- Postcoital bleeding.
- Dyspareunia (superficial/deep).

Menopausal symptoms: hot flushes, vaginal dryness, irregular periods, mood changes, concentration.
   If postmenopausal: what age did they go through the menopause?

Gynaecology history including smear history
- STD/pelvic inflammatory disease
- Contraception
- Smear:
  - Regular smears
  - Date of last smear
  - Past smears normal
- Past cervical procedures.

Need to know how to take a ...

Obstetric history
- Name.
- Age.
- Gestation.
- Gravidity and parity: miscarriages/terminations/stillbirths/other losses.

- Each pregnancy:
  - Antenatal/intrapartum/postnatal complications.
  - Age.
  - Weight.
  - Gestation at delivery.
  - How is the child now?
  - Blood relation to partner?
  - Mode of delivery.
  - Is it the same partner as previous pregnancies?
- Booking bloods:
  - Infection screen—syphilis, HIV.
  - Rubella immunity.
  - Rhesus status.
- Scans:
  - Booking.
  - Mid trimester.
  - Other, e.g. growth/uterine artery Dopplers/liquor/umbilical artery Doppler/middle cerebral artery.
- Down's syndrome screening:
  - Accepted.
  - Low/high risk.
  - Diagnostic tests, e.g. chorionic villus sampling/amniocentesis.
  - Results/counselling.

Plan of care at booking:
PC–HPC–pain (SOCRATES)
- Pre-eclampsia: headache, nausea and vomiting, oedema, blurred vision/flashing lights/epigastric pain.
- Diabetes: blood glucose levels.

Systems enquiry
- Urinary: dysuria, frequency, haematuria, loin tenderness, incontinence history.
- GI: appetite, nausea, vomiting, diarrhoea, constipation, PR bleeding, weight loss.
- CVS: chest pain (pleuritic), dyspnoea, palpitations.
- Respiratory: cough, sputum, wheeze.
- MSk: bone or joint pain, difficulty mobilizing.
- PMHx: diabetes, hypertension, renal disease, clotting disorders.
- Past surgical history (PSHx): especially abdominal surgery.
- Drug history (DHx): regular medications, allergies to medications or latex.
- Social history (SHx): smoking, ETOH, recreational drugs, home support, job.
- Family history (FHx): diabetes in first-degree relative, maternal pre-eclampsia.

Oncology

Oncology: overview

Cancer is one of the leading causes of death worldwide, accounting for >8 million deaths in 2012.[1] Age is a fundamental risk factor for the development of cancer. In the UK, cancer rates have risen by 23% in males and 43% in females since the mid 1970s with more than a third of new cancer diagnoses made in those aged ≥75. The burden of this disease will inevitably increase in ageing Western populations. Oncology is the medical specialty that deals with the diagnosis and management of solid cancers. Most management decisions take place in the outpatient setting and clinics will therefore form the basis of your attachment. However, you will see very little acute oncology here and it is vital that you also spend significant time on the specialist oncology wards and on-call to gain this experience.

Cases to see

The 'big four' tumour groups: breast, lung, prostate, and bowel cancer

You should have a basic understanding of the diagnosis and management of these four main tumour groups. This will best be done in outpatients. Follow-up clinics will not be useful to you so ask your consultant specifically about 'new patient' clinics. MDT meetings will also be beneficial as it is here that major treatment decisions are made.

Neutropenic sepsis

It is crucial you know how to manage this oncological emergency. Spend a couple of days shadowing the oncology SHO on-call and you should get good exposure to the cases that frequently present in the ED.

Honours

The Sepsis Six bundle

The 'Surviving Sepsis campaign' (⌘ www.survivingsepsis.org) was launched in 2002 with the aim of reducing mortality from severe sepsis and septic shock worldwide. The campaign saw the introduction of 'sepsis bundles', a selected set of evidence-based care elements which, when implemented, are designed to ensure the most effective management of the septic patient. 'The Sepsis Six' is a set of six interventions that can be delivered by any junior doctor in the acute setting to improve their patient's chance of sepsis survival:

- Administer high-flow oxygen.
- Administer broad-spectrum antibiotics.
- Start IV fluid resuscitation.
- Take blood cultures.
- Measure serum lactate and FBC.
- Measure hourly urine output.

Malignant spinal cord compression (MSCC)

Find out who the oncology registrar on-call is and ask them to call you when a case is referred. Suspected cases are relatively common so you should see a reasonable number.

Superior vena cava obstruction
Cases are rarer than MSCC but again, make the on-call registrar aware and you should be able to see at least one during your attachment.

Hypercalcaemia
A very common metabolic emergency in oncology patients. You will undoubtedly see numerous cases on the wards.

Tumour lysis syndrome (TLS)
Although more common in haematological malignancies, TLS is also seen in solid tumours. Ask the ward registrar to direct you to high-risk patients and pay close attention to their pre-chemotherapy protocols and blood results.

Procedures to see
External beam radiotherapy
Radiotherapy lists take place all day, every day. Find the department and liaise with the radiographers who will be able to take you through the set-up and the different aspects of treatment.

Places to visit
Chemotherapy day unit
It is worth spending some time on the day unit. Extravasation and anaphylactoid reactions are undesirable but inevitable consequences of chemotherapy and you will gain good experience here in their acute management. Chemotherapy nurses are arguably the best around when it comes to venous cannulation and there will be ample opportunity to practise. It is a great place to hone your practical skills away from the pressure of the wards.

The hospice
Palliative care forms a major part of oncology with symptom control and the emotional and psychological support of cancer patients being crucial to the holistic approach to their care. All specialist oncology units will have a palliative care team. Shadowing them and visiting a hospice should be easily negotiable and will give you a unique insight into the vital work they do.

Things to see
The oncology ward is perhaps one of the best places to see a number of things that will be useful to you both in exams and as a junior doctor. Signs include radiotherapy tattoos, radiation-induced skin changes, and clubbing (it does exist!). Devices include colostomies, pleural drains, ascitic drains, syringe drivers, Hickman/PICC lines, and portacaths. Patients with such devices *in situ* are a favourite for OSCE examiners as they provide an excellent discriminator in identifying those candidates who have actually spent time on the wards.

Reference
1. *Globocan 2012: Estimated Cancer Incidence, Mortality and Prevalence Worldwide in 2012.* Lyon: International Agency for Research on Cancer. ℘ www.globocan.iarc.fr/Default.aspx

Oncology: on the ward

Malignant spinal cord compression

Most commonly caused by direct pressure on the spinal cord/cauda equina from vertebral bone metastases. Prostate, lung, and breast cancers account for the majority of solid tumour cases. Any delay in diagnosis and treatment can have catastrophic neurological consequences thus a high index of suspicion is required. *Presentation*: the earliest manifestation is back pain. This may be followed by muscle weakness, loss of sensation, and bladder/bowel dysfunction. *Management*: high-dose dexamethasone should be commenced immediately and an urgent MRI scan of the whole spine arranged to occur within 24 hours. Patients with a good performance status and prognosis >3 months should be considered for decompressive surgery. All others can be treated with palliative radiotherapy. Treatment should commence within 24 hours of a positive MRI diagnosis.

Honours

Indications for surgical decompression

Decompressive surgery plus radiotherapy has been shown to have significantly improved outcomes in terms of regaining ambulation and pain control when compared to radiotherapy alone.[1] Common indications include:
- unstable spine
- cervical cord lesion
- solitary vertebral metastasis
- radioresistant tumour (e.g. melanoma, sarcoma)
- unknown primary (to obtain tissue diagnosis)
- previous radiotherapy
- neurological deterioration while having radiotherapy.

Superior vena cava obstruction

Due to compression or invasion of the SVC by tumour, thrombus, or mediastinal lymph nodes. Bronchial carcinoma and lymphoma account for the vast majority of cases. *Presentation*: onset is usually insidious over weeks with gradual development of shortness of breath, headache, facial swelling, and visual disturbance. *Signs*: distended thoracic veins and a raised JVP. *Pemberton's sign*: marked by facial congestion, dyspnoea, and cyanosis upon elevation of both arms. *Management*: supportive measures such as oxygen, analgesia, and high-dose dexamethasone for short-term symptomatic relief. Stenting is effective in >95% as a holding measure, providing relief within 48 hours. Chemotherapy is indicated in chemosensitive tumours (small cell lung cancer, germ cell tumours) and radiotherapy in all other solid tumours. Both may take up to 2 weeks to have their effect.

Hypercalcaemia

Defined by a corrected plasma calcium concentration of 2.6 mmol/L. Occurs as a result of direct destruction of the bone by metastases or consequent to circulating factors such as PTH-related peptide secreted by tumour cells. *Incidence*: highest in lung, breast, head, and neck and renal carcinomas. *Symptoms*: confusion, vomiting, constipation, abdominal pain, polyuria, and polydipsia. Left untreated, hypercalcaemia can progress to coma and death. *Management*: aggressive IV fluid administration forms the mainstay of treatment, ideally 3 L of crystalloid over 12 hours. Once adequately hydrated, IV bisphosphonates can be given and continued on a regular basis for maintenance.

Tumour lysis syndrome

Occurs due to excessive lysis of dying tumour cells, usually following chemotherapy, resulting in a huge release of intracellular contents into the systemic circulation. A series of metabolic derangements occur including hyperkalaemia, hyperuricaemia, hyperphosphataemia, and hypocalcaemia which can precipitate renal failure, arrhythmias, and seizures. Prevention is key to managing TLS. High-risk patients should be aggressively hydrated prior to chemotherapy and receive IV allopurinol—a xanthine oxidase inhibitor to reduce uric acid accumulation. Haemodialysis may be required if AKI still ensues.

Honours

Risk factors for tumour lysis syndrome

Identifying patients at risk is critical in preventing TLS. The following parameters are associated with a higher incidence of TLS:

- Highly proliferating tumour (leukaemia, lymphoma).
- Tumour highly sensitive to chemotherapy (small cell lung cancer, germ cell tumours).
- Bulky disease.
- Elevated LDH.
- Pre-existing renal impairment.
- Dehydration.
- High-intensity chemotherapy.

Reference

1. Patchell RA, Tibbs PA, Regine WF, et al. (2005). Direct decompressive surgical resection in the treatment of spinal cord compression caused by metastatic cancer: a randomised trial. *Lancet* 366(9486):643–8.

Oncology: in the emergency department

Neutropenic sepsis

Defined as a fever > 38°C and neutrophil count <500 cells/μL. Neutropenia means patients may not present with routine manifestations of sepsis such as tachycardia, sweating, and localized signs, so it may be easily missed. Have a high index of suspicion in all patients receiving chemotherapy. Broad-spectrum IV antibiotics must be commenced within 60 min of pyrexia, together with IV fluids. There is high potential for sudden deterioration into septic shock requiring aggressive resuscitation and rapid escalation of care. A full 'septic screen' should be performed including cultures (blood, sputum, etc.), blood tests, urinalysis, and CXR, but *antibiotics are the priority—do not delay their administration while obtaining investigations!* Ideally antibiotics, fluids, and paracetamol should be administered within <1 hour of presentation.

Symptom control

This is fundamental in the management of oncology patients. Patients may present to the ED with symptoms related to their disease, or side effects from either chemotherapy or radiotherapy.

Pain

This can be notoriously difficult to control, and cancer patients may require strong opioid analgesia at doses which you may not be experienced in prescribing. Patients attending the ED with intractable pain should be admitted and advice sought from the on-call palliative care team as soon as possible.

Nausea and vomiting

These are common side effects of both chemotherapy and radiotherapy. However, this is a diagnosis of exclusion and a full assessment of the patient is required to rule out all other possible causes first. Common underlying pathologies include sepsis, bowel obstruction, hypercalcaemia, and raised ICP secondary to brain metastases. Patients with severe N&V will most likely be dehydrated. Having excluded other organic causes, they should be admitted for symptom control in the form of IV fluid resuscitation and IV antiemetics. 5HT antagonists (e.g. ondansetron) are the preferred choice in chemotherapy-induced N&V.

Diarrhoea

As with N&V, diarrhoea is a common side effect of both chemotherapy and radiotherapy. Radiation colitis is the most severe form of the latter. Patients may again present significantly dehydrated. Infective causes should be excluded and patients should then be admitted and managed with aggressive IV fluid resuscitation and antidiarrhoeal agents such as loperamide.

Oncology: in clinic

While it is all too easy to sit and observe consultations from the safety of the corner of the clinic room, you will learn far more and gain invaluable points with your consultant if you see a patient first and present the case. No one will expect you to come up with a definitive treatment plan but taking an adequate history of both the patient and the tumour will allow for a sensible discussion as to how best to manage the case. When assessing the patient, take into consideration their presenting symptoms, risk factors, and importantly, their comorbidities. Surgery, chemotherapy, and radiotherapy can be intense treatments and not all patients will be fit enough to tolerate them.

Performance status

An impressive way for you to quantify a patient's fitness would be by quoting their 'performance status' (Table 24.1).

Staging and grading

When assessing the tumour, you should record both the histological diagnosis and the stage of the cancer. Histology will usually include the tumour type (e.g. adenocarcinoma, squamous cell carcinoma), the tumour grade, and the degree of differentiation. High-grade, poorly differentiated tumours tend to be associated with poorer prognoses. Staging describes the anatomical extent of the disease and is best defined using TNM staging. Each tumour group will have its own criteria for TNM staging, the minutiae of which you will not be expected to remember. A broad understanding of the principles of the system as described below should suffice (Table 24.2 and Table 24.3).

Table 24.1 The European Cooperative Oncology Group (ECOG) Performance Status scale

Grade	ECOG Performance Status
0	Fully active, able to carry on all pre-disease performance without restriction
1	Restricted in physically strenuous activity but ambulatory and able to carry out work of a light or sedentary nature, e.g. light house work, office work
2	Ambulatory and capable of all self-care but unable to carry out any work activities. Up and about more than 50% of waking hours
3	Capable of only limited self-care, confined to bed or chair more than 50% of waking hours
4	Completely disabled. Cannot carry on any self-care. Totally confined to bed or chair
5	Dead

Oken MM, Creech RH, Tormey DC, et al. (1982) Toxicity and response criteria of the Eastern Cooperative Oncology Group. *Am J Clin Oncol* 5(6):649–55

Table 24.2 The TNM classification of malignant tumours

Parameter	Description
T	The size of the primary tumour and its invasion into local tissue (T1–T4)
N	The extent of regional lymph node spread (N0–N3)
M	The presence of metastases to distant organs (M0–M1)

Table 24.3 Generic grading system for many types of cancer

Grade	Description	
Grade X	Grade cannot be assessed	
Grade 1	Low grade	Well differentiated
Grade 2	Intermediate grade	Moderately differentiated
Grade 3	High grade	Poorly differentiated
Grade 4	High grade	Undifferentiated

Tumour markers

Circulating tumour markers produced by cancers may serve as a useful adjunct to the histological diagnosis and staging of tumours and should be noted. However, tumour markers should be solely relied on since there is a high risk of giving false positives and hence causing anxiety to patients. There has to be a strong reason to request these and in some hospital, permission from consultants must be sought before ordering these investigations. They may be helpful in predicting prognosis and in monitoring response to treatment (e.g. cancer surveillancing). You may find yourself quizzed on the most clinically relevant tumour markers (Table 24.4).

National cancer screening

Programmes

Breast, lung, prostate, and bowel cancer together account for over half of all new cancer diagnoses per year. Cancers diagnosed at the earliest stage are those most amenable to cure. Cancer screening programmes are designed to try and identify disease in individuals in a population prior to the development of signs and symptoms, enabling earlier intervention and reducing the risk of mortality. There are currently three NHS cancer screening programmes in the UK: those for *breast cancer, bowel cancer, and cervical cancer*. There are currently no screening programmes for lung or prostate cancer. A successful screening programme must be robust, viable, cost-effective, and appropriate. WHO guidelines known as Wilson's criteria[1] were introduced in 1968 and these form the basis of the criteria used to justify the introduction of new screening programmes today.

Table 24.4 Common tumour markers and their associated cancers

Tumour marker	Cancer
PSA (prostate-specific antigen)	Prostate
CEA (carcinoembryonic antigen)	Colon
CA15-3	Breast
CA19-9	Pancreas
CA125	Ovarian
AFP (alpha-fetoprotein)	Hepatocellular, testicular
β-HCG (beta-human chorionic gonadotrophin)	Testicular, ovarian germ cell
LDH (lactate dehydrogenase)	Testicular, lymphoma

Wilson's criteria for screening

1. The condition should be an important health problem.
2. The natural history of the condition should be understood.
3. There should be a recognizable latent or early symptomatic stage.
4. There should be a test that is easy to perform and interpret, acceptable, accurate, reliable, sensitive, and specific.
5. There should be an accepted treatment recognized for the disease.
6. Treatment should be more effective if started early.
7. There should be a policy on who should be treated
8. Diagnosis and treatment should be cost-effective.
9. Case-finding should be a continuous process.

Prostate cancer

This accounts for ~30% of all cancers in men and is second only to lung cancer as the commonest cause of male cancer deaths. There is no national screening programme. *Presentation*: early-stage disease is often asymptomatic, but symptoms of 'prostatism' consequent to obstruction of urinary flow through an enlarged prostate may be present. Obstructive symptoms include hesitancy, terminal dribbling, poor or double stream, nocturia, and frequency. *Examination/diagnosis*: after taking a focused micturition history and performing a digital rectal examination, diagnostic investigations should include a PSA and transrectal ultrasound-guided prostate biopsy. Bear in mind that the PSA may be elevated in patient after performing a digital rectal examination so PSA can be tested beforehand. Staging investigations should include an MRI of the pelvis to assess local spread and a radionuclide bone scan to look for metastasis. *Management*: early stage, prostate-confined disease is managed with curative intent either with surgical prostatectomy or radical radiotherapy. Metastatic disease is treated with anti-androgen therapy and chemotherapy.

Honours
Gleason grading system
Prostate cancer is histologically graded using the Gleason system. This is based on the degree of glandular differentiation with grade 1 being well differentiated and grade 5 being the most poorly differentiated. The Gleason grades of the two most common histological patterns found within the tumour are summated to form the overall Gleason score, giving a range from 2 to 10. The higher the Gleason score, the more aggressive the cancer and the higher the risk of recurrence and mortality:
- Gleason < 7: low risk and favourable prognosis.
- Gleason = 7: moderate risk and intermediate prognosis.
- Gleason > 7: high risk and poor prognosis.

Breast cancer
Accounts for 20% of all cancer diagnoses and there is a 1 in 9 lifetime risk for women. There is a National Screening Programme for breast cancer in the form of a 3-yearly mammogram offered to all women aged 50–70. *Risk factors*: age >60, early menarche and late menopause, nulliparity, hormone replacement therapy, the oral contraceptive pill, and family history. *Genetics*: ~5–10% of cases are thought to be hereditary arising from germline mutations in *BRCA1* or *BRCA2* genes. *Diagnostic investigations*: mammogram (or US) and fine-needle aspiration (FNA) for histology. Tissue is always tested for the presence of oestrogen (ER), progesterone (PR) and HER-2 receptors. *Management*: surgery, either wide local excision (WLE) or mastectomy forms the mainstay of treatment for early breast cancer and surgical staging of axillary nodes takes place during primary surgery. Preoperative staging investigations are not routinely performed in low-risk patients. Following WLE and in high-risk mastectomy patients, locoregional radiotherapy is indicated to reduce the risk of local relapse. ER/PR-positive tumours are treated with hormone therapy such as antioestrogens such as tamoxifen and HER-2-positive tumours with trastuzumab®. Both treatments have been shown to improve survival. Chemotherapy is considered for high-risk early-stage patients (high grade, nodal involvement, HER-2 positive) and in metastatic disease.

Honours
Sentinel lymph node biopsy
Surgical staging of the axilla is carried out in all patients with invasive disease. Previously, this was done by axillary clearance but sentinel lymph node (SLN) biopsy is now the gold standard:
- The SLN is the first draining lymph node from the breast, thus it is the first to receive tumour cells from the primary tumour.
- Methylene blue dye and a radioisotope are injected preoperatively to identify the SLN.
- SLN is removed and examined histologically for tumour cells.
- If SLN is –ve, no further surgery is required. Axillary clearance and its associated morbidity (lymphoedema, pain) is avoided.
- If SLN is +ve, axillary clearance or radiation may be required

Lung cancer

Accounts for ~15% of all cancer diagnoses. It is the commonest cause of cancer death in men and equals the breast cancer mortality rate in women. *Aetiology*: smoking is the primary cause and is responsible for 80% of cases. Smoking is the commonest carcinogenic factor and risk of cancer is correlated with the number of pack-years. One pack-year is equivalent to smoking 20 cigarettes per day, every day for 1 year. *Symptoms*: cough, haemoptysis, shortness of breath, chest pain, hoarseness, and dysphagia on a background of fatigue, weight loss, and recurrent chest infections. *Investigations*: diagnostic investigations include pleural fluid aspiration and cytology, bronchoscopic biopsy, or CT-guided biopsy, depending on the location of the tumour. Staging investigations will include bronchoscopy and CT of the chest and abdomen. *Types*: lung cancer is divided histologically into two distinct clinical entities: small cell and non-small cell lung cancer (NSCLC). *NSCLC*: staged using the TNM system and early-stage disease is treated with curative intent with either surgical resection or radical radiotherapy. *Small cell disease*: tends to be advanced at presentation and surgery is not usually an option. It is staged as either limited or extensive depending on whether the disease extends beyond one hemithorax. Chemotherapy is the standard treatment together with concurrent thoracic radiotherapy in limited-stage disease.

To ask the boss

Stereotactic ablative radiotherapy (SABR)

SABR is a specialized form of radiotherapy that can be used to treat small, early-stage NSCLC in patients whose comorbidities or preferences preclude surgery. Compared to conventional radiotherapy which involves giving daily low doses of radiation over numerous weeks, SABR uses thin, focused beams to deliver higher doses to the tumour in far fewer treatments, usually between three and eight.

Bowel cancer

Accounts for ~13% of all cancer diagnoses and is the third most common cause of cancer deaths in both men and women.

Genetics

~10–15% of cases can be attributed to underlying inherited genetic conditions such as HNPCC and familial adenomatous polyposis.

Symptoms

Depend on the location of the tumour but may include changes in bowel habit (alternating diarrhoea and constipation), PR bleeding, tenesmus, weight loss, and fatigue.

Investigations

Honours
Bowel cancer screening
The NHS Bowel Cancer Screening Programme was introduced in England in 2006:
- Screening is offered every 2 years to all men and women aged between 60 and 74.
- Those eligible are sent out a letter and a faecal occult blood (FOB) test kit with instructions for use.
- Once samples are received in the lab, the test is processed and results sent out within 2 weeks.
- Those with a positive result are offered a colonoscopy.
- Those with a negative result return to routine screening.

A systematic review of bowel cancer screening using the FOB test has shown to reduce the risk of mortality from the disease by 16%.

Colonoscopy plus biopsy is the gold standard diagnostic investigation. Those intolerant to endoscopy can be referred for CT pneumocolon. Staging is with CT of the chest, abdomen, and pelvis.

Management
Surgical resection is the mainstay of treatment for all except extensive metastatic disease where palliative chemotherapy can be considered. Palliative stomas can also be an option for pain resulting from distal tumour obstruction.

Reference

1. Wilson JMG, Jugner G (1968). *Principles and Practice of Screening for Disease*. Geneva: World Health Organization.

Oncology: in exams

History station

Being able to take an appropriate history from a patient with suspected malignancy is an absolute must for medical students and is therefore one of the most commonly examined scenarios in the history station.

History of presenting complaint

Know your red flags! If a patient presents with one, establish its details (duration, timing, exacerbating/relieving factors, etc.) and then ask about the rest associated with that tumour (Table 24.5). Follow this up immediately by enquiring about the systemic features of malignancy. So-called constitutional symptoms consist of weight loss (to cachexia), fatigue, and anorexia ± night sweats. Recurrent infections may also occur.

Past medical history

Ask generally and then about any previous history of malignancy. Certain medical conditions predispose to individual cancers, particularly those of the GI tract and the best candidates will enquire about them specifically where relevant (see Table 24.6).

Family history

Again, ask generally and then specifically enquire about any family history of malignancy. 5–10% of breast cancers and 10–15% of bowel cancers are hereditary.

Social history

Smoking and alcohol are risk factors for numerous cancers so accurately quantify previous and current habits. Occupation is also important to establish any prior exposure to carcinogens.

Examination

Malignancy will form part of the differential diagnosis for a number of cases that may arise in the clinical exam. It should be considered in the patient with jaundice, ascites, pleural effusion, hepatomegaly, splenomegaly, and lymphadenopathy.

Table 24.5 'Red flag' symptoms for specific tumour groups

Cancer	'Red flag' symptoms
Colorectal	Change in bowel habit (diarrhoea/constipation), painless PR bleed, tenesmus, abdominal mass, mucoid discharge
Upper GI (stomach, oesophagus)	Dysphagia, dyspepsia, melaena, haematemesis, epigastric mass
Lung	Haemoptysis, chronic cough, recurrent pneumonia, chest pain, hoarseness, shortness of breath
Urogenitary (prostate, bladder, renal)	Painless haematuria, frequency, nocturia, urinary retention, poor stream, hesitancy

Table 24.6 Medical conditions predisposing to GI cancers

Cancer	Predisposing medical condition
Colorectal	Ulcerative colitis, Crohn's disease
Oesophageal	Barrett's oesophagus, coeliac disease, GORD
Stomach	Pernicious anaemia

Lung cancer

The one tumour group that may present as the primary diagnosis in the clinical exam. *Look for the thoracotomy scar!* So often missed as it may be subtle and well-hidden posterolaterally, its presence suggests a previous pneumonectomy or lobectomy and puts lung cancer right at the top of your differential. With the deal pretty much in the bag, you can then go on to confidently elicit any associated signs such as clubbing, cachexia, nicotine staining, Horner's syndrome, radiotherapy tattoos, and cervical lymphadenopathy. Ask about lifestyle factors that ↑ the risk of cancer (alcohol and smoking). More information is available for breast examination and prostate examination.

Final quick tips

Bear in mind that patients with cancer, a chronic process, can present late and may result in exudative effusions which can be massive before symptoms present, since there has been time to compensate (e.g. pleural effusion, ascites, etc.). Don't let this throw you. Finally, just remember, 'cancer' can be a highly emotive word and you should always take care to maintain sensitivity when presenting in front of patients in the clinical exam. *'Mitotic lesion'* or *'neoplasm'* are acceptable alternatives.

Ophthalmology

Ophthalmology: overview

Ophthalmology is the speciality concerned with diseases of the eye, the visual pathways of the CNS, ocular movements, and the adnexae (eyelids and orbits). It is a highly practical speciality with microsurgery, laser interventions, and minor operations forming a significant proportion of the workload. Patients of every demographic are seen from premature babies with retinopathy of prematurity to the very elderly with age-related macular degeneration (AMD) and glaucoma. The eye casualty offers the richest environment for learning about acute ophthalmic presentations (red eye/visual loss). Aim to spend at least two or three sessions here if possible. (See Fig. 25.1 and Fig. 25.2 for anatomy.)

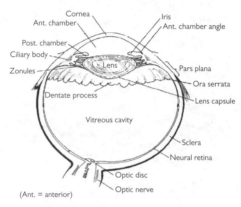

(Ant. = anterior)

Fig. 25.1 Anatomy of the eye. Reproduced with permission from Dodson, Paul, *Diabetic Retinopathy: Screening to Treatment* 2008, Oxford University Press.

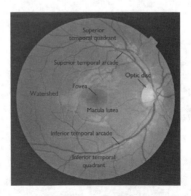

Fig. 25.2 Anatomy of the fundus. Reproduced with permission from Dodson, Paul, *Diabetic Retinopathy: Screening to Treatment* 2008, Oxford University Press.

Cases to see

Acute eye disease

Eye casualty offers many opportunities to see examples of acute ophthalmology such as trauma, chemical injuries, orbital cellulitis, corneal foreign bodies, microbial keratitis, acute iritis, acute glaucoma, retinal vascular disease, optic neuropathies (ischaemic/demyelinating), ocular motility disorders (compressive and microvascular cranial nerve disorders), and central causes of visual loss (migraines, TIAs, stroke, CNS tumours, etc.). Ensure you gain experience in distinguishing causes of red eye and visual loss on clinical assessment.

Chronic eye disease

The following four disorders form the majority of the ophthalmic outpatient workload. Try to gain an appreciation of how referrals are made, patients are assessed, treatments are delivered (including the timescales of urgency in each case), and progress assessed.

Age-related macular degeneration

AMD is the most common cause of blindness in the elderly. Dry (atrophic) AMD may require visual rehabilitation and risk of progression reduced with vitamin supplements and smoking cessation. Wet (exudative) AMD is treatable and involves regular visits for treatment with intravitreal injections and assessing response to therapy.

Cataract

Cataract is a common cause of reversible visual impairment. It is usually age related but accelerated by trauma, diabetes, and steroids.

Glaucoma

Glaucoma is a major cause of world blindness and remains asymptomatic until late. Intraocular pressure (IOP) is the major modifiable risk factor, lowered by drops or by surgery to prevent progressive, irreversible visual field loss.

Diabetic retinopathy

Diabetic retinopathy remains the commonest cause of blindness in the working population, either through complications of proliferative diabetic retinopathy (more common in type 1 DM), or diabetic macular oedema (more common in type 2 DM).

Procedures to see

Phacoemulsification cataract surgery

This is the most commonly performed operation by the NHS with >350,000 operations annually.

Laser procedures

YAG (yttrium aluminium garnet) capsulotomy is performed for patients with posterior capsular opacification (clouding of the lens capsule) as a late complication following cataract surgery (Fig. 25.3—note the clear central visual axis created by an opening produced by the YAG laser in the posterior capsule) and YAG peripheral iridotomy to create a small hole in the iris and break an attack of acute angle-closure glaucoma (see ➔ p. 503 and Fig. 25.5). Pan-retinal photocoagulation is used to treat patients with proliferative diabetic retinopathy (note the circular white/black laser scars which vary in appearance depending on laser uptake and interval following laser in

Fig. 25.4) and macular laser therapy may be used to treat macular oedema secondary to diabetes or retinal vein occlusion.

Trabeculectomy

This is an operation for patients with advanced or rapidly progressing glaucoma. The operation aims to create a communication between the anterior chamber and the subconjunctival space, to achieve long-term control of IOP without the need for drops.

Vitrectomy

Vitrectomy is an operation commonly performed for retinal detachment in which the vitreous gel is removed, the retina is flattened, and the retinal break is sealed.

Strabismus surgery

Squint surgery involves adjusting the length and insertion of the extraocular muscles in children to improve binocular visual development and treat amblyopia, and in adults to alleviate diplopia and improve cosmesis. It often requires a GA.

Intravitreal injections

These are commonly required to deliver biologic drugs (commonly against vascular endothelial growth factor (VEGF)) into the vitreous cavity for the treatment of wet (exudative) macular degeneration, retinal vein occlusion, or diabetic macular oedema. Antibiotics and anti-inflammatory agents can also be delivered by this route.

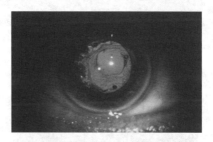

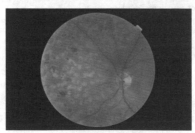

Figs 25.3 and 25.4 Ocular appearance following different forms of laser treatment. Photos courtesy of Mr. Martin Leyland.

Ophthalmology: in eye casualty

Red eye

Red eye is one of the most common acute presenting complaints in ophthalmology. Careful clinical assessment (history and examination) will identify the cause and appropriate management strategy.

- Unilateral red eyes with pain and visual loss require urgent ophthalmic referral suggesting potentially sight-threatening pathology
- Bilateral red eyes without pain and unaffected vision may be treated in the community

Acute angle-closure glaucoma

This is an *ophthalmic emergency*, an acute severe rise in IOP results from obstruction of the drainage angle of the eye.

Symptoms

Include unilateral severe pain/headache, nausea/vomiting, haloes, and reduced vision (secondary to corneal oedema) and may be provoked by poor light environments/prone posture.

Signs

An ovoid, mid-dilated pupil may be observed (ischaemic iris; Fig. 25.5). IOP may be 60–80 mmHg (normal IOP <21 mmHg). Bimanual palpation of an eye through a closed eyelid will reveal a unilateral hard eye.

Treatment

Intensive topical antihypertensive drops, topical steroids, pilocarpine to open the drainage angle, and systemic acetazolamide (Diamox®).

'ABC & Ps'

Management options include *a*lpha agonists (apraclonidine), *b*eta antagonists (timolol), *c*arbonic anhydrase inhibitors (oral acetazolamide or topical dorzolamide), *p*arasympathomimetics (e.g. cholinergic agents like pilocarpine), and *p*rostaglandin analogues (latanoprost). Once IOP is reduced, corneal oedema should resolve and clear the view for YAG iridotomy laser to be performed. This is the definitive treatment which must be performed on both eyes to prevent contralateral angle-closure glaucoma. The anterior segment appearance following laser iridotomy is shown in Fig. 25.5.

Risk factors

Age, female sex, hypermetropia, and those of Central or South-East Asian origin.

Bacterial keratitis

Bacterial keratitis in contact lens wearers necessitates urgent treatment to prevent corneal ulceration, which may → corneal perforation in extreme cases. Always ask about contact lens use in any patient with a (usually unilateral) red eye.

Symptoms

Include pain and photophobia, and vision may be reduced if the infection results in axial corneal opacity or secondary inflammation.

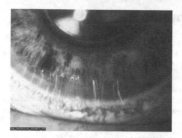

Fig. 25.5 The appearance of a laser peripheral iridotomy opening following acute angle-closure glaucoma. Image courtesy of Mr. Imran Yusuf.

Signs

Note the corneal infiltrate (opacity) typical of bacterial keratitis (Fig. 25.6), and the advanced corneal ulcer with large central ring infiltrate, corneal thinning, and hypopyon seen in advanced bacterial keratitis with a very inflamed eye (Fig. 25.7).

Management

May require a diagnostic corneal scrape before treatment with broad-spectrum topical antibiotics. Quinolones (ofloxacin) are typically used to cover *Pseudomonas* spp., an important cause of contact lens-related keratitis; chloramphenicol has no action against this organism and should not be used. Treatment is typically hourly drops for 48 hours, tailored according to clinical response and microbiology Gram stain/sensitivities.

Anterior uveitis (iritis)

Anterior uveitis commonly causes recurrent red eye, pain, photophobia, and reduced vision in susceptible patients.

Signs

The pupil may be irregular due to iris adhesions (Fig. 25.9) with appearance of an irregularly shaped pupil and a hypopyon (fluid level of sterile pus in the anterior chamber: Fig. 25.8) may be visible. White blood cells can be visualized directly with the slit lamp, IOP is measured and dilated fundoscopy performed to exclude posterior uveitis.

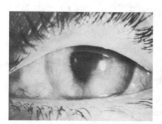
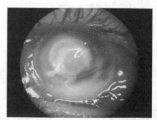

Figs 25.6 and 25.7 Examples of the clinical appearance of microbial keratitis Photos courtesy of Mr. Martin Leyland.

Genetics

The HLA-B27 haplotype (typical of seronegative spondyloarthropathies) predisposes to recurrent iritis which is often more severe.

Systemic associations

With sarcoid, IBD, etc. may be excluded by serum assays and imaging (CXR) if iritis is recurrent, bilateral, or severe.

Treatment

Is with frequent topical steroid drops, tailored over 4–6 weeks depending on severity. Topical steroids, in any context, must not be used for >4 weeks without monitoring by an ophthalmologist: secondary glaucoma or herpes simplex keratitis may progress undetected and cause permanent visual loss. Posterior uveitis (TB, syphilis, toxoplasmosis, etc.) is often sight-threatening and may require vitreous sampling, oral or intravitreal treatments, and a more aggressive diagnostic workup.

Endophthalmitis

This is the most devastating complication of any intraocular procedure (cataract surgery, trabeculectomy, vitrectomy, intravitreal injection, etc.).

Postoperative infective endophthalmitis

Results from bacterial entry into the eye, commonly *Staphylococcus. epidermidis, Staph. aureus*, and *Streptococcus* spp.

Endogenous endophthalmitis

Describes haematogenous seeding of bacterial/fungal/protozoal infection into the eye often in immunosuppressed patients. Treatment is of the underlying cause, but a careful search for a systemic focus may be required (blood culture, echocardiography, etc.) as directed by history, examination, and suspected causative organism.

Presentation

Is typically with red eye, grossly reduced vision, relative afferent pupillary defect (RAPD), and hypopyon visible in the anterior chamber, with vitritis.

Management

Urgent diagnostic sampling of vitreous ± anterior chamber fluid is required with intravitreal injection of antibiotics (commonly ceftazidime and vancomycin), topical steroids, antibiotics and dilating drops, with oral antibiotics (typically quinolones), sometimes with use of oral steroids after 24 hours.

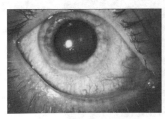 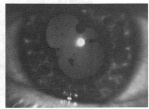

Figs 25.8 and 25.9 Clinical appearance of anterior uveitis with hypopyon (left) and posterior synechiae (right). Photos courtesy of Mr. Martin Leyland.

Early vitrectomy is advised if vision or light perception or worse to remove pus/cytokine soup from the vitreous cavity.

Scleritis

Scleritis causes unilateral red eye with deep pain (like toothache) which may wake the patient up at night.

Examination

Reveals injection of deep scleral vessels, and may reveal scleral thinning with appearance of darker hue due to exposure of underlying choroid. Scleritis is vasculitis of the sclera and systemic vasculitides are associated (e.g. RA, polyarteritis nodosa, granulomatosis with polyangiitis (formerly known as Wegener's granulomatosis) must be excluded with serum assays.

Management

Topical steroids and oral NSAIDs are required; rarely scleral thinning and perforation may occur. Referral to a rheumatologist is advised for treatment of the underlying systemic disorder.

Ulcerative keratitis

This may also cause red eye in patients with connective tissue diseases. Corneal perforation may occur if inappropriately managed.

Conjunctivitis

Conjunctivitis may be allergic, bacterial, viral (commonly adenovirus), or have another cause. Enquire about recent history of URTI or affected contacts—adenoviral conjunctivitis is highly contagious. Although this may present unilaterally, typically the second eye may become affected 2–3 days later (Fig. 25.10). Dryness/grittiness is typical and it is usually a self-limiting condition. The treatment is symptomatic (regular lubricants). Photophobia suggests secondary keratitis, which requires topical steroids. Bacterial conjunctivitis is more purulent and commonly unilateral.

Ophthalmia neonatorum

Describes conjunctivitis within the first week of life and is an emergency: corneal scarring may result. *Chlamydia* and gonococcal conjunctivitis may affect teenagers/young adults who are sexually active; specific treatment and genitourinary medicine referrals are mandatory. *Allergic conjunctivitis*: commonly causes bilateral itching with red eyes with chemosis (conjunctival oedema),

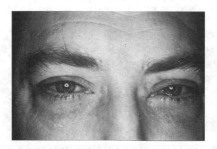

Fig. 25.10 Bilateral viral conjunctivitis. Photo courtesy of Mr. Martin Leyland.

typically in atopic patients (history of asthma, eczema, etc.) and may be seasonal. Follicles are often demonstrated on the tarsal conjunctiva. Eversion of upper lid may reveal flat-topped lesions—papillae—a sign of severe allergy. Any corneal involvement is sight-threatening and requires topical steroids. Topical and oral antihistamines/mast cell stabilizers are often sufficient.

Dry eye/blepharitis

Evaporative dry eye is very common and may result in mild conjunctival hyperaemia. It occurs due to blockage of Meibomian glands, with secondary reduced lipid content within the tear film and consequent rapid tear film evaporation. Gritty/burning eyes are the presenting symptoms.

A Meibomian cyst (chalazion) may occur intermittently secondary to viscous Meibomian gland secretions blocking the Meibomian ducts.

Examination

May reveal crusting around the base of the eyelashes, and fluorescein examination may reveal multiple, tiny epithelial erosions secondary to rapid evaporation of the tear film.

Treatment

Is regular lubricants and lid hygiene to unblock the Meibomian gland ducts and encourage physiological secretions to restore the composition of the tear film.

Subconjunctival haemorrhage

Is a typically unilateral, harmless collection of blood under the conjunctiva.

Presentation

It appears uniformly red (Fig. 25.11), and may cause mild ocular discomfort if large.

Risks

If spontaneous, BP measurement is required to exclude systemic arterial hypertension. Patients on anticoagulant and antiplatelet therapies are also at higher risk. Topical lubricants are often sufficient to alleviate discomfort if present. Traumatic subconjunctival haemorrhages require a complete examination to exclude associated ocular injuries (hyphaema, orbital blowout fracture, etc.).

Visual loss

The visual system is best considered from the tear film anteriorly to the primary visual cortex posteriorly with cornea, anterior chamber, lens, vitreous, retina, optic nerve, optic chiasm, and optic radiations between them. Pathology of *any* aetiology (infection, inflammation, neoplasia, etc.) affecting *any* of these structures can result in acute visual loss. Keep your differential appropriately broad, and use information from history and examination and knowledge of the visual pathways to determine the structure(s) affected and the underlying pathology.

Painless, unilateral visual loss

Determine whether visual loss is unilateral or bilateral, painful or painless.

Central retinal artery occlusion

Causes a dramatic, unilateral, painless, severe loss of vision due to retinal infarction.

Examination

Visual acuity is often reduced to counting fingers or worse with a dense RAPD. Retinal examination reveals retinal pallor and a 'cherry red spot'

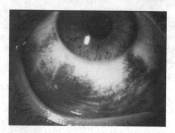

Fig. 25.11 Subconjunctival haemorrhage. Photo courtesy of Mr. Martin Leyland.

at the macula due to an intact choroidal circulation. A Hollenhorst plaque (cholesterol embolus) may be demonstrated in a proximal vessel secondary to rupture of atheromatous plaque from the ipsilateral carotid artery. A branch retinal artery occlusion occurs when only a branch of the retinal artery is occluded, with retinal pallor/oedema visible in the distribution of the occluded retinal arteriole manifesting as partial visual field loss.

Management

Acute treatment (<6 hours after the onset of symptoms) may involve dislodging the embolus (with drops, ocular massage, hyperventilation, etc.) into a smaller arteriole. Irreversible visual loss is the rule, which may be altitudinal if the embolus affects only a branch retinal artery rather than the central retinal artery.

Risk factors

Contributory systemic cardiovascular risk factors must be addressed: TIA clinic referral and carotid Dopplers/echocardiogram are required.

Associations

Giant cell arteritis must be excluded with ESR/CRP if >50 years of age. Amaurosis fugax describes transient monocular visual loss, and is considered a TIA variant affecting the central retinal artery.

Central retinal vein occlusion

Results in acute-onset unilateral visual loss, although vision may be relatively preserved in comparison to central retinal artery occlusion. A RAPD may be present.

Risk factors

Include atherosclerosis (retinal vein is compressed by a rigid adjacent retinal artery), or hypercoagulable states (myeloma, Waldenström's macroglobulinaemia, dehydration, etc.)—recall Virchow's triad.

Fundoscopy

Reveals retinal haemorrhages in all quadrants (if central) or sectoral (if branch of retinal vein only), with cotton wool spots and optic disc swelling. Visual loss is due to macular oedema and/or retinal ischaemia.

Treatment

Involves addressing cardiovascular risk factors, reducing IOP with topical drops if elevated. Retinal laser is required if new vessels are present

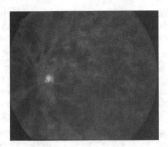

Fig. 25.12 Typical appearance in central retinal vein occlusion. Photo courtesy of Mr. Imran Yusuf.

or there is retinal ischaemia. Macular oedema may be treated with laser, intravitreal steroid, or anti-VEGF injections.

Anterior ischaemic optic neuropathy

Is usually non-vasculitic (i.e. caused by atherosclerosis rather than temporal arteritis). Typically occurs over the age of 55 with males and females being equally affected.

Signs

A RAPD is often present, and colour vision lost proportionally to visual acuity. Optic disc swelling with haemorrhages are often present acutely. Visual field defects may be altitudinal (respecting horizontal meridian).

Treatment

Is to exclude temporal arteritis by performing ESR/CRP as clinically indicated, control modifiable vascular risk factors (BP, cholesterol, blood glucose, etc.), and exclude contributory hypotensive drugs. Steroids may provide some benefit, although evidence is not conclusive. Disc swelling typically lasts 6–12 weeks, followed by optic atrophy. There is a significant risk of fellow eye involvement.

Vitreous haemorrhage

Causes sudden severe loss of vision in patients with new blood vessel formation (neovascularization) that occurs most commonly in patients with proliferative diabetic retinopathy or following ischaemic central retinal vein occlusion. New vessels grow into the vitreous from the retina and bleed, causing recurrent vitreous haemorrhage. The red reflex is lost when attempting fundoscopy. Retinal detachment may coexist and B-scan US is important to exclude this.

Management

Often involves waiting for the haemorrhage to clear before undertaking pan-retinal photocoagulation laser. A non-clearing vitreous haemorrhage (>3 months) may necessitate vitrectomy to restore a clear ocular media. Acutely, the most important step is to exclude a retinal detachment.

Macular haemorrhage

Bleeding or exudate from a choroidal neovascular membrane is the cause of acute visual loss in patients with wet (exudative) AMD which presents with acute central visual loss and distortion. The fovea is relatively avascular;

however, haemorrhage in front of the macula (premacular haemorrhage) may occur due to bleeding from a retinal vessel during the Valsalva manoeuvre when central venous pressure (and → retinal venous pressure) is acutely elevated.

Retinal detachment (RD)

Presentation
Is with 'flashing lights' (vitreoretinal traction) and 'floaters' (vitreous haemorrhage), which often do not occur in the above-mentioned disorders. Visual field loss (often described as a dark curtain) may exist.

Signs
Reduced visual acuity suggests that the macula has detached (poorer prognosis: Fig. 25.13), although acuity is spared in macula-on detachment.

Posterior vitreous detachment
Occurs in every healthy eye, typically between 40 and 60 years of age as the vitreous liquefies but may occur earlier in myopes (short-sighted patients). Posterior vitreous detachment does not cause significant visual loss but may create a retinal break in ~5% of patients; progressive recruitment of fluid in the subretinal space (via the break) causes retinal detachment. A localized break is treated with laser photocoagulation to prevent retinal detachment; therefore, all patients with flashes and floaters should undergo retinal examination.

Management
Urgent (same or next day) vitrectomy in macula-on cases and within a week for macula-off cases. Other forms of retinal detachment include tractional retinal detachment in diabetic patients, or exudative retinal detachment due to inflammatory or malignant disorders of the choroid/retina.

Painless, bilateral visual loss

Cerebrovascular disease
May present exclusively with visual field loss (particularly posterior circulation strokes which may result in occipital infarction, affecting the primary visual cortex). Middle cerebral artery strokes (anterior circulation) will likely cause sensory/motor deficits. Confrontation visual fields are therefore mandatory in the assessment of patients with visual loss.

Transient ischaemic attack
May present with transient visual loss (typically lasting <1 hour) and may be associated with systemic symptoms (motor deficits) depending on the affected

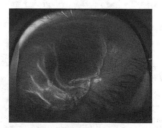

Fig. 25.13 Macula-off retinal detachment. Photo courtesy of Mr. Imran Yusuf.

cerebral artery. Management of TIAs may include neuroimaging (CT/MRI depending on timing of presentation), TIA referral for cardiovascular risk factor assessment, ECG/echocardiography, and carotid Dopplers. Remember that posterior circulation strokes stem from vertebrobasilar artery insufficiency so carotid Dopplers may therefore not identify the responsible pathology.

Migraine

Commonly presents with visual aura produced secondary to CNS vasospasm resulting in 15–30 min of evolving, bilateral scotomas which typically enlarge before disappearing. Scintillations (zigzags), flashing lights, and other 'positive' visual symptoms may exist. In classical migraine, a headache follows secondary to sequential CNS vasodilatation. This is not invariable and acephalgic migraines describe those without headache. Differentiating migraine from TIA relies on a careful history.

Painful visual loss

Painful visual loss associated with a red eye (acute angle-closure glaucoma, microbial keratitis, iritis, etc.).

Giant cell arteritis causing anterior ischaemic optic neuropathy

Is an important disease in that it is treatable, yet failure to do so can result in irreversible visual loss. Large vessel vasculitis of the short posterior ciliary arteries causes infarction of the optic nerve.

Symptoms

It affects patients aged >50 with symptoms including temporal headache, scalp tenderness, jaw claudication, systemic upset (weight loss, night sweats, etc.) Visual symptoms may be present: it can present as anterior ischaemic optic neuropathy (most common, with disc swelling and haemorrhages), central retinal artery occlusion, or rarely, isolated sixth nerve palsy. Management is urgent with high-dose systemic steroids. Raised inflammatory markers (ESR/CRP) are typical. Temporal artery biopsy is diagnostic to support long-term steroid use, although it is not 100% sensitive due to 'skip lesions'. Temporal artery ultrasound may prevent the need for biopsy.

Optic neuritis

Occurs secondary to demyelination typically affecting young females, often unilaterally.

Symptoms

Include central scotoma, pain on eye movements, and signs include reduced visual acuity, RAPD, and reduced red saturations or colour vision.

Examination

Fundoscopy reveals disc swelling in ~20%, although 80% have demyelination behind the optic nerve head (retrobulbar neuritis) and therefore have a normal funduscopic appearance.

Investigation

Gadolinium-enhanced MRI can demonstrate lesions separated in space and time and therefore can be diagnostic of MS (McDonald criteria, 2010) in the setting of an acute isolated demyelinating episode.

Management

Disease-modifying drugs (alemtuzumab, natalizumab) may prevent disability if started early. Referral to neurology is therefore considered appropriate.

Ophthalmology: in clinic

Cataract

Cataract describes opacity of the crystalline lens. It is associated with ↑age, but may form earlier in patients with diabetes, steroid use, associated syndromes (such as myotonic dystrophy), radiation, or patients with a history of skin disease. *Baby checks must include an examination of red reflexes:* loss of the red reflex suggests either congenital cataract or retinoblastoma, which if missed may result in blindness or death, respectively.

Symptoms

Include reduced vision and glare (particularly with posterior subcapsular cataract). Patients are often referred from optometrists through their GP.

Clinical assessment

Is required to confirm that cataract is the principal cause of visual loss (Fig. 25.14), particularly to check that the disc and macula are healthy.

Management

Most patients undergo phacoemulsification surgery under local anaesthetic. Sedation/GA may be required in some cases (head tremor, poor patient cooperation). To select the appropriate intraocular lens (IOL) implant power, corneal measurements and axial length of the eye are taken to plan the refractive outcome.

Postoperatively

Patients are typically seen at 2 weeks with measurement of visual acuity and refractive error. Only one eye operation is performed in most cases on a single day due to the risk of endophthalmitis (contaminated drugs/instruments would otherwise affect both eyes).

Glaucoma

Glaucoma is a major cause of irreversible blindness worldwide. It describes a group of diseases whose endpoint is damage to the optic nerve with loss of retinal ganglion cells, progressive visual field constriction, and blindness. The central acuity is preserved until late and consequently, most forms of glaucoma are asymptomatic until significant field loss is present.

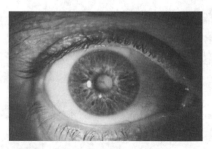

Fig. 25.14 A significant cataract in the right eye of a patient. Photo courtesy of Mr. Martin Leyland.

Clinical assessment

Includes a history (including family history of glaucoma), risk factors (trauma, steroid use, vasospasm such as migraine/Raynaud's phenomenon), measurement of IOP, assessment of optic disc appearance, and automated visual field testing (perimetry), increasingly supplemented with optic nerve imaging studies (e.g. optical coherence tomography of optic disc).

Fundoscopy

Optic discs demonstrate progressive optic disc cupping in glaucoma (the cup—a depression in the centre of the optic disc—becomes deeper and wider; Fig. 25.15). The neuroretinal rim becomes progressively thinner with irreversible loss of retinal ganglion cells and consequent visual field loss. Patients with raised IOP but no visual field loss and normal appearing optic discs have 'ocular hypertension': they are at ↑risk of glaucoma and require monitoring.

Intraocular pressure

Is the major modifiable risk factor in patients with glaucoma, and treatment is aimed to reduce the IOP to a level at which no further visual field loss occurs. Normal IOP is <21 mmHg (measured by tonometry), but target IOP may need to be kept lower in glaucoma as every mmHg drop in IOP confers a protective effect.

Management

Topical drops are often used initially, but laser treatments (trabeculoplasty) and surgical procedures (trabeculectomy) to ↑ outflow of aqueous may be required if medical treatment is not adequate.

> **Top tip**
>
> Glaucoma clinics are an excellent setting for practising direct ophthalmoscopy. Examine optic discs through undilated pupils if possible; try to draw the optic disc (practise interpretation) and compare it with the ophthalmologist's drawing.

Age-related macular degeneration

AMD is the leading cause of blindness in the retired population. Central visual loss occurs, with preservation of the peripheral visual field, even in advanced AMD.

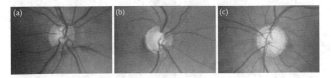

Fig. 25.15 Progressive cupping of the optic nerve in glaucoma. Photos courtesy of Mr. John Salmon.

Dry (atrophic) AMD

Describes the accumulation of drusen at the macula and atrophy of the retina (Fig. 25.16). Treatment is with high-dose vitamins (lutein/zeaxanthin) if drusen are large, and visual rehabilitation with magnifiers/lights to assist in reading and activities of daily living.

Wet AMD

Is the result of leakage from the choroidal neovascular membrane that forms under the macula. Leakage of fluid (blood/exudate) results in distortion and loss of vision (Fig. 25.17). Amsler's charts are provided to patients with dry AMD to identify new distortion that may herald the onset of wet AMD, and prompt timely referral for investigation/treatment.

> #### Honours
>
> *Treatment of wet age-related macular degeneration*
> Intravitreal injection of biologic drugs that inactivate VEGF are effective treatments in wet AMD, reducing leakage and stabilizing/improving vision. Drugs used include Lucentis® (ranibizumab), Eylea® (aflibercept), and rarely Avastin® (bevacizumab). The CATT and IVAN studies proved non inferiority of Avastin® compared with Lucentis® with no statistically significant differences in serious adverse events. However, Lucentis® and Eylea® are licensed in AMD, and are often used. Eylea® requires less frequent dosing and may be cost-effective due to reduced hospital visits for each patient.

Diabetic eye disease

Is the most common cause of blindness in the working population. It is asymptomatic until advanced; annual screening for diabetic patients >12 years of age is provided by the NHS with screening photographs. Patients with visually threatening changes are referred to the eye clinic.

Diabetic retinopathy

Is graded as background (dot/blot haemorrhages, exudates), pre-proliferative (cotton wool spots/venous changes), or proliferative diabetic retinopathy (new blood vessels on the retina, optic disc, or iris; see Fig. 25.18). New vessels result in vitreous haemorrhage, tractional retinal detachment, or rubeosis iridis (new vessels occlude the drainage angle causing raised IOP).

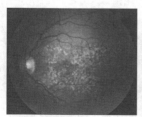 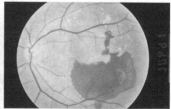

Figs 25.16 and 25.17 Typical appearance of dry (left) and wet (right) AMD. Photos courtesy of Mr. Imran Yusuf.

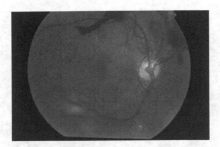

Fig. 25.18 Proliferative diabetic retinopathy with pre-retinal haemorrhages and neovascularization of the optic disc head. Photo courtesy of Mr. Imran Yusuf.

Background diabetic retinopathy

Multiple dot (small microaneurysms), and blot haemorrhages (large with indistinct edges). Blot haemorrhages are indicative of ischaemia if multiple and are a poorer prognostic sign (Fig. 25.19).

Proliferative diabetic retinopathy

Neovascularization in diabetic retinopathy occurs due to retinal ischaemia secondary to microvascular disease. This is demonstrated in the fluorescein angiogram: dark regions represent ischaemia (capillary non-perfusion) with enhancing (hyperfluorescent) areas representing leakage from adjacent new, pathological blood vessels. New vessels may also proliferate at the optic disc with collections of pre-retinal blood visible (see Fig. 25.18).

Pan-retinal photocoagulation is required in these patients to reduce production of VEGF from the ischaemic retina which may result in regression of new vessels.

Diabetic maculopathy

Characterized by haemorrhages or exudates at the macula (Fig. 25.20) causing chronic visual loss. Any pathology at the macula must be referred promptly as visual loss occurs early. Visual acuity is partly a function of macula integrity. Any pathology affecting the macula affects visual acuity early. Diabetic macular oedema typically affects type 2 diabetics, and results in chronic visual loss. Signs include exudates at the macula, and haemorrhages (Fig. 25.20). Microvascular non-perfusion (ischaemic maculopathy) may occur, demonstrated on the fluorescein angiogram with capillary non-perfusion (hypofluorescence) at the fovea. The patient in Fig. 25.20 can be expected to have reduced visual acuity.

Treatment

Treatment of diabetic eye disease must address systemic risk factors (blood glucose, BP, cholesterol, smoking, weight). Management of proliferative diabetic retinopathy is pan-retinal photocoagulation laser which aims to reduce the oxygen demand from an ischaemic peripheral retina at the expense of visual field loss. Treatment is titrated (new blood vessels regress leaving fibrous tissue behind) to reduce loss of visual field which may threaten driving vision. Patients not responding despite laser coverage may require

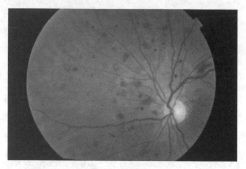

Fig. 25.19 Severe background diabetic retinopathy with multiple blot haemorrhages visible in a single quadrant. Photo courtesy of Mr. Imran Yusuf.

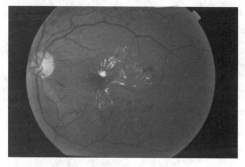

Fig. 25.20 Macula exudates in diabetic maculopathy. Photo courtesy of Mr. Imran Yusuf.

vitrectomy which removes existing VEGF by removing the vitreous in which it is contained although ongoing ischaemia may produce VEGF thereafter. Vitrectomy also removes the scaffold for new vessels. Patients with macula oedema may benefit from macula laser (avoiding the perifovea), or anti-VEGF agents/steroids if oedema is recalcitrant.

Honours

Glycaemic control on progression of diabetic retinopathy

The Diabetes Control and Complications Trial (DCCT) was a landmark longitudinal study identifying that intensive glycaemic control (HbA1c <6%) in diabetic patients was associated with a huge reduction in risk of diabetic retinopathy, nephropathy, and neuropathy over the 6-year study period. BP should be limited to 130/80 mmHg in diabetic patients, and 125/75 mmHg if microalbuminuria coexists.

Ophthalmology: investigations

Digital photographs

These are excellent for photo documentation of retinal or optic nerve pathology, for assessing response to treatment or identifying disease progression, or for medicolegal purposes such as documentation of retinal haemorrhages in abusive head trauma (non-accidental injury). Wide-field retinal imaging (with documentation of the retinal periphery) is now possible through an undilated pupil (Optomap®). Handheld retinal cameras are available for infants and supine/anaesthetized patients (RetCam®). In addition to optic nerve and retinal photographs, digital photography is used in oculoplastic surgery to document lid position, eyelid lesions, and evaluating the success of surgical intervention.

Optical coherence tomography

Optical coherence tomography provides rapid, non-invasive images using infra-red light to acquire cross-sectional images of the macula for assessment of wet AMD or macular oedema (in which fluid/exudate appears as focal cysts or subretinal fluid secondary to diabetic maculopathy, retinal vein occlusion, or following cataract surgery). Degenerative changes can be seen in dry AMD. It is now widely used in ophthalmology and an integral part of care in AMD.

Ocular ultrasound

B-scan US is useful to rule out retinal detachment in the presence of media opacity (dense cataract or vitreous haemorrhage), to measure the depth of choroidal naevi/melanomas, or to demonstrate fluid in posterior scleritis. Anterior segment US can delineate the configuration of the drainage angle.

Fundus fluorescein angiography

Fluorescein angiography is useful in the diagnosis and management of retinal vascular disease such as AMD, proliferative diabetic retinopathy (to highlight new vessels and ischaemic retina amenable to laser), wet AMD, retinal vein or artery occlusion, or where diagnostic uncertainty exists. Fluorescein is injected intravenously, passing progressively through the retinal arterial tree, capillaries, and venous system. Shellfish allergy is a contraindication; anaphylaxis is rare otherwise.

Ophthalmology: in theatre

During your ophthalmology placement, you may have the opportunity to attend an ophthalmic theatre list. There are >350,000 cataract operations performed in the UK annually and you should aim to observe two or three phacoemulsification and IOL procedures.

Phacoemulsification and IOL insertion

Phacoemulsification describes emulsification of the crystalline lens with US energy through a small incision through which the residual lens matter is aspirated. It is commonly performed with local anaesthetic (topical only (anaesthetic drops), under Tenon's capsule (subTenon)), although sedation/ GA is sometimes used.

Iodine is used to clean the periocular skin and sterilize the ocular surface, and a sterile drape is applied to remove the eyelashes from the surgical field. Typically, two or three small clear corneal incisions (bloodless) are used for bimanual manipulation within the eye (main corneal incision: Fig. 25.21a). A circular hole is fashioned in the lens capsule (capsulorrhexis: Fig. 25.21b) to allow access to the lens, which is dissected from the capsule with saline (hydrodissection). The phacoemulsification probe is introduced into the eye, and the nucleus is typically divided into four before aspirating each in turn (Fig. 25.21c). Soft lens matter is aspirated with smaller probes, before the capsular bag is filled with viscoelastic and the IOL is commonly injected through a small wound and placed within the capsular bag (Fig. 25.21d). Intracameral (into the anterior chamber) cefuroxime has reduced the incidence of postoperative endophthalmitis (bacterial infection of the eye) sevenfold. Wounds are hydrated rather than sutured in most cases. Patients are given topical steroids and antibiotics to prevent postoperative infection and inflammation.

Trivia

The invention of modern phacoemulsification cataract surgery

Charles Kelman (1930–2004) considered that US energy used by dentists to clean teeth could be used to emulsify a cataract and remove it through small wounds. Cataract had traditionally been removed whole which requires large wounds and a long rehabilitation period, and results in significant astigmatism. He pioneered modern phacoemulsification surgery, in which the lens is divided within the eye and emulsified using a probe manipulated in the eye through a small incision of ~2 mm. This has permitted more predictable refractive outcomes and cataract surgery to be performed as an outpatient procedure. Over 100 million individuals have benefitted from phacoemulsification cataract surgery worldwide to date.

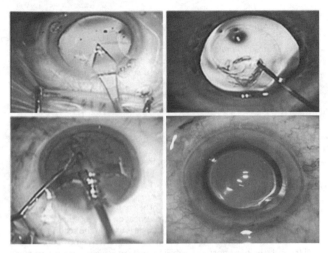

Fig. 25.21 Intraoperative appearances during phacoemulsification cataract surgery. Photos courtesy of Mr. Imran Yusuf.

To ask the boss

Intraocular lens choice

An IOL is implanted following removal of the cataract to replace the focusing contribution of the lens to the eye. The lens power predicted to produce distance vision (emmetropia) is calculated by measuring the corneal curvature and axial length. Some patients may be kept myopic for unaided reading vision if they are used to this. More than 6000 IOLs have been designed, differing in material, shape, and where in the eye it may be safely implanted. The first IOL was made from PMMA, as it was observed that shattered PMMA plastic from airplane windshields did not excite an inflammatory reaction in the eyes of affected pilots. Most commonly, an IOL is implanted in the capsular bag once the cataract within it has been removed.

Trabeculectomy

Trabeculectomy describes the surgical fashioning of a communication between the anterior chamber and the subconjunctival space to permit an accessory pathway for aqueous humour to drain from the eye. This is created superior to the cornea, under the upper eyelid. It commonly reduces IOP to 10–15 mmHg without the need for topical drops, and may last for decades. In young patients, scarring can close the surgical communication and the procedure may be augmented with mitomycin C to eliminate subconjunctival fibroblasts which mediate fibrosis.

A diamond knife is used to fashion a scleral flap once the conjunctiva is dissected. The anterior chamber is then entered; a punch is used to remove a small piece of sclera from the base of the flap. A peripheral iridectomy (seen as a triangular defect in the iris; Fig. 25.22) is performed to prevent the iris from occluding drainage before the scleral flap is sutured back and conjunctiva sutured to prevent leakage (and passage of infection into the eye). A drainage bleb of conjunctiva is formed under the upper eyelid where it is hidden (Fig. 25.22). Intensive topical steroids are used for 3 months postoperatively to reduce the likelihood of scar formation. There is a risk of high or low pressure in the immediate postoperative period which needs to be closely observed and managed appropriately.

Vitrectomy

Vitrectomy entails surgical removal of the vitreous gel in order to gain access to the retina to peel membranes (for treatment of macular hole and epiretinal membranes), remove traction (retinal detachment), and clear ocular media (non-clearing vitreous haemorrhage). A surgical lens is mounted onto the operating microscope to permit a direct view of the retina. Surgical ports (typically three) are created in the pars plana 3.5–4 mm behind the limbus (junction of cornea and sclera) to safely enter the eye without damaging the lens or retina. Irrigation is secured to one port to maintain the pressure of the eye. A light pipe is used in the second port, and the vitrector (a guillotine with a high cut rate) is used to remove the vitreous gel through the third port. Dyes may be used to visualize fine retinal membranes to facilitate their removal. Laser and cryotherapy may be used to secure retinal breaks. Heavy gases may be used to create an endotamponade, taking several weeks to absorb. Silicone oil creates a stable long-term tamponade but may cause raised IOP. Vitrectomy ↑ the risk of cataracts.

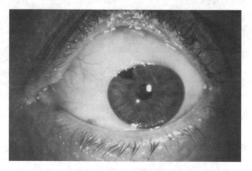

Fig. 25.22 The appearance of the eye following trabeculectomy surgery demonstrating a peripheral iridectomy and shallow bleb superiorly. Photo courtesy of Mr. John Salmon.

We wish to thank *Mr John F. Salmon*, Consultant Ophthalmologist at the Oxford Eye Hospital for being the senior reader for this chapter and for providing some of the presented images; *Mr Martin Leyland*, Consultant Ophthalmologist at the Royal Berkshire Hospital, Reading, for kindly providing many anterior segment photographs; and medical students *Daniel Fitzgerald* and *Stuart Faragher* for their valued feedback.

Paediatrics

Paediatrics: overview

Welcome to one of the toughest but also one of the most rewarding specialties there is! The range is mindboggling: from the ventilated, 500 g premature baby on the neonatal unit to the 11-year-old who weighs considerably more than you do and who is attending clinic for childhood obesity (and full marks if you thought of the Barker hypothesis and the '*thrifty phenotype*' to link the two cases[1]).

Considered the last general hospital specialty, paediatrics has become increasingly specialized as a greater number of children with multisystem disorders survive into adulthood. In the age of the Internet, parents are better informed, demands on paediatric services are rising, while healthcare staff, from primary to tertiary settings, are having to adapt to ever greater patient complexity. The UK is getting better at looking after children, having pulled itself up from last place on the UNICEF league table for child health in developed countries in 2001 to 16th (out of 29 countries) by 2013.[2] We are also the advocate for child health globally since many are working towards the UN's Sustainable Development Goal 3 ('by 2030, end preventable deaths of newborns and children aged <5 years, with all countries aiming to reduce ... under-5 mortality to at least as low as 25/1,000 live births') (℠ http://www.un.org/sustainabledevelopment).

You cannot possibly do the whole of paediatrics in a 4–6-week rotation but you will get a pretty good idea if you recognize opportunities. Leap at the chance to take histories and examine children and thereby learn to communicate with them and their families—good communication is *the foundation of paediatrics*. Take a deep breath, and jump in!

Emergency department and the ward

Anything and Everything (A&E) will come through the door. This is your chance to observe a full-blown resuscitation, take the first history of a breathless child (?asthma ?DKA, ?foreign body inhalation, ?metabolic, ?anaemia, ?pneumonia) and learn not only how to manage a fractured femur but how to negotiate the thorny path of non-accidental injury (NAI) that it could be associated with. Try to follow-up children you have seen in the ED who have been admitted to the ward to appreciate the outcomes of management. Also, find out about play specialists, clowns, and hospital schools on the ward.

Neonatal unit

The hi-tech end of paediatrics most readily available to you. Here you can get to learn about management of premature babies, ventilation, jaundice, hypoglycaemia, and infection.

Clinics

Learn about the management of bread-and-butter paediatrics: constipation, asthma, primary nocturnal enuresis (bed-wetting), and poor growth. Most 'general' paediatricians now have their own specialty clinics and these are good opportunities to see how chronic conditions such as diabetes and epilepsy are managed. Specialist paediatricians will also hold clinics as satellites of tertiary centres, looking after children with conditions such as cystic fibrosis and leukaemia and where you will get to see Hickmann lines, portacaths, and percutaneous endoscopic gastrostomy tubes.

Honours

Top tips

Make friends with the nursing staff and do not get under their feet. They know the children and families better than the medics and will help you find a good time to take a history or examine a child. You will also learn a huge amount from specialist nursing staff in the neonatal intensive care unit or at their own specialist asthma/epilepsy/diabetes/enuresis/constipation clinics. Also, try and get to morning handover. This is where you will hear how cases are presented and where our bosses comment on the management and to hear how child protection cases are managed. And winter—'cough! cough!'—is better than summer for seeing acute paediatrics.

Community paediatrics

A different pace but this is where you will learn child development rather than trying to memorize lots of milestones. You will get time to take histories and examine children with cerebral palsy (and see what a vast array of different presentations there are for this unsatisfactory catch-all term), Duchenne's muscular dystrophy and other neuromuscular disorders, watch children being assessed for autism spectrum disorder, learn about looked-after children, and see children with Down's syndrome at their routine follow-up. This is the specialty par excellence of MDT collaboration, where you will see the magic of physiotherapy, occupational therapy, speech and language therapy, and community nursing.

A career in paediatrics

If you are thinking about a career as a paediatrician, try and choose a set of jobs which includes some paediatric experience. There is a useful overview on paediatric careers on the Royal College of Paediatrics and Child Health website (℘ www.rcpch.ac.uk/careers). And talk to paediatricians, both trainees and consultants—they are an approachable bunch and will give you excellent advice. Good luck!

References

1. Hales CN, Barker DJ (2013). Type 2 (non-insulin-dependent) diabetes mellitus: the thrifty phenotype hypothesis. *Diabetologia* 35(7):595–601.
2. UNICEF Office of Research (2013). *Child Well-Being in Rich Countries: A Comparative Overview.* Innocenti Report Card 11. Florence: UNICEF Office of Research.

Paediatrics: neonates

Neonatal units vary from basic, level-one special care baby units (SCBUs), where the little ones are mostly *'feeding and growing'*, to tertiary-level neonatal intensive care units (NICUs). Neonatologists can be found on the maternity wing as they also attend high risk deliveries (to be on hand to resuscitate the baby if necessary) and trouble-shooting minor problems on the postnatal ward.

Neonatal resuscitation

A small percentage of babies at both high-risk deliveries (e.g. existing maternal medical condition, instrumental delivery, meconium, multiple births) and at low-risk ones take a bit of time *'to get going'* (i.e. the baby has to quickly clear her lungs of fluid), sending the circulation a different way while trying to cope with a sudden fall in temperature and nutrients. The majority of babies who are given a bit of gentle stimulation by being wrapped and quickly dried do fine and should be handed straight to mum for skin-to-skin care. A baby with a hearty cry at delivery is a happy baby! Some babies need help to oxygenate their lungs and this is when paediatricians step in. They assess the baby's tone, colour, breathing, and HR, which will go towards the Apgar score (see Table 26.1). Based on this, paediatricians follow the newborn life support protocol with inflation breaths to oxygenate the lungs. Often, gentle stimulation and airway manoeuvres are sufficient for the baby to adapt to extrauterine life.

Honours

If the fetus is hypoxic, its oxygen-starved brain will stop breathing and the baby enters primary apnoea. The HR slows down, anaerobic metabolism takes over, and the baby becomes acidotic. Some babies almost certainly resuscitate themselves as primal reflexes take over and cause the baby to gasp every 10–12 sec. If this fails to reverse the hypoxia, the baby enters secondary apnoea after approximately 20 min, the acidosis worsens, and the heart stops beating. However, even at this late stage, timely resuscitation with bag-mask ventilation can reverse this process. The first sign of improvement is usually an ↑HR.

Skin-to-skin care is evidenced based: 'The intervention appears to benefit breastfeeding outcomes, and cardio-respiratory stability and decrease infant crying, and has no apparent short- or long-term negative effects.'[1]

Prematurity

Babies born at 23 weeks' gestation are resuscitated at some tertiary units. Remember, the main block to pushing back the age at which premature babies can be resuscitated is lung immaturity. Most babies <28 weeks are given surfactant (via ETT direct to the lungs) to help overcome surface tension and expand the lungs. There is a move away from prolonged intubation of premature babies (less barotrauma). Along with immature lungs, premature babies can have problems with their eyes (retinopathy of prematurity), brains (intraventricular haemorrhage), gut (necrotizing enterocolitis), and infection. Ask the neonatal nurses to take you on a tour of an incubator.

Table 26.1 Apgar score out of 10, with scores made at 1, 5, and 10 min of life

Sign	0	1	2
Heart rate	Absent	<100	>100
Respiratory rate	Absent	Weak, irregular	Good, crying
Muscle tone	Flaccid	Arms and legs flexed	Well flexed
Reflex irritability	No response	Grimace	Cough/sneeze
Skin colour	Blue, pale	Hands and feet blue	Completely pink

Honours

Survival in premature babies

The EPICure studies, 1 and 2 (♒ www.epicure.ac.uk), looked at survival of neonates born between 22 and 26 weeks' gestation (extremely preterm) in the UK. EPICure 2 in 2006 found the number of premature babies admitted to neonatal units had ↑ by 44% compared to EPICure 1 in 1996. Survival improved, with 53% of babies born at 24–25 weeks surviving to discharge (40% in 1996). Developmental outcomes also improved but the study showed that 66% of surviving extremely premature babies have developmental problems.

Jittery babies

Nursing staff have noted the baby is '*jittery*', or shaking. Your main differentials are hypoglycaemia, hypocalcaemia, seizure (?hypoxic ischaemic encephalopathy), normal Moro reflex. Babies have less glycogen stores and it takes little to drop their sugars—hypothermia, poor feeding. After ABC, 'Don't Ever Forget Glucose'.

Feeding problems

WHO recommends exclusive breastfeeding for the first 6 months of life which is at 1% in the UK (♒ www.unicef.org.uk). Breast milk protects against infections (borrowing the mother's immunoglobulins), eczema, and obesity later in life. Also associated with lower rates of breast and ovarian cancer in mothers. Watch the breastfeeding counsellor on the ward.

Jaundice

Many causes in newborns, the main cause being physiological (i.e. normal) in babies. All jaundice in babies <24 hours old is pathological until proven otherwise (main causes are infection and haemolysis secondary to ABO incompatibility). Jaundice is treated by careful feeding and phototherapy (blue light breaks down bilirubin, the product from old RBCs that causes jaundice). At high levels, bilirubin is neurotoxic and a few babies need an exchange transfusion, where twice the circulating blood volume is replaced.

Rashes

Learn to recognize the ominous-sounding but benign erythema toxicum in neonates. Also, milia, Mongolian blue spots (often mistaken as a bruise from NAI), and neonatal acne.

Baby checks

The *only* way to learn what is normal in babies. Learn how to perform these on the postnatal ward.

Procedures

You might get to see ...

Intubation

Becoming less common as less invasive ventilation (e.g. CPAP) is being used.

Lines

Newborns can have both a venous central line and arterial line (not so easy) placed through the umbilical cord (which normally has one vein and two arteries).

Cranial ultrasound

A view into the neonatal brain via the anterior fontanelle, used mainly as means of screening for and grading intraventricular haemorrhage, which has implications for subsequent development.

Reference

1. Moore ER, Anderson GC, Bergman N, et al. (2012). Early skin-to-skin contact for mothers and their healthy newborn infants. *Cochrane Database Syst Rev* 5:CD003519.

Paediatrics: in the emergency department and on the ward

Over 3 million children attended the ED in 2006–2007. This ↑ to 4.5 million attendances in 2010–2011 (accounting for 25–30% of all ED attendances).[1] As more children with complex needs survive, EDs are having to cope with more than coughs, colds, bumps, and bruises. Only a fraction get admitted. In recognition of this, paediatric emergency medicine is now a subspeciality in its own right, with its own training programme. The atmosphere can be challenging when crowds of children and their anxious parents are waiting to be seen. But this is the best place to see and hear pathology and learn how acutely ill children are managed, from a simple cold to a cardiac arrest. Follow children you have seen who have been admitted to the ward (also a good place to clerk patients and be pointed to good signs)—paediatricians quite often do not have a firm diagnosis until they have observed, tried a bit of this and that, and had test results back. Also, some hospitals have regular resuscitation scenario training—ask if you can watch.

Be helpful—answer telephones, look for X-ray forms, etc. and the frontline medics will take time to go over your histories and watch you examine. And watch the experienced paediatric ED nurses at work, who have a sixth sense when it comes to spotting the sick child (check out ♒ www.spottingthesickchild.com). A very useful set of paediatric ED guidelines from the Royal Children's Hospital, Melbourne, is available at ♒ www.rch.org.au/clinicalguide. Also, have fun—you will make a scared kid having their head glued a lot happier if you are prepared to sing 'Incey, wincey spider' along with mum.

'All grown-ups were once children—although few of them remember it.'
The Little Prince, Antoine de Saint Exupery

The following list covers common paediatric medical presentations, in descending order for the top five, according to a recent study from the busy Nottingham ED[2] (37% of all paediatric attendances—the rest were injuries). *Always have a wide differential diagnoses!*

Difficulty in breathing (20.1%)

With the return to school in September, wheezing season starts. Is it asthma (reversible bronchoconstriction)? Viral-induced wheeze in a pre-schooler? Bronchiolitis (in the under ones)? You may come across different and sometimes conflicting management advice, evidence that we have still got a lot to learn about wheeze in children. However, this is your best chance to see respiratory distress: *count the respiratory rate* and listen to the whistles, wheezes, snap, crackle, and pop of the paediatric chest. Get to know your hospital guidelines for bronchiolitis and the British Thoracic Society's asthma guideline for children (♒ www. brit-thoracic.org.uk/). Children get pneumonia too so do not forget to ask about fever. Look at lots of CXRs—is that right upper lobe focal consolidation in a toddler actually a bit of normal thymus? And learn from the nurses how to give inhalers via a spacer—a core skill (and tricky with a grumpy 2-year-old).

To ask the boss

Steroids for wheeze?
To give steroids or not to give steroids for pre-school wheeze? The move is away from steroids for the under-fives with wheeze.[3]

Fever (14.1%)

Paediatricians wish they had a quick, reliable test to sort out the child with a mild viral infection from the one with a life-threatening bacterial infection (rarer, thanks to immunization). When seeing a child with fever, find a focus. Best to see and examine the child once she has had paracetamol. Full history, including immunizations, foreign travel (have they returned from an area endemic for malaria, dengue, or Ebola?), infectious contacts. A 2-month-old child with fever (or hypothermia) will usually earn themselves a full septic screen—bloods (including culture), urine dip, CXR, and LP. Always examine the ears and throat, except if you suspect upper airway obstruction (i.e. croup, epiglottitis). Think about joint infections. Is the fontanelle bulging? Full exposure for rashes. And remember the differential: this could be a rheumatological or oncological presentation. Many children perk up after some paracetamol but the skill is in spotting the child with a serious infection or who is about to crash with overwhelming sepsis before it happens. See NICE's traffic light system for identifying serious illness in children (🖱 www.nice.org.uk/nicemedia/pdf/CG47QuickRefGuide.pdf). Also, know your country's vaccination schedule (🖱 www.mvec.vic.edu.au/immunisation-references/vaccine-schedule-by-country).

Diarrhoea and vomiting (14%)

The majority of children can be managed with oral rehydration salts and in rich-country settings, with dilute apple juice.[4] Important to take a good

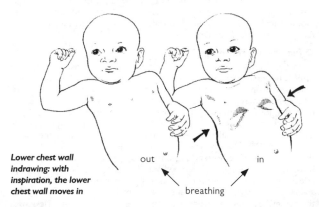

Lower chest wall indrawing: with inspiration, the lower chest wall moves in

out   in

breathing

Fig. 26.1 Signs of respiratory distress—chest wall indrawing. Reproduced with permission from *Pocket Book of Hospital Care for Children* 2e, WHO 2013, p87.

history (do not forget tropical travel) and perform a thorough examination as young children often vomit for a variety of different reasons and blood in the stool might be IBD—again, a wide differential. Many children start to drink when approached with a NG tube.

Honours

Rotavirus vaccine

A live, attenuated, oral vaccine against rotavirus, the commonest culprit for D&V, has been introduced for babies at 2 and 3 months of age. The vaccine has saved many lives in the developing world and its success has seen norovirus take over as the main cause of D&V in the US. Contraindicated in babies >3 months because of the very small association with intussusception in older children.

Rash (8.6%)

There is much anxiety around rashes because of meningococcal septicaemia, decreasing in the UK thanks to vaccination. But all children who are unwell with fever need full exposure to look for the tell-tale non-blanching petechial or purpuric rash. Dermatology atlases do help but by seeing rashes you can build up your own mental atlas so you can confidently differentiate them.

Cough (6.7%)

Viral URTI? Croup ('Doctor, she barks like a seal!'—know about your hospital's croup score)? Or is there a history of a toddler playing with his older sibling's Lego and a concomitant choking episode (inhaled foreign body)? Or a child with fever, night sweats, weight loss, and several courses of antibiotics (TB—ask families about TB contacts and know how to recognize a BCG scar)? Know how to examine ears and throat (and when *not* to examine the throat, e.g. croup, or in the toxic-looking child with possible epiglottitis—has the child had all his vaccinations, including HiB?)

Other common presentations

Crying baby

Surgical emergency? Sepsis? Reflux? Cow's milk protein intolerance? Colic? Are the parents coping? Crying is the commonest trigger for physical abuse in infancy.

Headache

Viral illness? Too much screen time? Meningitis? Brain tumour? Bullied at school? Migraine (check for a family history)? A wide differential, a detailed history, and thorough examination are essential in evaluating headache in children.

Self-harm

About 10% of children between the ages of 13–17 years presenting to the Nottingham ED attended with self-harm. You might not clerk a child presenting with self-harm but listen out for how they were managed in handover, particularly the importance of medical care (overdose? cutting?), psychiatric management, and child protection.

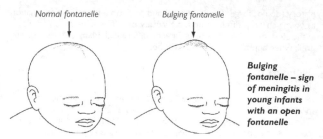

Fig. 26.2 Bulging fontanelle in infant with meningitis. Reproduced with permission from *Pocket Book of Hospital Care for Children* 2e, WHO 2013 p56.

Abdominal pain/vomiting

Similar approach to headache, both organic and functional (again, ask about family history of migraines). As for adults, a wide differential but also think about the lower lobe pneumonia or otitis media (mesenteric lymphadenitis, a diagnosis of exclusion) masquerading as tummy pain. Remember surgical causes—?appendicitis, which does not always present classically with RIF pain and can present with a limp—and to ask about bilious vomiting (?obstruction—intussusception, malrotation volvulus, incarcerated inguinal hernia).

Safeguarding (child protection)

The on-call registrar usually sees children with safeguarding concerns under the main categories of NAI, neglect, emotional abuse, or sexual abuse. Safeguarding is an important part of the paediatric surgical sieve (has the baby in resuscitation collapsed from sepsis, a cardiac anomaly, a metabolic problem, or has he been shaken by his parents?). Useful resources are the modules for level 1 and 2 safeguarding at ℘ www.e-lfh.org.uk/programmes/safeguarding-children/. Think of medical causes in suspicious presentations, such as osteogenesis imperfecta ('brittle bones') and bleeding disorders (e.g. haemophilia). Always ask whether the patient is known to the child protection registry or social services, even if it was in the past.

Trauma, including head injury

About half of most ED attendances are injuries. Broken bones are usually managed by the ED doctors or orthopaedics but head injuries, especially moderate to severe injury requiring urgent CT and neurosurgical referral, are usually managed first by paediatrics. Major trauma is usually managed by a paediatric major trauma centre. Be aware of children's growth when viewing plain films—the developing epiphysis can look like fractures to the uninitiated! A common presentation and evolving surgical orthopaedic emergency is supracondylar fracture of the distal humerus. The ossification centres of the elbow are outlined in Table 26.2.

Table 26.2 Ossification centres of the elbow

	Ossification centre	Age of fusion (years)
C	Capitellum	1
R	Radial head	4
I	Internal (medial) epicondyle	6
T	Trochlea	8
O	Olecranon	10
L	Lateral epicondyle	12

Top tip

More tips on paediatric elbow radiology can be found at ℬ www.
radiologymasterclass.co.uk/tutorials/musculoskeletal/x-ray_trauma_
upper_limb/elbow_fracture_x-ray.html.

Acute limp: golden rules

Limping in children is usually of benign origin (eg irritable hip) but more
serious diagnoses (eg septic arthritis) need to be ruled out. It is a common
exam case too so be mindful of the following:
- Beware labelling a limp traumatic. History of trauma may be
  coincidental and unrelated. Patients discharged with a diagnosis of
  trauma should be told to expect improvement in their symptoms and
  advised to seek help if their symptoms worsen or fail to settle.
- Remember referred pain. In any child with knee or thigh pain an
  underlying hip condition should be considered.
- Consider NAI or you may miss an at-risk child.
- Do not be falsely reassured by normal plain radiographs. Changes of
  osteomyelitis may not be evident for 7–10 days.

History

Age, fever, constitutional symptoms, pain worse on waking and eases with
activity (i.e. rheumatological diagnosis), nocturnal pain, rest pain, history of
trauma and mechanism of injury, weight-bearing status, and family history
(of rheumatological, haematological, or neuromuscular disorder).

Examination

Temperature, gait/weight bearing/position of limb at rest, examine the
joint and compare to the opposite side and examine a joint above and
below, focused neurological examination, and examine spine.

Investigations

FBC, CRP, ESR, sickle cell screen, blood cultures if pyrexia, X-ray, US in joint
effusions, urine dipstick (e.g. Henoch–Schönlein purpura, SLE, appendicitis,
salpingitis), and stool sample if diarrhoea (*Salmonella* and *Yersinia*).

Table 26.3 Kocher scoring

Score	Likelihood of septic arthritis
0	0.2%
1	3%
2	40%
3	93%
4	99%

Kocher criteria (differentiating transient synovitis from septic arthritis)

1. History of fever >38.5°C.
2. Non-weight bearing.
3. ESR >40 mm/hour.
4. White blood cell count >12 × 10^9/L.

Differentials

- Developmental dysplasia of the hip
- Trauma (eg toddler's fracture)
- Infection (septic arthritis, osteomyelitis)
- Neoplasia
- Irritable hip
- Perthes, Slipped Upper Femoral Epiphysis

References

1. Royal College of Paediatrics and Child Health (2012). *Standards for Children and Young People in Emergency Care Settings*. London: RCPCH.
2. Sands R, Shanmugavadivel D, Stephenson T, et al. (2012). Medical problems presenting to paediatric emergency departments: 10 years on. *Emerg Med J* 29(5):379–82.
3. Panickar J, Lakhanpaul M, Lambert PC, et al. Oral prednisolone for preschool children with acute virus-induced wheezing. *N Engl J Med* 360(4):329–38.
4. Freedman SB, Willan AR, Boutis K, et al. (2016). Effect of dilute apple juice and preferred fluids vs electrolyte maintenance solution on treatment failure among children with mild gastroenteritis: a randomized clinical trial. *JAMA* 315(18):1966–74.

Paediatrics: in clinic

Choose clinics with a learning objective and try and get time to clerk the patients yourself. Clinic is the place to get a good idea of how chronic illnesses affect children and their families. Clinic is also where you will get to meet the MDT—specialist nurses, dietitians, physios, etc.

Obesity

One-third of British 10–11-year-olds are obese or overweight and the WHO sees childhood obesity as a major public health problem. These children are ↑risk of type 2 DM, asthma, MSk problems, CVD, and mental health problems (bullying, low self-esteem). See ℬ www.hekint.org/life-at-the-table.html for a reflection on the Mediterranean diet and Weiss et al.[1]

Poor growth

At the other end of the spectrum is 'weight faltering' (the term which has replaced 'failure to thrive'), where there are concerns about a child's growth (in the under fives). The majority of growth problems are caused by inadequate calorie intake but the differential diagnosis is wide. In older children, common concerns are delayed puberty. This is where to learn about plotting weight, height and head circumference on a growth chart (you must know how to do this!), estimating adult height by calculating mid-parental heights, and knowing about Tanner charts and orchidometers for staging puberty.

Constipation

Be familiar with macrogols (the mainstay of treatment for both disimpaction and maintenance treatment) and do not forget the psychosocial side—one candidate failed a history taking station in the Royal College of Paediatrics and Child Health membership exam for missing that the child's soiling from overflow diarrhoea had forced the child to move schools because of bullying.

Allergies

Where demand vastly outweighs supply of paediatric allergists. Learn how to use an adrenaline (epinephrine) auto-injector for anaphylaxis and observe skin-prick testing. See ℬ www.itchysneezywheezy.co.uk.

Cardiorespiratory

Learn about the management of more complex asthma and cystic fibrosis (a multisystem disorder). A chance to see lung function testing in older children. The paediatric cardiology clinic is a gold mine for murmurs.

Diabetes mellitus

Type 1 DM is commonest in children but type 2 is increasing. This is a chronic disease which becomes particularly challenging during the teenage years. Learn how very young children give their own insulin injections, cope with complex insulin pumps, and where delivery of care is delivered by a specialist paediatric diabetes team 24/7.

Reference

1. Weiss R, Dziura J, Burgert TS, et al. (2004). Obesity and metabolic syndrome in children and adolescents. N Engl J Med 350(23):2362–74.

Paediatrics: in the community

Paediatrics for children outside hospital. It is important to contact the community paediatricians early in a placement and provide a wish-list as space can be limited and clinics often take place in schools (much of the community paediatrician's role is to help integrate children into the school system). Check with your paediatric educational supervisor as some medical schools allocate specific weeks in the community during your attachment. This is also a great opportunity to see physiotherapists, occupational therapists, speech and language therapists, and audiologists at work.

Developmental delay

A wide differential, including cerebral palsy, neuro-, genetic, and metabolic diagnoses. Your main aim should be to have a systematic approach to evaluating the main areas of childhood development: gross motor ('*When did he start walking?*'), fine motor and vision ('*How does he hold a crayon?*'), speech and hearing ('*When did he start babbling?*'), and social ('*Does he play with other children?*').

Down's syndrome

Children with Down's syndrome have MDT follow-up for medical problems (at greater risk of cardiac/GI/cervical spine/thyroid problems, and leukaemia), for monitoring and help with development, vision, and hearing (glue ear). See the Down's Syndrome Medical Interest Group website (⊕ www.dsmig.org.uk). Children with Down's syndrome have specific growth charts.

Autism spectrum disorder

A disorder of social interaction and communication and known as 'autistic spectrum disorder' as there is great variation in how children are affected (it now incorporates Asperger's syndrome). There is no blood test or scan to make the diagnosis, which is made on a thorough history taken from both parents and teaching staff and on careful observation of the child, usually by community paediatricians and speech and language therapists.

Honours

Measles, mumps, and rubella (MMR)
Know about the MMR vaccine controversy, where a now widely debunked piece of research linking the MMR vaccine to autism led to low uptake and the resurgence of measles in the UK. Research shows overwhelmingly no link between MMR and autism.[1]

Red book

The Personal Child Health Record (also known as the PCHR or 'red book') is a national standard main record of a child's health and development including vaccinations. There is also an online version. Always ask the patient's parents to present the red book to obtain a collateral history of treatment and development to date.

Table 26.4 UK vaccination schedules

Timing	Vaccination	Dose
8 weeks	• 6-in-1 (single jab) against: diphtheria, tetanus, pertussis, polio, Hib, hepatitis B	1
	• PCV + rotavirus + Men B vaccines	1
12 weeks	• 6-in-1 + rotavirus vaccines	2
	• 6-in-1 vaccines	3
	• PCV + Men B vaccines	2
1 year	• Hib	4
	• PCV + Men B vaccines	3
	• Men C + MMR vaccine (single jab)	1
2–8 years	• Children's flu vaccine	Annual
3 years, 4 months	• MMR vaccine	2
	• 4-in-1 pre-school booster against: diphtheria, tetanus, pertussis and polio	1
12–13 years (girls)	• HPV vaccine (against cervical cancer)—2 injections given 6–12 months apart	1–2
14 years	• 3-in-1 teenage booster against: diphtheria, tetanus, polio	1
	• Men ACWY vaccine against: meningitis A, C, W and Y	1

Men, meningococcal; PCV, pneumococcal conjugate vaccine.

Growth charts

See Fig. 26.3. This one shows inadequate calorie intake but growth charts can gives important pointers for a wide range of pathologies in children, from poor weight gain secondary to an undetected cardiac problem to an abnormally large head circumference pointing to hydrocephalus. Know how to plot and interpret these.

Congenital heart disease (CHD)

Is common, with 0.8% of live births affected. Genetic (such as Noonan syndrome), chromosomal (such as trisomy 21 and DiGeorge syndrome), and environmental influences (such as lithium or maternal diabetes) are described but most cases (>80%) are sporadic with no identifiable cause CHD is only diagnosed in 40–50% of infants by 1 week of age, ↑ to 50–60% by 1 month of age. You should know the basic changes to the fetal circulation at birth and common lesions.[2]

Fetal circulation

In utero, oxygenated blood from the placenta bypasses the lungs by flowing from the right atrium through the foramen ovale to the left atrium and out through the aorta or directly from the pulmonary artery to the aorta via a patent (open) ductus arteriosus. At birth, the baby's first breaths see a drop in pulmonary vasculature resistance, ↑ pressure in the left atrium, which in turn closes the foramen ovale. At the same time the increase in

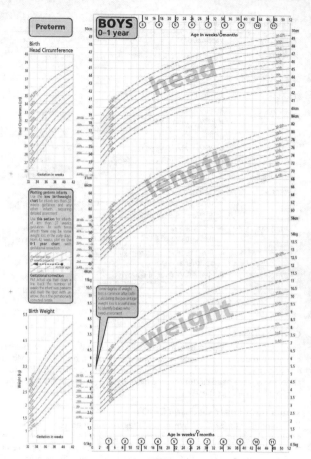

Fig. 26.3 Growth chart. Reproduced with permission from Royal College of Paediatric and Child Health, © DH Copyright 2009.

blood oxygen alongside lowering of prostaglandin levels (with the placenta removed from the circulation) causes the ductus arteriosus to close. Both the closure of the foramen ovale and the ductus arteriosus ensure blood flows through the lungs before being entering the systemic circulation. (See Fig. 26.4.)

Knowledge of the fetal circulation will help you understand treatment of the collapsed neonate with a cardiac cause. *IV prostaglandins* up to ~1

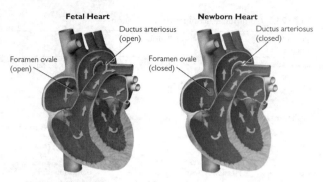

Fig. 26.4 Fetal versus newborn heart. Image reproduced from Wikimedia Commons, released free of copyright.

week of age help to keep the ductus open, allowing for a temporary mixed circulation until definitive treatment of a duct-dependent lesion. Likewise, balloon atrial septostomy to widen a hole in the foramen ovale will allow oxygenated and deoxygenated circulations to mix for a neonate born with transposition of the great arteries.

Neonates can present with
- a murmur
- collapse
- cyanosis
- tachypnoea
- absent femoral pulses
- gallop rhythm, enlarged liver, and wet lungs of heart failure.

Be watchful for more subtle signs
- Poor feeding, sweating when feeding.
- Poor weight gain (CHD uses up lots of calories → poor growth).
- Tachycardia (?heart failure, ?SVT, myocarditis).

Chest pain and faints
In older children are common presentations and are often benign (e.g. a MSk problem). However, you must take a cardiac history, with questions on exercise tolerance, family history of CHD, and a perinatal history (is the mother diabetic?). An ECG should be performed for a child with a murmur, an unexplained tachycardia (?SVT, ?myocarditis), and for a child who has fainted or had a first seizure, to rule out long QT syndrome (a cause of sudden cardiac death due to mutations in cardiac Na^+/K^+ channels and screened for on ECG by calculating the corrected QT interval).

Cardiac examination
- Growth chart.
- From the end of the bed: pale, cyanotic, anaemic, breathless, sternotomy/drain scars, dysmorphic features (e.g. Down's syndrome).

Table 26.5 Common heart murmurs by location

Site of loudest volume	Timing	Radiation	Pathology
Apex	Pansystolic	To axilla	Ventricular septal defect (VSD)
Lower left sternal edge	Early systolic	Does not radiate	Innocent murmur
Pulmonary area	Pansystolic Ejection systolic	To the back	Patent ductus arteriosus (PDA); atrioventricular septal defect (AVSD); pulmonary stenosis
Aortic area	Ejection systolic	To carotid arteries/back	Coarctation of the aorta; aortic stenosis

- Hands: clubbing, splinter haemorrhages.
- BP: cuff should cover >two-thirds of the upper arm and measurements compared to age-specific charts.
- Chest palpation: situs inversus (e.g. heart on right side—in OSCEs so always examine for the apex beat, and whether displaced, on both sides of the chest), thrills/heaves.
- Auscultation: murmur (see Table 26.5),[3] including timing with pulse, where loudest and grade of murmur (1 = very quiet, 2 = quiet, 3 = easily heard, 4 = loud with thrill, 5 = very loud with thrill but still need stethoscope, 6 = heard without stethoscope).
- Oedema: pulmonary, peripheral, hepatomegaly

Cardiac investigations
- Pre- and postductal oxygen saturations. Oxygen saturations must be <85% to spot visually. Some centres screen newborns for low saturations but a national screening programme is absent. A difference in saturations measured on the right hand—preductal—and on a foot—postductal—can give a clue to pathology (e.g. higher pre-ductal sats in aortic coarctation/interruption/hypoplastic left heart syndrome/critical aortic stenosis and higher post-ductal sats in transposition of the great arteries with either PPHN or coarctation).
- Blood gas in unwell children (raised lactate).
- Cardiac catheter (spend time in cath lab to understand anatomy).
- CXR—heart size, lung fields—oligaemic with ↓pulmonary blood flow (tetralogy of Fallot), congested (total anomalous pulmonary venous drainage).
- FBC, U&E, Ca^{2+}, and Mg^{2+}
- ECG
- Echocardiogram
- Cardiac MRI.

Congenital lesions

Is the lesion *cyanotic* (i.e. right-to-left shunt meaning some/all the blood bypasses the lungs)? Remember the *5 Ts*:

Transposition of the great arteries

Aorta arises from right ventricle, pulmonary artery from left ventricle, with neonates dependent on PDA and balloon atrial septostomy until switch procedure (3–5%). The condition is not compatible with life. See Fig. 26.5.

Truncus arteriosus

Single arterial 'trunk' overrides both ventricles and supplies pulmonary and systemic circulations, with VSD (1–2%).

Tricuspid valve anomalies

1–2%.

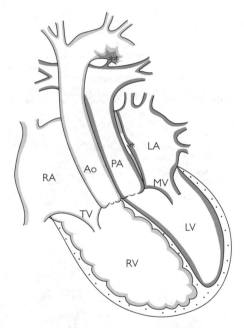

Fig. 26.5 Complete transposition of the great arteries. The pulmonary and systemic circulations are completely separate once the arterial duct and foramen ovale close. Ao, aorta; LA, left atrium; LV, left ventricle; MV, mitral valve; PA, pulmonary artery; RA right atrium; RV right ventricle; TV, tricuspid valve; *, patent arterial duct; **, patent foramen ovale. Reproduced with permission from Warrell, D.A. et al, *Oxford Textbook of Medicine*, 2010, Oxford University Press.

Total anomalous pulmonary venous drainage
Pulmonary veins do not drain into the left atrium but elsewhere (e.g. right atrium, 1–2%).

Tetralogy of Fallot
Pulmonary stenosis, over-riding aorta, VSD, right ventricular hypertrophy (5–7%). See Fig. 26.6.

Others
Prolonged pulmonary hypertension can reverse a left-to-right shunt, causing cyanosis (*Eisenmenger's syndrome*).

Acyanotic lesions
Left-to-right shunt with some blood 'looping' or bypassing the systemic circulation, with volume/pressure overload leading to heart failure.

Patent ductus arteriosus (PDA)
Ductus remains open, with left-to-right shunting that can cause heart failure (6–8%). See Fig. 26.6.

Coarctation of the aorta
Congenital narrowing of the aorta where the ductus arteriosus inserts (5–7%). The classic sign in newborns is absent femoral pulses confirmed by a >20 mmHg differential between the upper and lower limbs (hence the request for a '*four-limb BP*'). Neonates with coarctation present with collapse and shock from pressure overload when the ductus starts to close. See Fig. 26.6.

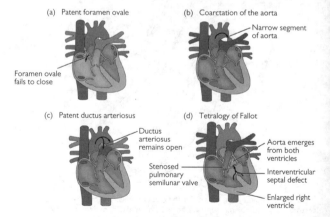

(a) Patent foramen ovale

Foramen ovale fails to close

(b) Coarctation of the aorta

Narrow segment of aorta

(c) Patent ductus arteriosus

Ductus arteriosus remains open

(d) Tetralogy of Fallot

Aorta emerges from both ventricles

Stenosed pulmonary semilunar valve

Interventricular septal defect

Enlarged right ventricle

Fig. 26.6 Congenital lesions. *Reproduced from Anatomy & Physiology*, Connexions Web site. http://cnx.org/content/col11496/1.6/, Jun 19, 2013. Creative Commons Attribution 3.0 Unported license.

Atrial septal defect (ASD)
Left-to-right shunt from blood flowing through defect in septal wall, from left atrium to right atrium (6–8%). See Fig. 26.7.

Ventricular septal defect (VSD)
Left-to-right shunt the commonest congenital heart lesion (30–35%). (See Fig. 26.8.) Around 30–35% of small defects in the ventricular septum close on their own by the second year of life. A small defect is more likely to have a louder murmur than a large defect. Residual higher atrial and pulmonary artery pressure in newborns mean large VSDs are often not picked up until 6 weeks of life when infants can present in heart failure from volume overload. These larger lesions are corrected surgically to treat heart failure and prevent pulmonary hypertension and resultant Eisenmenger's Syndrome.

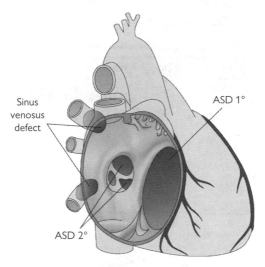

Fig. 26.7 Atrial septal defect (ASD) 1° denotes primum ASD; ASD 2° denotes secundum ASD. Reproduced with permission from Singh, A., Loscalzo, J., *The Brigham Intensive Review of Internal Medicine*, 2014, OUP.

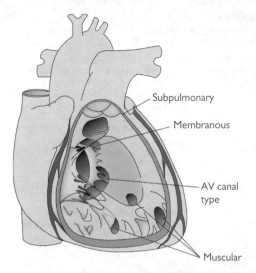

Fig. 26.8 Ventricular septal defects. AV, atrioventricular. Reproduced with permission from Singh, A., Loscalzo, J., *The Brigham Intensive Review of Internal Medicine*, 2014, OUP.

References

1. Madsen KM, Hviid A, Vestergaard M, et al. (2002). A population-based study of measles, mumps, and rubella vaccination and autism. *N Engl J Med* 347:1477–82.
2. Kliegman RM, Stanton BF, St Geme JW III, et al. (2016). *Nelson's Textbook of Pediatrics*, 20th ed. Philadelphia, PA:
3. Brugha R, Marlais M, Abrahamson E (2013). *Paediatric Clinical Examination*. London: JP Medical.

Paediatrics: in exams

The art—and the fun—of paediatrics is how to maintain a systematic approach when chaos reigns. Your examiners will look hard at your communication skills and your interactions with children and their families. Allowances will always be made if you are presented with a tired, grizzly child (unlikely), but it shows if you have not put in the time on the wards (see ➲ pp. 527–32). Paediatrics can be a vastly rewarding and fun speciality, but most students despite enjoying their rotations develop big anxieties when thinking about the exams. The key to success is to spend time developing skills in engaging and examining children of different ages and developing an appropriate approach to assessment. Clerk as many children as you can and you will become confident in the differences in history taking, examining children, and key conditions/presentations that may guide your further reading. You need to have an idea about growth charts, their likely development, and therefore how you might engage them during the OSCE—this will only really come by seeing lots of children.

Be prepared

Read the module handbook and the curriculum and their associated learning outcomes, which should give you a good idea of what the examiners are hoping to assess you on. Pay attention to the structure of the examinations and proportion of marks for each section. This information should be freely available and will help you to make the best preparation possible.

Some things are likely to be the same wherever you study
- There will be a written exam paper to test your overall knowledge of paediatrics (MCQ, EMQ, SBA, etc.)
- An OSCE-style practical examination, usually covering some or all the following elements:
  - A history taking station.
  - A counselling station.
  - One or more systems examination stations.
  - A child development station.
- Remember, the 'patients' might be real patients, actors, or children of staff.
- The exam will often focus on areas that are different from adult medicine. Good attention to growth, development, and safeguarding is crucial to success.

Top tip: NAI signs

TEN-4 bruising rule: Torso, Ears, Neck or bruising anywhere on a child <4 months old is a strong indicator of abuse. Other presentations can be found at ℬ www.fpnotebook.com/mobile/Prevent/Abuse/ChldAbs.htm. Learn to differentiate between a brief resolved unexplained event (BRUE) versus an apparent life-threatening event (ALTE).

OSCE stations

For most medical students, it is the OSCE-style examination in paediatrics that fills them with dread. The idea of being faced with a potentially screaming, spitting toddler or vomiting child is fairly terrifying, but the reality is usually very different. It will soon be evident if you have not seen that many children and this will ↑ your anxiety during the exam accordingly! How you interact with both the child and their parents is vastly more important than if you miss a few points during your examination. Remember, if the child is very upset or difficult to examine, allowances will be made. It is your approach that is important—observe how paediatricians deal with this on the wards and in clinic.

> **Top tips**
> * Communicate with both the child as well their parent(s). Try and introduce yourself to the child first, especially if they are >5 years of age.
> * *Be observant.* You can get vital marks before even touching the child— even more key in paediatrics.
> * *Use the parents.* E.g. positioning on their lap, pretend to listen to their chest before the child if needed
> * *Be flexible and adaptable.* Get auscultation in early on (if needed) and leave things that might upset the child until later.
> * *Get down on their level.* You can always tell a paediatrician by looking at the worn knees on their trousers!
> * *Tools to engage.* Notice the character on their top, a favourite toy, or what is on their socks and use this to try and engage them. Listen to their teddy's heart first!
> * *Growth.* Say you will plot the child's height and weight on a growth chart (and head circumference for infants).

Try not to get too bogged down with the complexity of some of the rarer paediatric conditions—these are not your specialist postgraduate paediatric exams. You need a good grounding in common paediatric conditions and an awareness of how key, rarer conditions (e.g. CHD), may present.

> **Honours**
> Do not just concentrate on the ins and outs of medical treatment. Emphasize the impact of illness on the whole family, development and growth, education, and psychosocial well-being of the child. This will score you much more marks than knowing the details of a particular treatment.

The OSCE examination station might be in any system and it is worth practising different systems examinations on the wards. Likely cases are going to involve patients with long-term, chronic conditions, as others are much more difficult to put into the exam.

Patients with conditions such as cystic fibrosis, cerebral palsy, CHD, and chronic liver disease are possible cases. One station that you are likely to get is *development*. Practise developmental examination by playing with children on the wards, in outpatients, and on relatives' and friends' children—wherever an opportunity arises. When doing the development station, see what the child is doing when you walk in and start with that area. Then try to examine development with some sort of structure, sticking broadly within each of the four developmental areas where possible (*gross motor, fine motor, speech and language, social*). Find the stage that they have achieved and one that they have not in order to find their level. Ensure you present their developmental age for each area of development.

Examination

The baby is fast asleep, explain that you are going to do the quiet bits first and, with great stealth, undo the baby's gown and listen to the heart sounds, observe and auscultate the chest, and gently palpate the abdomen and the femorals. Then fully expose to check for rashes, and gently assess tone—remember, a neurological examination in babies and toddlers is different to adults and older children.

Things you should practise beforehand

Know how to plot a growth chart and how to measure a head circumference. Know how to look up a drug and calculate a weight-based dose from the *BNFC*. Be able to perform a baby check.

History taking station

Use as much as possible the child's or parent's own words. When a mother tells you, '*When my baby was lying on my chest, I felt her heart going impossibly fast!*' you might not get the possible diagnosis, but someone in the paediatric team will immediately consider supraventricular tachycardia. Clerk lots of patients, if possible before the doctor and before reading the notes. Practise forming an impression and a plan of investigations and management. Use the parent's/child's own words and clarify points that you do not understand clearly. Practise questioning parents/children clearly; open questions, as well as more focused questions for clarification. Do not ask two questions in one go, as that is likely to lead to confusion.

Remember the importance of
• feeding and growth
• birth history and development
• family history, including consanguinity
• social history, including school/education, psychosocial concerns, and social worker involvement
• immunization status.

Counselling station

The counselling station is another potential way of examining your communication with children and parents and is potentially easier to organize for undergraduate staff such as using actors, doctors posing as parents, or real parents/children—there are many options! Verbal and non-verbal communication skills are both important, the latter forming much more of your communication with the child. Do not make things up if you do not know, admit your uncertainties and explain what you are going to do to clarify. Look for the underlying psychosocial concern, there is usually one there!

Possible topics might include
- explanations of common conditions or treatments, e.g. constipation, asthma (e.g. inhaler technique), and diabetes
- a medication error or mistake in treatment
- exploring why a teenager is not taking her antiepileptic medication.

The bonus here is that you can practise on your peers, as well as real families. Remember to make appropriate adjustments for development when counselling children, making explanations age appropriate.

MCQ exam

A MCQ exam in paediatrics is common to most medical school examinations and is one of the easiest ways for medical schools to assess your overall knowledge of paediatrics as a specialty. Many conditions, especially acute conditions or rare presentations, are difficult to examine via an OSCE-style exam.

Certain topics lend themselves to the MCQ style exam and it is worth considering the likely topics when revising. Common topics include the following:
- Conditions where there are clear diagnostic criteria (e.g. Kawasaki's disease and neurofibromatosis).
- Those areas more unique to paediatrics (e.g. vaccinations, syndromes, childhood cancers or CHD).
- Safeguarding will almost always feature somewhere in the paediatric MCQ paper—these questions can be more difficult, requiring a significant amount of judgement. See safeguarding cases on the ward or discussions at handover to get an idea of approach.

Useful texts

Avoid postgraduate door-stoppers. What you want is a good overview:
- Brugha R, Marlais M, Abrahamson E (2013). *Paediatric Clinical Examination*. London: JP Medical (excellent short guide to paediatric history and examination).
- South M, Isaacs D (2012). *Practical Paediatrics*, 7th ed. Edinburgh: Churchill Livingstone/Elsevier.
- WHO (2013). *Pocket Book of Hospital Care for Children*, 2nd ed. (℘ www.who.int/maternal_child_adolescent/documents/child_hospital_care/en/—essential reading for paediatric electives in developing countries—free to download.

Palliative medicine

Palliative medicine: overview

Palliative medicine is a medical speciality that aims to provide fully holistic care to those with life-limiting illness, throughout their time with that illness. The focus is on quality of life rather than simply its prolongation. This is achieved through excellent symptom control, for symptoms including pain, nausea, breathlessness, and many more; and extends to spiritual, social, and psychological care and care of the relatives of the patient too. Palliative medicine also provides individualized patient care at the end of life. The speciality was originally associated with cancer care, but in fact the specialty cares for anyone with a life-limiting illness regardless of underlying aetiology. All acute hospitals have palliative care teams, but the specialty is mainly based in the community providing both inpatient care in hospices and community services, allowing patients to be cared for at home if they choose.

The palliative care team

Palliative care teams are truly multidisciplinary. In a hospice, the MDT will often consist of most of the following:
- Medical staff
- Clinical nurse specialists
- Inpatient nursing staff
- Physiotherapist
- Occupational therapist
- Psychologist
- Chaplain
- Social worker
- Benefits/advocacy specialist
- Bereavement team.

> ### Honours
> *Good palliative care introduced early helps patients live longer and better.*
> The SUPPORT trial, published in the *New England Journal of Medicine* in 2010, randomized 151 patients with newly diagnosed, metastatic non-small cell lung cancer to standard care, or standard care plus an early review by a palliative care team. Not only did the patients who received a palliative care review have better symptom control and quality of life scores, they also lived longer (11.6 months vs 8.9 months, $p = 0.02$).

In the hospital

The palliative care team usually reviews and advises on the management of patients being looked after by other clinicians. The team are experts in holistic care including symptom control and end of life care. They routinely have excellent communications skills and are often asked to help discuss difficult aspects of care with patients and their families. During your training, you will witness sensitive conversations that have not been handled as well as they could have been—watching the palliative care team is a great opportunity to see these conversations done well. Try to reflect on the differences between those you see which went well and those that you felt did not.

Trivia

The first modern hospice was St Christopher's, founded in 1967 in Sydenham, London, by Dame Cicely Saunders. Originally training as a nurse and then as a medical social worker, Dame Cicely then trained as a physician and spent a career focusing on the care of the dying. She founded St Christopher's with the aim to provide excellent clinical care alongside research and education. She died in 2005 in the hospice she helped to found.

In the hospice

Hospices are the specialist inpatient units for palliative care. The most common reason for admission is for symptom control, where there has been a symptom that has been difficult to control at home. Once the symptom is under better control, the patient will be discharged home again. Patients are also admitted for end of life care. Some people choose to die in the hospice, while others require admission because it is no longer possible to meet their care needs in their current location. Finally, hospices sometimes offer respite admissions for patients, while their family or carers may be away for example. Most hospices also run a 'day hospice'. This is an area where patients can come 1 day a week and access hospice services such as psychology or physiotherapy, often while giving respite to carers.

What to do in the hospice

Try to spend time with the more senior hospice doctors and watch them clerk if you can. Pay attention to the way they ask some of the more sensitive questions during the consultation. Learning how to discuss a prognosis, do-not-resuscitate (DNAR) forms, and ceiling of treatment decisions with patients and their families is a career-long process, but get a head start by watching hospice clinicians who have these conversations every day.

In the community

Community palliative care teams are often based in hospices, but can be based on their own in some areas. It is in the community that the bulk of patients known to palliative care are cared for. This care is rarely delivered on its own; rather, the specialty works in close quarters with GPs and district nursing teams as well as other community services, e.g. community matrons or community outreach teams.

Cases to see

In hospitals, patients receiving palliative care input are nearly always under the care of a primary clinical team related to the underlying diagnosis. Try to see a hospice MDT in action. These will be much more holistic than in most other settings and you will notice that the most significant discussion will not be led by the doctors, but instead the nurses, social workers, psychologists, and chaplaincy.

Palliative medicine: symptom control

Palliative care is focused on providing holistic care to patients with life-limiting illnesses. It is far more than the management of specific medical issues, just as patients are much more than a collection of symptoms and conditions. Care therefore is multifaceted as described below:

Symptom control

The focus of palliative care is to try to improve the quality of life of the patients in whichever way the patient feels is important to them. One major way this is achieved is through the relief of unpleasant symptoms. The first symptom people tend to think of is pain, but others such as breathlessness, N&V, constipation, or anxiety can be equally debilitating.

Pain

This is a common symptom experienced by patients with many conditions. There are many possible ways to control pain and it is important to take a full history to try to identify the nature of the pain the patient has. It is important to note that they may have several different pains at the same time, e.g. a neuropathic pain in distal limbs from chemotherapy, a visceral pain from a specific tumour, and liver capsular pain from liver metastases. Analgesia (pain relief) needs to be tailored to the pain, or pains, the patient is experiencing. The choice of treatment should relate to the underlying cause of the pain. Some causes of pain can be better treated for the long term in a non-pharmacological manner, e.g. painful bone metastases can respond very well to radiotherapy.

WHO analgesic ladder

The WHO has developed a three-step ladder for prescribing in cancer pain:
- Level 1: non-opioids (aspirin and paracetamol) ± adjuvant.
- Level 2: mild opioids (codeine) ± non-opioid ± adjuvant.
- Level 3: strong opioid (e.g. morphine) ± non-opioid ± adjuvant.

The use of adjuvants will be determined by the type and cause of the pain experienced by the patient.

Nociceptive pain

This is a common type of pain associated with the activation of nociceptors in different organs and tissue throughout the body.

Neuropathic pain

This is pain that derives from damaged nerve fibres and can be difficult to treat with simple analgesia and opioids alone. It can be caused by direct invasion of nerve fibres, compression of nerve roots, or systemic causes for nerve damage such as chemotherapy.

Often it is necessary to start targeted neuropathic agents to help control it, such as gabapentin and pregabalin.

Incident pain

This pattern (rather than type) of pain can be challenging to manage as it is transient in nature and only present in certain circumstances. Commonly it is voluntary movement related. Quick-acting opioids such as sublingual fentanyl can help manage this if given prior to known triggers—such as dressing changes, personal care, and toileting.

Honours

Total pain

The concept of total pain is important in palliative care. Dame Cicely Saunders recognized that pain is often far more complex than a simple visceral event. Taking a thorough history can identify other sources of distress for the patient such as spiritual, social, or psychological pain and these can all influence the patient's overall (total) experience of pain. Addressing these other important factors via the MDT may provide much more effective reductions in pain than simply ↑opioid doses.

Nausea and vomiting

These are often thought of as vomiting being an extension of the nausea, but it is possible to have vomiting without protracted nausea and so they should be thought about separately. When taking a symptom history for nausea, it is important to try to identify the underlying cause. Some causes are reversible and the most effective relief of the nausea can be achieved through direct management of the cause, e.g. dexamethasone to reduce raised intracranial hypertension.

Antiemetics

These have different physiological mechanisms and it is good to initially try to match the mechanism of action to the underlying cause of the nausea. For example, metoclopramide promotes gastric motility and can be useful when there is delayed gastric emptying. Most antiemetics were not originally developed as such, some are antihistamines and others older typical antipsychotics. For example, haloperidol is a potent antiemetic, particularly useful for opioid-induced nausea—if you see this on a drug chart it is not because the clinicians think the patient is psychotic. Commonly prescribed antiemetics include metoclopramide, cyclizine, haloperidol, and levomepromazine.

Breathlessness

This can be an extremely debilitating and unpleasant symptom. As with other symptoms, there are a range of pharmacological and non-pharmacological management strategies. Acute and chronic breathlessness can have both physical and psychological causes and consequences and so, as with everything in palliative care, it is important to address the underlying exacerbating factors, wherever they may lie. Examples include correcting a severe anaemia or draining a malignant pleural effusion. For patients without easily reversible causes, many find opioids helpful and there is good evidence for opiate use for breathlessness. In addition, there is a role for benzodiazepines. The short-acting benzodiazepine lorazepam quickly dissolves under the tongue and has a short half-life making it very good at helping to manage acute episodes of breathlessness, or related panic attacks. Non-pharmacological interventions that help include providing an airflow, through an open window or the use of a fan for example, and are also evidence based. Breathlessness support groups are often run in hospices by physiotherapists and give patient other practical ways of managing acute episodes. Simply telling someone who is experiencing a panic attack to slow their breathing down is unlikely to work, try telling them to concentrate on breathing out slowly. Oxygen can be helpful too, but much less often than some might imagine. In addition, the practicalities of arranging oxygen to be delivered to a person's house can delay discharge and so need to be thought about in advance.

Anorexia

This is common in most advanced illnesses. Encourage frequent, small meals. Review medications that can cause nausea or anorexia, e.g. opiates. Provide good mouth care and inspect regularly since there are often mouth ulcers or oral candida that can be missed.

Constipation

Bowel disruption is another very common problem with advanced illness. Constipation can be very uncomfortable and the pain can mimic more serious intra-abdominal pathology. Poor oral intake, immobility, weakness, and multiple types of medication are just some of the possible causes. Common in palliative care, the use of opioids is quite constipating and laxatives should be started at the same time—90% of patients on opioids will need a laxative. There are different classes of laxatives—osmotic, stimulant, faecal softeners, bulk forming—that can be used and it is good to have an understanding of their different mechanisms of action. Sometimes a more direct approach is needed and suppositories and enemas are used.

Diarrhoea

This can equally be distressing to patients and carers. The most common type seen is 'overflow diarrhoea'. This is actually a symptom of constipation and the treatment is, slightly counterintuitively on first thought, laxatives. Sometimes it can be difficult to convince a patient of the need for laxatives in this situation. Often overflow is described as 'gritty' by the nurses. It is important to check for other causes of diarrhoea and so take a normal history as you would for a gastroenterology patient. Is there blood or melaena? Have they been on antibiotics recently? Are they on laxatives currently? If the diarrhoea continues to be a problem then sometimes drugs such as loperamide and codeine can be helpful.

Excess secretions

Use hyoscine butylbromide/hydrobromide, or glycopyrronium, usually subcutaneously but sometimes topical patches have a role.

Dehydration

Dying patients will inevitably drink less but may not feel thirsty. Good mouth care and keeping the mouth moist helps. The role of artificial hydration at the end of life should very much be decided on an individual patient basis.

Bowel obstruction

Predominantly found in malignancies that have areas of abdominal disease, worsening constipation can also be a sign of impending bowel obstruction. As you may imagine, this is an unpleasant condition, often marked with vomiting, abdominal distension, and pain. Some patients may be suitable for surgical intervention, but often this is not appropriate. In the acute phase, conservative management and bowel rest may be tried.

Sometime a trial of high-dose dexamethasone (6–16 mg/24 hours) may be helpful to try to reduce any oedema present. If this fails, the aim of care is to minimize the distress to the patient. Depending on the cause and the individual patient this may require a varying combination of analgesia, antispasmodics such as hyoscine butylbromide, antiemetics, and antisecretory agents that work in the bowel, such as octreotide. Sometimes a patient will benefit from a NG tube to help decompress the GI tract, but this is very much an individual decision.

Lymphoedema

While worldwide the most common cause is filariasis, in the UK the most common cause is secondary to treatment for cancers. Lymphoedema is the collection of fluid in the limbs due to a disruption of the lymphatic drainage channels, often following surgical dissection or radiotherapy. Lymphoedema is managed in specialist clinics which are often based in cancer centres or more commonly hospices. The primary aims of treatment are excellent skin care, exercise and movement, manual lymph drainage techniques, and support bandaging.

Itch

A complex and deeply unpleasant symptom for some patients. There are many different approaches, many topical and skin related, others more systemic such as drug reactions (~30% of patients will itch with morphine—it is solved by rotating to another opioid). Look for changes in the skin—is it wetter or dryer than usual? Has it changed colour? If appropriate, try local methods first such as emollients. If these aren't working then often more systemic methods are considered.

Spiritual care

Holistic care of the patient involves a broader focus than simply their medical condition. For many patients approaching the end of life, there can be religious, spiritual, or general existential questions and/or worries. A palliative care history should involve a spiritual assessment. Many patients like to have chaplaincy input during their admissions and without asking during the history you will not identify this care need. Some religions have specific requirements about care of the body after death, or timings of burials, and it is important to know this in advance. Spiritual distress is one of the dimensions of total pain (see ➔ p. 551).

Psychological care

Anxiety and depression are commonly underdiagnosed in both patients and their carers. It is important to explore a patient's psychological state during a palliative care clerking. Often, if there are signs of depression, more formal exploration of this is required, including an evaluation of any suicidal ideation that may be present. Treating an undiagnosed depression can markedly help improve many other symptoms. Hospices often have clinical psychologists and counsellors on site and some hospices can offer an outreach service. Patients can often undergo a range of psychological interventions from counselling to cognitive behavioural therapy. Anxiolytics and antidepressants also have a role.

Family and carers

Good holistic care of a patient also involves looking after the needs of their family, those important to them, and their carers. They will have their own psychological, spiritual, and existential care needs. Psychological morbidity is extremely common amongst carers. Often carers feel left out of the medical process as all the attention frequently has been on the patient in busy clinics and their hospital admissions. This is a very important part of holistic care, not least because many patients are worried about their relatives, sometimes worried about the burden being placed on them, or possibly what will happen after their death. Special consideration needs to be taken when there are children involved. The palliative care MDT team is able to help with things such as creating memory boxes for children, helping with explanations about what is happening to a patient's younger children, or liaising with a child's school. This can help ensure the school understands what is going on and can monitor for behavioural changes and liaise with their own educational psychologists as needed. The hospice teams will often help with benefits, arranging the creation of wills and other important financial matters towards the end of life. They also not uncommonly help to arrange a wedding at short notice.

Bereavement care

Palliative care teams have access to bereavement care which concentrates on care of family and carers after a patient's death. If a death has been particularly traumatic or difficult for a family member, it is good practice to let the bereavement team know so they can follow up the family appropriately. In some cases this will be with the help of the GP. Often hospices will have services of remembrance, commonly around times of year more focused around family. Relatives will return to remember their loved ones and benefit from the mutual support on offer. Many families return year after year. If you are in a hospice and one of these is held, then make an effort to see it. It highlights that our patients are people, not just collections of pathology.

Care of the dying patient

In hospital placements, you may well be attached to teams that are caring for actively dying patients and it is here you are more likely to learn the beginning of these skills. Good care at the end of a person's life is important for both that person and their family. Family members will often remember the care their relatives received as they were dying for the rest of their own lives.

The aim of good end of life care is to provide only those interventions that are beneficial to the patient. Every patient is an individual and so all management at the end of life should be bespoke. This is achieved through the use of various medications used to respond to symptoms as they develop. This is often referred to as anticipatory prescribing. Typically they will be administered by the SC route as swallowing may be becoming more difficult or impossible.

The anticipatory medication is chosen using the same attention to underlying cause as in symptom control. If repeated doses are required, then often they administered via a continuous SC infusion, often called a 'syringe driver' that lasts for 24 hours. This allows for a constant dose of symptom-relieving medication to be administered via a reliably absorbable route. The doses are reviewed on a daily basis as the patient and their symptoms change, and this allows for responsive dose changes. Multiple medications can be combined in a single pump, and 'as-needed' doses can often be given through the same line if more modern connectors are used.

Terminal restlessness

This is sometimes seen in the few days before death. It is a heightened level of agitation in the days before death. This can be well controlled once recognized. It is important to differentiate terminal agitation from other cases of agitation such as urinary retention, or hypoxia, as these can often be more effectively managed in other ways, e.g. a urinary catheter.

Holistic review

Other important aspects when caring for a dying patient is to consider the interventions currently in place and use clinical judgement to decide whether they should be continued or altered. Some examples of this are non-invasive ventilation, antibiotics, artificial fluids, and nutrition.

There are no fixed rules on stopping interventions, rather each should be considered individually, and rationales discussed with the patient, or their family if the patient is unable to have these conversations. These conversation need to be undertaken with sensitivity, they are by their nature likely to be upsetting. Communication is not a one-off process. Rapport and effective communication will develop and continue over time.

Morphine shortens life—a medical myth

It is a commonly held belief among the general public and a significant number of health professionals that administering morphine in a palliative care setting shortens the patient's life, usually through a suppression of respiratory drive.

This is a medical myth. Opioid prescribing as used by palliative care teams does not shorten life. Inappropriately large doses will do, of course, but appropriate dose titration and ongoing review will achieve good symptom control without shortening life.

In exams

Palliative care patients are rarely used for OSCEs and so the stations will normally have an actor/simulated patient.

Often they will focus on a specific area as taking a generalized history would take too long for a standard OSCE station slot. Communication skills are therefore often tested. The key is, as always, establishing rapport early, elicit the patient's concern, and dealing sensitively with them.

Remember that silence can be extremely useful, especially if you are slightly unsure where to go next—the actor will often guide you if they feel you are genuinely listening. Another tip is to be careful with your active listening cues. Avoid getting into the habit of saying 'good' as a cue for example, as it makes you sound like you are not listening when the actor has just told you they have a terminal illness and are worried about dying!

Skills to practise

Communication is the most prominent skill in palliative medicine. It is through communication that the palliative care clinician elicits the symptoms, troubles, hopes, goals, and fears of their patients and their families.

Breaking bad news is a part of palliative medicine, although do not forget that the diagnosing and treating teams are the ones who tell the patient their diagnosis.

Pathology

Pathology: overview

Pathology is the scientific study of disease, while clinical pathology is about integrating the morphologic, biochemical, and molecular analyses with the clinical information provided to achieve a definite diagnosis. Its major subdivisions include histopathology, cytopathology, haematopathology, chemical pathology, and medical microbiology. Other disciplines include medical genetics, immunology, virology, toxicology, and forensic pathology.

Clinical pathology is predominantly a consultant-delivered service and is a hidden speciality which is largely based in the clinical laboratory where pathological specimens are received, examined, and reported. It accounts for ~85% of patient diagnosis. In general, there is limited clinical contact with patients. Therefore, your exposure to clinical pathology depends largely on your medical school curriculum and your placement as pathology services have become increasingly centralized. But above all, pathology exposure depends on your enthusiasm and interest, therefore discuss with your local department to arrange for pathology shadowing if it is not routinely done.

Histopathology

Is a key speciality of clinical pathology that deals with the tissue diagnosis of disease based on biopsy material taken from the patient in the clinic, ward, and theatre or during postmortem examination. It plays a crucial role in patient care especially those with cancer by differentiating between benign and malignant neoplasms and establishing the primary origin of metastatic tumour. It is not only about diagnosis but also includes prevention and reducing the incidence and mortality from cancer through the cancer screening programmes. Some histopathologists also perform autopsies.

Chemical pathology

Or clinical biochemistry involves the investigation and interpretation of biochemical tests of bodily fluids (e.g. blood, urine, and CSF) to diagnose biochemical disorders, especially metabolic diseases. There is some direct patient contact in the clinic where biochemical investigations are usually requested such as metabolic bone disease and cardiovascular risk prevention clinics. In addition, metabolic diseases will be featured in other clinical rotations including clinical medicine, endocrinology, and paediatrics.

Cytopathology

Involves examination of cells. This is subdivided into gynaecological cytology (cervical Pap smears) and diagnostic cytology (e.g. cavity fluid, FNA, CSF, and urine).

Haematopathology

Involves the diagnosis of haematological disorders and malignancies derived from myeloid and lymphoid cells usually through a lymph node or bone marrow biopsy and peripheral blood smear. Ancillary techniques such as immunohistochemistry, molecular genetic/FISH, and flow cytometry play significant roles in supporting the diagnosis.

Medical microbiology

Does not only involve the investigation and diagnosis of infectious diseases, but also controls the spread of infection and provides advice on antimicrobial treatment. You will meet a consultant/registrar microbiologist regularly during some clinical ward rounds (e.g. intensive care).

Forensic pathology

Involves the investigation of deaths provided by the coroners and police (in England and Wales), where a forensic pathologist performs a detailed postmortem examination of criminal law cases (e.g. homicides, violent, death in custody, or suspicious deaths). You will have limited or no exposure to forensic cases.

Honours

Staging and grading

Are crucial in management and prognosis.

- *Grading* is based on the histological appearances of the tumour cell and how much different it looks from the tissue of origin (e.g. well, moderately, poorly, or undifferentiated). In addition to Gleason grading for prostate carcinoma, another good example is grading of breast tumour based on Tubule formation (T), nuclear Pleomorphism (P), and Mitotic count (M).
- *Staging* is based on clinical, radiological, surgical, and pathological criteria including tumour size, vascular invasion, and lymph nodes or distant metastases. Tumours are staged using the TNM staging system based on three measurements: extent of primary tumour (T), regional lymph node metastasis (N), and distant metastases (M). Other staging systems include the Dukes staging system for colorectal cancer and FIGO staging system for gynaecologic cancers.

Cases to see

You will be exposed to a huge variety of cases from different surgical and medical specialities. The following are some examples and diagnostic features of important surgical specimens. Please refer to individual specialty pages for clinical presentation and management.

GI specimens

Are usually small biopsies taken during endoscopy or colonoscopy. Look for chronic idiopathic inflammatory bowel disease: Crohn's disease versus ulcerative colitis.

Hepatobiliary specimens

Gallbladder removed for gallstones and/or chronic cholecystitis is the commonest specimen. Histology shows chronic inflammation, Rokitansky–Aschoff sinus formation and fibromuscular hypertrophy.

Liver specimens are largely medical liver biopsies but you will also see liver biopsies for focal liver lesion, metastatic tumour, and cirrhosis (end-stage of chronic liver disease characterized by irreversible fibrosis and diffuse nodules formation). You should be aware of different causes of cirrhosis including alcoholic liver disease, viral hepatitis, PSC, PBC (positive anti-mitochondrial antibody serology), haemochromatosis, α1-antitrypsin deficiency, Wilson disease, and drugs. Complications include liver failure, portal hypertension, and ↑risk for hepatocellular carcinoma.

Steatohepatitis is characterized by fatty changes with ballooning degeneration of hepatocytes and Mallory body formation with variable degrees of fibrosis ± lobular neutrophils. This could be alcoholic (ASH) or non-alcoholic steatohepatitis (NASH) secondary to obesity, DM, hypertension, and hyperlipidaemia. Correlation with clinical biochemistry and microbiology results is essential for infectious (especially viral hepatitis B, C) and autoimmune liver disease. For instance, autoimmune hepatitis will show high titres of anti-ANA, smooth muscle antibodies, and liver kidney microsomal antibodies.

Gynaecological specimens
• Include cytology (Pap smear, peritoneal washings) and surgical biopsies or resections.
• Hysterectomy for fibroids (leiomyomas) will be your commonest specimen in the gynaecological cut-up (well-circumscribed benign tumours; white-tan, whorled cut surface; interlaced smooth muscle).
• Different types of benign and malignant ovarian tumour using ovarian tumour FIGO staging. Advanced ovarian cancers have ↑CA125 in the blood.
• Understand the risk factors for cervical intraepithelial neoplasia (CIN) such as early age at first intercourse, multiple sexual partners, and high-risk HPV infection. You will get brownie points by showing knowledge of the NHS cervical screening programme and HPV testing.
• A cervical cytology report will indicate with a result code whether the samples are inadequate (code 1), negative (2), or abnormal: mild dyskaryosis (3), moderate dyskaryosis (7), severe dyskaryosis (4), ?invasive (5), ?Glandular (6), and borderline nuclear changes (8).

Urological specimens
Specimens for adult renal neoplasm could be either partial or radical nephrectomies. Renal cell carcinoma represents ~90% of renal neoplasm. Risk factors include family history (association with von Hippel–Lindau disease), smoking, obesity, and long-term renal dialysis. The commonest carcinoma is clear cell carcinoma (70–80%) with macroscopically variegated (yellow/red/white) cut surface. Prognosis depends on Fuhrman nuclear grading and TNM staging which incorporates tumour size, vascular invasion, and extrarenal extension.

Wilms tumour (nephroblastoma) is the commonest (85%) paediatric renal tumour with triphasic components: stromal, epithelial, and blastemal (small blue round cells). The tumour is WT1-positive and associated with genetic defects on chromosome 11.

Honours

Cancer screening programme

In the UK, these currently include cervical, breast, and colorectal screening programmes.

- In *cervical screening*, free cervical smear tests take place every 3 years (age 25–49) or every 5 years (age 50–64).
- In *breast screening*, women aged 50–70 are invited for a mammogram every 3 years.
- In *colorectal screening*, men and women from the age of 50 will be invited for screening every 2 years. The initial phase is based on a clinical chemistry test called faecal occult blood (FOB) test, where positive results are followed by a colonoscopy. Here, the endoscopist will biopsy any polyps seen and these are examined by the pathologist aiming to detect early bowel cancer.

Haematopathology specimens

- Investigations for lymphoma and leukaemia include blood film, FNA, bone marrow trephine biopsy, and core and excisional lymph node biopsies.
- Two groups of lymphomas are recognized, Hodgkin lymphoma (HL) and non-Hodgkin lymphoma (NHL), which both have different behaviours, prognosis, and treatment. Macroscopically, there is a homogeneous, white, cut surface of the enlarged lymph node.
- HL is characterized by presence of Reed–Sternberg cells which have multiple nuclei with prominent nucleoli and are positive for CD30 and CD15. The commonest subtype (75%) is nodular sclerosis.
- The majority of NHLs are of B-lymphocyte origin in which follicular lymphoma is the commonest type in adults (40%). Neoplastic cells express BCL2, CD10, and CD20. A characteristic translocation is t(14;18). Other important translocations to remember are t(11;14) in mantle zone lymphoma which express cyclin D1, and t(8;14) in Burkitt lymphoma involving the *MYC* gene on chromosome 8.

Skin specimens

- During skin cut-up, you will encounter different biopsy types including punch, curetting, shave, incisional, and excisional ellipse biopsies. Try to see examples of basal cell carcinoma, squamous cell carcinoma, and melanoma which are the commonest malignant skin tumours.
- Grossly, a malignant melanoma can be a nodular or ulcerated pigmented lesion but non-pigmented melanomas also exist. If the morphology is unusual, the diagnosis can be confirmed by S100, HMB45, and Melan-A staining.
- Beware of prognostic factors as well as parameters that should be included in the pathology report. These include melanoma type, growth phase (radial/vertical), Breslow thickness, ulceration, lymphovascular invasion, regression, mitotic rate, and excision margins.
- Also keep up to date with the recent targeted therapy for melanoma. As half of the patients have changes in the *BRAF* gene, drugs that target this gene (e.g. vemurafenib) can be used for treatment of *BRAF* mutation-positive melanoma.

Diagnostic cytology specimens

- Samples include urine, FNA, CSF, and serous cavities (pleural, peritoneal, and cardiac fluid).
- Pleural fluid from an elderly male with a history of asbestos exposure can confirm malignant mesothelioma which shows cellular sample containing 3D clusters of mesothelial cells with nuclear enlargement and macronucleoli.
- Urothelial carcinoma or carcinoma *in situ* can be diagnosed from a urine sample but correlation with cystoscopy findings is essential. Urine with BK (polyoma) virus is seen mainly in renal transplant patients.
- Thyroid FNA is useful to differentiate between benign lesions (Thy2), follicular neoplasm (Thy3), or papillary carcinoma (Thy 5). Inadequate sample is classified as Thy1 and suspicious for malignancy sample as Thy4. FNA from papillary thyroid carcinoma are usually highly cellular and composed of papillary groups with irregular nuclear membrane, nuclear overlapping, nuclear grooves and intranuclear inclusions.
- A BAL sample can differentiate between small cell carcinoma and non-small cell carcinoma (SCC or adenocarcinoma). In immunocompromised and HIV patients, a fungal (Grocott) stain of BAL can identify *Pneumocystis jirovecii* cysts within amorphous proteinaceous casts.
- Synovial fluid samples are useful to identify rhomboid-shaped calcium pyrophosphate crystals in pseudogout or needle-shaped uric acid crystals in gout.
- CSF results should be correlated with clinical and microbiological findings for the diagnosis of bacterial or viral meningitis.

Pathology: in the pathology laboratory

Clinical pathology is largely based on macroscopic and microscopic visual skills, so familiarize yourself with the use of the light microscope. During your rotation in the histopathology department, you are likely to shadow a histopathology registrar. After pathology specimens get booked at the reception you will observe specimen dissection or cut-up, which involves gross examination of organs and tissues taken from patients for diagnosis, during which representative sections (tumour, polyps, resection margins, lymph nodes, etc.) are processed to slides for microscopic examination. Later, you will do examination of tissue sections under the light microscope not only for determining the type of disease, but also for characterizing its severity and extent to ensure that patients receive the appropriate treatment (e.g. determining severity in IBD and degree of hepatic fibrosis in hepatitis C). After finishing your allocated cases, you will have one-to-one teaching with a senior registrar or a consultant to discuss the cases and finalize reporting. A portion of the samples that you will examine are cytology specimens and these include pleural and ascitic fluid, urine, cervical smears, as well as breast, thyroid, salivary gland, and lymph node aspiration cytology. In addition to patient information, the histopathology report will include macroscopic and microscopic descriptions, diagnosis, and comments to clinicians.

Honours

Clinicopathological correlation (CPC)

Part of your shadowing will be centred on liaison with other clinicians mainly through CPC and MDT meetings, in which the diagnosis and clinical management of patients (especially malignant cases) are discussed in a multiprofessional setting. You must attend some of these meeting or even present an interesting case in CPC meeting after discussing it with your supervising consultant.

Ancillary studies in pathology

In addition to light microscopy for morphological diagnosis, you will notice that pathologists might also use additional diagnostic techniques to assist in reaching a final diagnosis. These include some recent advances in clinical investigative science which you should understand for their clinical application. The technical aspect is generally performed by biomedical scientists and interpreted by pathologists. In addition to shadowing pathologists, try to spend some time in the pathology lab with biomedical scientists to understand the principles and clinical applications of ancillary studies, including the following:

Special stains

Are very useful in liver and renal medical biopsies (e.g. reticulin, silver stain) and detection of microorganisms (e.g. periodic acid–Schiff for fungi, Gram for bacteria).

Immunohistochemistry

Involves the use of labelled antibodies which stain specific proteins in tissue sections (see Table 28.1). Immunohistochemistry helps to identify tumour type including the origin of metastasis (e.g. melan A in metastatic melanoma, CD45 in lymphoma, and cytokeratin in carcinoma), to determine prognosis and treatment (e.g. oestrogen receptor in breast cancer), identifications of organisms (e.g. HSV, CMV, *Pneumocystis*), and lymphoma subtypes (e.g. cyclin D1 and CD5 in mantle cell lymphoma).

Immunofluorescence

Is used for evaluation of some inflammatory skin diseases (e.g. bullous pemphigoid and dermatitis herpetiformis) and renal biopsies for glomerular disease (e.g. lupus nephritis and IgA nephropathy) by detection of antibodies or immune complexes.

Flow cytometry

Is used for cell counting and sorting cell types in a suspension. It plays a crucial role in lymphoma and leukaemia subclassifications.

Electron microscopy

Will be available in large university hospitals. Electron microscopy is mainly used in evaluation of glomerular disease in renal biopsies.

Molecular biology

Identifies cytogenetics for undifferentiated tumours or difficult cases, predominantly chromosomal translocations associated with sarcomas, leukaemias, and lymphomas (e.g. t(9;22) in chronic myeloid leukaemia, t(X,18)in synovial sarcoma). It is also important to test for clonality in lymphomas. FISH is used for detection of HER-2 in breast cancer. PCR plays an increasingly revolutionary role in clinical pathology, especially the diagnosis of infectious disease (viruses and *Pneumocystis*).

Honours

See Table 28.1.

Table 28.1 Differential diagnosis of undifferentiated tumour

Key immunohistochemistry/ special stain	Key immunohistochemistry/special stain
Carcinoma	CK, EMA, mucin stains (Alcian blue)
Lymphoma	CD45, CD3 (T-cells), CD20 (B-cells)
Melanoma	Melan A, S100, HMB 45, Fontana–Masson stain
Sarcoma	Actin/desmin/myogenin (muscle), S100 (neural), CD34 (vascular)
Neuroendocrine	Synaptophysin, chromogranin, CD56
Mesothelioma	Calretinin,WT1,CK5/6
Germ cell tumour	PLAP, CD117

Pathology: in exams

As clinical pathology highlights the diagnostic and prognostic aspects of diseases, pathology questions can be integrated within exams of other specialities, where you might be asked about laboratory investigations, serology, and pathological features. Most pathology exams are based on topics covered during clinical pathology tutorials and lectures as well as during your departmental rotation. There will be no real patients and the examiners should be consultants from different pathology disciplines. Exam questions could include MCQs, an essay, photos, and viva which are mainly problem-solving oriented. As pathological specialties are mainly visual, you should practise during your rotation to describe the gross and microscopic appearance of different specimens you see in the pathology laboratory. For instance, describing a caecal adenocarcinoma in a right hemicolectomy specimen and understanding the prognostic factors that affect patient management; these include lymph node metastasis, extramural lymphovascular invasion, and completeness of excision. Knowing the principles of tumour staging, different tumour markers, and advances in diagnostic techniques are important components of the viva.

You should also enhance your virtual skills by reviewing pathology websites. For example, ℘ http://library.med.utah.edu/WebPath provides excellent collections of microscopic and macroscopic pathology images, exam questions, and tutorials. Recently, the Royal College of Pathologists established a new eLearning project of pathology specimen podcasts (℘ e-pathpots.org.uk) which includes a wide range of gross appearances of diseases to support teaching medical students using virtual pots. Many thanks to the Leeds Virtual Pathology website (℘ http://virtualpathology.leeds.ac.uk) which provides a rich collection of virtual slides. These are high-resolution digital scans that can be viewed and navigated online using a computer-based program.

Honours

Reasons for referring death to the coroner

- The cause of death is unknown or unnatural or an unidentified body.
- The patient was not attended by a doctor during the last illness or was not seen within the last 14 days prior to death.
- The death occurred within 24 hours of admission to hospital.
- The death occurred during an operation or before recovery from the effect of an anaesthetic or related to the anaesthetic.
- Death in custody or shortly after release.
- Death is related to an abortion.
- Accident-related death or due to industrial disease or related to patient's employment.
- Question of negligence.
- Suicide or homicide.

Psychiatry

Psychiatry: overview

The history of modern psychiatry began in the 1800s, and over the twentieth century biological theories around mental illness, psychological ideas, and psychopharmacology grew into the basis of what exists today. Psychiatric illnesses are classified in the ICD-10 (used in the UK, developed by the WHO) and the fifth edition of the *Diagnostic and Statistical Manual of Mental Disorders* (*DSM-5*) (developed by the American Psychiatric Association). The classifications are periodically reviewed as new evidence emerges. The ICD-11 (currently being prepared for implementation) has classified gaming disorder, and reclassified gender incongruence from mental health to sexual health.

Psychiatry: the placement

The three rules

1. *Be curious*: ask questions to staff and patients alike.
2. *Be respectful*: when assessing patients, do not push your agenda.
3. *Be safe*: the wards can sometimes be chaotic and patients can quickly become agitated.

Most placements are general adult or older adult subspecialties with a mix of inpatient/outpatient experience, or attached to a psychiatry liaison team covering a general hospital. There may be options to access various subspecialties.

Observations

Observations (or 'obs') in psychiatry is different from a general hospital and refers to how often a member of the nursing team should check on a patient. Standard obs are hourly, and patients with ↑risk are managed on 15 min and 1:1 or 1 min (i.e. a nurse is present with the patient at all times). Psychiatric care is heavily reliant on a MDT:

- *Consultants and junior doctors*.
- *Community psychiatric nurses (CPNs)*: these nurses hold caseloads in the community, managing the patients with input from the psychiatrists and other members of the MDT. Social workers and occupational therapists also hold caseloads when working with the community teams.
- *Registered mental health nurses (RMNs)*: all mental health nurses are RMNs, but the term is used commonly when requesting 1:1 obs on the general wards.
- *Approved mental health practitioners (AMHPs, formally approved social worker)*: required to coordinate and facilitate Mental Health Act (MHA) assessments and to submit the paperwork.
- *Occupational therapists (OTs)*: within a mental health unit, OTs run various groups for inpatients, may do 1:1 work around improving living skills, facilitate access to voluntary placements, and aid patients in accessing employment upon discharge.
- *Psychologists*: may provide individual cognitive behavioural therapy (CBT) on wards and in the community. In Child and Adolescent Mental Health Services (CAMHS), there may be psychologists providing family therapy, group therapy, or other forms of individual work. The wards may have art/music/drama therapists.
- *Independent mental capacity advocates (IMCA)*: act as advocates for the patient, by liaising with the patient prior to a meeting (e.g. ward round) and relaying the patient's opinions and concerns.

Psychiatry: mental health and mental capacity acts

Mental Health Act (MHA)

The MHA came in to effect in 1983, and was amended in 2007, with the aim of enabling detention and treatment of those suffering with mental illness without their consent, due to risk to themselves or others. A MHA assessment is carried out by an AMHP and two section 12-approved doctors who all have to agree that a patient has a mental illness of sufficient degree and nature to warrant being placed under section of the MHA.

Some important sections to the MHA

- *Section 2*: lasts for up to 28 days for assessment and treatment of a mental illness
- *Section 3*: lasts for up to 6 months, for assessment and treatment for a mental illness. After 3 months, the patient will be asked for consent to continue treatment. If this is refused and treatment is deemed necessary, a second opinion-appointed doctor will review.
- *Section 5(2)*: used in both general hospital and mental health units, the admitting team (i.e. not necessarily the psychiatry team) can detain a patient for up to 72 hours if there are concerns that their mental state is deteriorating and the patient is a risk to self or others. Section 5(2) cannot be used in the ED. The use of section 5(2) will trigger a MHA assessment
- *Section 12*: approves a doctor on behalf of the Secretary of State as having special expertise in the diagnosis and treatment of 'mental disorders'.
- *Section 136*: lasts up to 72 hours; under this section the police can bring a patient into a place of safety for a MHA assessment if they are concerned about the mental state of a patient. The use of a section 136 will trigger review by an AMHP or doctor to assess whether there is evidence of mental illness

Mental Capacity Act (MCA)

Legislation was produced in 2005 to enable clinicians to determine whether a patient is able to make an informed decision about their treatment. This applies to all specialties in medicine, not just psychiatry. It is commonly used for patients with:

- a mental health condition
- learning disability
- dementia
- traumatic brain injury.

Honours

Capacity

The MHA is, in part, used to treat mental health conditions with pharmacological interventions; however, inpatients often suffer with co-morbid physical health conditions, e.g. cardiovascular disease. These cannot be treated under the MHA, and instead the Mental Capacity Act should be used.

The clinician administering the proposed treatment plan should assess capacity.

The information provided must be in a language the person can understand (i.e. may require the use of an interpreter and the use of layman's terms is important) and the communication does not have to be spoken (i.e. it can be written).

Honours

Five guiding principles to assessing capacity

1. The person is assumed to have capacity until it is established that they do not.
2. The person must be given appropriate help to make the decision.
3. A person is not treated as lacking capacity merely because the decision they make is considered unwise.
4. A decision made under this act for someone who lacks capacity must be in the person's best interests.
5. Any decision made should be the least restrictive option.

Honours

Four criteria to be met to determine capacity

1. The person is able to understand the information provided.
2. The person is able to retain the information provided.
3. The person is able to weigh up the pros and cons.
4. The person is able to communicate this decision.

Psychiatry: on the ward

There are plenty of learning opportunities on an inpatient ward. It is a chance to assess patients who are acutely unwell and review their progress during your rotation. It is important to follow safety procedures on the ward, which includes informing someone of your whereabouts at all times, and if appropriate, carrying a personal alarm or familiarizing yourself with the fixed alarms on the walls.

Cases to see

- Schizophrenia
- Bipolar affective disorder
- Depression
- Emotionally unstable borderline personality disorder.

Honours

Psychosis is seen in organic and psychiatric disorders. Common organic causes for psychotic symptoms are:

- a brain tumour
- alcohol misuse
- side effect from Parkinson's medication
- CNS infection (e.g. syphilis, HIV)
- autoimmune conditions affecting the CNS system (e.g. SLE, MS).

Psychosis

Is the term describing a constellation of symptoms affecting a person's perception of their surrounding environment. The symptoms typically fall into two categories:

1. *Hallucinations*: a change in the perception by the senses (e.g. hearing voices of people who are not there which is the most common hallucination). It can affect all given senses.
2. *Delusions*: a disordered belief system that when examined are obviously untrue (e.g. believing that the FBI are spying on you through your chimney).

Disorders with psychosis as a feature you may see on the ward include:

- schizophrenia
- bipolar disorder
- severe (psychotic) depression
- postpartum psychosis
- drug-induced psychosis (cannabis, ketamine, LSD, psilocybin, etc.).

Schizophrenia

This is characterized by a range of symptoms affecting a person's perceptions and thoughts. It is typically a long-term diagnosis, requiring anti-psychotic medication to treat the symptoms and improve a patient's daily functioning. The symptoms of schizophrenia were documented by Kurt Schneider (known as Schneider's first rank symptoms).

Schneider's first-rank symptoms

- Auditory hallucinations:
  - Thought echo (hear own thoughts spoken aloud).
  - Running commentary (of actions).
  - Third-person auditory hallucinations (two or more voices conversing).
- Thought:
  - Insertion (thoughts being placed in own mind).
  - Withdrawal (thoughts being removed from own mind).
  - Broadcasting (believing others know own thoughts).
- Made:
  - Feelings (belief that feelings are not own but have been imposed by an external force).
  - Impulses (experiences impulses that are not own but believed to be imposed by an external force).
  - Actions (experiences actions and will are controlled by external force).
- *Somatic passivity* (believing that an external agent is manipulating own body e.g. twisting intestines).
- *Delusional perception* (linking normal perceptions with bizarre meanings, e.g. hearing a car horn means the Queen has summoned you).

These listed symptoms would be considered *positive symptoms* of schizophrenia. Other positive symptoms of schizophrenia include:
- *knight's move thinking* (thinking that is difficult to follow due to loosening of association of ideas)
- *delusional mood/atmosphere* (a sudden perceived change in the environment which may be linked to a specific meaning)
- *persecutory delusions*
- *word salad* (confused, garbled speech that is difficult to follow).

Negative symptoms are more subtle and associated with a worse prognosis:
- disturbance in sleep
- social isolation
- changes in mood
- blunting of affect
- poverty of thought content
- slowness of thought, speech, and movement (psychomotor retardation).

Honours

Exam revision

Be clear in your own mind the definitions of each of the listed symptoms. A top student will be able to differentiate each of the symptoms when taking a history so it is important to source a number of examples of each until you feel confident.

Ask the boss
The most common subtype of schizophrenia is paranoid schizophrenia. Ask your consultant about other subtypes such as hebephrenic and residual schizophrenia.

Management of psychosis/schizophrenia
The management of all mental health conditions considers the:
- biological
- psychological
- social aspects of the disease.

Honours
Exam revision
The most common symptom in people with schizophrenia is lack of insight into their mental illness.

Immediate management of acute psychosis is with antipsychotics and benzodiazepines (to reduce agitation).

Honours
Antipsychotics
Antipsychotics come in two classes—first and second generation. First-generation drugs have a more parkinsonian side effect profile (e.g. tremors, stiffness) and sedation. Second-generation drugs have a less pronounced parkinsonian side effect profile but can cause significant weight gain (↑appetite) and sedation among others.
   Tip: side effect profile can affect medication compliance.

Mood disorders
Are the spectrum of disorders that encompass symptoms of:
- *elated* (manic and hypomanic)
- *depressive* (mild, moderate, and severe) moods.

The most commonly seen in an inpatient unit are manic episodes or severe depressive episodes.

Bipolar affective disorder
Is a condition of both mania and depression. There are several differentiations:
- *Bipolar 1* diagnosed after at least one manic episode lasting 1 week. A patient may only present with mania, but may have experienced preceding subclinical depressive episodes or develop subsequent depressive episodes.
- *Bipolar 2* consisting of hypomania and moderate/severe depressive episodes.
- *Cyclothymia* with elated plus low moods that do not meet the threshold for bipolar affective disorder.
- *Rapid cycling* with four or more mood swings within a 12-month period.

Symptoms of mania/hypomania

- Persistently elevated mood, quick to become irritable.
- ↓Sleep.
- ↓Appetite.
- High energy levels/always on the go.
- Highly distractible.
- Inflated self-esteem, grandiosity.
- Pressured speech.
- Difficulty following thoughts—flight of ideas.
- ↑'Risky' behaviour: promiscuous behaviour, reckless spending, unawareness of personal safety (e.g. running across the road).
- Mood-congruent psychotic symptoms can occur.

Honours

Mania

For a diagnosis of mania, the symptoms have to be present for *7 days*. For a diagnosis of hypomania, the symptoms should be present for *4 days* and should not be severe enough to significantly impact daily functioning.

Hypomania may be seen in outpatient clinics but a manic episode is most often managed as an inpatient admission. Immediate management is with sedatives (benzodiazepines) and mood stabilizers (e.g. sodium valproate or lithium).

Honours

Lithium toxicity

Lithium toxicity can occur due to overdose, dehydration, or abnormal renal function. Symptoms include diarrhoea, vomiting, drowsiness, and muscle weakness.

Depression

Depressive episodes are classed as mild, moderate, and severe depending upon the number of symptoms present. The core triad of symptoms are:
- low mood
- low energy
- anhedonia (loss of enjoyment of activities previously enjoyed).

Ask the boss

Risk management in mania can be ethically complex such as:
- Should you remove a patient's smartphone and tablet if you are aware they are spending online beyond their means?
- Should you prevent a patient having contact with another patient on the ward they are attracted to?

Beck's triad (Fig. 29.1) forms the cognitive theory of depression consisting of the following negative thoughts:
1. Hopeless
2. Helpless
3. Useless/worthless.

There are additional biological and psychological features (See Table 29.1):
• *Mild*: at least one of the core symptoms and four in total.
• *Moderate*: two or more core symptoms and up to six in total.
• *Severe*: two or more core symptoms and seven or more in total or associated mood congruent psychotic symptoms.

Immediate management is with antidepressants and ↑levels of observation dependent upon levels of risk. Consider previous use of antidepressants and reasons behind non-compliance prior to commencement. CBT for depression should also be offered.

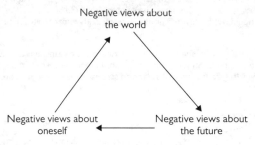

Fig. 29.1 Beck's triad. Reproduced from Wikimedia commons under the Creative Commons Attribution-Share Alike 3.0 Unported license

Table 29.1 Biological and psychological features of Beck's triad

Biological	Psychological
Poor sleep (especially early morning waking)	Low self-esteem/self-worth
Poor appetite	Poor concentration
Loss of libido	Feelings of guilt/blame/hopelessness
Psychomotor retardation	Suicidal ideation

Diagnosis of depression (symptoms should be present for >4 weeks).

Emotionally unstable borderline personality disorder

Is the most common personality disorder seen on the acute psychiatric ward. Symptoms include extreme, intense, and volatile emotions, impulsivity, fear of abandonment, and feelings of emptiness. Patients are often admitted following an episode of deliberate self-harm or with suicidal ideation. A short admission or intensive work with the home treatment team can help to contain the risk during the crisis.

Following deliberate self-harm or with ongoing suicidal ideation, a patient may be placed on 1:1 obs which are reviewed daily. Medication is not often used in acute crises except if the patient becomes a risk to themselves or others (e.g. extreme agitated behaviour). The patient may already be on medication in the community, which should be continued through admission as appropriate. The patient should be actively encouraged to engage in the therapeutic process and work with the MDT to resolve the crisis.

Things to do on the ward

- Morning handover between staff is a good way to learn about new patients on the ward and decide with the staff who would be best for you to assess that day.
- Most wards will have a morning meeting with the patients, which can be useful to attend to observe the staff/patient dynamics and find out about OT-run groups that day.
- A ward round occurs once or twice a week.
- Other reviews such as CPA meetings with a care coordinator occur on an ad hoc basis
- Try shadowing the on-call doctor to experience ward emergencies, how to assess new admissions, walk-in patients, and patients brought in under section 136

Seclusion

Some inpatient sites will have a seclusion room. The seclusion room is a last resort to managing an escalating patient on the ward (e.g. if a patient becomes violent towards staff or other patients, and rapid tranquilization has failed to calm them down). Attend a seclusion review if possible. The team will re-assess risk and conclude whether the patient is settled enough to return to an open ward or may move to a psychiatric intensive care unit (PICU).

PICU

Is a single-sex locked ward with a higher staff-to-patient ratio to manage high-risk patients. The aim is to stabilize the patient on medication, reducing the risk in order to transfer them to an open ward. Patients from open wards can be escalated to a PICU. If a PICU bed is not available, patients can be managed on an open ward with two or more staff members providing continuous obs.

Electroconvulsive therapy (ECT)

Is used as a treatment for severe treatment-resistant depression, a protracted manic episode, and catatonia. It involves placing the patient under sedation and providing a muscle relaxant, and then inducing seizure activity via electrodes placed on the temples. The procedure lasts a matter of minutes and is repeatedly weekly or twice weekly for a number of sessions (usually up to 12).

Ask the boss
The rationale behind unilateral ECT versus bilateral ECT.

Trivia
ECT was developed in the 1930s and prior to electricity, seizures were induced by chemical agents such as metrazol and camphor.

Side effects of ECT
Short-term amnesia, drowsiness, headache, confusion, loss of appetite, aching muscles, and risk of anaesthetic.

Honours
Catatonia
Catatonia is defined as a state of neurogenic motor immobility and behavioural abnormality. It is rarely seen these days but can be a manifestation of schizophrenia, bipolar affective disorder, depression, and post-traumatic stress disorder. Symptoms include immobility (stupor), rigidity, posturing (waxy flexibility is the maintenance of a given position), echolalia, and echopraxia (mimicking speech and actions).

Psychiatry: in clinic

Outpatient clinics are a good place to assess patients diagnosed with anxiety disorders and review patients who are managing with schizophrenia in the community. It may also provide the opportunity for home visits.

Anxiety disorders

Are more likely to be seen in clinic if the patient is on medication (typically SSRIs). Many are offered CBT through a GP or self-referral service known as IAPT (improved access to psychological therapies). When taking the history, it is important to elicit:
- when the symptoms started
- whether the symptoms have worsened
- whether anything makes the symptoms improve
- whether there were any significant life changes prior to the symptoms
- how the symptoms affect daily functioning.

Generalized anxiety disorder (GAD)

Is often experienced as a free-floating anxiety with constant chronic worrying about all aspects of daily life. Sufferers feel constantly on edge. To be diagnosed, the anxiety must be present for at least 6 months. They will catastrophize events (e.g. if their spouse has not arrived home from work, they will fixate on the cause being a fatal accident). GAD affects concentration and sleep. It may impact the ability to maintain employment and affect relationships with others.

Panic disorder

Is defined as experiencing panic attacks without an apparent trigger. A panic attack is a physiological response to a stressful situation ($\uparrow$HR, sweating, breathlessness, chest pain). Often the symptoms of a panic attack will further cause anxiety, which can further perpetuate the symptom and can be a frightening experience. The person may avoid situations which trigger the panic attack (e.g. a crowds or tight spaces). Those who suffer with panic disorder can become extremely anxious about suffering another panic attack, as they fear the frightening experience.

Obsessive–compulsive disorder (OCD)

The patient will experience obsessions and associated compulsions. Obsessions are intrusive thoughts or images, which are negative in nature (e.g. a belief that something deadly will happen, images of people dying, a fear of paedophilic thoughts). The patient may experience compulsions which, when carried out, can provide some immediate but not long-standing relief from the symptoms. The compulsions can start to affect daily living, intruding on time and ability to function in employment.

Examples of OCD
- A fear of contracting a deadly infectious disease (obsession) may result in compulsive hand-washing (compulsion).
- A belief that something bad will happen to love ones (obsession) may result in a switching the light switches on and off 33 times (compulsion).

Hypochondriasis/health anxiety

Is the obsessional idea that the sufferer has an undiagnosed medical condition, often cancer or HIV, and will repeatedly request investigations to assess for the specific condition, only being temporarily satisfied with a negative result. Sufferers may also believe they have a serious illness with the experience of symptoms (e.g. experiencing a headache will precipitate the worry of a brain tumour). The anxiety experienced may cause physical symptoms which further perpetuate the idea that there is a serious medical issue.

Somatization disorder

Is the physical manifestation of psychological phenomenon where the patient experiences variable physical symptoms (GI, dermatological, cardiovascular such as chest pain, breathlessness, etc.) with no confirmed medical diagnosis. The symptoms must be present for at least 2 years. Often the sufferer will seek medical help or self-medicate to alleviate the symptoms. The difference between somatization disorder and hypochondriasis is that in somatization disorder, the sufferer does not fixate on a specific diagnosis.

Schizophrenia in the community

Patients diagnosed with schizophrenia in the community attend outpatient appointments regularly to manage their medication and side effect profile. Those on depot medication will attend either fortnightly or monthly for their depot and will be reviewed by a CPN. They should also have annual blood tests and a physical health screen either by the CMHT or their GP.

Honours

Treatment-resistant schizophrenia

A person is diagnosed with treatment-resistant schizophrenia if they have tried two different antipsychotic medications at a therapeutic dose for 6 weeks or more and their symptoms are still uncontrolled. Clozapine is an antipsychotic medication that can be used in these cases.

Psychiatry: the specialties

There are subspecialties within psychiatry that you should experience.

Older adult

The older adult wards treat older adults diagnosed with psychosis and mood disorders similar to those present in the general adult population. The older adult service also aids with diagnosis and management of dementia. See Table 29.2.

There are several formal cognitive assessments to assess for dementia. The ward staff will have access to the assessment templates including the MMSE, Addenbrooke's Cognitive Examination III (ACE-R), clock drawing test, and frontal lobe tests. Practise on each other for fluency and then assess patients.

Table 29.2 Types of dementia

Dementia	Pathological Characteristics	Symptoms
Alzheimer's disease	Protein build-up in brain to form plaques and tangles	Short-term memory loss—forgetting appointments, forgetting location of day-to-day items (e.g. keys), forgetting recent events
Vascular dementia	Reduced blood supply to areas of brain through small strokes	Memory loss occurs later in comparison to Alzheimer's Impairment of executive function
Frontotemporal dementia	Atrophy of frontal and temporal lobes over time	Significant behavioural/personality changes Progressive language difficulties Difficulties with comprehension
Dementia with Lewy bodies	Deposits of Lewy body protein in cortical areas	Impaired executive function Fluctuating alertness/attention over the course of the day Visual hallucinations Eventual motor coordination symptoms as in Parkinson's
Parkinson's dementia	Linked to deposits of Lewy bodies in brainstem	Differs from dementia with Lewy bodies as motor impairment occurs first Memory loss Loss of executive function Emotional volatility Visual hallucinations
Posterior cortical atrophy PCA (Honours)	Similar to Alzheimer's affecting posterior region of the brain	Initially problems with recognizing faces/objects but persevered memory. There may be issues with literacy
Progressive supranuclear palsy (PSP) (Honours)	Linked to tau protein deposits.	Problems with balance/steadiness Frequent falls Supranuclear ophthalmoplegia

Liaison psychiatry team

Is based in general hospitals and consist of psychiatrists and psychiatric liaison nurses who will review inpatients on the general wards with regard to their mental health. These may be patients who have comorbid mental health issues but are being treated for their physical health or patients who have been admitted for a mental health issue (e.g. deliberate self-harm) but require medical input first. The psychiatric liaison nurses will review patients presenting to the ED with mental health problems.

Home treatment team

(Sometimes known as the crisis team.) Is staffed by psychiatrists and psychiatric nurses, who deliver intensive care for weeks in the community. They provide a 24-hour community service, and will review patients once a day administering medication and monitoring their mental state. The inpatient teams may refer to the home treatment team to monitor a patient being discharged, or CMHT may refer a patient whose mental state deteriorates with the aim that intense community input will prevent admission.

Child and Adolescent Mental Health Services (CAMHS)

The optimal outcome is to be able to sit in on an assessment with a family but this may not occur due to the age of the child or refusal of the family.

Learning point: diagnosis and management of …
- attention deficit hyperactivity disorder (ADHD)
- autistic spectrum disorder (ASD)
- deliberate self-harm in the community (keeping the young person safe at home and school).

Eating disorders

There may be opportunity to attend an inpatient or day patient service.

Learning points
- Familiarize with diagnostic criteria for anorexia nervosa and bulimia.
- Re-feeding syndrome.
- Psychotherapeutic interventions available (group therapy, cognitive analytical therapy).

Honours

ASD assessment considers the following areas:
- Communication
- Reciprocal social interaction
- Creativity/imagination
- Repetitive/restrictive behaviour.

ADHD is a constellation of symptoms of inattention, hyperactivity, and impulsivity. The symptoms must be present for 6 months and onset before the age of 7 years.

Trivia
In the ICD-10, ADHD does not exist as a diagnosis, rather it is known as hyperkinetic disorder.

Learning disability
A half-day/day placement in the learning disability inpatient or outpatient service is rare as often a trust will have one team covering a large area.

Learning points
- Management of agitation/behavioural changes.
- Management of comorbid psychosis.

Substance misuse services
As well as addictions outpatient services, detoxing patients may also be seen on acute inpatient wards or with the psychiatry liaison team in general hospital.

Learning points
- Familiarize with common medications used in detox such as chlordiazepoxide (Librium®), acamprosate, and methadone.
- Use of CIWA scale to monitor effects of alcohol withdrawal.
- Questionnaires to assess for harmful alcohol use (e.g. AUDIT questionnaire).

Honours
Eating disorders
Anorexia nervosa
- Intentional weight loss (BMI <17.5 kg/m^2).
- Disturbed perception of body image.
- Morbid fear of obesity.
- Physical signs: include dry yellow skin, fine blonde hairs (lanugo), bradycardia, hypotension, anaemia, and complications of recurrent vomiting (hypokalaemia, alkalosis, and poor dentition). Russel sign is calluses on the back of the hand from repeated and chronic self-induced vomiting.

Bulimia nervosa
- Binge eating sessions (>2000 kcal).
- Excessive compensatory behaviour (e.g. diuretics, laxatives, fasting or exercise).
- Morbid fear of obesity.

Psychiatry: in exams

Taking a history

General advice

A good history is the backbone of psychiatric diagnosis, with the bulk of clinical examination and investigations used to rule out organic causes. The history is comprehensive and relies on collateral history from family, previous discharge summaries, and from the patient's GP.

Psychiatric assessment

Mode of admission

How the patient presented to hospital (e.g. under section 136 or as a walk-in).

History of presenting complaint

- What symptoms have caused the patient to present—explore each in depth considering length of symptom and current impact on patient's life, e.g. are they able to continue working, have they stopped eating?
- Triggers that may have caused the admission, e.g. significant life event, non-compliance with medication.

Past psychiatric history

- Previous admissions to hospital—informal or under section.
- Previous treatment options—oral medication, depot medication, ECT.
- Previous therapies—CBT, individual psychotherapy, group therapy.

Past medical history

- Any current/past medical conditions.
- Usually confirmed by the GP.

Medication history

- Any current medication use.
- Usually confirmed by the GP.
- Any medication allergies.

Family history

- Family history of mental health conditions.
- Usually gained through collateral history from family members.

Personal history

- Developmental history (including pregnancy, reaching developmental milestones—may require input from family members or GP).
- Educational history.
- Family circumstances during childhood.
- Significant relationships.
- Employment history.

Social history

- Current housing situation.
- Current employment situation.
- Current relationship status.
- Any dependent children.

Alcohol and substance use
- Current alcohol use (quantify units per week, binge-drinking).
- Any physical symptoms secondary to long-term alcohol misuse.
- History of substance use (quantify amount used per week).
- Previous history of attending rehabilitation facilities (e.g. inpatient, Alcoholics Anonymous).

Forensic history
- Any arrests or time served in prison—note the dates and history of allegations or convictions.
- Note specifically history of violence to others.

Premorbid personality
- Usually provided by family members or the GP.

The history is concluded with a mental state examination, risk assessment, and summary/formulation. The mental state examination (MSE) provides a snapshot of how the patient is at the moment of assessment. This can help in the future to identify deterioration or assess improvement. Do not confuse the *MSE* with the *MMSE* (Mini-Mental State Examination)!

Mental state examination (mnemonic ASEPTIC)

- *Appearance/behaviour*: provide a snapshot of what the patient looked like at that moment. Comment on their ethnicity, general appearance (clothes, are they well-kempt?), and the quality of the interaction: was the rapport good, did they maintain good eye contact, were they agitated, pacing, violent, drowsy, etc.?
- *Speech*: describe the tone, rate, and volume of speech, e.g. angry tone, pressured speech (suggestive of a manic state) or slow (depression), loudly or quietly.
- Emotion/*Mood and affect*: consider both subjective mood and objective affect.
  - *Subjective*—in patient's own words, how would they describe their mood, what is their mood between 1 (the worse it has ever been) and 10 (the best it has ever been)?
  - *Objective*—how do you perceive the patient's mood: low, elated—and their affect—flattened or labile?
- *Thoughts*: comment on whether there is formal thought disorder. Consider the content of the thoughts (are they paranoid, grandiose, suicidal, delusions, obsessions?). Is there any thought possession (withdrawal, insertion or broadcasting)?
- *Perceptions*: is the patient experiencing any perceptual abnormality—comment on the nature of hallucinations (auditory, somatic, visual).
- *Cognition*: is the patient orientated to time, place, and person? Consider doing a MMSE or further cognitive testing if appropriate.
- *Insight*: assess the patient's insight. Do they understand why they are in hospital? Do they believe they have a mental illness? How do they feel about taking medication? Assess their judgement and ability to problem-solve.

The risk assessment is dynamic and levels of risk change over time. The assessment provides a summary of historic and current concerns around risk.

Risk assessment

- *Risk to self*: has the patient had an episode of self-harm/suicide attempt in this admission? Has the patient harmed themselves or attempted suicide in the past? It is important to give details of the suicide attempts. Does the patient currently express suicidal ideation?
- *Risk to others*: has the patient been violent to staff/other patients/ family members/strangers during this admission? Is there a past history of violence towards anyone? Has the patient ever been admitted to the PICU for violent behaviour? Do they have any criminal convictions following violence in hospital? Does the patient have any children or vulnerable adults in their care?
- *Risk from others*: is the patient particularly vulnerable? Has there been neglect from carers? Is the patient at risk of manipulation from others (e.g. financially)?
- *Risk of neglect*: has the patient been caring for themselves? Are they malnourished? Do they have any significant medical conditions that have been neglected?
- *Risk of absconding*: has the patient absconded during this admission? Does the patient have a history of absconding? Have they been admitted to PICU due to their persistent attempts at absconding?

The assessment is concluded with a summary or formulation of the presenting problem, ongoing stressors, and current risk.

Honours

Formulation

Consider the following for the current presentation:

- *Predisposing factors*: what predisposes the individual (e.g. genetic, environmental etc.)?
- *Precipitating factors*: what triggered the episode?
- *Perpetuation factors*: what ongoing issues contribute (e.g. homelessness, substance misuse)?
- *Protective factors*: what helps the individual/prevents worsening (e.g. supportive family, good relationship with CPN)?

Tips for exams

Clinical examination

- Be sure to use lots of open questions.
- Consider 'why now', as in why has the patient attended now or why have the symptoms precipitated now?
- Be sure to ask about compliance with medication.
- Ask about alcohol and substance use.
- Ask about any significant life events.
- Ask about how the patient feels about their diagnosis (insight) and what help they hope to gain from attending hospital/clinic.

See Tables 29.3–29.5 for common drugs and side effects.

Table 29.3 Antidepressants

Class	Drug	Common side effects
SSRI (selective serotonin reuptake inhibitors)	Fluoxetine Sertraline Citalopram Paroxetine	GI symptoms, dizziness, insomnia, weight gain, tremor, sweating
SNRI (serotonin-norepinephrine reuptake inhibitors)	Venlafaxine Mirtazapine	Fatigue, weight gain, dry mouth, blurred vision
TCA (tricyclic antidepressants)	Amitriptyline Clomipramine	GI symptoms, sun sensitivity, difficulty passing urine, blurred vision

Table 29.4 Antipsychotics

Antipsychotic	Side effects
First generation	
Chlorpromazine	Severe sedative effects, moderate EPSEs
Haloperidol	Pronounced EPSEs, moderate sedative effects
Sulpiride	Moderate sedative, antimuscarinic and EPSEs
Second generation	
Olanzapine	↑Appetite and weight gain, drowsiness, GI symptoms
Quetiapine	Dry mouth, drowsiness, GI symptoms, ↑appetite
Risperidone	Dizziness, EPSEs, restlessness
Amisulpride	Drowsiness, GI symptoms, weight gain, dry mouth
Aripiprazole	Dizziness, GI symptoms
Clozapine	Weight gain, GI symptoms, hypersalivation Neutropenia (incidence 2%) Agranulocytosis (incidence 0.8%)

EPSE, extrapyramidal side effect.

Table 29.5 Mood stabilizers

Drug	Common side effects
Lithium	GI symptoms, fine tremor, thirst, frequent urination, fatigue
Sodium valproate	GI symptoms, ↑appetite, hair loss
Carbamazepine	GI symptoms, dry mouth, drowsiness, unsteadiness

Respiratory medicine

Respiratory medicine: overview

Respiratory medicine is a medical speciality dealing with disorders of the respiratory system. The predominant population are patients with chronic lung disease often related to smoking.

Cases to see

In clinic

COPD

Such patients are not hard to find—in fact they can be found almost everywhere. These patients are usually managed by their GP in the community, but may be referred to clinic if difficult to treat and for ↑frequency of exacerbations.

Asthma

Much like COPD, asthmatic patients can be found almost anywhere. While most are managed by the GP in the community, patients with more severe asthma can be followed up in clinic. You may also see acute asthma attacks and refractory cases presenting to ED who will need at least admission if not further intervention such as intubation.

Cancer

Lung cancer is managed by a MDT so you may find it more useful to attend thoracic clinics to learn about the non-operative and operative interventions offered by the oncologists and surgeons respectively.

Interstitial lung disease/occupational pneumonitis

These patients are distinctively shared by the respiratory team as well as an immunologist to identify their triggers. You will find these patients in clinic with long-term follow-up.

Sleep apnoea

This is becoming an increasingly common problem due to obesity rates in developed countries. You can find these patients in respiratory clinic with consultations with bariatric surgeons and sleep study suites.

Bronchiectasis

You can find these patients in clinic as long-term follow-up. This disease is commoner in adults including those with recurrent pneumonia, auto-immunity, and extraintestinal features of IBD. Children with cystic fibrosis and those immunocompromised (e.g. AIDS → recurrent pneumonia → destruction of elastic tissue → scarring) are also susceptible.

Cystic fibrosis

Patients are going to be children and adolescents followed up both in the community and the clinic. Since most patients are children, most exacerbations will be admitted onto paediatric ward. Extrapulmonary manifestations (e.g. endocrine, GI, subfertility) are also followed up in respective outpatients.

In the ED

Respiratory failure

There are two types: type 1 (hypoxic and known as 'pink puffers') and type 2 (hypoxic and hypercapnic also known as 'blue bloaters'). Patients with chronic failure are managed by the GP but are also followed up in clinics with specialist respiratory nurses and physicians. Acute exacerbations present to ED where patient ought to be thoroughly investigated for reversible causes.

Pneumonia

Depending on the extent of dyspnoea, pyrexia, and dehydration, patients may require admission for IV antibiotics and hydration especially if there is another respiratory comorbidity such as asthma or COPD. Otherwise, community-acquired pneumonias are frequently treated in the community.

Acute exacerbations asthma and COPD

You will see patients (children with asthma and adults with COPD who smoke) with acute dyspnoea from either infective or non-infective causes who almost always require at least monitoring on the wards for a few days if not antibiotics and steroids. Refractory asthma attacks (status asthmaticus) is a medical emergency and may need sedation, intubation and ventilation on the ITU.

Pulmonary embolism

This is a medical emergency in which not only does the treatment need to commence immediately, but any underlying disease or reversible causes need to be addressed to prevent further propagation of clots. Patients will present with dyspnoea, pleuritic chest pain, and possibly haemoptysis.

Pulmonary oedema

You will encounter patients with dyspnoea, a wet persistent cough, and fluid overload who cannot manage their symptoms with oral medication (e.g. diuretics) at home. The underlying cause is often cardiac and/or renal failure or hypoalbuminaemia. Patients need to be admitted for offloading and (sometimes invasive) monitoring.

Pleural effusion

Moderately sized effusions will present as ↑severity of dyspnoea. As well as treatment, the underlying disease/cause ought to be investigated and treated. Beware of chylothorax (lymph fluid) or haemothorax (blood) in trauma patients with penetrating injuries (e.g. stab).

Pneumothorax

Leakage of air into the pleuritic space can be disastrous! Tension pneumothorax where the mediastinum and trachea shift away is a medical emergency. May either be primary (spontaneous) or due to trauma (e.g. penetrating injury).

Procedures and investigations to see
CXR
These are ubiquitous in any speciality and you will undoubtedly be expected to present them at ward rounds and in clinics.

Bronchoscopy
You will be able to attend theatre lists of bronchoscopy conducted either by the respiratory or the cardiothoracic teams. You will be expected to know about the procedure, its indications, contraindications, and complications, to consent a patient confidently in your exams.

Chest drain
You will be able to see these inserted on the ward for stable patients or in a resuscitation bay for trauma patients with haemo/pneumothorax.

Pneumothorax/fluid aspiration
Pleurocentesis is a procedure that can save lives but it is important to understand the key anatomical landmarks for doing one to avoid iatrogenic injury. These often be seen in a resuscitation bay with tension pneumothorax. Fluid aspirations diagnose content of pleural effusions.

Spirometry
This is also known as pulmonary function tests and depicts spirograms of flow (litres per second) against volume. Flow–volume loops may also be another option. Differences in loop shapes are observed between restrictive and obstructive pulmonary diseases as well as acute obstruction. This investigation is usually conducted in the outpatient clinic. (See Fig. 30.1.)

Computed tomography pulmonary angiogram (CTPA) and ventilation (V)/perfusion (Q) mismatch scans
Rule out pulmonary embolism. CTPA may be contraindicated in pregnancy in which the older V/Q scan modality is suitable. You can also discuss which modality is optimal in various clinical scenarios.

Non-invasive ventilation (NIV)
Is usually seen on either the respiratory ward or HDU/ITU.

Pleurodesis
In refractory cases of pleural effusions, obliterating the pleural space with tetracycline, bleomycin, or talcum powder.

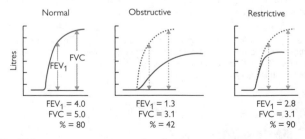

Fig. 30.1 Spirometry. Reproduced with permission from Wilkinson, Ian, et al, *Oxford Handbook of Clinical Medicine* 10e, 2017: Oxford University Press.

Respiratory medicine: in clinic

Lung disease causing shortness of breath is classified into obstructive or restrictive disease, strictly based on spirometry.

Obstructive

Most commonly asthma and COPD (forced expiratory volume in 1 sec (FEV_1)/FVC <0.8, FEV_1 <80% predicted) causing reduced airflow due to bronchoconstriction or obstruction (mucosal inflammation and ↑mucus).

Restrictive

Intrinsic lung fibrosis (most commonly interstitial pulmonary fibrosis) or extrinsic chest wall disease (e.g. myasthenia gravis, Guillain–Barré; FEV_1/FVC >0.8) leads to a chest which is difficult to expand.

Asthma

Is typified by reversibility of airway obstruction, diurnal variation in symptoms/PEFR (worse in mornings), associated with atopy (eczema, hay fever, allergy), occasionally with clear precipitants (e.g. allergens, cold air, smoking). In the clinic, emphasis will be on optimizing disease control, utilizing a stepwise escalation in medication beginning with short-acting beta agonists (SABAs, e.g. salbutamol) and inhaled steroids (e.g. beclometasone) to long-acting beta agonists (LABAs, e.g. salmeterol) and oral steroids. Aminophylline and anticholinergics (e.g. ipratropium) may also be added (see British Thoracic Society (BTS) guidelines: ℘ www.brit-thoracic.org.uk).

Obstructive sleep apnoea

Is intermittent pharyngeal collapse in the obese. There is a characteristic history of snoring (and apnoeic episodes described by patients' partners) and daytime somnolence. Treatment includes weight loss, CPAP, and surgery as a last resort.

COPD

Is a spectrum of lung disease due to smoking which encompasses chronic bronchitis (defined clinically) and emphysema (defined histologically). Elements of both are likely to be present. There is little or no reversibility of airway obstruction, minimal diurnal variation, and greater association with sputum production, chronic dyspnoea, and older age of onset (>35 years). Clinical presentation consists of persistent cough/sputum on most days for 3 months for 2 consecutive years. Manifestations of COPD as type 1 and type 2 respiratory failure are described as 'pink puffer' (normal/low PCO_2 due to ↑ventilation) and 'blue bloater' (cyanosis, hypercapnia with hypoxia driving ventilation) respectively. You will see these patients being managed in the ED following acute exacerbations, often infective, or end-stage in decompensated respiratory failure/cor pulmonale. Medical management is similar to asthma using bronchodilators and inhaled steroids, and stratified by severity as per BTS guidelines, with long-term oxygen therapy considered in later disease for some patients. (See Fig. 30.2.)

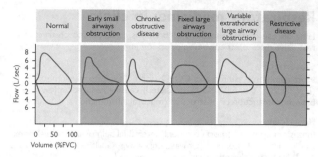

Fig. 30.2 Flow volume. Reproduced with permission from Jonathan Wilkinson et al, *Thoracic Anaesthesia*, 2011, Oxford University Press.

Sarcoidosis

A multiorgan (pulmonary, neurological, cardiac, GI, cutaneous, etc.) syndrome of unknown cause resulting in granulomas. Pulmonary symptoms include dry cough, reduced exercise tolerance, and progressive dyspnoea. CXR may show bilateral hilar lymphadenopathy ± infiltrations, bullae, cysts, and fibrosis). Patients may also present with symptoms related to hypercalcaemia. Blood test shows elevated calcium and angiotensin-converting enzyme concentrations. Treat with immunosuppression (steroids, antimetabolites, biological, and chemotherapy, etc.).

Cystic fibrosis

Involves a mutation of the *CFTR* gene on chromosome 7 (incidence 1:2000, autosomal recessive). The pathology involves thick alveolar secretions → chronic infection → bronchiectasis. Complex cases may be managed in tertiary centres, receiving multidisciplinary respiratory support (antibiotics, mucolytics, bronchodilators), GI support (pancreatic enzyme replacement and nutritional supplementation), and fertility support, and may eventually require lung or liver transplant. Look for extrarespiratory signs.

Interstitial lung disease

Is a general term describing diffuse inflammation and/or fibrosis of the lung interstitium (i.e. space between alveoli). This restrictive pathology is most commonly idiopathic or can be associated with connective tissue disorders (SLE, RA), environmental exposure (asbestosis, bird droppings), and drugs (nitrofurantoin), etc. Regardless, the principles of treatment are similar: trigger avoidance, supplemental O_2, and a trial of corticosteroids.

Lung cancer

Is classified histologically into small cell (20%) or non-small cell (80% squamous, adenocarcinoma, large cell), and is primarily due to smoking. Presentation results from tumour mass (cough, wheeze, dyspnoea), local invasion (chest pain, haemoptysis, hoarse voice), and metastatic (bone pain) and paraneoplastic features (e.g. Cushing's, hypercalcaemia). Attend the radiology MDT to observe imaging (CT, PET/CT, bone scan) and biopsy list in theatres (lung/lymph node where possible—bronchoscopic or transthoracic). These results assist with assessment and planning treatment. In general, most lung cancers have poor prognosis with small cell lung cancer generally disseminated at presentation, and relapse after chemotherapy with 3-month median survival (cf. 8 months for stage IV non-small cell lung cancer). Rarer cancers include malignant mesothelioma (related to asbestosis).

Bronchiectasis

Is also a chronic obstructive airways disease, characterized by permanent dilatation of the bronchi due to destructive/inflammation from infection. Less common congenital causes include cystic fibrosis and those with primary immunodeficiencies. You can expect to see treatment with similar medications as COPD/asthma, with antibiotics for exacerbations. (See Fig. 30.3.)

Investigations

CXR

Plain radiographs of the chest provide important information and is a low-risk non-invasive investigation. The radiation dose is equivalent to 3 days' worth of background radiation. Views include posteroanterior (PA) which

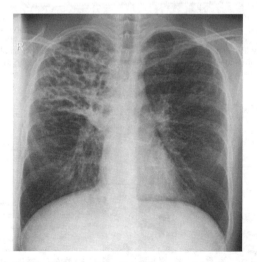

Fig. 30.3. CXR showing abnormal dilatation of the airways of the right upper lobe. Appearances are that of bronchiectasis. The fine background reticular lung pattern may indicate interstitial lung disease. Reproduced with permission from Wilkinson, Ian, et al, *Oxford Handbook of Clinical Medicine* 10e, 2017: Oxford University Press. Image courtesy of Nottingham University Hospitals NHS Trust Radiology Department.

is the most common, followed by anteroposterior (AP) which is usually done if the patient is too ill and supine, and lateral which is uncommon but helpful in delineating size and location of loculations for drainage under image guidance. These can be presented using the **ABCDE** method (see Fig. 30.4.)

Bronchoscopy

Endoscopy of the bronchial tree for diagnostics (malignancy, interstitial lung disease), and therapeutic purposes (aspiration mucus plugs). Most commonly flexible, but rigid under GA for retrieving a large foreign body and electrocautery for massive haemoptysis. The lung may be biopsied under image guidance (e.g. CT) transbronchially, percutaneously, or at video-assisted thoracic surgery (see ➜ pp. 643–4). *Complications*: infection, bleeding and perforation.

Chest drain

A tube into the pleural space to remove air/fluid/pus. You may see large-bore 'surgical' drains (e.g. trauma or draining haemothorax), while the respiratory ward is more likely to site Seldinger chest drains. Chest drain swinging—fluid in tube moving back and forth subtly with respiration—meaning the drain is in communication with the pleural space. Analysis of the fluid obtained—transudate vs exudate (including empyema) and Light's criteria (pathology).

Peak flow

It is useful to have practised this first. Refer to a copy of predictive values to get an appreciation of numbers. This measures FEV_1 values which are compared on a graph adjusted for age, height, and sex. Peak flow is often used to establish a rudimentary baseline of respiratory function and to observe effect of inhalers and nebulizers. Please find a suitable patient on the ward who is willing to perform one for you.

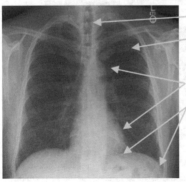

A – *airway* – exclude tracheal deviation in tension pneumothorax
B – *breathing* – exclude pulmonary oedema, pneumothorax, consolidations, coin lesions and pleural effusions from both lung fields
C – *circulation* – look for size and shape of heart and aortic knuckle
D – *diaphragm* – exclude blunting of cardiophrenic + costophrenic recesses
E – *everything else* which are easily missed but may be catastrophic to the patient. These include rib fractures, subcutaneous surgical emphysema and ensure to exclude a pneumothorax again which is a medical emergency.

Fig. 30.4 Chest radiograph. Amended from Wikipedia under creative commons license.

V/Q mismatch scan

This is not a common investigation. However, if you have spare time during your block you may wish to find out if any are being conducted at your nuclear medicine department.

Spirometry

There will be a respiratory investigations department where spirometry takes place, typically for new diagnoses of lung disease and preoperative assessments. Familiarize yourself with the typical appearance of obstructive and restrictive flow loops. The most important values are FEV_1—speed of flow (impaired in obstructive), FVC (reduced in restrictive disease); the FEV_1/FVC ratio is ↑ in restrictive disease (reduction in FVC >>FEV_1) and vice versa with obstructive disease.

ABG

Most students qualify without being able to confidently perform arterial blood for analysis. This will cause you many wasted hours stressed on-call without fulfilling a basic requirement of a junior doctor. Use this rotation to ensure you do not find yourself in this position as many respiratory patients require multiple arterial samples. Try to see arterial punctures in multiple locations (radial >femoral). Before arterial sampling of the wrist, perform *Allen's test*.

CTPA

You will never be required to state definitively whether a CTPA shows evidence or not of a PE; albeit, you might be interested and ask your consultant to point out key features of the CT (origin and path of the pulmonary artery) as it is relatively simple to see deficits representing embolus to impress your bosses in future.

Non-invasive ventilation

Comes in two basic forms: CPAP continuous pressure support for type 1 respiratory failure represents splinting airway open (e.g. pulmonary oedema), and BPAP (bilevel positive airway pressure or non-invasive positive pressure ventilation) with IPAP pressure applied during triggered breaths and expiratory positive airway pressure (EPAP) (continuous positive pressure) between breaths.

Respiratory medicine: in the emergency department

Respiratory failure

- *Airway*: assess and manage airway using manoeuvres/adjuncts.
- *Breathing*: assess respiratory effort, 15 L/min O_2, if no respiratory effort → arrest team.
- *Circulation*: capillary refill time, pulse, BP, if no pulse → arrest team.

Respiratory failure is failure of ventilation or gas exchange. Hypoxia can be due to V/Q mismatch (commonest), hypoventilation (+raised CO_2), abnormal diffusion, right–left cardiac shunt. VQ mismatch may be due to inadequate ventilation (e.g. pneumonia) or inadequate perfusion (e.g. PE).
- *Type I failure*: PaO_2 <8 kPa, $PaCO_2$ <6 kPa
- *Type II failure* PaO_2 <6 kPa, $PaCO_2$ >6 kPa.

Pneumonia

Implies infection within the airways. As a junior doctor, it is one of the pathologies that you will frequently encounter in ED/wards and should be familiar with assessment and management. Community-acquired pneumonia is commonly caused by *Staphylococcus aureus* and *Streptococcus pneumoniae*; hospital-acquired pneumonia is commonly caused by Gram-negative organisms; while aspiration pneumonia is commonly secondary to anaerobes. It is worth practising using the CURB-65 score as a guide to determine which patients should be admitted for treatment, and looking at the CXR of these patients (comparing them to previous CXRs). Also take blood samples, blood cultures, ABG (if hypoxic), sputum sample, and urinary antigens (pneumococcal and *Legionella*). Treatment is with oxygen (keep sats >94%), antibiotics, and hydration as well as steroid in asthma/COPD as per local protocol. Admit if CURB-65 score >2, hypoxic, septic, comorbidities, requiring IV antibiotics, or unable to cope at home. A repeat CXR is indicated 6 weeks afterwards which is the time it takes for radiological resolution to occur. (See Fig. 30.5.)

CURB-65

Is a simple, validated scoring system. See Table 30.1 and Table 30.2.

Acute exacerbation of asthma

Is characterized by the inability of complete full sentences, tachypnoea, PEFR <50%, with normal $PaCO_2$. Beware of silent chest! You must elicit whether the patient has ever been intubated or admitted to ITU before. Also, look to exclude any triggering allergens and foreign travel. Triggers can be remembered as **SAUCES**:
- Stress
- Allergy
- URTIs
- Cold air
- Exercise
- Smoke.

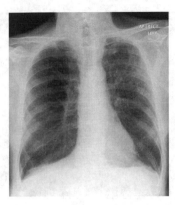

Fig. 30.5 Air space heterogeneous shadowing in the left upper zone with air bronchograms demonstrating a consolidation likely to represent pneumonia. However, since this is non-specific, you ought to rule out other differentials from a history and clinical examination. Reproduced with permission from Wilkinson, Ian, et al, *Oxford Handbook of Clinical Medicine* 10e, 2017: Oxford University Press. Image courtesy of Nottingham University Hospitals NHS Trust Radiology Department.

Table 30.1 CURB-65 scoring

C	Confusion—abbreviated mental test ≤8/10	1
U	Urea >7 mmol/L	1
R	Respiratory rate ≥30/min	1
B	BP <90 mmHg systolic and/or 60 mmHg diastolic	1
65	Age ≥65 years	1

Table 30.2 CURB-65 scoring results

Score	Mortality risk 30 days	Management
0–1	Mild (<3%)	Home treatment possible
2	Moderate (9%)	Hospital therapy
≥3	Severe (15–45%)	Severe pneumonia—consider ITU support

Radiological signs include hyperinflation and diaphragm flattening but other pathologies such as pneumothorax, pneumomediastinum, and pneumonia ought to be excluded swiftly. (See Fig. 30.6.)

The BTS has guidelines for each of these (⅏ www.brit-thoracic.org.uk). Do not forget oxygen is a drug and should be prescribed, including flow rate, target SpO_2, and mode of delivery (e.g. nasal prongs/face mask). Decide

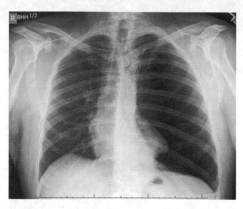

Fig. 30.6 Acute exacerbation of asthma. Reproduced with permission from Scott Moses, MD, www.fpnotebook.com.

Table 30.3 Asthma

Moderate	Severe	Life-threatening	Near fatal
Increasing symptoms	*Any 1 of:*	*Any 1 of:*	↑PaCO₂ and/or requiring mechanical ventilation with ↑inflation pressures
PEFR >50–75% best or predicted	PEFR 33–50% best or predicted	PEFR <33% best or predicted	
No features of acute severe asthma	Resp. rate ≥25/ min	SpO₂ <92%	
	HR ≥110/min	PaO₂ <8 kPa	
	Inability to complete a sentence in one breath	Normal PaCO₂ (4.6–6.0 kPa)	
		Silent chest	
		Cyanosis	
		Poor respiratory effort	
		Arrhythmia	

if the exacerbation is mild, moderate, severe, life-threatening, or near fatal (see Table 30.3).

Be on the lookout for exhaustion as time goes by whereby the patient struggles to breathe more and more. Since younger patients have a greater physiological reserve whereby they can compensate for longer compared to the elderly, they can also deteriorate much more rapidly once decompensation occurs. If you struggle, it is best to call the on-call or crash team anaesthetist sooner rather than later. NIV followed by intubation may be the last resort but still takes time to prepare and set up before it could become too late.

Treatment can sometimes be very difficult as it may not always work. This is when you think of **OH SPIT MAN** (Table 30.4).

Table 30.4 OH SPIT MAN

O	Oxygen (aim for SpO2 94–98%)
H	Hydration (IV fluids)
S	Salbutamol nebulizers (5 mg back-to-back if necessary)
P	Prednisolone (30–40 mg PO) or hydrocortisone (200 mg IV)
I	Ipratropium bromide (Atrovent®) nebulizers (5 mcg 4–6-hourly)
T	Transfer to HDU/ITU (if suspecting life-threatening asthma)
M	Magnesium sulfate
A	Aminophylline (antibiotics if infective cause)
N	NIV and intubation if tiring

A classic exam scenario is the management of an asthmatic patient who deteriorates due to the development of a pneumothorax. Consider discharging patients whose PEFR is >75% best or predicted 1 hour after initial treatment. Give a 5-day course of prednisolone (30–40 mg once daily), check inhaler technique, and advise GP follow-up within the next 48 hours or to return to hospital if symptoms recur.

Acute exacerbation of COPD

Consider the diagnosis in smokers >35 years with exertional breathlessness, chronic cough, regular sputum production, frequent winter 'bronchitis', or wheeze. Spirometry can support the diagnosis (FEV_1/FVC ratio <0.7). An exacerbation is a sustained worsening of symptoms which is beyond normal day-to-day variations, and is acute in onset. Symptoms include worsening breathlessness, cough, ↑sputum production, and change in sputum colour. Patients with COPD are at higher risk of acute deterioration, which is most commonly secondary to infection. Patients with asthma/COPD may benefit from specific antibiotics to cover certain organisms, as well as optimization of their chronic disease. Treatment is similar to asthma exacerbation with a few exceptions:

- Target SpO_2 88–92% initially. If $PaCO_2$ is normal adjust target to 94–98% (unless there is a history of NIV/intermittent positive pressure ventilation) and recheck ABGs after 30–60 min
- Nebulizers: salbutamol and ipratropium. If a patient is hypercapnic or acidotic the nebulizer should be driven by compressed air, not oxygen (to avoid worsening hypercapnia). Oxygen can be given simultaneously by nasal cannulae if needed.
- Prednisolone 30 mg PO for 7–14 days. Consider osteoporosis prophylaxis in patients requiring frequent courses of oral corticosteroids.
- NIV for persistent hypercapnic ventilatory failure despite optimal medical therapy. Before starting NIV, the ceiling of therapy should be agreed (i.e. is invasive ventilation appropriate?).

To ask the boss

Relative merits of steroids in exacerbations of chronic lung disease
- Consider the anti-inflammatory effect on chronic lung disease.
- Doubling steroid supplementation in steroid-dependent septic patient at risk of Addisonian crisis.
- Immunosuppressive effect in infections.

Pulmonary embolism

Describes an embolus thrombus in the pulmonary vasculature impairing gas exchange. Sudden-onset dyspnoea and pleuritic chest pain in the presence of type 1 respiratory failure. Other signs include syncope, haemoptysis, and even cardiac arrest in large PEs. Virchow's triad describes risk factors for all VTEs including PEs. Practise calculating two-level Well's scores[1] to aid your diagnosis; <4 is unlikely and D-dimer may be used to rule out PE (sensitive not specific). (See Table 30.5.)

Investigations

- *ABG*: may initially present with respiratory alkalosis from hyperventilating before decompensating (towards metabolic acidosis).
- *ECG*: may be normal or show sinus tachycardia, p pulmonale, AF, right bundle branch block, right axis deviation ('S1'), Q wave and inverted T in III ('Q3, T3'), T inversion in V1–4. S1Q3T3 on ECG is said to be *pathognomonic* but it is rare, and you are more likely to see a sinus tachycardia, right axis deviation, or right bundle branch block indicating right heart strain.
- *CXR*: to exclude other causes.
- *FBC, INR, APTT, U&E*: WCC may be high.
- *CTPA*: the gold standard; V/Q mismatch scan may be considered in pregnancy to avoid contrast and radiation.

Table 30.5 Two-level PE Wells score

Clinical feature	Points
Clinical signs and symptoms of DVT (minimum of leg swelling and pain with palpation of the deep veins)	3
An alternative diagnosis less likely than PE	3
HR >100 bpm	1.5
Immobilization for >3 days or surgery in the previous 4 weeks	1.5
Previous DVT/PE	1.5
Haemoptysis	1
Malignancy (on treatment/treated in the last 6 months/palliative)	1
Clinical probability simplified scores	
PE *likely*	>4
PE *unlikely*	<4

- *PE likely*: immediate *CTPA* or if not available, parenteral anticoagulation followed by CTPA. Consider a proximal leg vein US scan if the CTPA is negative and DVT is suspected.
- *PE unlikely*: D-dimer, and if positive → CTPA.

Management

Usually consists of treatment dose of anticoagulation (LMWH/ fondaparinux) within 24 hours for 5 days until warfarinized and INR ≥2; rarely haemodynamic instability necessitates unfractionated heparin and thrombolysis (know the contraindications). Warfarin needs to be continued for at least 3 months for first time VTE, extended therapy duration for second recurrence (if risk of bleeding is low), and indefinitely if recurrent VTEs with irreversible risk factors (deficiency in antithrombin III, protein S and C, factor V Leiden mutation, or the presence of antiphospholipid antibodies). If warfarin is unsuitable then consider rivaroxaban (factor Xa inhibitors). Thrombolectomy and vena cava filters are reserved as a last resort (especially if anticoagulation is contraindicated or recurrent PEs occur despite INR target of 3–4).

Aetiology

Causes for PE/VTE consist of **I STOP OCPs** (or **I POST COPS**):

I	Immobility
S	Surgery
T	Thrombophilia
O	Obesity
P	Pregnancy
O	Oral contraceptive pill (OCP)
C	Cancer
P	Previous VTE
S	Smoking.

Pleural effusion

Is fluid (blood (haemothorax), lymph fluid (chylothorax), pus (empyema)) within the pleural space. You will be expected to know about ten different causes for your finals but to sound slick remember to always 'classify or die' (Table 30.6). The effusion is either a transudate (mainly intrinsic organ failure from increasing hydrostatic and reduced osmotic pressures) or exudate depending on the protein content. Light's criteria will determine samples in between 25-30 g/dl of protein content.

Pneumothorax

Is air leaking into the pleural space. Spontaneous (primary) in young, tall, thin males, secondary to asthma/COPD (from bullae) and traumatic from penetrating injury (e.g. subclavian lines). Presentation is variable, and treatment depends on symptoms and size of pneumothorax with decompression pleurocentesis followed by chest drains. It is important for you to identify the admitted patients on the ward with treated pneumothoraces to appreciate the pre- and post-decompression plain films. (See Fig. 30.7.)

Table 30.6 Pleural effusion

Transudative	Exudate
• Serum protein <25 g/dL	• Serum protein >30 g/dL
• Fluid:serum protein <0.5	• Fluid:serum protein >0.5
• Fluid:serum LDH <0.6	• Fluid:serum LDH >0.6
Failure: heart/kidney/liver/pancreas/thyroid	Always exclude malignancy first
Meig's syndrome—benign ovarian tumour	Autoimmunity (e.g. rheumatoid arthritis)
Hypoalbuminaemia—nephrotic syndrome	Infection—'parapneumonic effusion'
Myxoedema	PE or pulmonary infarction

Light's criteria (exudate if the following present):

• High protein + LDH = exudate
• Pleural fluid:serum protein >0.5
• Pleural fluid:serum LDH >0.6
• Pleural fluid level >2/3 of upper value for serum LDH
• Serum albumin − pleural fluid albumin <1.2 g/dL

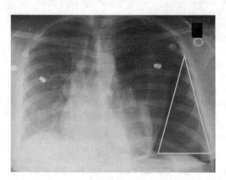

Fig. 30.7 Left tension pneumothorax. Note delineated area with absent lung markings, the tracheal deviation, and movement of the heart away from the affected side. Amended from Wikimedia under creative commons licence.

Management is determined by the size as measured at the level of the hila (large >2 cm, small <2 cm) and whether there is dyspnoea (see Fig. 30.8 for BTS guidelines).

Pulmonary oedema

Is fluid accumulation in the interstitium and air spaces. It is often cardiogenic and always resulting from damage to the vasculature and/or lung parenchyma. Management is ensuring adequate oxygenation (e.g. supplemental oxygen and positive pressure) and other treatments include glyceryl trinitrate (to reduce venous return) and loop diuretics (to offload fluid). (See Fig. 30.9.)

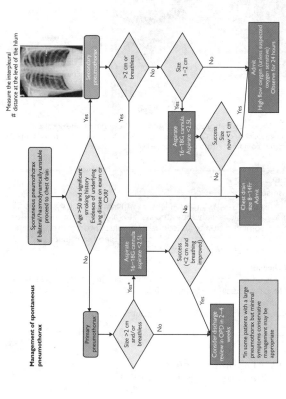

Management of spontaneous pneumothorax

Measure the interpleural distance at the level of the hilum

Spontaneous pneumothorax if bilateral/haemodynamically unstable proceed to chest drain.

Age >50 and significant smoking history. Evidence of underlying lung disease on exam or CXR?

— Yes → **Secondary pneumothorax**

— No → **Primary pneumothorax**

Secondary pneumothorax

>2 cm or breathless

— Yes → **Chest drain size 8–14Fr Admit**

— No → **Size 1–2 cm**
  - Yes → **Aspirate 16–18G cannula Aspirate <2.5L**
    - **Success Size now <1 cm**
      - Yes → **Admit High flow oxygen (unless suspected oxygen sensitive) Observe for 24 hours**
      - No → **Chest drain size 8–14Fr Admit**
  - No → **Admit High flow oxygen (unless suspected oxygen sensitive) Observe for 24 hours**

Primary pneumothorax

Size >2 cm and/or breathless

— Yes* → **Aspirate 16–18G cannula aspirate <2.5L**
  - **Success (<2 cm and breathing improved)**
    - Yes → **Consider discharge review in OPD in 2–4 weeks**
    - No → **Chest drain size 8–14Fr Admit**

— No → **Consider discharge review in OPD in 2–4 weeks**

*In some patients with a large pneumothorax but minimal symptoms conservative management may be appropriate

Fig. 30.8 BTS guidelines on managing spontaneous pneumothorax. Reproduced with permission from MacDuff, Andrew, et al. Management of spontaneous pneumothorax: British Thoracic Society pleural disease guideline 2010, *Thorax*, 2010, Vol 65 Supp. II.

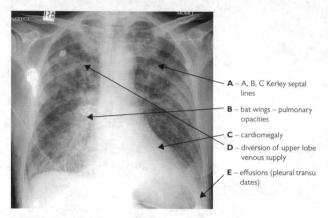

A – A, B, C Kerley septal lines

B – bat wings – pulmonary opacities

C – cardiomegaly

D – diversion of upper lobe venous supply

E – effusions (pleural transudates)

Fig. 30.9 Widespread reticulonodular shadowing showing both interstitial and alveolar pulmonary oedema. Classic signs include *ABCDE*. Amended from Wiki-media under creative commons Attribution-Share Alike 3.0 Un-ported license.

Honours

V/Q mismatch

Leads to hypoxia which can be explained by the dissociation curves for O_2 and CO_2: OxyHb is already saturated at >90% and therefore there is little 'space' for compensation by functional lung units. In comparison, greater amounts of CO_2 can be exchanged from the blood into functional lung units, → normal CO_2 levels.

Raised D-dimer

D-dimer is a breakdown product of a thrombus (e.g. DVT) but may be raised (e.g. false positives) in the **LIMPS**:
• Liver disease
• Infection and Inflammation (including autoimmune)
• Malignancy
• Pregnancy
• Surgery.

Bilateral hilar lymphadenopathy (BHL)

Causes include sarcoidosis, lymphoma, and TB.

Pulmonary tuberculosis

There was a time when every baby was inoculated with BCG after birth. Then came a time where only high-risk populations were vaccinated (e.g. Indian sub-continent and African origins). With an increasing migrant population, there has been a resurgence of TB. The *Mycobacterium tuberculosis* infection may be latent and present with systemic symptoms. Pulmonary symptoms include cough/sputum, pleurisy, haemoptysis, pleural effusion with constitutional symptoms including anorexia, weight loss, malaise, and night sweats. CXRs may show consolidations, fibrosis, and calcifications which may represent the hallmark pathology of caseating granulomas known as Gohn's focus/complex. Miliary TB results from haematogenous spread and shows up as widespread millets on both lung fields. At least three sputum samples need to be sent to the lab to test for acid–fast bacilli (AFB), and culture and sensitivity. Other immunological tests consist of tuberculin skin test, QuantiFERON TB Gold® and T-SPOT®.TB tests which have replaced the older Mantoux testing. While waiting for the lab results, quadruple drug therapy is instigated in two phases.

See Table 30.7 and Table 30.8.

All four drugs are given for 8 weeks and then only rifampicin and isoniazid are continued for another 16 weeks. Pyridoxine (vitamin B6) should be supplemented to counteract isoniazid toxicity.

Table 30.7 Pulmonary tuberculosis: side effects of drugs

Drug	Side effects
Rifampicin	Hepatitis, orange-staining of tears and urine
Isoniazid	Hepatitis, neuropathy, agranulocytosis
Pyrazinamide	Hepatitis, arthralgia
Ethambutol	Optic neuritis (colour vision first)

Table 30.8 Recent studies in respiratory medicine

Details	Trial	Comments
2003 JAMA N = 314	Reduction in the Use of Corticosteroids in Exacerbated COPD (REDUCE)	A 5-day course of glucocorticoids is non-inferior to a 14-day course for treating acute COPD exacerbations and preventing further exacerbations
2003 JAMA N = 401	PneumA (randomized, controlled trial)	Equivalent mortality in ventilator-associated pneumonia treated with 8 vs 15 days of antibiotic therapy, except for Pseudomonas aeruginosa
2006 NEJM N = 824	Prospective Investigation of Pulmonary Embolism Diagnosis (PIOPED	83% sensitivity and 96% specificity with CT angiography in detecting acute PE including strongly correlating with pre-test probability with Well's score
2011 NEJM	National Lung Cancer Screening (NLST)	Low-dose screening CT scans reduce lung cancer mortality compared to CXR

Reference

1. Wells PS, Anderson DR, Rodger M, et al. (2000). Derivation of a simple clinical model to categorise patients' probability of pulmonary embolism: increasing the model's utility with the SimpliRED D-dimer. Thromb Haemost 83:416–20.

Respiratory medicine: in exams

Exam tips

Most respiratory patients are stable and chronically unwell and in abundant supply for medical school examinations.

History station

Common symptoms reported will be progressive shortness of breath, coughing up sputum/blood, and chest tightness. Again, a focused history is key for you not to waste time chasing red herrings. Also remember that respiratory symptoms may also originate from cardiogenic (e.g. cardiogenic asthma) and GI (e.g. dyspepsia, GORD) causes. Make sure you ask about previous need for intubation or ITU admission for asthmatic/COPD patients to give you an idea of how severe their disease is. Key elements to check include travel history, pet exposure, occupation, smoking, and allergies/atopy.

Examination

In all respiratory examinations expect paraphernalia around the bed—inhalers, oxygen cylinders, etc. There are more things to see at the end of the bed looking at a respiratory patient than most other patients. Practise this on every ward round.

Pneumonectomy/lobectomy

This requires you to do your examination thoroughly. A good inspection for previous scars especially around the back is crucial. Remember sensible suggestions in finals (i.e. tension pneumothorax less than likely).

The art of a good percussion note

Practise your percussion on the respiratory ward; you should practise 'feeling' the difference between stony dull effusion, dull consolidation, resonant normality, and hyper-resonance in asthma and pneumothorax. Ask your partner to stand at the other side of the bay and also listen to the percussion note. The quality of medical students can sometimes be judged by bizarre indicators and a strong percussion note is indicative of this.

Look towards constellation of signs

For instance, look for the barrel-chested obese patient with inhalers by the bedside, be open to hyperexpansion on palpation and hyper-resonance on percussion.

Warn the patient

Always mention to patients what you are going to be doing next and warn them when they may feel discomfort (e.g. feeling for the trachea).

Rheumatology

Rheumatology: overview

Rheumatology (Greek rheuma—river) is the study of rheumatic conditions involving the joints, soft tissues, bones, connective tissue disorders, vasculitides, and a number of autoimmune conditions.

Cases to see

- Rheumatoid arthritis (RA)
- Spondyloarthropathy
- Systemic vasculitides
- Osteoporosis
- Crystal arthritis: gout and calcium pyrophosphate disease (CPPD)
- Polymyalgia rheumatica (PMR) and giant cell arteritis (GCA)
- Systemic lupus erythematosus (SLE)
- Antiphospholipid antibody syndrome
- Other autoimmune disorders:
  - Polymyositis and dermatomyositis
  - Systemic sclerosis (SSc)
  - Sjögren's syndrome
  - Mixed connective tissue disease/overlap syndromes.

Patterns of rheumatological disease

Rheumatology is a specialty driven by pattern recognition. Disease labels often describe a constellation of associated and overlapping features. This can make accurate diagnosis very difficult. The first question is usually '*Is this inflammatory disease?*' The cardinal sign of inflammatory disease is stiffness, particularly in the morning, of at least 30–45 min duration which contrasts with the few minutes of stiffness reported in OA.

Inflammatory vs non-inflammatory

There is no one feature that distinguishes between inflammatory and non-inflammatory conditions. The diagnosis is often led by clinical experience taking into account the whole clinical picture (see Table 31.1).

Regional vs generalized features

Regional symptoms suggest regional aetiology—unilateral shoulder pain and restriction is far more likely to be due to '*frozen shoulder*' or cervical nerve root irritation than primary muscle disease.

Patterns of joint involvement

- *Monoarthritis*: suggests crystal arthritis (hot, red, very painful), septic/infective (hot, red, very painful) spondyloarthropathy/seronegative arthritis, monoarticular presentation of polyarticular disease (e.g. rheumatoid, lupus, vasculitis).
- *Oligoarthritis* (≤4 joints): spondyloarthropathy, rheumatoid, infections, sarcoid, Behçet's disease.
- *Polyarthritis*: RA, seronegative inflammatory arthritis, SLE.
- *Location of involved joints*: first metatarsophalangeal joint (MTPJ) involvement is most likely to be due to gout. First carpometacarpal joint involvement is typical of osteoarthritis. Distal interphalangeal joint involvement is most likely due to osteoarthritis, psoriatic arthritis, or gout.

Table 31.1 Inflammatory versus non-inflammatory disease

Favours inflammatory disease	Favours non-inflammatory disease
Early morning stiffness >45 min	Short-lived stiffness
Worse in morning (and sometimes evening as well)	Worse after exertion/in the evening
Systemic symptoms (malaise, fatigue, fevers, sweats, anorexia, weight loss)	No systemic symptoms
Raised inflammatory markers (depends on stage of disease and joints involved—normal inflammatory markers do not exclude inflammatory disease), normocytic anaemia, thrombocytosis	Normal inflammatory markers (erythrocyte sedimentation rate (ESR) and CRP)
Widespread symptoms (caution in pain syndromes, e.g. fibromyalgia)	Regional symptoms (but see text, e.g. monoarthritis)

Reproduced from NICE CKD Guidelines 2014. Adapted from Kidney Disease: Improving global outcomes (KDIGO) CKD work group. KDIGO 2012 clinical practice guideline for the evaluation and management of chronic kidney disease, *Kidney Intern. Suppl.* Vol 3:1 (1.Jan.2013) pp 1–150.

Symmetrical vs asymmetrical

- *Symmetrical*: most likely rheumatoid.
- *Asymmetrical*: psoriatic arthritis, other spondyloarthropathy/seronegative arthritis.

Most rheumatological diseases are treated with a predictable stepwise series of anti-inflammatory and immunosuppressive treatments:
- NSAIDs: a class of drugs with a self-explanatory name.
- Glucocorticoids.
- Disease-modifying anti-rheumatoid drugs (DMARDs): methotrexate, azathioprine, mycophenolate mofetil, hydroxychloroquine, sulfasalazine, leflunomide.
- Biological agents: anti-TNF, e.g. infliximab.

Honours

Methotrexate toxicity

Inappropriate prescribing of methotrexate has led to deaths. It is only given weekly for rheumatological disease and should never be co-prescribed with trimethoprim and co-trimoxazole. The risk is of bone marrow suppression and subsequent sepsis.

Rheumatology: in clinic

There are hundreds of rheumatological diseases, but the good news is that you can complete a whole medical career without knowing much about most of them. However, there are a small number of extremely important diseases that you will encounter throughout your career. For this reason, they are high yield both for medical school assessments and afterwards.

Rheumatoid arthritis

RA is the most common autoimmune inflammatory joint disease, and is characterized by a synovitis, which unchecked → limitation of movement, joint damage, deformity, and destruction, with subsequent loss of function. It is a symmetrical polyarthropathy (affecting multiple joints), usually affecting the small joints first, and is associated with elevated rheumatoid factor/anticitrullinated protein antibody.

Radiological features include LESS (loss of joint space, erosions, soft tissue swelling, soft bones [osteopenia]), panniculitis, and chondrolysis (see Fig. 31.1). Extra-articular features (lung fibrosis, pleural effusion, vasculitis, scleritis/scleromalacia) are rare at presentation. Long-term complications are disability, cardiovascular disease, amyloid, and myelopathy from atlanto-axial subluxation.

The last two decades have seen a paradigm shift in treatment of RA, both in the use of the DMARDs that were previously available and the introduction of new biological therapies. Methotrexate is the first-line drug, and may be combined with sulfasalazine and/or hydroxychloroquine. If a patient does not respond to these first-line DMARDs then the next step is

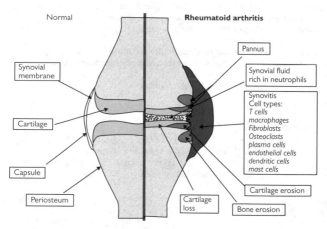

Fig. 31.1 The pathology of rheumatoid arthritis: normal joint (left) and rheumatoid joint (right). Reproduced with permission from Warrell, D. et al, *Oxford Textbook of Medicine*, 2010, Oxford University Press

biological therapies (anti-TNF, rituximab, tocilizumab, abatacept). NSAIDs are also helpful adjuncts for short-term flare-ups, as are steroids.

Spondyloarthropathy

The spondyloarthropathies are a group of conditions characterized by sero-negativity (i.e. rheumatoid factor negative) in the presence of inflammatory arthritis involving the spine (spondylo-), peripheral joints, and entheses (site of ligament, tendon, and capsule insertion into the bone). They can be classified as axial or peripheral, and include:

- ankylosing spondylitis (AS) & Non-radiographic spondylarthritis
- psoriatic arthritis
- reactive arthritis
- arthritis/spondylitis associated with IBD (enteropathic)
- undifferentiated spondyloarthropathy.

Ankylosing spondylitis

AS is the typical disease of the spondyloarthropathies, affecting the sacroiliac joints and spine resulting in progressive joint stiffness. AS was typically associated with HLA-B27 affecting mainly men in their 30s who present with persistent lower back or alternating buttock pain (sacroiliitis), and early morning/inactivity stiffness which improve with exercise but not with rest. These patients are often described as having a 'question mark' posture, and the best students will spot this typical posture from the bedside. If you are shown a plain radiograph of a spine in the rheumatology clinic the answer may well be bamboo spine with syndesmophytes (new bone formation) of AS. Non-radiographic SpA includes patients with inflammatory back pain that have MRI changes not visible on plain radiographs. Treatment is similar to RA in the form of exercise, NSAIDs, DMARDs, and anti-TNF-α agents to reduce symptoms and improve function, but they do not prevent bony progression.

Psoriatic arthritis

Typically includes a personal or family history of psoriasis (not essential), nail changes, dactylitis, and/or radiological evidence of new bone formation in the hands or feet. There are a number of clinical patterns of psoriatic arthritis described, including distal interphalangeal joint disease, symmetrical polyarthritis similar to RA, asymmetrical oligoarthritis, spondylitis, and arthritis mutilans. The pattern may alter with time.

Reactive arthritis

Reactive arthritis is an aseptic arthritis triggered by an infectious agent outside the joint, usually occurring 1–4 weeks following urethritis (*Chlamydia, Ureaplasma* spp.) or dysentery (*Campylobacter, Salmonella, Shigella,* or *Yersinia* spp.). There may be polyarticular features, mucocutaneous lesions, conjunctivitis, and enthesitis. Attempts should be made to identify the causative organism including the aspiration and culture/histopathological evaluation of an involved joint to guide antibiotic treatment.

Enteropathic spondyloarthropathy

These occur with concomitant ulcerative colitis and Crohn's disease, and can manifest as peripheral or axial disease, enthesitis, mucocutaneous disease, and anterior uveitis.

Gout

The most common cause of inflammatory arthritis, associated with the deposition of monosodium urate crystals within joints and soft tissues. Most commonly presents as recurrent, self-limiting attacks of acute, severe arthritis.

Typical history

Onset within a few hours (often overnight) of a hot, red, swollen, very painful, and tender joint. The first MTPJ is the most common site (but can affect other limb joints). Look for (and aim to correct) common triggers: heavy alcohol intake, dehydration (especially with diuretic use), joint trauma, surgery, other medical illness, and high-purine diet (beer, spirits, meat, seafood, sugary drinks, fructose). Address metabolic factors (BP, diabetes etc.).

Examination

Temperature can be raised in severe attack. One or more warm, red, tender joints. Check for gouty tophi (chalky deposits of urate crystals found on the pinna of the ear or overlying the joints).

Diagnosis

Gold standard is the finding of negatively birefringent, needle-shaped crystals under polarized light microscopy, in a sample of tissue or synovial fluid for cytology. Serum urate may be normal or low during an acute attack, so normal levels do not exclude an attack. Gout and joint sepsis may be clinically indistinguishable, so a sample should be sent for Gram stain and culture as well.

Management

Acute attack: NSAIDs (contraindications: elderly, CV disease, kidney disease, GI bleed)/colchicine/oral, IM or intra-articular steroids. Recurrent or chronic gout: urate-lowering drug e.g. allopurinol (xanthine oxidase inhibitor). Co-prescribe colchicine (for up to 6 months) or NSAIDs (e.g. naproxen for 6 weeks) when initiating urate-lowering therapy. You should remember that urate-lowering drugs can precipitate/exacerbate an acute flare of gout, therefore they should not be started during an acute flare.

Pseudogout (CPPD)

Pseudogout has a similar presentation to gout, the difference is biochemical, with positively birefringent analysis on crystal analysis.

Osteoporosis

Osteoporosis is the most common metabolic bone disease, in which low bone mass and alteration of bone architecture → fractures. Bone is a dynamic tissue, with a turnover of up to 10% at any one time; this process is driven by osteoblasts which lay down the bone matrix and mineralize it, and osteoclasts which promote resorption. Risk factors can be non-modifiable (age, female, family history, collagen disorders), or modifiable (smoking, alcohol, early menopause, steroids).

Mnemonic: risk factors for osteoporosis (MESSAGE)

- Menopause
- ETOH
- Smoking
- Steroids
- Age
- Gender
- Ethnicity.

Osteoporosis is clinically silent until a fracture occurs. Particularly with vertebral fractures, it is important to check for other causes of fragility fracture such as malignancy or metabolic bone disease. The five 'B's describe some of the most common cancers which metastasize to bone—'Breast, Bronchus, B(k)idney, B(t)hyroid, B(p)rostate'. Prostate are more likely to be sclerotic while myeloma are classically the lytic tumours. Osteoporosis is categorized by the presence or absence of fracture, and the T-score reported on a dual-energy X-ray absorptiometry (DXA) scan (see Table 31.2). The T-score reflects the patient's bone mass density (BMD) compared to bone mass at peak density, while the Z-score reflects BMD compared to age- and sex-matched controls. In younger patients, the Z-score is used. Treatment is based on identifying patients at risk prior to development of osteoporosis/fracture, e.g. DEXA scans for patients on long-term steroids, modifying risk factors, and using antiresorptive bisphosphonates (e.g. oral alendronate, IV zoledronate). See Table 31.2.

Honours

Antiresorptive therapies

These may cause marked hypocalcaemia; ensure that the patient is calcium and vitamin D replete prior to treatment. Osteonecrosis of the jaw has also been reported with bisphosphonates. Long-term bisphosphonate use (>5 years) has been linked with an ↑ risk of atypical (subtrochanteric) femoral fractures.

Table 31.2 . WHO definitions for osteoporosis—postmenopausal women and men ≥50 years old

Definition	Bone mass density measurement	T-score
Normal	BMD within 1 SD of the mean bone density for young adult women	≥ –1
Low bone mass (osteopenia)	BMD 1–2.5 SD below the mean for young-adult women	Between –1 and –2.5
Osteoporosis	BMD ≥2.5 SD below the normal mean for young-adult women	≤ –2.5
Severe or 'established' osteoporosis	BMD ≥2.5 SD below the normal mean for young-adult women in a patient who has already experienced ≥1 fractures	≤ –2.5 (with fragility fractures)

SD, standard deviation.

Polymyalgia rheumatica

PMR, the most common inflammatory rheumatic disease in the elderly, is characterized by widespread muscle pain and stiffness, particularly affecting the shoulder and hip girdle. The overwhelming majority of patients are treated with steroids. If the patient does not report a rapid improvement (≥70% improvement within 1 week), then the diagnosis is something else. DMARDs are reserved for refractory cases.

Giant cell arteritis

GCA is a granulomatous large/medium vessel vasculitis which classically affects the extracranial arteries, hence the alternative name, temporal arteritis. GCA can result in permanent blindness if untreated. For this reason it is important, both because you must not miss the diagnosis as a doctor, and you are likely to be grilled on the subject as a medical student. It is characterized by headache, jaw claudication, visual disturbance, and scalp tenderness (e.g. pain on brushing hair, usually in an elderly lady). The most important thing to know is that GCA should be treated (with steroids) as soon as it is suspected and certainly before investigation (e.g. positive biopsy or ESR >50). There is also an association with PMR.

Systemic lupus erythematosus

SLE is a multisystem connective tissue disease, characterized by immune complex formation and deposition. It is one of the 'great imitators' as it can present in countless ways and affect many organ systems. Constitutional symptoms (malaise, fatigue, weight loss, etc.) are extremely common. Textbook signs of SLE include malar rash, discoid rash, photosensitivity, oral ulcers, neuropsychiatric features, and a positive ANA. Other types of lupus (not SLE) include discoid (chronic skin disorder), drug induced (similar symptoms to SLE but reversible), and neonatal (associated with complete heart block).

Antiphospholipid antibody syndrome

Typically this presents as recurrent miscarriages in young females. It is a hypercoagulable state that may be diagnosed by a single clinical event and positive blood tests (anticardiolipin, lupus anticoagulant) on 2 occasions at least 12/52 apart. Treatment is with anticoagulation, e.g. warfarin (not in pregnancy—causes craniofacial defects), LMWH, and aspirin.

Vasculitis

Vasculitis (literally 'inflammation of blood vessels') is an umbrella term covering a group of heterogeneous multisystem diseases.

Honours

The Chapel Hill Consensus Conference (1994) classified vasculitides by vessel size, although there may be overlap between sizes of affected vessels:

- Large vessel: e.g. Takayasu's arteritis, GCA.
- Medium vessel: polyarteritis nodosa, Kawasaki disease.
- Small vessel: microscopic polyangiitis (MPA), granulomatous polyangiitis (GPA, previously known as Wegener's granulomatosis), eosinophilic granulomatous polyangiitis (EGP, previously known as Churg–Strauss syndrome), immunoglobulin A vasculitis (Henoch–Schönlein purpura), and antineutrophil cytoplasmic antibody-associated vasculitis.
- Variable vessel: Behçet's disease can affect any size of vessel

There is significant variability in severity, from isolated skin rash to multiorgan failure and death, even within groups of patients with the same disease. The consequences of vasculitis are vascular stenosis which may progress to occlusion, and aneurysmal dilatation, with subsequent vessel rupture. Treatment is stepwise immunosuppression.

Polymyositis and dermatomyositis

These are poorly understood connective tissue diseases characterized by inflammatory changes within skeletal muscles causing myalgia and muscle weakness. Classical symptoms of dermatomyositis include skin rash (heliotrope periorbital rash, Gottron's papules on the knuckles), and symmetrical proximal muscle weakness. Polymyositis has a similar constellation of features without the skin signs. Investigations include an elevated CK and autoimmune antibodies (anti-Jo-1), and attempts should also be made to exclude a concurrent malignancy.

Systemic sclerosis

SSc is a multisystem connective tissue disease, in which vascular endothelial damage and subsequent fibroblast proliferation and accumulation occur. SSc is classified into limited SSc and diffuse SSc (involving GI, cardiovascular, respiratory, renal systems). Limited SSc has previously been known as CREST because of a constellation of Calcinosis, Raynaud's, (o)Esophageal dysmotility, Sclerodactyly, and Telangiectasia. In an exam the characteristic appearance plus blood tests showing anaemia should prompt consideration of GI telangiectasiae (microcytic) or bacterial overgrowth (macrocytic).

Sjögren's syndrome

Often found in middle-aged females, who will have dry mucous membranes and various other glandular and MSk symptoms. Autoantibody associations (e.g. anti-Ro/La), but definitive diagnosis is biopsy. These patients have a 5–10% lifetime risk of lymphoma and this might be an opportunity to practise your lymph node examination.

Rheumatology: in exams

History station

The most likely scenario in a history taking station will be of a new-onset inflammatory arthritis. Use the principles outlined at the start of this chapter to establish the presence of inflammatory disease, and then drill down to what type. PMR or GCA may also be found in history stations.

History of presenting complaint

'SOCRATES' is useful (see ➋ p. 148–9), but be prepared to ask about stiffness (duration, timing, etc.) If back pain is reported, again try to differentiate inflammatory from non-inflammatory pain; ask about radiation—alternating buttock pain is the classical description of sacroiliitis. If back pain is present then always check for 'red flag' symptoms—bladder/bowel dysfunction, saddle anaesthesia, progressive neurology, night pain, history of malignancy or immunosuppression, systemic symptoms.

Past medical history

Ask about psoriasis or skin problems that might suggest psoriasis, even if the patient has not had a diagnosis. Check for inflammatory bowel symptoms, uveitis ('Have you ever had a red, painful eye?'). Think about connective tissue disease and ask about thrombosis, miscarriage, photosensitivity, rashes, and migraine. Take a travel and sexual history if reactive arthritis is possible.

Family history

Try to discern whether this is inflammatory or degenerative. Patients often do not distinguish between OA and RA although the distinction is important. They will often know OA as 'wear and tear' arthritis. If inflammatory arthritis is being queried, ask specifically about family history of psoriasis.

Drug history

Do you take any medications? Do you have any allergies? Ask what drugs the patient has tried for their symptoms.

Social history

Smoking, alcohol, and impact on life (how do you get around normally? How has this affected you day to day? What sort of things are you struggling to do at home or at work?). Functional status is very important to the patient. The easiest way to assess function is to ask the patient what they can do—it is surprising what people with marked hand deformities are still able to do!

Hand examination

Hands are the most common joint in medical school exams, and knees are also common, but you may be asked to examine any joint. If faced with an unfamiliar joint, return to first principles—look, feel, move (active first, then passive), and 'special tests', e.g. anterior draw test or McMurray's test for knees. There are many different systems for examining the hands; the smoothest and most professional of these approaches is described as follows. As with all physical examinations there is a theatrical component, and you should rehearse the steps with colleagues and patients as many times as is necessary for fluency.

Approach

Inspect as you approach the patient—look for signs of systemic disease, e.g. the facial changes of SSc or obvious psoriatic plaques.

Exposure

Ensure the patient is exposed enough for you to see the area of interest (many people use the 'expose up to one joint above and one joint below' approach). In any hand examination, make a show of examining the elbows and then resting the patient's hands on a pillow (ask your examiner for one), and ask whether they are comfortable—this is the first of your communication marks in case you forget to win some more later on.

Examination

Inspection is an important part of examining the hands—do not be worried about looking at all aspects of the hands (including elbows) as the examination will be over very quickly if you do otherwise. One systematic method is to work distally to proximally on each hand. First inspect the hand as a whole and look for gross bony deformities (symmetrical/asymmetrical, fixed/reversible). Then look in turn at nails (pitting, onycholysis, nail bed infarcts), distal interphalangeal joints (DIPJs) (Heberden's nodes, gouty tophi), proximal interphalangeal joints (PIPJs) (Bouchard's nodes), metacarpophalangeal joints (MCPJs), and muscle wasting (Fig. 31.2). Check for skin changes (scleroderma, telangiectasiae, vasculitic lesions, steroid purpura).

Feel the joint with the back of your hand—is it warm (if so, likely to be tender, so proceed carefully), beginning from DIPJ, PIPJ, dorsum of hand,

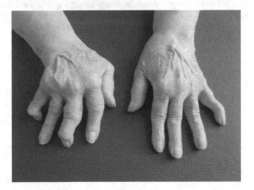

Fig. 31.2 Patient with RA presenting with a radial deviation (right wrist), swan-neck deformity with hyperextension of the PIPJs and flexion of DIPJs (digits 3 right and 5 on both sides) and boutonnière deformity with flexion of the PIP and hyperextension of DIP joints (digit 2 right). Reproduced from Richard A. Watts, *Oxford Textbook of Rheumatology* (4 ed.), 2013, Oxford University Press.

and wrist. Then palpate each of the joints distally to proximally for structural abnormalities and tenderness. Make a request to the patient that you wish to turn their hands over as you gently supinate their hands. Inspect first for muscle wasting (thenar, hypothenar eminences reflecting median or ulnar nerve deviation respectively) and carpal tunnel scar (longitudinal scar across the wrist). Depending on the case you could consider special tests for carpal tunnel syndrome (e.g. Tinel's). Inspect the patient's forearm up to the elbows (extensor rash of psoriasis, rheumatoid nodules).

You should then check the following movements. Wrist flexion/extension, finger flexion/extension/abduction, and thumb abduction/opposition (feeling for thenar muscle bulk for wasting). Finally, you should perform a functional assessment of grip strength (around your middle and index finger), pincer grip (around index finger), and ask them to pick up a small object such as a coin. Finish off your exam by offering to perform a full neurovascular exam.

Once you have finished, think about the examination in context. If the patient has Raynaud's and digital ulceration, are there any other signs of SSc or SLE? Does the patient with apparently rheumatoid hands have any nail dystrophy or psoriasis that might alter your differential diagnosis? Most students are easily able to recognize RA, but often struggle to describe it; if you can produce a smooth, sequential presentation supporting your diagnosis, you will please the examiner.

Honours

Clinical signs of RA

(See Fig. 31.2.) The most likely case is a rheumatoid hand. Students are very good at identifying a rheumatoid hand (severe cases are obvious) but often struggle to describe its features. Learn a list of features which are almost always present together and mentally check these when examining the patient. Once you have confirmed all are present, you can recite the clinical signs confidentially and firmly. Clinical signs include:

- swan neck deformity
- Boutonniere's deformity
- Z deformity of thumb
- Bouchard's nodes (PIPJ)
- Heberden's nodes (DIPJ, first MCPJ)
- finger ulnar deviation (MCPJ)
- wrist radial deviation and subluxation.

Part 3

Clinical surgery

Breast surgery

Breast surgery: overview

Cases to see

Breast lumps

You will see these repeatedly in the breast clinic so make sure you develop a system for how to approach this finding. Other presentations (e.g. nipple discharge, breast pain) will also frequently appear in the breast clinic so establish a system for these symptoms.

Procedures to see

Mammography

Uses ionizing radiation to create images of breast tissue looking for characteristic masses and microcalcifications. It is also used as the primary breast cancer screening tool in the UK.

Ultrasound

Is often used for younger women as their breasts are more dense, which makes mammography less effective. US and mammography will sometimes take place in the same patient.

Core needle biopsy

Uses a small hollow needle to remove breast tissue that can be analysed to obtain a histological diagnosis.

Operations

Include mastectomy, wide local excision, breast reconstruction, axillary clearance, and sentinel lymph node biopsy.

Things to do

Learn to assess the patients and plan appropriate investigations. (See Table 32.1)

Table 32.1 Regional anatomy of the breast

Arteries	*Internal mammary* (most), lateral thoracic, thoracoacromial, posterior intercostal
Veins	Axillary, subclavian, intercostal, internal thoracic
Lymphatics	Axillary, parasternal, inferior phrenic nodes
Nerves	4th–6th intercostal nerves
Breast boundary	Clavicle superiorly, latissimus dorsi laterally, sternum medially, and inframammary fold inferiorly
Axillary boundary	Axillary apex superiorly, axillary fascia basally, pectoral muscles anteriorly, latissimus dorsi/teres major/subscapularis posteriorly, serratus anterior + first four ribs medially, humeral bicipital groove + biceps laterally
Axillary contents	Axillary artery/vein/lymph nodes, intercostobrachial + long thoracic nerves, infraclavicular part of brachial plexus' to 'thoracodorsal nerve

Breast surgery: in clinic

Most patients with breast symptoms are referred to the breast clinic. Beware: patients with query breast cancer are referred to the one-stop breast clinic under the 2-week rule pathway.

History

Key features of the history include duration and timing of symptoms. You will certainly be expected to know about the risk factors for developing breast cancer: History ALONE:

- History of breast cancer/family history (*BRCA* genes)/HRT ± oral contraceptive pill.
- Age (↑risk).
- Late menopause.
- Obesity.
- Nulliparity.
- Early menarche.

Ask about family history in a first-degree relative (including the age at which they were diagnosed). These risk factors all heighten exposure to oestrogens (→ breast cell proliferation → risk of cancer).

Triple assessment

Most patients in the breast clinical will undergo the 'triple assessment' of *clinical examination, radiological imaging*, and *histological investigation*. It is rare that a GP or even a breast specialist will consider a defined breast lump as warranting anything less than a full triple assessment.

Examination

Every breast examination should be performed with a chaperone present regardless of the examiner's sex and patient's age. Patients are typically anxious so be extra cautious to remain respectful throughout the examination. The patient should be positioned ideally at 45° with their arm above their head. The reason for this position is that it reduces the distance between the examiner's hand and the chest wall therefore making it easier to detect any abnormal areas. The breast tissue is examined with the most sensitive part of the hand, the fingertips. Following examination of breasts, it is essential to examine both axillae.

Examination findings should be documented on a scale of 1–5 with the prefix 'E':

- E1: no finding.
- E2: benign finding.
- E3: indeterminate.
- E4: probably malignant.
- E5: malignant finding.

Clinical presentation

It is highly likely that you will encounter patients in clinic who are found to have a new diagnosis of breast cancer. The most common presentation is a solitary lump. Note its size, consistency, and fixation. Typically the cancer is a firm mass, which demonstrates tethering to the skin. It may also present with features of local advancement demonstrating skin ulceration, erythema, puckering, dimpling, or peau d'orange. Nipple changes include retraction, discharge, and dry scales. It is essential that if you find such a mass, an examination of the axilla is performed to identify any axillary nodes. The alternative method of presentation is detection of cancer in the screening programme.

Imaging

Following examination, the patient will proceed to have a mammogram ± target US to the area of concern or a target US only if <35 years of age. This is because mammograms are not typically performed due to the density of the breast tissue in the <35 age group, rendering the mammogram of limited value. The mammogram consists of two views: mediolateral oblique (MLO) view and the craniocaudal (CC) view. The mammogram and US are classified 1–5 with the prefix M and U for mammogram and US respectively (i.e. M5 signifies a malignant tumour on mammogram). In certain cases the breast tissue is further evaluated with MRI. This is useful for assessing indeterminate breast masses, breast lumps post previous surgery to distinguish between scar tissue and breast tumours, and for screening women at high risk (i.e. those with a strong family history).

Biopsy

Lesions of concern are biopsied using the core biopsy technique. This involves cores of tissue being removed from the area of concern through a 14 G needle connected to a mechanical gun. Similarly to the other components of the triple assessment, the biopsy is classified from 1 to 5 with the prefix B. The alternative to core biopsy is FNA of the lesion. This is performed less frequently but is able to differentiate between a solid or cystic lesion. This involves a 21 G needle attached to a syringe being introduced into the lesion with suction applied. The aspirate from the lesion is then sent for cytology. The cytology of the lesions is again classified from 1 to 5 but on this occasion with the prefix C.

Pathophysiology

Breast cancer is the second most common cancer in females accounting for 31% of all new cases of cancer in females and affects 1:9 women. Breast cancer is derived from the epithelial cells lining the ducts and from the acini forming lobules. Therefore the most common form is invasive ductal followed by invasive lobular carcinomas. If the cancer does not breach the basement membrane, this is an *in situ* carcinoma such as DCIS (ductal carcinoma *in situ*).

Genetic

These account for 5–10% of breast carcinomas with 60% of these associated with breast cancer genes: BRCA1 and BRCA2. These are tumour suppressor genes located on chromosome 17q and 13q respectively. If either of these genes is mutated, this results in an ↑risk of developing breast cancer.

Grading

You will encounter the description of the grade of the tumour in the pathology report from the biopsy and will hear about this in the MDT meeting. The grade of the tumour relates to the degree of differentiation of the tumour cells. This is dependent on the degree of tubule formation, nuclear pleomorphism, and the mitotic count. In simplistic terms, the lower the tubule formation, the greater the nuclear pleomorphism and the higher the mitotic count can all contribute towards a higher grade. The pathologist then derives these features from the specimen and classifies the tumour according to a grade:

Grade 1: well differentiated.
Grade 2: moderately differentiated.
Grade 3: poorly differentiated.

Receptor status is in reference to the receptors on the surface of breast cancer cells. This refers to the oestrogen (ER) and progesterone receptor (PR) status, and the c-erbB2 receptor status (HER2). This description will subsequently guide further treatment for the cancer.

Staging

The stage is according to the TNM classification. This consists of the size of the tumour (T), whether the tumour has spread to the lymph nodes (N), and whether the tumour has metastasized (M). This is then incorporated into the Union for International Against Cancer Control (UICC) classification to stage the tumour.

Treatment

Options include both surgical and medical treatment with the main decision regarding treatment decided in the MDT meeting.

Adjuvant therapy

Chemotherapy

Is not essential for all patients and the MDT team will determine its use, for each individual patient. Typically patients with high-grade disease, axillary or distant metastatic disease will be a candidate for cytotoxic agents. Combination therapy is required for these patients as cancer cells within metastasis may be at different stages of their cell cycles. The common combination therapy is referred to as *FEC*. This consists of (1) 5-fluorouracil (antimetabolite), (2) epirubicin (anthracycline), and (3) cyclophosphamide (alkylating agent). These agents can also be used as neoadjuvant to reduce the tumour size or in metastatic disease. Alternative agents such as paclitaxel (taxane) can also be used in metastatic disease particularly in disease that is resistant to anthracyclines or in relapse of disease post anthracycline treatment.

Radiotherapy

Should be administered to all patients who have undergone breast-conserving surgery and is also an option for axillary disease.

Hormonal treatment

Tamoxifen
Is a hormonal agent that acts by binding to ERs to block the effect of endogenous oestrogen on disease progression. Tamoxifen displays benefits in both pre- and postmenopausal women with maximum benefit from a daily dose given for 5 years.

Aromatase inhibitors
Prevent the aromatization of androgens to oestrogen in peripheral tissue such as the adrenal cortex and adipose tissue. Hence, it is only of value in postmenopausal women as the majority of oestrogen is derived from the ovaries in premenopausal women. The most common aromatase inhibitors you will encounter are anastrozole or letrozole.

Trastuzumab
Is commonly known as Herceptin®, a monoclonal antibody and is used in HER2-positive cancers. It can be used in metastatic disease in combination with taxanes.

Follow-up
Patients who have had breast-conserving surgery are at risk of developing recurrence. Patients who have had a mastectomy are also at risk of developing breast cancer on the contralateral side. Follow-up typically includes an annual mammogram with routine breast examination. Other investigations are only performed if a patient complains of symptoms that could be suggestive of metastatic disease.

Benign breast disease
In the breast clinic, the main purpose is to identify any new cases of breast cancer. However, in the majority of patients this is frequently excluded following triple assessment. The following are some differentials you ought to know about.

Fibroadenomas
Typically develop from whole breast lobules and present as a painless solitary mass. They are frequently encountered in women aged <25 years. Treatment options include leaving them alone or excision depending on patient choice/symptoms. Their sizes may correlate with menstrual cycles and grow/shrink during the month.

Breast cysts
Are distended and involuted lobules that are most common in perimenopausal women. Patients frequently complain of breast pain and tenderness over the site of the cyst. These cysts can be aspirated with or without US guidance and re-examined to ensure resolution.

Duct ectasia
The subareolar ducts can dilate and result in persistent nipple discharge. Duct ectasia can be treated conservatively. If the nipple discharge is particularly troublesome then ducts can be excised.

Breast pain

Can typically be cyclical or non-cyclical (i.e. dependent on the menstrual cycle). If the patient's assessment has not identified any underlying pathology, the patient can be reassured regarding the findings. Evening primrose oil may improve symptoms.

Breast abscess

Frequently a patient with a breast abscess may present in the ED. Depending on the level of sepsis (fever, inflammatory markers (CRP and WCC)) the patient may require admission for IV antibiotics or for potential drainage as an emergency. Alternatively, they may be referred to the next clinic appointment within the next few days. Breast abscesses may be lactational or non-lactational. A lactational breast abscess is predominantly caused by *Staphylococcus aureus* whereas a non-lactational breast abscess is associated with smoking. The optimal management is recommendation of the cessation of smoking, antibiotic therapy, and US evaluation. Following this, the breast abscess should be drained repeatedly via US guidance until resolution. If possible, incision and drainage of a breast abscess should be avoided unless necessary due to scarring of the breast and the risk of developing a mammary duct fistula.

Phyllodes tumour

The aetiology of these rare tumours is frequently unknown. They are predominantly benign breast tumours but can be malignant on occasion. Their typical age of onset is after the age of 40. They may present with rapid growth resulting in venous engorgement and potentially ulceration of the breast. The aim of management is to remove them with a clear macroscopic margin.

Fat necrosis

This can occur following trauma to the breast. Fat necrosis of the breast can produce a mass, which can appear similar on examination to a breast cancer. It is therefore important to proceed with imaging and not be dismissive of any bruising. The vast majority of cases are treated conservatively and it is predominantly a self-resolving condition.

Breast surgery: in theatre

Mastectomy

Involves the removal of all the breast tissue with an ellipse of skin and the nipple. This is typically indicated for patients who would prefer a mastectomy, tumours ≥4 cm, central tumours, and for those with multi-focal disease. Preoperative counselling is required since this can psychologically affect patients. Those with genetic risks may also want to pursue prophylactic bilateral mastectomies which require multiple consultations.

Wide local excision

Includes the removal of clinically palpable tumours with an appropriate (ideally ≥10 mm) margin of normal breast tissue. The mainstay of this treatment is that the removal of the cancer will leave an appropriate cosmetic appearance of the breast after the surgery.

Wire-guided wide local excision

For clinically impalpable tumours it is necessary for the radiologist to place a wire into the tumour either by US or mammography guidance. A subsequent incision is then made close to the wire and breast tissue encompassing the tumour is removed.

Axillary surgery

Sentinel lymph node biopsy

You will see this procedure combined with breast surgery (i.e. mastectomy or breast-conserving surgery) or in isolation. This is a diagnostic procedure and not a therapeutic one. The basis of this is to identify the draining lymph node of the breast cancer. Prior to the procedure, a radioactive substance tagged with technetium-99m is injected in proximity to the tumour. Following this before the start of the operative procedure, patent blue dye is injected close to the previous injection site. The purpose of the sentinel lymph node biopsy is to find the draining lymph node either via visual inspection (the draining node will be blue) or through a gamma probe. Upon removal of the node, this sentinel node will be sent to the pathology laboratory to establish whether it is positive for axillary nodal disease. If further treatment will be required then the patient will be booked for an axillary clearance.

Axillary dissection

Again, this is a procedure you will encounter during the breast surgery attachment. This involves the removal of all of the axillary nodes and is also termed a level III axillary clearance. The axillary nodes are described in relation to the pectoralis minor muscle in the axilla (see Fig. 32.1).

• *Level I*: inferolateral to pectoralis minor.
• *Level II*: posterior to pectoralis minor.
• *Level III*: superomedial to pectoralis minor.

It is imperative that you learn the local anatomy of the axilla because you need to be aware of possible complications (e.g. injury to intercostobrachial nerve (T1–T2) → posteromedial paraesthesia of proximal arm/axilla/shoulder).

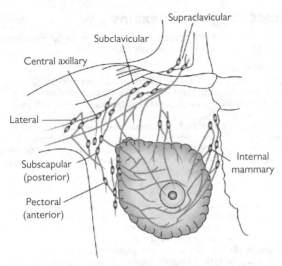

Fig. 32.1 Axillary lymph nodes and regional anatomy. Reproduced from Selden, David L. and Corbett, Siobhan, *Lachman's Case Studies in Anatomy*, 2013, Oxford University Press.

Breast reconstruction

Breast reconstruction following mastectomy can be performed at the time of the oncological clearance (immediate) or months to years later after completion of any adjuvant therapy (delayed). Reconstruction aims to reduce both the aesthetic as well as the psychological morbidity associated with breast cancer. Reconstruction of the breast can be implant based (e.g. using a silicone prosthesis, similar to that used for aesthetic augmentations), which is placed under the muscle to rebuild a breast shape. This is currently one of the most common forms of breast reconstruction. However, on the increase is a sought-after form of breast reconstruction using the patient's own tissue to form a new breast, which may have a more natural feel or consistency; this is known as autologous reconstruction. This can be achieved by using either a (1) free flap (i.e. using microsurgery to connect the blood vessels, also known as microvascular free tissue transfer) such as a deep inferior epigastric artery perforator (DIEP) or transverse rectus abdominus myocutaneous (TRAM) flap taken from the abdomen and consisting of skin and fat, or (2) pedicled flap (i.e. microsurgical anastomosis of vessels is not required, rather the flap and its main blood supply are moved into the defect) such as the latissimus dorsi (LD) flap (muscle and overlying skin) taken from the side of the back.

Breast surgery: in exams

Breast surgery does not present too frequently in formal examinations. However, it can appear in the following contexts:

Communication skills

- *Taking a history*: in this format it is important to be succinct, by establishing the presenting complaint and the associated features. It is then imperative to ask about the risk factors, which demonstrates knowledge of them.
- *Explaining to a patient they require triple assessment and what this entails*: for it is important to be able to explain the imaging procedures in simple terms and what is involved. For this scenario, it would be sensible for you to practise with a non-medic to ensure the information being explained is well understood.

Examination

Breast examination tends to be restricted to OSCEs. It is typical for you to encounter a synthetic breast model, which may or may not be attached to an actor. Although actual female actors may also be present! In either scenario, it is important to treat this as a real patient.

- Introduce yourself, wash hands, and always request a chaperone.
- Ensure that the patient's dignity is always covered with a sheet.
- *Inspection*: inspect the breasts at eye level, so kneel down, and put your hands behind your back to avoid any embarrassing gestures!
- Ask the patient to sit up and inspect for scars, skin changes, nipple dimpling, nipple discharge, asymmetry, masses in four positions: (1) arms by their side, (2) leaning forward, (3) hands behind their head, and (4) hands on their waist (tensing pectoralis).
- *Palpation*: position the patient at 45° with the ipsilateral hand behind their head; expose one breast at a time, examine the normal breast first using the flats of your fingers in a clockwise direction in four quadrants and describing findings using a clock face (Fig. 32.2)
- If a mass is found, then describe it thoroughly.
- *Nipple*: allow patient to express discharge (blood (?cancer) vs pus).
- *Axillary tail (of Spence)*: palpate where most cancers occur.
- *Lymphadenopathy*: support patient's arm on your shoulder. Palpate all axillary lymph node groups as well as the supraclavicular fossa.
- *Exclusion of metastases*: palpate liver for masses ± hepatomegaly. Ask patient to lean forward and feel for spinal tenderness.
- Thank the patient, cover her up with a sheet, hands behind your back, and report your findings.
- See Fig. 32.3 for anatomy of breast.

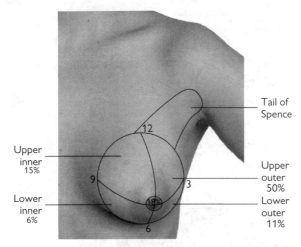

Fig. 32.2 Breast quadrants and frequency of cancers. Amended with permission from Thomas, James, Monaghan, Tanya, *Oxford Handbook of Clinical Examination and Practical Skills* (2 ed.), 2014: Oxford University Press.

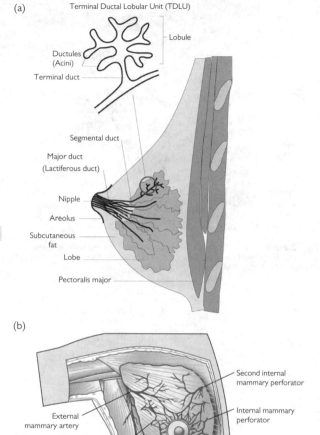

(a)

Terminal Ductal Lobular Unit (TDLU)

Lobule

Ductules
(Acini)

Terminal duct

Segmental duct

Major duct
(Lactiferous duct)

Nipple

Areolus

Subcutaneous
fat

Lobe

Pectoralis major

(b)

Second internal
mammary perforator

External
mammary artery

Internal mammary
perforator

Anterolateral
intercostal perforator

Anteromedial
intercostal perforator

Fig. 32.3 Anatomy of breast. Reproduced from Harvey, James et al, *Breast Disease Management: A Multidisciplinary Manual*, 2013, Oxford University Press.

Cardiothoracic surgery

Cardiothoracic surgery: overview

Cardiothoracic surgery encompasses all aspects of disease that can be managed surgically within the thorax. This includes primarily conditions of the heart, thoracic aorta, lungs, tracheobronchial tree, and conditions of the chest wall. Transplantation of the heart and/or lungs and mechanical circulatory support also fall under the remit of the speciality.

Cardiothoracic surgery is a highly specialized field and despite the extent of anatomical coverage, it is a small speciality with a relatively small body of consultants in the UK, with further divergence within the specialty to subspecialize either into cardiac or thoracic surgery. Within each subspeciality there are opportunities to further super-specialize. Due to the nature of the speciality, cardiothoracic surgery has always remained within a tertiary referral centre and commonly one that is also a major trauma centre. In the UK occasionally, a thoracic surgical unit may be at a different geographical location to a cardiac surgical unit. Therefore depending where you are posted, you may not necessarily see the full gamut of the speciality. In addition, a cardiothoracic surgical placement may not be part of your standard surgical rotation and extra effort may be required to organize such a placement (i.e. special study module, optional attachment, taster weeks). Therefore, if you are placed in a regional tertiary referral centre make the extra effort during your surgical attachments to organize some time within the cardiothoracic department. It may be your only exposure. You will gain the most from this during your later stages of surgical training, once you have mastered the generality of undergraduate surgical training.

Cases to see

Ischaemic heart disease (IHD)

This is the most common condition that is referred to a cardiac surgeon by a cardiologist. This referral may take place once medical therapy has failed and the patient remains symptomatic, or the extent/pattern of IHD warrants an early cardiac surgical referral. In addition, this may be either before or after an ACS or following an admission to hospital with unstable angina.

Valvular heart disease

Valvulopathy can affect any valve but commonly affects the left-sided valve (aortic and mitral). It can either be stenotic, regurgitant, or mixed. Valvular heart disease is the second most common pathology that is referred to the cardiac surgeon and therefore is a prevalent condition. Patients with mixed valvulopathy may have one valve with mixed pathology or more than one valve being affected at the same time.

Disease of the aorta

There is a large spectrum of disease that can affect the aorta but commonly this takes the feature of aortic ectasia where the aorta becomes aneurysmal. Connective tissue diseases (i.e. Marfan's disease, Ehlers–Danlos syndrome, mixed connective tissue disease) ↑ the risk of aneurysmal change in the aorta. It is this aneurysmal change that causes greatest harm and ↑ the risk of aortic rupture. Once diagnosed, surveillance is paramount and surgical intervention is warranted if the patient is symptomatic. In the ascending aorta, if the diameter is >5 cm in a patient with connective tissue disease, female, or of South Asian ethnicity or >5.5 cm otherwise, elective surgery is indicated. This threshold is lower if the patient is undergoing a cardiac procedure for a different pathology (i.e. aortic valve replacement for AS). The threshold ↑ to >5 – 6 cm if the aortic arch is aneurysmal and >6.5 cm with an aneurysmal descending thoracic aorta.

Lung cancer

Thoracic surgeons are referred patients that are deemed operable or have a type and/or pattern of lung cancer than is amenable to surgical treatment. This is usually decided in an MDT, which takes place before the referral for surgical review. Lung cancer surgery is the brunt of the thoracic surgical workload and mostly includes tumours of the lung and also includes tumours of tracheobronchial tree and chest wall.

Benign thoracic disease

This encompasses all benign conditions of the tracheobronchial tree, lungs, mediastinum, and chest wall and includes conditions such as surgical management of tracheal strictures, pneumothoraces, pleural effusions, and empyemas.

Investigations and procedures to see

Coronary angiography

The best place to see how this is done and understand the technique is the cath lab in the cardiology department. The interventional cardiologists perform this procedure routinely. It assesses the two-dimensional (2D) anatomy and degree of stenosis within the coronary arteries. While you are in the cath lab you may also see some coronary angioplasties and coronary stenting. Angioplasty simply means restoring the patency of the blood vessel but stenting maintains patency. Once you understand the technique of acquiring these images, they can be viewed offline for each patient having a cardiac operation.

Transthoracic echocardiogram

This is a 2D representation of the heart and its structures. It allows for the assessment of valvular and ventricular function and through this the extent of valvular disease can be quantified.

Lung function tests

These provide an assessment of the patient's baseline pulmonary lung function. They measure the FEV_1 and the FVC, which are used to calculate the ratio of FEV_1/FVC to assess the degree of lung disease (i.e. obstructive or restrictive) (see ➲ Chapter 30). It also plots flow–volume loops.

CT thorax

A CT scan is a common tool for radiological diagnosis and is mandatory in the diagnosis of lung tumours. Visit the radiology department to see how this is performed and then get familiar with the lung, mediastinal, and bone windows (which you can switch between), which allow for greater clarity to view the different tissue densities.

Operations to see

In addition to the operations listed in the next section, depending on the expertise of the unit, try to observe surgery of the aorta, trachea, and bronchial tree as well as cardiac and lung transplantation. Chest wall surgery is not common but can be graphic if it entails a large resection. Transplantation usually happens overnight and if it is during the day, do not miss the opportunity to witness it. Aortic surgery is complex and therefore can be a long, all-day case; be prepared for this, especially if it is descending thoracic or thoracoabdominal surgery.

Intensive care

(See ◗ Chapter 9.) During your placement in this speciality, it is important not to miss the opportunity to visit the cardiac ITU and/or the thoracic HDU. All patients following a cardiac operation will spend the first day or two on the ITU, and this is an opportunity to familiarize yourself with the extent of haemodynamic and respiratory support that some patients require. Try to familiarize yourself with some of the common drug used (e.g. adrenaline (epinephrine), noradrenaline (norepinephrine)) and types of respiratory support (mechanical ventilation, CPAP, etc.). Once you have spent some time on the cardiac ITU, you will find that most patients will recover very quickly and be transferred to ward. In thoracic surgery, most patients will be transferred to HDU mainly for postoperative monitoring. These patients are at high risk of developing early complications hence more intensive monitoring is required for a day or two.

Cardiothoracic surgery: in clinic

Attending a cardiac outpatient clinic will provide the best opportunity to hone your skills of obtaining a focused cardiovascular history and examination. In a thoracic outpatient clinic, you will be able to practise taking a respiratory history and perform examinations. Invariably, a patient with a valvular lesion or IHD will attend a cardiac clinic and one who has been diagnosed with a lung tumour will attend the thoracic clinic. In addition, this is a good opportunity to review patients post major cardiac and thoracic surgery, as you will get an opportunity to see follow-up patients. Preoperative assessment clinic is a good opportunity to practise your history and examination as well as review all the preoperative investigations prior to surgery.

Cardiac history

Within the HPC, if it is related to pain follow the *SOCRATES* scheme. If there is angina or dyspnoea, confirm exactly when they come on and what the patient was doing at the time they get the symptoms. Is it reproducible? Confirm if there is evidence of rest or night pain, which indicates more unstable and severe angina. Establish symptoms of heart failure such as orthopnoea or paroxysmal nocturnal dyspnoea and confirm any history of peripheral oedema especially towards the end of the day. Key features in a cardiac history should include the risk factors the patient has for developing a cardiac condition. *Common risk factors*: include diabetes, smoking, hypercholesterolaemia, hypertension, male sex, age, IHD, and significant family history of heart disease. Within PMHx, with valvular heart disease establish if they have had *rheumatic fever* as a child. Establish their *respiratory status* by specifically asking them about asthma, COPD/emphysema, and TB. Within the SHx, try and establish their capabilities of independence and activities of daily living. Clarify the extent of help they receive with these tasks and also address their mobility and overall frailty.

Thoracic history

Lung cancer is common, and the PC may usually be as simple as shortness of breath (SOB). Pain is not a common association. In the HPC try to tease out other associated symptoms such as duration and progression of *dyspnoea, cough, haemoptysis*, and constitutional symptoms including weight loss, anorexia, and night sweats. Also, identify *risk factors* such as history of smoking (calculated the number of pack-years smoked), and type of occupation (miners and those who have worked in the heavy dye industry may have been exposed to carcinogenic chemicals dyes, etc.) The PMHx follows the same criteria as a cardiac history. In the SHx, again identify the extent the condition impinges on activities of daily living and through this, assess their *general state of health* (are they physically capable to undergo a major operation?).

Cardiothoracic surgery: in the emergency department

When a patient presents to the ED with a cardiothoracic problem, it is likely to be a life-threatening emergency in the resuscitation unit.

Stanford type A aortic dissection

This is a cardiac surgical emergency. A tear in the intima creates a dissection plane between the intima and media of the aortic wall and blood traverses through this plane, creating a false lumen. A type A dissection is one that originates anywhere between the aortic valve and the left subclavian artery and hence within the pericardium. The dissection can progress from the point of origin proximally or distally and can involve the entire aortic vasculature. Depending on the extent of the tear, complications include cardiac tamponade, aortic valve incompetence, MI (involving the coronary ostia), stroke, rupture into the pleura, or compromise of any of the aortic branches. Branch compromise can → stroke, upper limb arterial insufficiency, paraplegia, lower limb ischaemia, renal ischaemia, or mesenteric ischaemia.

Risk factors for an aortic dissection include hypertension and connective tissue disorders. Patients with a bicuspid aortic valve are known to have a higher incidence of aortic dissection. A CT aortogram aids in accurate diagnosis of an aortic dissection. However, subtle feature may include widening of the mediastinum on CXR. In addition, a TOE can assess the aortic valve, exclude tamponade, and confirm a dissection. At times, a dissection is only diagnosed in the cath lab during a coronary angiogram for a suspected coronary event. (See Fig. 33.1.)

Surgery is indicated for all patients with a type A dissection and the goals of surgery are to re-establish the true lumen, obliterate the false lumen, maintain aortic valve competence, and re-establish coronary arterial blood flow.

Chest trauma

Chest trauma is common and can either be blunt or penetrative. Life-threatening injuries can be remembered by **ATOM FC**:

- Airway disruption
- Tension pneumothorax
- Open pneumothorax
- Massive haemothorax
- Flail chest
- Cardiac tamponade.

Each patient assessed in the resuscitation department needs to be done systematically as per the Advanced Trauma Life Support® (ATLS®) principles. You will also see thoracostomy tubes (chest drains) inserted.

Potentially life-threatening injuries can be remembered by **PODCAST**:

- Pulmonary contusion
- Oesophageal disruption
- Diaphragmatic tear
- Cardiac contusion
- Aortic disruption
- Sternal and rib fractures
- Tracheobronchial disruption.

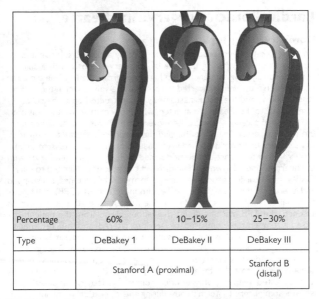

Percentage	60%	10–15%	25–30%
Type	DeBakey 1	DeBakey II	DeBakey III
	Stanford A (proximal)		Stanford B (distal)

Fig. 33.1 Aortic dissection. Reproduced from https://en.wikipedia.org/wiki/ Aortic_dissection. Image licensed under the Creative Commons Attribution-Share Alike 3.0 Unported license.

Traumatic disruption of the aorta occurs in any type of deceleration injury (i.e. road traffic accident or a fall). Oesophageal injures and diaphragmatic tears[1] can be difficult to diagnose. With all chest trauma one should have a high index of suspicion for these injuries. One of the most dramatic scenes in the resuscitation departments in trauma centres is clamshell thoracotomies done in absolute emergencies. The procedure exposes both thoracic cavities to allow access to the heart for cardiac massaging and managing profound hypotension or cardiac arrest. These patients will need to be transferred to theatre imminently.

Reference

1. Wilson E, Metcalfe D, Sugand K, et al. (2012). Delayed recognition of diaphragmatic injury caused by penetrating thoraco-abdominal trauma. *Int J Surg Case Rep* 3(11):544–7.

Cardiothoracic surgery: in theatre

Coronary artery bypass graft surgery

This is the commonest procedure performed by a cardiac surgeon and essentially involves bypassing the area of coronary stenosis with a suitable conduit, usually long saphenous vein harvested from the leg. The direction of flow within the vein is inverted (to prevent the valves within the vein restricting flow) and the distal anastomosis is constructed onto the coronary artery distal to the area that is affected, with the proximal anastomosis onto the proximal ascending aorta. Therefore blood flow is re-established from the proximal ascending aorta, beyond the coronary stenosis to a myocardial territory that previously had inadequate blood supply (i.e. ischaemia).

Surgery on the heart can be performed with the heart beating or with the heart stopped. However, beating heart operations are limited to mainly CABG. Most cardiac procedures are performed while the heart is stopped and therefore the role of the cardiopulmonary bypass (CPB) machine is essential to keep the patient alive during the length of the procedure. In essence, the CPB machine drains the venous blood from the patient, the blood is temperature controlled, oxygenated, filtered, and then returned to the arterial system. During cardiac surgery, an optimum operating environment is when there is a motionless and bloodless operative field, in which the heart needs to be arrested. A cross-clamp is placed across the ascending aorta proximal to the arterial return from the CPB machine. The heart is then arrested with a potassium-rich solution called 'cardioplegia'. This is then administered intermittently during the operation to maintain diastolic arrest which reduces the metabolic demands of the heart. Following cardioplegia, the heart regains its intrinsic activity on reperfusion when the aortic cross-clamp is released at the end of the main procedure. The patient is gradually weaned off the CPB machine, and the work of the heart and lungs are gradually transferred from the machine back to the patient.

Aortic valve replacement

This is one of the most common open-heart operations. An open-heart operation is one where one or more chambers of the heart are opened to the atmosphere as part of the procedure and therefore the patient is liable to have an air embolism if the chambers of the heart are not de-aired at the end of that segment of the procedure. The aortic valve is routinely replaced but aortic valve repair is also susceptible to pathologies. During valve replacement, a biological (e.g. bovine or porcine) pericardial tissue valve or a mechanical valve can be implanted. The ascending aorta is opened to access the native aortic valve. The valve is debrided and explanted off the aortic annulus and the new valve is stitched in place. Finally the aorta is closed, the heart is de-aired, and the aortic cross-clamp is removed.

Mitral valve repair/replacement

The mitral valve is repaired whenever possible. A repair maintains part of the valvular apparatus, which includes the chordae tendineae and papillary muscles. The type of repair depends on the extent and type of the underlying pathology. When a repair is not suitable, the mitral valve too can be replaced with a tissue or mechanical valve.

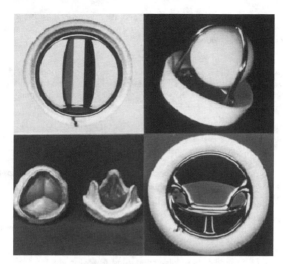

Fig. 33.2 Common types of heart valve prostheses (from top left clockwise): St Jude's Medical™ bileaflet valve, Starr–Edwards ball and cage valve, Björk–Shiley tilting disc valve, stented porcine prosthesis. Reproduced with permission from Punit Ramrakha and Jonathan Hill, *Oxford Handbook of Cardiology* 2e, 2012, Oxford University Press.

The approach to the mitral valve can be transseptal or directly into the left atrium through Sondergaard's groove.

Lobectomy

This refers to the surgical removal of one or more lobes of the lung that has a lung tumour within it. Preoperative planning will identify which lobe the tumour is in and if there is any invasion into another adjacent lobe or if there is any local spread to surrounding tissue or lymph nodes. The right lung consists of three lobes and the left has two lobes. The left lung lacks a middle lobe but has a smaller lobe called the lingula. The lobes are separated by inter-lobar fissures. These fissures aid in excision of an entire lobe, as the surgical plane follows the inter-lobar fissures and dissection continues down into the hilum to identify the lobar bronchus, veins, and pulmonary arteries that supply the lobe that is to be excised. Once the lobectomy is complete, a series of lymph nodes are sampled for pathological stages of the tumour.

Video-assisted thoracic surgery (VATS)

This refers to the equivalent of laparoscopy surgery but in the chest, and is a form of minimally invasive surgery. Ideally three incisions are made and access gained through appropriate intercostal spaces; the camera port is placed through one and surgical equipment through the other two ports. Procedures commonly performed using VATS include lobectomy, wedge resections, pleurectomy, bullectomy, and lung biopsies for diagnosis. VATS offers a better view of the anatomy and surgical procedure being performed compared to one that is accessed via a thoracotomy, due to the restricted space provided.

Bronchoscopy

This is a key skill and is performed in every patient prior to undertaking the main operation. It allows for visual assessment of the tracheo-bronchial tree in case of tumour invasion. Brush cytology and biopsies can be sampled for microscopic diagnoses. (See Fig. 33.3.)

Cervical mediastinoscopy

This is a procedure that is performed mainly for diagnostic purposes. It is performed through a small transverse incision 1–2 cm above the suprasternal notch. Dissection is made down to the trachea and a mediastinoscope is placed in the pretracheal plane. It allows for multiple lymph node biopsies to be taken for diagnosis and staging of tumours.

Intercostal chest drain insertion

This is a common surgical procedure and every doctor should know the principles of this procedure and be familiar with it. It is performed in the safe triangle—the area between latissimus dorsi, pectoralis major, apex of the axilla, and fifth intercostal space within the anterior axillary line. The procedure is performed by blunt dissection using artery forceps and a key step is digital palpation after penetrating the pleural cavity to push the lung away. This protects the lung from penetrative trauma as the chest drain advances into the pleural cavity. An appropriately sized drain is placed to the apex (for air) or to the base (for fluid) and secured with an external suture.

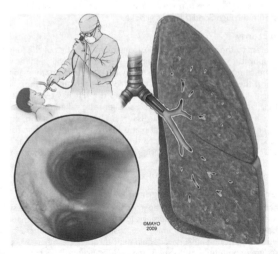

Fig. 33.3 Bronchoscopy. Reproduced with permission from Eelco F. M. Wijdicks, *The Practice of Emergency and Critical Care Neurology* (2 ed.), 2016. Oxford University Press.

Cardiothoracic surgery: in exams

As cardiothoracic surgery is a specialized field, you will not get examined extensively on this speciality per se. However, the medical conditions that warrant referral to cardiothoracic surgery will certainly get examined and these are what you should be confident about (i.e. angina, AS, AR, lung cancer, pneumothorax, pleural effusions). In the history stations, it is common to have a PC of chest pain or SOB. With chest pain you should go down the cardiac history route, but with SOB it could either be cardiac or respiratory in origin. You may also get a history on palpitations so remember to ask about frequency, duration, preceding events, and associated symptoms (i.e. SOB, chest pain, and associated PMH such as TIA/stroke). Be confident with a full CVS and respiratory examination and their separate components. It is highly likely in an OSCE that you will be asked to examine the chest or precordium. The clue to which system you need to examine will be in the question, where you may be offered a short history. There are plenty of patients with asymptomatic murmurs and they are commonly asked to attend an OSCE, so be confident in identifying a systolic from a diastolic murmur (it is likely to be a systolic murmur). Practise the additional manoeuvres you can perform to elicit clearer heart sounds or murmurs (i.e. roll the patient into the left decubitus position for mitral murmurs, sit the patient upright and lean them forward for AR, left-sided murmurs are enhanced on expiration and right-sided murmurs are enhanced on inspiration). See Table 33.1.

Table 33.1 Recent research trials

Year	Trial	Comments
2009 NEJM N = 2368	Bypass Angioplasty Revascularization Investigation 2 Diabetes (BARI 2D)	Patients with T2DM + stable CAD that are CABG candidates, CABG + OMT reduced the rate of CV events compared to optimal medical therapy (OMT) alone, but no difference in the PCI cohort
2011 NEJM N = 1212	Surgical Treatment for Ischemic Heart Failure (STICH)	In ischaemic cardiomyopathy with LV ejection fraction ≤35%, CABG (added to OMT) only reduces cardiovascular-related deaths after 5 years and all-cause mortality after 10 years
2012 NEJM N = 1900	Future Revascularization Evaluation in patients with Diabetes Mellitus: Optimal Management of Multivessel Disease (FREEDOM)	Among diabetic patients with multivessel CAD, CABG reduces the rate of death + MI compared to PCI, but causes ↑rate of stroke
2013 JAMA N = 1021	Mitral Regurgitation International Database (MIDA)	Retrospective study: in chronic flail MR, early surgery was associated with improved survival compared to medical management

Cardiovascular system examination

(See ➋ 'Cardiovascular examination' pp. 900–4.) Concentrate on practising a complete CVS exam. There is enough time in clinic to do this especially if you are seeing a new patient. A full CVS examination should include the assessment of the patient from the end of the couch, assessment of their peripheries (capillary refill time, peripheral warmth, and examination of their hands to identify features of cardiovascular disease) before moving onto examining the chest. You can conclude your CVS examination by examining the peripheral arteries and assessing for signs of heart failure (i.e. peripheral and/or sacral oedema and auscultating the lung bases for crepitations). If you are asked to examine the chest, then this should include the inspection, palpation, percussion, and auscultation (IPPA) model of the chest only and not a full CVS exam. Examination of the chest should be limited to the CVS and not be overlapped with the respiratory system. You may be specifically asked to examine the precordium.

In examining the precordium, do not rush through inspection (looking at chest deformities, i.e. pectus excavatum and carinatum), previous incisions, and visible pulsations. Palpate and show that you are confirming the position of the apex beat (by counting from the manubriosternal joint). Also take time in palpating for heaves or thrills (palpable murmur). Being able to palpating a thrill is not common but look out for it, as once you have felt it, it is indistinguishable. On auscultation, first identify which heart beat corresponds with the pulse by palpating the carotid artery at the same time (the pulse corresponds with the first heat beat). If you then hear a murmur, identify if this in the systolic phase or the diastolic phase of the cardiac cycle. Once this is established, try to identify if its ejection is systolic (AS), pansystolic (MR), early diastolic (AR), or late diastolic (MS). The latter two are more difficult to identify. Right-sided valve lesions are less common and tend to coincide with congenital abnormalities.

Respiratory examination

(See ➋ 'Respiratory examination' pp. 905–9.) The complete respiratory examination is a full assessment of the patient as per the CVS examination, which includes assessment from the end of the couch, examination of the hands, examination of the neck for cervical lymphadenopathy (indicative of lymph node involvement/metastases) and palpation for the trachea (displacement and tracheal tug), before focusing on the chest. Examination of the peripheral arteries is not necessary. To be more focused on the chest, examination includes the IPPA model.

Do not forget to examine both the anterior and posterior chest including the axilla. The thoracic clinic will allow you to assess patients post major thoracic surgery and may have patients with a previous thoracotomy scar. Some patients may have had lobectomies, whereas others may have had a pneumonectomy (complete resection of the lung on one side). These patients have interesting and rare clinical signs so look out for them.

Colorectal surgery

Colorectal surgery: overview

Colorectal surgery is the branch of surgery primarily concerned with the colon, rectum, and anus. Colorectal surgeons (along with upper GI surgeons) are the closest descendants of the 'general' surgeon, who would have previously operated on any acute surgical complaint (e.g. ruptured abdominal aortic aneurysm, testicular torsion) prior to the appearance of specialities. A large amount of colorectal surgery is centred on non-operative management, and it is a useful skill to try to gain a feel for when the acute abdomen can be managed conservatively.

Cases to see: elective

- *Colorectal cancer*: PR bleeding (DD IBD, diverticulitis, dysentery, angiodysplasia, etc.).
- *IBD*: operations including strictureplasty.
- *Hernias*: inguinal, femoral, etc.
- *Perianal pathology*: haemorrhoids, fissure-in-ano, pilonidal sinus, fistulas, rectal prolapse.

Cases to see: trauma/emergency

- 'Acute abdomen' etc. including mesenteric ischaemia.
- Acute appendicitis.
- Bowel obstruction:
  - Mechanical:
    — *Aetiology*: volvulus, stricture, hernia, etc.
    — *Management*: flatus tubes.
    — *Complications*: hernia (including Richter's hernia).
  - Pseudo-ileus.
- Acute diverticulitis.

Investigations/operations/procedures to see

- Appendicectomy: US scanning.
- Colectomy: hemi, transverse, sigmoid, anterior resection (see Fig. 34.11).
- Abdominoperineal resection, Hartman's procedure.
- Operations/stomas.
- Acute abdominal investigations: plain AXR (± erect CXR), CT abdomen/pelvis, MRCP/ERCP.
- Hernia repair including pantaloon.

Things to do

- Examining the 'acute' abdomen.
- Rectal examination.
- Proctoscopy in clinic.

Colorectal surgery: in clinic

Colorectal cancer

This is the third commonest cancer, associated with:
- Familial syndromes (e.g. HNPCC/familial adenomatous polyposis).
- IBD (UC > CD).
- Low-fibre diet.
- Smoking.
- Neoplastic polyps (esp. >2 cm/villous > tubulovillous > tubulous).

Cancers may present with localizing symptoms, particularly left sided:
- PR bleeding.
- Changed bowel habit.
- Tenesmus.

While right-sided present more insidiously with:
- anaemia (iron deficiency)
- constitutional symptoms (weight loss, lethargy, anorexia, sweats).

Presentation
In general, weight loss (unintentional 10% loss in past 6 months) in the context of cancer should always trigger a suspicion of lymph node involvement of distant metastases. Remember to look out for colorectal cancer in the ED, presenting emergently as perforation, obstruction, or even appendicitis (caecal tumours in the elderly!).

Imaging
CT, MRI (for rectal cancers), and PET are used to stage the colorectal cancer—look for lymphadenopathy and haematogenous spread to liver, lung, and bone (spine).

Management
Surgery ± radio/chemotherapy can be used palliatively or curatively. The precise surgery depends on presentation and tumour location ± its extent.

Staging
Colorectal cancer staging has moved on from the well-known Duke's classification to the more universally accepted TNM as in most cancers. With TNM, it is not as easy to give a prognosis as the Duke's system but the TNM is more precise and gives more information during decision-making on future management of the cancer (see Table 34.1).

Ask the boss ...
Consider the appropriateness of curative surgery in your patients after accounting for their comorbidities. When is symptomatic management (e.g. stenting) appropriate?

Bowel cancer cases:
percentage distribution by anatomical site

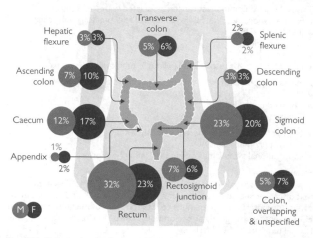

Fig. 34.1 Colorectal cancer locations. Reproduced with permission from www.cruk. org/cancerstats. Accessed February 2018.

Honours

- *Radiotherapy tattoos*: may be identified for preoperative treatment for rectal cancer prior to surgery (as opposed to colon cancers). Since it lacks a mobile mesentery, we can target a fixed area of bowel beforehand. Radiotherapy is associated with higher rates of fistulization, VTE, and pathological fractures (from osteonecrosis).
- *(Neo-)Adjuvant therapy*: to improve the chances of curative surgery, neoadjuvant therapy can debulk the tumour size with preoperative radiotherapy for instance. Adjuvant therapy (e.g. radio/ chemotherapy) is administered postoperatively to kill any metastatic disease that was not amenable to surgical resection.

Cancer pathway

All new colorectal cancer presentations must go through a local cancer MDT weekly meeting. Historically, any metastatic disease found at the time of diagnosis meant poor survival and contraindication to surgical treatment. While many colorectal cancers present as multiple metastases, single liver metastasis and subsequent liver resection can improve 5-year survival to ~40%.

Table 34.1 Colorectal cancer staging

Primary tumour		Lymph node (LN) status		Metastasis	
T0	No evidence of primary tumour	N0	No LN involved	M0	No distant metastases
T1	Tumour invades submucosa	N1	1–3 local LNs	M1a	Metastases confined to 1 site (e.g. lung, liver)
T2	Tumour invades muscularis propria	N2	4 or more LNs	M1b	Metastases to >1 site
T3	Tumour invades through muscularis propria into pericolonic tissue				
T4	Tumour penetrates surface of peritoneum or invades adjacent organs				

Honours

Suspected cancer pathway

As with most specialties there is a suspected colorectal cancer pathway known as the *2-week wait (2WW)* pathway. GPs can refer patients via a fast-track system if they fit certain criteria known as *red flags* (e.g. rectal bleeding, change in bowel habits, or iron deficiency anaemia). Once referred, surgeons must expedite all reviews, investigate, and either (1) make a diagnosis of cancer and commence treatment within 62 days of referral or (2) remove the patient from the pathway after excluding malignancy.

Inflammatory bowel disease

IBD is primarily managed medically by gastroenterologists (see ⊃ pp. 310–11), although surgical intervention (Table 34.2) may be necessary in the following cases:

Acute presentations

(More common in *UC, **CD.)

- Perforation in UC (acute flare-ups), in CD secondary to strictures.
- Toxic megacolon (bowel >6 cm with shock, refractory to maximal medical management).*
- Obstruction secondary to strictures.**
- Fistulae/abscesses** presenting with intra-abdominal sepsis.
- Massive haemorrhage.

Elective

- Failure to respond to medical therapy (e.g. remains symptomatic, unacceptable side effects, exacerbations affecting growth in children, ongoing nutritional challenges).
- Pre-malignancy (high-grade dysplasia)/malignancy of colon.

Table 34.2 IBD surgical options

UC	CD
• Pan-proctocolectomy (colon, rectum, anus) + end ileostomy	• Deal with complications, e.g. sepsis, obstruction with aim of preserving bowel
• Proctocolectomy leaving the anus for an ileoanal pouch later	• Crohn's mass, abscess, symptomatic fistula
• Total abdominal colectomy (colon only) + ileostomy (leaving rectum/anus in the unwell)	• Strictureplasty

Abdominal wall hernias

Protrusion of a viscus from its body compartment to another through a normal or abnormal opening. (See Fig. 34.2.) This is one of the most common conditions referred to any general or colorectal surgeon. Most common types include:
• inguinal (direct vs indirect)
• paraumbilical
• epigastric/ventral
• femoral
• incisional
• spigelian
• recurrent (previously repaired).

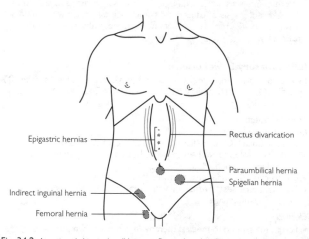

Fig. 34.2 Anterior abdominal wall hernias. Reproduced with permission from Callaghan Chris, *Emergencies in Clinical Surgery*, 2008: Oxford University Press.

Examination

Examine hernias with the patient standing up as well as supine. Assess the defect where the hernia arises and try to reduce the hernia back to the abdomen through the defect. Note the difference between *direct* (arising *medial* to the inferior epigastric artery) and *indirect* hernias (arising *lateral* to the inferior epigastric artery and enter the inguinal canal at the deep ring). Establishing whether a hernia is femoral is crucial as this carries a higher risk of strangulation (constriction and loss of blood supply to the contents of hernia) due to the narrower neck of the femoral canal.

> **Top tip**
> - Differentiating femoral hernias from inguinal is done by looking at the position relative to pubic tubercle—femoral hernias are *inferolateral* and inguinal are *superomedial*.
> - GPs may send in elderly patients with a query hernia but in fact the diagnosis may be '*divarication of recti*' muscles due to age-related muscular weakness. There is no treatment required here besides reassurance.

Differentials for lumps in the groin
- Femoral hernia
- Hydrocele
- Spermatic cord lipoma
- Lymph node swelling
- Abscess
- Saphena varix
- Varicocele
- Bleeding
- Undescended testis
- Femoral artery aneurysm
- Psoas mass/abscess
- Femoral neuroma.

Investigations

Straightforward hernias do not require investigation prior to operation if the diagnosis is obvious from the history and clinical examination. Imaging for anatomical delineation is reserved for unusual hernias (e.g. spigelian) and complex incisional hernias.
- *Dynamic US*: first-line imaging for assessing difficult hernias.
- *CT scan*: useful for incisional and complex abdominal wall defects.
- *MRI*: good for assessing groin hernias where US has not been clear and still high degree of suspicion.
- *Herniogram*: contrast injected into peritoneum and X-rayss taken to assess its spread into possible sites of herniation. This technique has largely been superseded by cross-sectional imaging.

Operations

Hernias are most commonly repaired openly with a mesh traditionally. Laparoscopic repair has become much more common in the past decade;

yet, studies have concluded little difference between both techniques. In fact, there may be a slightly higher risk of complications overall with laparoscopic repair.

Honours
Conditions for choosing laparoscopic repair over open technique
- Bilateral groin hernias.
- Recurrent groin hernias where the initial operation was open (if the initial operation was laparoscopic then open should be attempted for the re-do).

Diverticular disease
Encompasses *diverticulosis* (without inflammation) and *diverticulitis* (with inflammation from infection). It is a condition where outpouchings exist in the colonic wall at weak points where blood vessels traverse. This is usually confined to the sigmoid colon although diverticula can occur throughout the colon. Acute diverticulitis ± abscess may present with:
- change in bowel habit
- left-sided abdominal pain
- bleeding
- bloating
- flatulence.

Examination
If a patient has acute left-sided tenderness or any signs of peritonism, this should prompt hospital admission or at the very least urgent outpatient imaging to exclude acute diverticulitis and its complications which may need urgent treatment. Complications to keep in mind:
- Stricturing
- Fistulae
- Perforation
- Abscess formation.

Investigations
With the symptoms being relatively vague and many in common with colorectal malignancy, the priority is to exclude cancer.
- Colonoscopy should be first line if the patient is fit, but it is contraindicated in acute episodes of diverticulitis (risk of perforation).
- CT cologram/'virtual colonoscopy' is carried out with oral contrast, bowel preparation, and CO_2 insufflation in the CT scanner. It is indicated where colonoscopy has failed due to acute angulation, stricturing, or narrowing at the affected areas which the scope cannot pass.
- CT abdomen ± pelvis will confirm the diagnosis, but it will not exclude underlying polyps or cancers, so is reserved for acute episodes.
- If a CT scan occurred during the acute episode which has now settled, they should be reviewed in clinic at 6–8 weeks and colonoscopy arranged to exclude any underlying cancers or polyps.

Management
Avoidance of constipation should be advised to avoid flare-ups. There is no evidence for dietary restrictions at present.

Definition

Fistula

An abnormal tract or connection between two epithelialized surfaces. In diverticulosis, the most common site is *colovesical* (between the colon and urinary bladder).

Surgical options

Where young patients (<60s) have presented with multiple episodes of diverticulitis, careful consideration can be given to sigmoid colectomy. Symptomatic strictures may also prompt a discussion for surgical management. If severe diverticulosis is confined to this area, removing the sigmoid colon will avoid future problems but is of course not without risk as a major operation. Patients may also develop symptomatic colovesical fistulae and present with recurrent UTI, pneumaturia (gas in the urine), or in extreme cases pass feculent matter in the urine. Operations can be difficult as there has usually been chronic inflammation and possibly previous localized perforation making tissue planes difficult to see let alone dissect. Options include sigmoid colectomy and primary anastomosis, Hartman's, or simple proximal diversion with stoma. A urologist will be present to protectively stent the ureters and repair in case of damage intraoperatively.

Proctology

Applied anatomy

The anorectal junction forms a distinct angle due to the puborectalis muscle. The anus is lined by squamous epithelium, while the rectum is lined by columnar epithelium.

This transitional area is known as the mucocutaneous junction representing the fusion of the embryological hindgut and the ectoderm. The internal sphincter is a continuation of the inferior aspect of the circular smooth muscle of the rectum, whereas the external sphincter is derived from striated muscle surrounding the anal canal. Both muscles function to assist defaecation and continence. The autonomic afferents from the pelvic splanchnic nerves of S2–S3 are responsible for the sensation of rectal distension. The pudendal nerve supplies the levator ani muscles and the external sphincter. The internal sphincter receives innovation from both sympathetic and parasympathetic fibres with the parasympathetic nerves being responsible for keeping high intra-anal pressure and closure of the anal canal. (See Table 34.3.)

Examination of the anorectum

Digital rectal examination (DRE)

Ensure adequate privacy and dignity for the patient with a chaperone. Obtain verbal consent for the examination after a full explanation.

- Lie the patient in the fetal position (hip and knee flexed to 90°) on their side.
- Equipment: glove, lubrication, light.
- Inspection: part buttocks carefully and inspect skin of anal verge. Look for excoriation/rashes/stool/mucus/pus/blood/scarring/external openings/swellings—haemorrhoids/warts/polyps/prolapse/fissure. Ask patient to cough to examine contraction of sphincter and to bear down looking for prolapse.
- Palpation: after placing lubricating gel, place pulp of index finger of right hand over the anus. Assess perianal skin circumferentially for scarring, openings, induration (sepsis/malignancy). Note resting tone of sphincter where ↑tone may signify a fissure/local sepsis.

Table 34.3 Anatomical differences above and below the anorectal junction

Above the junction	Below the junction
• Rectum has autonomic sensation	• Anal skin has somatic sensation
• Arterial blood supply from mesenteric vessels	• Arterial supply from iliac vessels
• Venous blood drains into portal circulation	• Drains venous blood into iliac veins
• Drains lymph → mesocolic + para-aortic lymph nodes	• Drains lymph nodes → inguinal lymph nodes

- Examine each quadrant carefully for masses, pain, tenderness, and feel for the smooth rectal mucosa. Assess mass if identified—ulcerated, within or outside wall, mobile fixed, position according to clock face. Note the contents—faeces, blood, mucus. Assess the squeeze pressure. Other areas to examine include pouch of Douglas, cervix, prostate (surface, smooth, enlarged, irregular).
- Check gloved finger at the end.

Endoscopic examination

Sigmoidoscopy
Illuminated tube total 20 cm in length inserted into the rectum for inspection. Rounded obturator, a lens, and a bellow for insufflation. No bowel preparation required; position as per DRE. Use insufflation to separate rectal walls and negotiate Houston's valves to rectosigmoid junction depending on faecal amount present. Biopsies can be taken.

Proctoscopy
Short illuminated tube for inspecting anal canals. Used for managing haemorrhoids where banding or injection can be applied.

Other anorectal investigations
Sepsis/fistula in ano
- MRI scan: identification of fistula tracts, localized sepsis.

Malignancy
- MRI scan: staging of rectal/anal lesions.
- Endoanal US: staging of rectal lesions.

Pelvic floor
- Proctography (MRI): assists in diagnosing obstructed defaecation.
- Endoanal ultrasound: assesses sphincter damage during childbirth.
- Anorectal physiology: assesses anal pressures/volumes and sensation.

Haemorrhoids
Are engorgements of the venous plexuses within the anal canal.

Pathophysiology
Anal cushions are submucosal fibrovascular structures with arteriovenous communications involving the haemorrhoidal arteries, typically found in three classical positions at 3, 7, and 11 o'clock. Straining and passing hard stools → the descent of the anal cushions following degeneration of the connective tissue matrix. Compromise of the venous return causes ↑congestion and subsequent inflammation with the risk of trauma.

Incidence
4.4%.

Risks
Poor fibre intake, constipation, and raised intra-abdominal pressure (e.g. pregnancy, pelvic tumours, etc.).

Types
External haemorrhoids originate from the inferior haemorrhoidal plexus below the dentate line supplied by somatic pain drivers. Internal haemorrhoids originate from superior haemorrhoidal plexus above the dentate line with an *insensate* columnar epithelial. (See Table 34.4.)

Symptoms
On defaecation, little bright red bleeding usually on the tissue paper or in the pan, mucus/faecal discharge, pruritus ani, prolapse, and acute thrombosis.

Investigations
Assessments (1) to exclude malignancy via endoscopy, (2) of evacuation difficulties including anorectal physiology in incontinence. Proctoscopy confirms diagnosis.

Treatment
Conservative (first degree)
Dietary advice, ↑water intake, avoidance of straining and constipation. Topical creams (i.e. local anaesthetics and steroids) for symptomatic relief.

Rubber band ligation (second/third degree)
Success rate up to 80% where bands can be positioned at the base of the internal haemorrhoid at least 1 cm above the dentate line to minimize discomfort.
   Risks: bleeding pain and pelvic sepsis.

Injection sclerotherapy (second/third degree)
Using 5% phenol in almond oil into the anorectal junction. This causes intravascular thrombosis followed by fibrosis. Success rate is lower than rubber band ligation and may require repeated injections.
   Risk: iatrogenic prostatitis.

Haemorrhoidectomy (second/third degree)
Staged (if bulky) vs total excision.
   Risks: anal stenosis, pain (metronidazole may help), bleeding (up to 6 weeks), pelvic sepsis, incontinence.

Transanal haemorrhoidal dearterialization (second/third degree)
This method uses a proctoscope (incorporating a Doppler) to identify and disrupt the superior haemorrhoidal artery (located together with mucosal plication) → less postoperative pain than traditional haemorrhoidectomy.

Table 34.4 Classification of internal haemorrhoids

Degree	Signs
First	Bleeding but no prolapse
Second	Prolapsing but spontaneously reducible
Third	Prolapsing requiring manual reduction
Fourth	Chronic, irreducible prolapse

Stapled haemorrhoidopexy (third/fourth degree)
Restores relationship of the haemorrhoids to the anal canal while disrupting the superior rectal artery → markedly reduced pain/discharge and faster return to normal function. However, there is an ↑ in postoperative faecal urgency, more significant risks of rectal perforation or severe sepsis.

Anal fissure
Is a linear split in the anal mucosa → pain on defaecation.

Aetiology
Most cases are idiopathic, or commonly associated with constipation/repeated diarrhoea. Fissures can also be associated with other conditions such as CD, sarcoid, TB, or drugs such as nicorandil. A majority of fissures are posterior, with anterior fissures more commonly found in postpartum.

Presentation
Self-remitting severe sharp pain on defaecation ± fresh rectal bleeding (noted on wiping). Other symptoms are mucus discharge and perianal itching.

Examination
↑Internal anal sphincter tone and visible mucosal split. Simple fissures heal within a few days, while others persisting for >6 weeks turn chronic, with induration, a sentinel pile (associated skin tag) and visible fibres of the internal anal sphincter. Sepsis can be associated with fissures developing into superficial fistulae. Fissures identified at other sites around the anal circumference or with atypical features should be assessed urgently (often under anaesthetic) to exclude sexually transmitted or malignant ulcers.

> **Honours**
> *Other sources of anorectal ulceration*
> • Malignancy: squamous/basal cell carcinoma.
> • IBD.
> • Perianal haematoma.
> • Infection: syphilis/herpes simplex/TB.
> • Sarcoidosis.
> • Nicorandil ulcers.

Management
Conservative measures such as treatment of constipation, analgesia, and local anaesthetic ointment. A regular bowel habit with the passage of soft stool is central to all treatment pathways with the assistance of both an ↑fibre and ↑fluid intake and stool softeners. Medical therapies reduce anal tone and stimulate healing by ↑ the blood flow. Both topical glyceryl trinitrate and diltiazem for 6 weeks report healing rates of 65–70% (but warn of the risk of headaches due to cranial venous dilatation). Botulinum toxin can be injected into the internal anal sphincter providing relaxation for 3 months. Surgical intervention is a last resort. The commonest form is the lateral sphincterotomy with higher healing rates of 90% reported, although

a risk of minor incontinence is documented in 20–30%. The procedure involves developing a plane in the inter-sphincteric space followed by a controlled partial division of the internal sphincter fibres.

Treatment of anal fissure

Normalization of bowel habit
- ↑Fibre and fluid.
- Stool softeners.

Conservative measures
- Topical ointment: glyceryl trinitrate/diltiazem.

Surgical intervention
- Lateral sphincterotomy.
- Anal advancement flap.

Rectal prolapse

This is an intussusception of the full thickness of the rectum through the anal verge. Most commonly occurs in elderly females likely secondary to pelvic floor weakness and pudendal neuropathy. There is a clear association with incontinence and constipation.

Presentation

Swelling around the anal verge which may either reduce spontaneously or require manual reduction. This is often associated with pain and fresh rectal bleeding together with symptoms of incontinence/tenesmus and constipation. In adults, associations are made with parity and connective tissue disorders together with neurological abnormalities. In children, the commonest association is with cystic fibrosis, chronic constipation, and Hirschsprung's disease.

Diagnosis

Surrounds distinguish a full thickness rectal prolapse from a mucosal prolapse or prolapse of haemorrhoidal disease. One important distinction is the concentric folds demonstrated on a full thickness prolapse, compared with the radial markings of a mucosal prolapse.

A coexisting genital prolapse can be identified in 10–20% of cases.

Investigations

Pelvic floor disorders require a MDT approach including urogynaecologists, radiologists, physiologists, gastroenterologists, and physiotherapists. This warrants an endoscopy to exclude neoplasms, IBD, and solitary rectal ulceration through biopsy. Evacuatory disturbance can be investigated with colonic transit studies to distinguish between a more global picture (pancolonic slow transit constipation) rather than localized to the anorectum (pelvic outlet obstruction), also confirmed by defaecography.

Management

Conservative measures (bulking agents and ↑fibre intake). Surgery via either an abdominal or perineal approach ± resection.

Perineal approach

Delorme's procedure strips the excess rectal mucosa and plication of the prolapsed muscle wall without any resection. It is tolerated well in the frail under spinal anaesthesia. Yet there is a high recurrence rate >25%. Altemeier's procedure involves opening the peritoneal cavity via the prolapse, performing a resection of the rectosigmoid and coloanal anastomosis. Lower recurrence rate but higher risk of anastomotic dehiscence → localized sepsis.

Abdominal approach

Laparoscopic vs open technique. A rectopexy involves mobilization and straightening of the rectum with fixation onto the sacrum with sutures or mesh ± resection. Lower recurrence rates but a higher incidence of defaecatory disorder.

Pilonidal disease

Is a condition affecting the natal cleft usually attributed with hirsute young adults (more in males). It refers to a mass of hairs found within the natal cleft region → subcutaneous abscesses and sinuses containing hair. An acquired disease resulting from a foreign body reaction caused by the frictional forces in the natal cleft region → infection → abscess.

Presentation

Is usually twofold either following formation of an acute abscess requiring either antibiotics or incision and drainage, or secondly with a chronic sinus (midline openings communicating by a granulation tissue lined track containing loose hair follicles). Differentials include hydradenitis suppurativa and complex fistula-in-ano.

Treatment

Incision and drainage of the cavity. The wound is left open and packed with regular dressings and healing rates of ~60% are described. In cases of recurrent disease, rotational flap techniques have been adopted with encouraging results.

Fistula-in-ano

Anal sepsis presents either in the form of an acute abscess or as chronic pain and discharge from an anal fistula. Multiple conditions are associated with anal sepsis including inflammatory bowel conditions such as CD, TB, skin conditions such as hydradenitis suppurativa, trauma or as a sign of malignancy, and a male predominance. Infection of the anal glands in the intersphincteric space is the likely cause of this disorder, where the spread of infection may occur in three directions: vertically (commonest → perianal abscess), horizontally, and circumferentially. Following acute inflammation, infected fluid from the abscess traverses the wall of the anorectal canal along the anal ducts to emerge from the mucocutaneous junction → generating internal + external openings with granulated tract. Endoscopic procedures such as proctoscopy and sigmoidoscopy should be performed in the outpatient clinic. The main areas to be identified as part of the assessment are the locations of the internal and external openings, the path of the primary tract, potential further tracts, and other associated disease. Assessment is complemented by an examination under anaesthesia allowing the probing of openings to confirm tracts. The mainstay of imaging for fistula-in-ano is the MRI scan given its high soft tissue resolution.

Honours

Park's classification of anal fistulae

See Fig. 34.3.

- *Intersphincteric*: tract medial to external sphincter.
- *Transsphincteric*: the primary tract crosses the external sphincter, with the external opening located lateral to the pigmented perianal skin.
- *Extrasphincteric*: often related to pelvic sepsis or after surgical intervention, with the tract lying away from the sphincter complex.
- *Suprasphincteric*: a high tract passing over the levator muscle.
- *Superficial (submucosal)*: limited to superficial tissue often with a skin bridge between openings.

Goodsall's rule is applied to the examination of anal fistula (Fig. 34.4). It states that:

- if the external opening of a fistula lies posterior to a line drawn from 9 to 3 o'clock, then it tracks around the anus laterally and opens into the midline posteriorly
- if the external opening lies anterior to this line, then it opens directly into the anal canal.

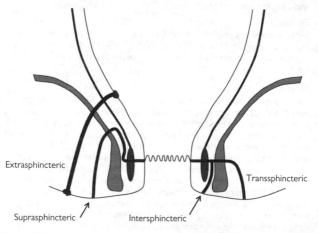

Fig. 34.3 Park's classification of types of anal fistulae. Reproduced with permission from MacKay, G.J. *Colorectal Surgery*, 2010: Oxford University Press.

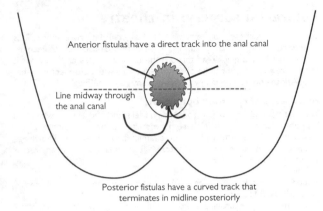

Anterior fistulas have a direct track into the anal canal

Line midway through
the anal canal

Posterior fistulas have a curved track that
terminates in midline posteriorly

Fig. **34.4** Goodsall's rule. Reproduced with permission from MacKay, G.J. *Colorectal Surgery*, 2010: Oxford University Press.

Management

Superficial and intersphincteric fistulae can often be laid open giving them the best chance for resolution. Treatment for transsphincteric and suprasphincteric fistulae can be more complicated, often requiring multiple procedures, focusing on preserving as much sphincter function as possible. In such cases, a loosely tied thread or seton can be placed through the tract. This serves the purpose of a marker of the exact position of the tract in relation to the sphincter, while allowing drainage of acute sepsis and local wound healing. This technique can be used as part of a staged fistulotomy aiming to reduce the amount of division of sphincter fibres. Over the years, other techniques such as core fistulectomy, injection of fibrin glue, insertion of collagen plugs, and more recently laser treatment have been introduced with variable results.

Colorectal surgery: in theatre

You will have a chance to see some technically difficult procedures so it is wise to revise the relevant anatomy and parts of the procedure to keep up. You should have a quick read through the patient's notes and know what procedure you are going to be observing/assisting with before entering theatre. Ask the doctors to take you through any relevant imaging (e.g. CT).

Basic steps of common operations

This will hopefully allow you to better understand and engage when you happen to observe/assist in these procedures during your surgical placements. It would be particularly useful to familiarize/refresh your knowledge of basic abdominal anatomy, e.g. anterior abdominal wall layers and rectus sheath (see Fig. 34.5 and Fig. 34.6):

1. Skin.
2. Superficial fascia comprising of (i) an outer fatty Camper's layer which overlies a (ii) fibrous layer (Scarpa's fascia).
3. A musculo-aponeurotic plane consisting of rectus abdominis, external oblique, internal oblique, and transversus abdominis.
4. Transversalis fascia.
5. Parietal layer of peritoneum.

Laparoscopic appendicectomy

Indication
Appendicitis.

Position
Supine + strapped to bed for tilting patient.

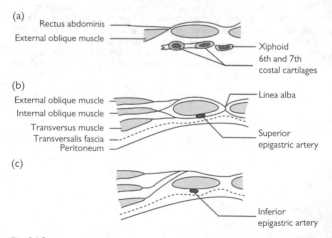

Fig. 34.5. Layers of rectus sheath. Reproduced with permission from Harold Ellis, *Clinical Anatomy* 13e, Wiley, 2013, figure 42, p66.

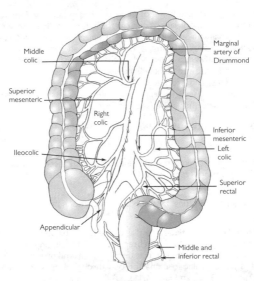

Fig. 34.6 Colonic vascular supply. Reproduced with permission from MacKay, G.J. *Colorectal Surgery*, 2010: Oxford University Press.

Procedure

Establish pneumoperitoneum using Hasson's open technique: carefully dissecting down to the linea alba and the cicatrix. Carefully incise 5 mm at this junction longitudinally and insert a blunt umbilical port under direct vision. Inset laparoscopic camera into abdomen. Insert ports into suprapubic and LIF allowing triangulation of instruments under direct vision and avoiding inferior epigastric artery. Identify appendix and apex of taeniae coli on caecum. Dissect mesoappendix and ligate appendicular artery safely. Skeletalize base of appendix using diathermy and then apply two endoloops to base and one above. Resect appendix above the second endoloop and place it in bag for removal from abdomen. Washout and close.

Lichtenstein hernia repair

Indication

Unilateral inguinal hernia.

Position

Supine.

Procedure

The principle of any hernia repair is to dissect out and define the hernial sac and defect, reduce the contents of the hernia sac, and complete a sound repair to reduce the risk of an incisional hernia. Incision is 1 cm above inguinal canal from level of superficial ring to two-thirds of length of inguinal canal. Incise Scarpa's and Camper's fasciae and ligate vessels encountered securely. Identify arching fibres of external oblique fascia and incise fascia 1 cm proximal to superficial ring and clip the external oblique. Self-retaining retractor to maintain wound open with ilioinguinal nerve preserved and protected. Insert finger down to pubic tubercle and hook finger to draw spermatic cord upwards—hold with rubber sling or hernia ring. Incise external spermatic fascia to identify hernial sac (of indirect hernia), open sac, explore contents, and proceed. Identify direct hernia (deficit in posterior wall/transversalis fascia) in relation to inferior epigastric vessels within Hesselbach's (inguinal) triangle (see Figs 34.7–34.9 and Tables 34.5–34.7)

Laparoscopic right hemicolectomy with primary anastomosis

Indication
Ascending colon/proximal transverse colon cancer/ascending colon diverticulitis complications/caecal volvulus.

Position
Supine, strapped for tilting. Establish pneumoperitoneum.

Procedure
Commence lateral to medial/medial to lateral mobilization of ascending colon. Identify right colic and right branch of middle colic and ligate arteries. Resect tumour through resection at terminal ileum and proximal transverse colon and perform ileocolic anastomosis through extension of umbilical wound (see Fig. 34.10 and Fig. 34.11).

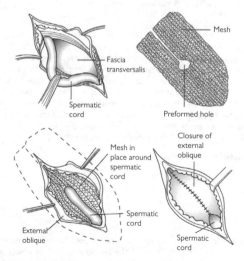

Fig. 34.7 Mesh repair of inguinal hernia—standard steps. Reproduced with permission from McLatchie GR and Leaper DJ. *Oxford Specialist Handbook of Operative Surgery* 2nd edition. 2006. Oxford: Oxford University Press, p.369, Figure 11.1.

Table 34.5 Extension of layers from abdominal wall to spermatic cord

Abdominal wall	Spermatic cord/testicle
Skin	Scrotum
Superficial fascia	Dartos fascia and muscle
External oblique aponeurosis	External spermatic fascia
Internal oblique muscle	Cremaster muscle
Transversalis fascia	Internal spermatic fascia
Peritoneum	(Processus) Tunica vaginalis

Table 34.6 Contents of the inguinal canal: *rules of 3*

Male—spermatic cord/female—round ligament (see also Fig. 34.11)

3 arteries	To the vas, testicle, cremaster
3 fascial layers	Cremaster, external + internal spermatic
3 other structures	Vas deferens, pampiniform venous plexus, genital branch of the genitofemoral nerve (L1/L2)

Table 34.7 Boundaries of the inguinal canal—*2 MALTs*

Roof (2 Muscles)	Muscle: internal oblique + transverse abdominus
Anterior	Aponeurosis: external + internal oblique
Floor (Lower)	Ligaments: inguinal + lacunar
PosTerior	Transversalis fascia + conjoint Tendon

Laparoscopic anterior resection

Indication

Tumour or diverticular complications of rectum or sigmoid colon.

Position

Lloyd Davis.

Procedure

Establish pneumoperitoneum. At the sacral promontory identify and ligate the inferior mesenteric artery, while identifying and protecting the left ureter and gonadal vessels. Continue with medial to lateral and lateral to medial dissection of rectal total mesenteric excision (TME) to reach beyond distal margin. Resect specimen distally with laparoscopic stapler. Extend suprapubic port to Pfannenstiel incision and retrieve specimen into wound and resect proximal margin. Mobilize splenic flexure if require extra length to reach tension-free anastomosis. Circular stapler from rectum and introduce anvil proximally to perform stapled anastomosis. Air leak test to check anastomosis integrity. Perform loop ileostomy to defunction anastomosis. (See Fig. 34.10.)

Stoma surgery

See Table 34.8 for indications.

Sites to avoid

Scars, skin folds, creases, bony prominences, umbilicus, belt/waistline, previous radiation sites

Reversibility

Loop (two lumens (proximal and distal limbs), defunctioning loop colostomy for bowel rest—elective reversal in months–years) vs end (one lumen, e.g. end colostomy, Hartmann's procedure—permanent usually but reconstructive options available). Double-barrelled stoma (Paul–Mikulicz) looks like a loop stoma (but severed into two separate lumens) and has only one functioning lumen excreting faeces.

Table 34.8 Indications of stoma (Greek for 'mouth/opening')

Type	Loop (temporary) vs end (permanent)
Feeding	Percutaneous endoscopic gastro-/jejunostomy
Decompression	Obstruction (e.g. colorectal cancer)
Diversion	IBD, ischaemia, fistulae, bowel perforation, trauma, protecting distal bowel anastomosis (temporary)
Exteriorization	Bowel perforation, low rectal cancers, permanent stomas (abdominoperineal resection), low bowel perforations

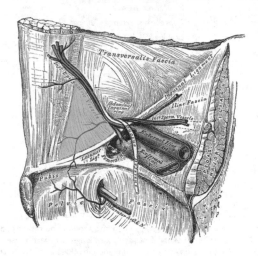

Fig. 34.8 Hesselbach's (inguinal) triangle (green). Reproduced from Häggström, Mikael (2014). 'Medical gallery of Mikael Häggström 2014'. *WikiJournal of Medicine* 1 (2). Public Domain.

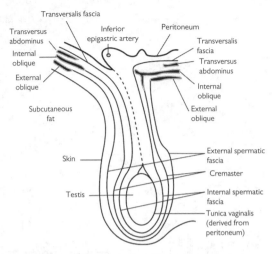

Fig. 34.9 Contents and coverings of inguinal ligament. Reproduced with permission from Agarwal, Anil, *Oxford Handbook of Operative Surgery* 3e, 2017: Oxford University Press.

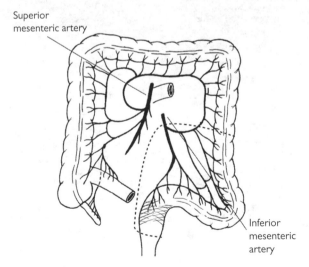

Fig. 34.10 Anterior resection. Reproduced with permission from McLatchie, G, and Leaper, D. *Operative Surgery* 2nd edition, Oxford University Press: 2006.

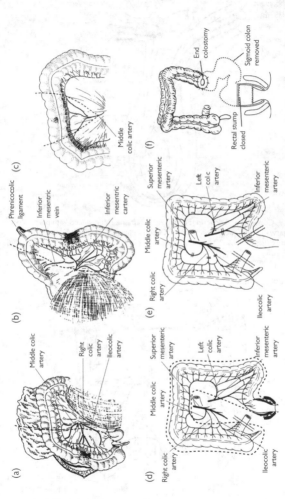

Fig. 34.11 Options for colectomies. A = right colectomy, B = left colectomy, C = transverse colectomy, D = abdominoperineal resection (APE), E = total colectomy, F = Hartmann's procedure. Reproduced with permission from McLatchie, G, and Leaper, D. *Operative Surgery* 2nd edition, Oxford University Press: 2006.

Colorectal surgery: on the ward

Anastomotic leak (AL)

This is failure of a surgical joint between two hollow viscera resulting in leakage of luminal content.

Incidence

Ranges from 2% to 25% following colorectal surgery and has an associated mortality as high as ~40%.[1] Typically occurring 5–7 days postoperatively, signs and symptoms can vary from subtle, tachycardia, low-grade pyrexia, prolonged ileus, to a septic patient with a rigid peritonitic abdomen with faecal matter present in surgical drains.

Risk factors

Poor nutrition, steroid use, perioperative blood transfusions, and importantly, the level of the anastomosis—with ↑risk of AL ≤7 cm from the anal verge.

Consequences

Intra-abdominal abscess, enterocutaneous fistula, and global peritonitis.

Management

High level of suspicion of an AL is required, with a low threshold to order a CT abdomen/pelvis; or take the patient urgently back to theatre for washout and proximal faecal diversion in the form of an ileostomy or colostomy. Air leak test can identify anastomotic leaks intraoperatively, and right-sided anastomoses have a lower AL risk than left ones (~1 vs 5%).

Wound dehiscence

This is failure of wound healing resulting in partial or complete re-opening of a surgical incision (see Table 34.9 for risk factors).

Incidence

Estimated at 0.5–3.4% of abdominopelvic surgeries and associated with a 40% mortality rate.[2]

Aetiology

Can be categorized as pre-, peri-, and postoperative. Initial signs can be ↑abdominal pain and pink wound discharge (blood-tinged peritoneal exudate); preceding complete wound dehiscence where abdominal viscera may protrude through the wound or be visible.

Management

If stable, urgent return to theatre for closure with tension sutures.

Honours

See Table 34.9.

Table 34.9 Risk factors for wound dehiscence

Factors contributing to wound dehiscence		
Preoperative	Perioperative	Postoperative
• Diabetes	• Poor surgical technique, e.g. suture placement or slip knots	• Chronic cough
• Smoking		• ↑Intra-abdominal pressure
• Vitamin K deficiency	• Wound contamination	• Wound infection
• Anaemia		
• Malignancy		

Postoperative ileus (POI)

This is disruption in normal peristalsis of the alimentary canal following surgery. It is considered an expected physiological response after handling bowel, lasting for hours (stomach/small bowel) and days for the colon.

POI is considered pathological when it extends beyond these periods and results in intolerance of oral intake, abdominal distension, and N&V.

Aetiology

Prolonged POI includes intra-abdominal sepsis, drugs (opioids), and electrolyte disturbances (K^+/Mg^{2+}). Longer duration of surgery and open technique (vs laparoscopy) ↑POI risk too.

Management

A NG tube should be passed if significant abdominal distension and repeated vomiting, with fluid resuscitation to match gastric output and fluid requirement. Parenteral nutrition should be considered if POI extends beyond 7–10 days. POI resolution is monitored through (1) reduced NG output, (2) abdominal distension, and (3) passing of flatus/stool.

Low postoperative urine output

Oliguria is defined as urine output <0.5 mL/kg/hour. *Causes*: categorized as (1) pre-, (2) renal, or (3) post-renal oliguria. Initial assessment should look to identify evidence of pre-renal causes—negative fluid balance or sustained periods of hypotension. Hypovolaemia may be caused due to fluid losses from haemorrhage, evaporation, and 'third spacing'.

Management

Fluid resuscitation guided by response to fluid challenges. Excessive fluid administration → ↑risks of complications (e.g. anastomotic leakage and bleeding). A common post-renal cause is a palpably distended bladder due to urinary retention. In the absence of pre/post-renal causes, intrinsic renal causes can be explored.

Investigations

Fluid challenges, flush urinary catheter, stop nephrotoxics, urine dip ± MSU, U&E, renal US.

Postoperative pyrexia

A low-grade fever is common in the first 24 hours following surgery due to the release of inflammatory mediators. Postoperative pyrexia can be indicative of a range of postoperative complications, which can be remembered as the 7 Cs:

• Chest (infection or PE)
• Catheter (infection)
• Cut (wound infection)
• Collection (subphrenic/pelvic)
• Cannula (infection)
• Central venous line (infection)
• Calves (DVT).

Further clues as to the source of the pyrexia could be taken from associated signs and symptoms—respiratory or irritative urinary symptoms and wound discharge. Pre-existing comorbidities → a higher risk of specific complications (e.g. COPD patient and pneumonia, or diabetics and wound infections). The nature and timing of onset of the pyrexia—intra-abdominal collections typically developing 4–10 days postoperatively and following a swinging pattern. *Management*: stabilize the patient with high-flow oxygen and IV fluids, septic screen including bloods ± cultures, ABG, CXR, urine dip ± MSU, wound/line swab, stool sample, CT, etc. *Treatment*: antibiotics, removal of infected lines/catheters or surgical wound clips to encourage draining of discharge and radiological/surgical drainage of abdominal collections.

Complications of stoma surgery

Early

• Bleeding.
• Infection—mostly candidiasis and *Staphylococcus aureus*.
• High output → dehydration, hypovolaemia, and electrolyte disturbance.
• Electrolyte disturbance (Na^+, K^+, Ca^{2+}, Mg^{2+}).
• Peristomal contact/allergic dermatitis (from ileostomy contents).
• Ischaemia/necrosis—dusky, dark, purple, and black appearance.
• Bowel obstruction (from constipation or parastomal hernia).
• Ileus (takes several days to resolve).

Late

• Prolapse (from high intra-abdominal pressure).
• Retraction (from excess tension) → peristomal dermatitis → leakage.
• Stomal stenosis/strictures (from chronic ischaemia).
• Parastomal hernia (from chronic comorbidities such as diabetes and immunosuppression → poor healing, high intra-abdominal pressure).
• Peristomal pyoderma gangrenosum (from ulceration in IBD).
• Fistula formation.

References

1. Murrell ZA, Stamos MJ (2006). Reoperation for anastomotic failure. *Clin Colon Rectal Surg* 19(4):213–6.
2. Shanmugam VK, Fernandez SJ, Evans KK, et al. (2015). Postoperative wound dehiscence: predictors and associations. *Wound Repair Regen* 23(2):184–90.

Colorectal surgery: in the emergency department

Acute abdomen

Is a surgical emergency and presents as *peritonitis*. Acute abdominal pain is commonly referred to the surgeons with a wide range of pathologies. Any viscus is susceptible to obstruction, inflammation, perforation, or ischaemia, and it is helpful to think about the differentials in terms of site of pain (i.e. organ involved) and these four mechanisms of pathology. (See Table 34.10.)

Ischaemic colitis

Left-sided abdominal pain, bleeding, and diarrhoea from ischaemia to the splenic flexure or descending colon in the area supplied by the marginal artery. Essentially this is the part of the colon with the poorest blood supply. *Pathology*: low-flow states or other significant medical issues can precipitate this condition. *Diagnosis*: can be clinically suspected based on abdominal CT scan. There is no acute occlusion here as in acute mesenteric ischaemia but CT could show end-organ ischaemia or simply colitis. If CT is unclear, endoscopy and biopsy can confirm the diagnosis. *Management*: supportive with fluids and optimization of cardiovascular status. Surgery and resection will be rarely required if there is complete necrosis, if the patient is peritonitic and in extremis. These patients are usually high risk as vasculopaths. Most times patients will stabilize with conservative measures.

Acute mesenteric ischaemia

Occurs with blockage of the superior mesenteric artery (a principal arterial supply of the GI tract) with an embolus. Associated mortality rate of 70% due to high risk of bowel perforation secondary to absolute ischaemia.

Table 34.10 Differentials for right lower quadrant pain

Organ	Inflammation	Obstruction	Perforation (local/generalized)	Ischaemia
Appendix	Appendicitis		Appendicitis	
Caecum	IBD	Bowel obstruction (with competent ileocaecal valve)		
Bowel	IBD	LBO/SBO	Ulcers LBO/SBO	Mesenteric ischaemia
Tubo-ovarian	Salpingitis/oophoritis Cyst		Ectopic pregnancy	
Ureter	UTI	Stone, tumour, clots	Iatrogenic (intraoperative)	

IBD, inflammatory bowel disease; LBO/SBO, large/small bowel obstruction; UTI, urinary tract infection.

Presentation
Classically with severe diffuse abdominal pain disproportionate to clinical findings (Fig. 34.12), bloody bowel evacuation, and the presence of new-onset AF. A high index of suspicion should be adopted in older arteriopathic patients with cardiovascular comorbidities.

Investigations
ABG—high lactate/metabolic acidosis. May also have high WCC, CRP and amylase in formal blood testing.

Management
Fluid resuscitate, correct dysrhythmias, antibiotics, followed by prompt CT angiography (if patient is stable) or exploratory laparotomy (if unstable/peritonitic) for resection of necrotic bowel.

Appendicitis

Is the most common abdominal surgical emergency, resulting in 40,000 admissions annually in England[1] and occurs after obstruction of the vermiform appendiceal lumen → inflammation → phlegmon/abscess or tissue necrosis/perforation.

Aetiology
Faecolith, lymphoid hyperplasia, and malignancy.

Peak incidence
Age 10–19 years.

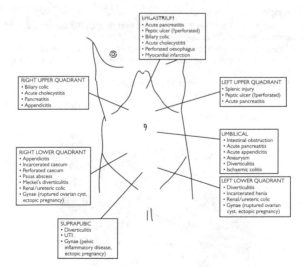

Fig. 34.12. Causes of abdominal pain according to each section. Reproduced with permission from Athanasios Kalantzis and Crispian Scully, *Applied Medicine and Surgery in Dentistry* (3 ed.) 2009, Oxford University Press.

Presentation

Classically a short history of initially intermittent, diffuse periumbilical pain, which migrates and evolves into a constant localized right lower quadrant pain days later, associated with N&V and anorexia.

Examination signs

Guarding and rebound tenderness at McBurney's point (one-third of the way between umbilicus and anterior superior iliac spine (ASIS)). (See Fig. 34.13.)

- Rovsing's sign (palpating left lower quadrant induces pain in right lower quadrant).
- Iliopsoas sign (pain on hip extension in retrocaecal appendix).
- Obturator (Cope's) sign (pain on hip internal rotation in pelvic appendicitis).
- Dunphy's sign (pain on movement and coughing).

The most common appendix tip location is retrocaecal.

Investigations

WCC (neutrophilia/left shift), urine pregnancy test (rule out ectopic pregnancy), and US in atypical cases where other differentials may be likely (e.g. ovarian pathology). *Diagnosis*: can be guided by scoring systems (Alvarado) and investigations, but the diagnosis is fundamentally clinical.

Management

Prompt antibiotics and laparoscopic appendicectomy with washout ± drain insertion if complicated appendicitis.

> **Top tips**
>
> - *Younger patients:* Be aware of those presenting with RIF pain as a sign of terminal ileitis (CD) as opposed to appendicitis.
> - *Males:* any male with abdominal pain *requires* a testicular exam.
> - *Child bearing age: always do a urinary pregnancy test to rule out an ectopic pregnancy!*
> - *Older patients:* at the other end of the age scale, right-sided colonic tumours may present as RIF pain mimicking appendicitis (or even causing it) and patients over the age of 50 should be investigated with an urgent CT scan prior to operation.

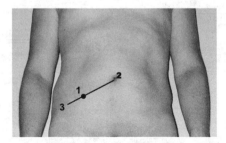

Fig. 34.13 McBurney's point. Reproduced from https://commons.wikimedia.org/w/index.php?curid=1211886 licensed under the Creative Commons Attribution-Share Alike 3.0 Unported license.

Diverticulitis

This is the presence of diverticulum (outpouching of the bowel wall) most commonly present in the sigmoid colon and is present in half the population ≥50 years. Diverticulitis occurs when faecal matter and bacteria congregate within these outpouchings resulting in inflammation.

Risk factors

Age, low-fibre diet (western diet), smoking, and obesity. *Presentation*: left lower quadrant pain, low-grade fever, less commonly PR bleeding, tender on PR.

Management

Conservatively with fluids and antibiotics. CT can (1) confirm the diagnosis, (2) see if it is amenable for radiological drainage of abscesses, and (3) identify any complications (e.g. perforation or fistulas). Extent of perforations can be classified using the Hinchey classification. Surgical management is required in one-third of patients who fail to respond to conservative treatment/perforation with faecal peritonitis—commonly a Hartmann's procedure with a colostomy. (See Fig. 34.14.)

Large bowel obstruction (LBO)

Is the mechanical blockage of the colon preventing the passage of colonic content → gross dilation → bowel perforation (if untreated). It is less common than small bowel obstruction (SBO), only accounting for 20% of bowel obstructions.

Aetiology

90% accounted for by colonic malignancy and diverticulitis. Other causes are volvulus (sigmoid/caecal), faecal impaction (especially in the elderly and secondary to opioids) and hernias. (See Fig. 34.15.)

Presentation

Initial colicky abdominal pain which becomes constant. Absolute constipation is where there is no passing of stool or flatus. Worsening pain on movement may imply bowel ischaemia/perforation. Vomiting is initially gastric → bilious → faecal. In LBO, vomiting is a late sign but vice versa in SBO. *Examination*: tympanitic abdomen, palpable abdominal mass, visible hernia, localized tenderness (ischaemic bowel segment), tinkling bowel sounds, PR rectal mass/empty.

Investigations

Lactate (to assess level of ischaemia); AXR/CXR—free air (pneumoperitoneum secondary to perforation), level of bowel dilatation, volvulus, concurrent small bowel loops suggests incompetent ileocaecal value; CT to demonstrate the level and cause of LBO.

Management

Varies according to the cause and associated complications (ischaemia/perforation). Treatments range from conservative '*drip and suck*' (keep patient nil by mouth, IV fluids plus NG tube) to surgery.

Top tip

Always examine hernial orifices in patients presenting with bowel obstruction.

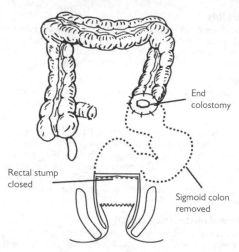

Fig. 34.14 Hartmann's procedure. Reproduced with permission from McLatchie, G, and Leaper, D. *Operative Surgery* 2nd edition, Oxford University Press: 2006.

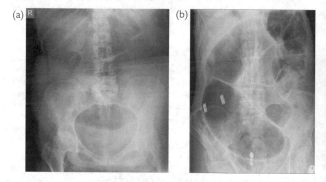

Fig. 34.15 AXR of caecal volvulus (left) and sigmoid volvulus (right). Reproduced with permission from Thomas, William E.G., et al, *Oxford Textbook of Fundamentals of Surgery*, 2016 Oxford University Press.

Reference

1. Simpson J, Samaraweera AP, Sara RK, et al. (2008). Acute appendicitis – a benign disease? *Ann R Coll Surg Engl* 90(4):313–6.

Colorectal surgery: in exams

History

Typical OSCE histories orientate around PR bleeding, change in bowel habit, and abdominal pain. Generally speaking you cover most of the same questions but ask increasingly focused questions depending on the actor's responses. Key focused questions:

- *PR bleeding*: blood on toilet paper/in toilet/around stool/mixed in stool. Was the blood fresh/clots/melaena? Amount of blood (teaspoons/cups)/frequency?
- *Change of bowel habit*: weight loss, anorexia, symptoms of anaemia (lethargy, sob, palpitations), tenesmus, family history.
- *Familiarize yourself* with common abdominal scars and what previous surgeries they represent (see Fig. 34.16). They may act as clues to what other clinical signs you may expect to find during the examination (e.g. laparotomy scar associated with a reversed stoma scar). Remember that one of the key differentiating features between a surgical abdominal examination vs a medical one is the addition of vascular clinical signs (abdominal aortic aneurysm and aortic/renal bruits). So if you find you finish your examination station with time to spare, just quickly consider whether you felt for an expansile and pulsatile mass (Table 34.11), and whether you only listened for bowel sounds instead of renal/femoral bruits. Common signs presenting in the surgical abdomen examination include hernia, stoma, hepato-/splenomegaly, and renal transplant (palpable mass in right lower quadrant).

Stoma examination

A stoma is a surgically created opening into a hollow viscus into the external environment. Stomas in exams are very common since it is a common procedure in colorectal surgery.

Introduction

Introduce yourself, wash your hands, and put on gloves. Lie the patient down at 45° and explain what you will be doing.

Inspection

- *Site*: colostomy usually in LIF vs ileostomy in RIF (but stomas can be anywhere—see Fig. 34.17).
- *Sprout*: ileostomy/urostomy are sprouted to avoid contact dermatitis (from alkaline/caustic content). Colostomy is flushed to the skin.
- *Content*: green/brown soft/liquid output in ileostomy. Formed faecal matter in colostomy. Urostomy contains urine.
- *Number of lumens*: single (end) vs double (loop).
- *Output*: ileostomy (500–1000 mL/day) > colostomy (<300 mL/day).
- *Complications*: retraction (obstruction), prolapsed (high output), infarction, parastomal hernia (risk of bowel strangulation), haemorrhage, excoriations, skin changes.

Palpation

Having removed the stoma bag:

- Palpate for stoma tenderness.
- Ask the patient to cough and palpate for parastomal hernia.
- Look at your finger tip to rule out blood, pus, and mucus.

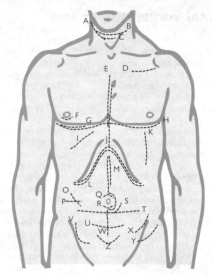

Fig. 34.16 Incisions of the neck, chest, and abdomen. A. Carotid incision B. Thyroidectomy incision C. Tracheotomy incision D. Subclavicular incision E. Sternotomy incision F. Infra-areolar incision G. Inframammary incision (either side) H. Clamshell incision I. Kocher/subcostal incision J. Mercedes Benz incision K. Paramedian incision (either side) L. Chevron incision M. Epigastric/upper midline incision O. McBurney's/Gridiron incision (right side only—for appendectomy) P. Rockey-Davis/Lanz incision (right side only—for appendectomy) Q. Supraumbilical incision R. Infraumbilical incision S. Pararectus incision T. Mayland incision U. Pfannenstiel/Kerr/pubic incision V. Gibson incision (either side, but conventionally left) W. Midline incision X. Inguinal incision Y. Femoral incision Z. Turner–Warwick's incision. Reproduced from Wikimedia commons, available under Creative Commons Public Domain.

Auscultate for bowel sounds

To rule out obstruction (high-pitched tinkling) and ileus (absent).

Hernia examination

Hernia is defined as a protrusion of (part of) a viscus through the walls of its containing cavity into an abnormal position. (See Fig. 34.18 and Table 34.12.)

Aetiology

Congenital (patent processes vaginalis), acquired (surgical incisions) defects in the abdominal wall or due to ↑intra-abdominal pressure (cough, straining, ascites). Hernias can present in clinic as a relatively asymptomatic lump or can present in the ED with pain and distension due to complications:

• Incarceration
• Obstruction
• Strangulation.

Table 34.11 Examining a lump or bump

Finding	Examples
Site	Local anatomy
Size	Width × length × depth
Shape	Round/oval
Surface	Smooth/lumpy
Surrounding skin	Erythema, bruise, sinus/fistula, lacerations/abrasions
Consistency	Soft/firm/hard/irregular
Compressibility	Yes (e.g. saphena varix or varicose veins)/no
Colour	Erythema, pigmentation
Tenderness	On palpation
Transillumination	Using pen torch (e.g. cyst/lipoma)
Tethering	E.g. to skin
Fluctuance	Yes with a fluid thrill (e.g. cyst/abscess)/no
Fixity/mobility	E.g. to deep structures like underlying muscles
Pulsatility	Yes (e.g. aneurysm)/no
Percussion	Resonant vs dull (e.g. in cystic and solid lesions)
Reducibility	Yes/no (e.g. reducible vs strangulated hernias)
Auscultation	?Bruit (e.g. aneurysm)
Edges	Smooth/nodular/defined borders/hard (e.g. cancer/bone)
Distal examination	Nerves, lymph nodes, pulses and capillary refill

The *sac* is a diverticulum of peritoneum, consisting of the mouth, neck, body, and fundus. It is covered by layers of the abdominal wall. Content normally consists of the omentum or bowel.

Inguinal hernias
These are the commonest hernia (prevalence of 4% >45 years and accounting for 75% of all anterior abdominal wall hernias). These usually appear in clinical exams so take every opportunity to examine these on the ward, in clinic, or in the ED. (See Table 34.13.)

Anatomy
The deep inguinal ring is at the *midpoint of the inguinal ligament* (halfway between *ASIS* and pubic *tubercle*). The superficial ring is just lateral to the pubic crest. Do not get confused with *mid-inguinal point* (halfway between *ASIS* and the pubic *symphysis*) which is the location of the femoral pulse. (See Fig. 34.19 and Fig. 34.20.)

Table. 34.12 Classification of hernias

Reducible	Contents can be returned to the abdomen
Irreducible	Contents cannot be returned to the abdomen
Obstructed	Bowel in hernia is obstructed but *not* ischaemic
Strangulated	Bowel in hernia is ischaemic → gangrene → perforation → peritonitis
Incarcerated	Bowel in hernial sac is blocked with faeces/adhesions
Reduction-en-mass	Reduction of the hernial sac together with its contents with the bowel still remaining incarcerated (rare form of acute bowel obstruction)

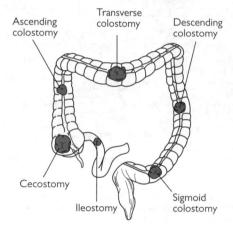

Fig. 34.17 Sites of stoma Reproduced from Lammon, Carol, et al, *Clinical Nursing Skills*, 1995, with permission from Elsevier.

Table. 34.13 Types of inguinal hernias

Dual/pantaloon/saddlebag	Concurrent direct and indirect inguinal hernias
Sliding (hernia-en-glissade)	Retroperitoneal organ is part of hernial sac
Richter	Partial circumference of the bowel is obstructed ± strangulated
Maydl	'W' hernia: hernial sac contains two loops of bowel with another loop of bowel being intra-abdominal
Littre	Meckel's diverticulum in hernial sac
Amyand	Appendix in hernial sac

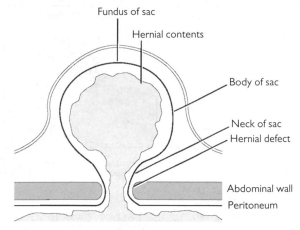

Fig. 34.18 Composition of a hernia. Reproduced with permission from Francis, David M.A., et al, *Textbook of Surgery* 3e, 2008, Wiley.

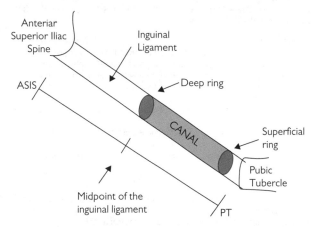

Fig. 34.19 Anatomical landmarks of the inguinal canal. Image reproduced from GeekyMedics.com, illustrated by Mr Robert Pearson.

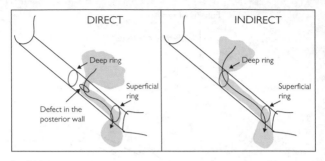

Fig. 34.20 Differentiating direct and indirect inguinal hernias. Image reproduced from GeekyMedics.com, illustrated by Mr Robert Pearson.

Steps of examination

1. *Introduction*: introduce yourself, wash your hands, gain consent.
2. *Inspection*: look for vomiting bowls and lie the patient down before standing the patient up to repeat the examination. Look for abdominal/groin lumps and ask the patient to cough (cough impulse).
3. *Palpation*: for scrotal contents + hernia orifices. Describe the lump and feel for a cough impulse. Gently reduce the lump and check for reducibility.
4. *Percuss*: for bowel in the hernial sac and examine the abdomen
5. *Auscultate*: the hernia for bowel sounds.

Reducibility

- *Direct* inguinal hernias occur through a defect in the posterior wall (transversalis fascia) of the inguinal canal at Hesselbach's triangle.
- *Indirect* inguinal hernias traverse via the inguinal canal—through the deep and out of the superficial ring (and often into the scrotum—i.e. inguinoscrotal)
- To differentiate between the two, reduce the lump, cover the deep ring, and ask the patient to cough.
- If the hernia returns, it is a *direct* inguinal hernia, and *indirect* if it does not.
- However, the true origin of a hernia can only be confirmed after surgery.

Femoral hernias

The femoral canal lies medial to the femoral vein and acts as a space for physiological expansion of the femoral vein. Femoral hernias can occur by passing through the femoral ring through the canal and out of the saphenous opening. Femoral hernias are more common in *women* due to the wider pelvic shape. The tightness of the femoral ring makes femoral hernias higher risk for *strangulation* than inguinal hernias (providing a more pressing need to operate) but may be managed conservatively with monitoring.

Ear, nose, and throat surgery

Ear, nose, and throat surgery: overview

Otolaryngology/head and neck surgery, or ear, nose, and throat (ENT) surgery as it is commonly known, is an incredibly diverse specialty. At least 50% of ENT is clinic based reflecting the large medical component of the specialty. Medical school ENT rotations are typically short which means you have to be particularly proactive.

Cases to see

Epistaxis

These patients usually present to the ED.

Acute tonsillitis and quinsy

Again, these patients usually present to the ED or are admitted directly onto the ENT ward. As well as seeing patients with acute tonsillitis, consolidate your learning with observing an elective tonsillectomy.

Head and neck cancer

If your ENT department has a head and neck service, it is best to spend time in the head and neck clinic to see a large volume of patients at different stages of their disease. Otherwise the neck lump clinic will provide an ideal opportunity to practise palpating thyroid and neck masses.

Otitis externa

Commonly referred to the ENT emergency clinic by the GP, these patients may require aural microsuction under a microscope, allowing you to view the ear under high magnification.

Airway emergencies

Due to the unpredictable timing, you may not be exposed to an airway emergency during your attachment.

Investigations/procedures to see

Flexible nasoendoscopy

Commonly performed in clinic, on the ward, or in ED to look for abnormalities with the internal nose, post-nasal space, pharynx, and larynx.

Pure tone audiometry

This is performed by audiologists in the audiometry department to assess hearing.

Operations

Aim to see the common operations for each of the main subspecialties of ENT: tonsillectomy, adenoidectomy, myringotomy and grommet insertion, functional endoscopic sinus surgery, septoplasty, myringoplasty, thyroidectomy, tracheostomy, and neck dissections.

Ear, nose, and throat surgery: in clinic

Otitis externa

Inflammation or infection of the external ear. Risk factors for this condition include swimmers, psoriasis, and diabetes. On examination there may be associated cellulitis of the pinna, a narrowed and oedematous external auditory canal (EAC), with foul smelling discharge and debris. Management includes advice on keeping the ears dry (i.e. no swimming), and regular aural toileting and antibiotic steroid ear drops. Aural microsuction is the mainstay of treatment. If the EAC is narrow, a pope wick can be inserted to reduce swelling. In diabetic patients it is important to exclude malignant otitis externa where classically there are granulations on the floor of the EAC. Treatment is with systemic and topical antibiotics.

Lower motor neuron seventh nerve palsy

A full cranial nerve exam should be performed, in order to determine if there are any other neurological signs and if the seventh nerve palsy is an upper or lower motor neuron lesion. In a lower motor neuron lesion, the entire ipsilateral face is affected, while in an upper motor neuron lesion, the forehead is spared. The ears should be examined and a neck examination should be performed to exclude any neck lumps. Causes of a lower motor neuron lesion include Bell's palsy, viral infections, cholesteatoma, cerebellopontine angle tumours, trauma, and malignancies of the parotid gland. When a cause for a lower motor neuron seventh nerve lesion cannot be found, it is termed Bell's palsy. The majority of Bell's palsy patients make a full recovery. This is managed with a course of oral prednisolone. Corneal ulceration can occur if there is incomplete eye closure so the patient should be given eye drops/ointment and advised to tape their eyelid closed at night. The presence of painful vesicles over the ear canal, on the tongue, and palate may suggest Ramsay Hunt syndrome, which is causes by herpes zoster infection. Aciclovir and prednisolone are the usual treatments.

Fractured nose

A patient with a fractured injury must be examined to exclude a head injury, another facial bone fracture, CSF leak, or septal haematoma. Otherwise they are usually seen in the ENT emergency clinic after 5–7 days once swelling has reduced. If the nose is deviated, and the patient is unhappy with their appearance, a manipulation under anaesthesia may be performed within 14 days of the injury, and certainly by 21 days at the latest.

Acute otitis media

An infection of the middle ear, which affects all ages but is very common in children. Often there will be history of a recent UTRI, followed by otalgia and fever. Discharge suggests a perforated ear drum. Management consists of analgesia. Antibiotics are not routinely indicated but may be beneficial if symptoms persist after 2 days, if there is systemic upset, or a particularly bulging tympanic membrane. (See Fig. 35.1.)

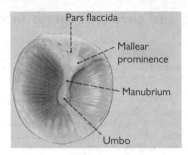

Fig. 35.1 Anatomy of the tympanic membrane. Reproduced from Baloh, Robert W., Honrubia, Vicente, et al., *Baloh and Honrubia's Clinical Neurophysiology of the Vestibular System* (4 ed.), 2011, Oxford University Press.

Vertigo

This is a hallucination of movement and needs to be differentiated from other symptoms such as lightheadedness and unsteadiness. It is important to probe about the character of the symptom and any triggers. Vertigo can be due to central or peripheral causes. Central vertigo is caused from an insult to brainstem vestibular nuclei that can result from CVA, MS, and tumours. The majority of vertigo is a result of peripheral causes.

Neck lump

Most neck lumps in children will be benign, but in adults a neck lump is considered malignant until proven otherwise. Red flag symptoms for head and neck malignancy are important to recognize and include a short duration of presentation with an enlarging lump, associated unilateral otalgia or nasal obstruction, dysphonia, dysphagia, and weight loss. These symptoms should raise the suspicion of either malignant lymphadenopathy or a primary malignancy. Ask about risk factors for malignancy. Weight loss and night sweats may suggest lymphoma. A recent URTI suggests reactive lymph nodes. A benign diagnosis is more likely for a neck lump with a longer history and without red flag symptoms. Clinic investigations include a full ENT examination, flexible nasoendoscopy, and blood tests. FNAC of the lesion may be performed to diagnose the neck lump. Imaging includes US, CT, or MRI of the neck. A CT chest or CXR can be used to exclude a second primary or distant metastasis. Panendoscopy is indicated if these investigations do not yield a diagnosis.

Honours
Risk factors for head and neck cancer
The biggest risk factors for developing head and neck cancers are smoking tobacco and drinking alcohol. If these risk factors are combined, then there is a synergistic ↑ in the likelihood of developing cancer. About 75% of head and neck cancers are related to tobacco and alcohol. Smaller risk factors include a positive FHx, previous radiotherapy, exposure to wood dust (paranasal sinus cancers), nickel, and asbestos. Infection with HPV subtypes 16 and 18 is now recognised as an important risk factor, and is responsible for the dramatic increase in oropharyngeal cancers.

Investigations
Pure tone audiogram
This is the standard hearing test performed by audiologists in a soundproof booth to determine the hearing sensitivities to tones with a set frequency (pure tones). The aim is to detect the extent of hearing loss. Frequencies vary from low pitches to high pitches. A button is pressed by the patient when they can hear the sound being played through the microphone, and the sound intensity is ↓ until it is no longer heard. The results are plotted on a chart, providing information on the severity of hearing loss, and whether the hearing loss is conductive, sensorineural, or mixed. The hearing test requires the cooperation of the individual, so it cannot be used on children under the age of 3.

US scan
Permits the rapid assessment of masses arising from the neck, thyroid gland, and salivary glands without the risks of radiation or contrast. It gives important information on whether a lesion is cystic or solid. When performed by an experienced operator in conjunction with FNAC it has high sensitivity and specificity for diagnosis. US scanning is limited by the skill of the operator, and is inappropriate for deeper structures.

MRI scan
The ability to define soft tissue makes MRI the gold standard for diagnosing vestibular schwannomas. It is important in evaluating the extent of head and neck tumours, and to look for any vascular involvement. Contraindicated in patients with metallic implants and cochlear implants.

Ear, nose, and throat surgery: in the emergency department

Epistaxis

Nosebleeds are very common and most cases are self-limiting. In more severe cases, blood loss has the potential to be significant necessitating prompt treatment. Causes are divided into local (e.g. idiopathic, nose picking, trauma, infection, tumours) and systemic (e.g. anticoagulation, hypertension, coagulopathy). The commonest site of bleeding is Little's area, (the Kiesselbach's) plexus of branches of the internal and external carotid arteries located at the anterior nasal septum. Less commonly, the source of bleeding is the posterior septum from Woodruff's plexus. Remember that anterior epistaxis is more common but posterior epistaxis can be more more serious. All patients requiring admission need a FBC and clotting screen and severe cases require a group and save. Interventions start with basic first aid (applying firm pressure and ice to the nose) and progressing in a stepwise manner to cauterization (silver nitrate sticks), anterior nasal packing (with tampons or bismuth iodine paraffin paste impregnated ribbon gauze), posterior nasal packing with a Foley catheter, electrocautery, ligation of artery, and embolization.

Acute tonsillitis and peritonsillar abscess

Tonsillitis is a very common condition. The condition presents with sore throat, pain and difficulty in swallowing, fever, tonsillar swelling and exudate, and earache. (See Fig. 35.2.) It is usually bacterial in origin but can occur after a viral infection. Patients who have difficulty swallowing enough fluids or severe pain usually require admission. Treatment consists of regular analgesia, oral or IV fluids, and penicillin antibiotics (ampicillin is not given due to a potential type IV hypersensitivity reaction, a pruritic maculopapular rash, in patients with glandular fever). Tonsillitis can be complicated with a peritonsillar abscess (quinsy) which presents as a swelling of the soft tissue between the tonsil and pharyngeal constrictor with uvular deviation. Incision and drainage or aspiration using a wide-bore needle and IV antibiotics is required.

Airway emergencies

Airway emergencies are uncommon, but potentially life-threatening when they occur. Senior help is mandatory and management should be joint with anaesthetics and in children, the paediatric team. Stridor is an important sign that you need to witness. It is caused by a narrowed airway, and is a late alarm sign for airway obstruction. Acquired causes include croup, epiglottis, supraglottitis, foreign body, trauma, or a deep neck space infection. The priority is to decide whether intervention is needed to secure the airway and this is based on careful assessment of the patient to look for any respiratory distress. In children, it is important not to cause further distress, so that means do not examine their throat, no cannulas, and no radiographs. Medical management involves high-flow oxygen, nebulized adrenaline (epinephrine), IV steroids, and antibiotics if the cause is infective. Definitive airway interventions begin with endotracheal intubation, and if this fails a cricothyroidotomy or tracheostomy is indicated.

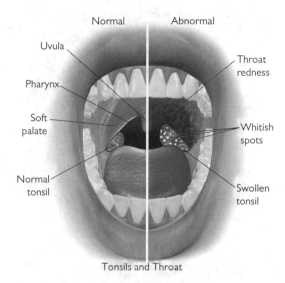

Fig. 35.2 Anatomy of the tonsils and throat. Reproduced from Blausen.com staff (2014), 'Medical gallery of Blausen Medical 2014'. *WikiJournal of Medicine* 1 (2). Free to use under CC BY 3.0 license.

Airway assessment

- *Look* for drooling, cyanosis, intercostal recession, assessor muscle usage, respiratory rate, nasal flaring, oxygen saturation, and fever.
- *Listen* for stridor, cough, voice, and difficulty in finishing full sentences.

Stridor vs wheeze

Wheeze is heard on expiration and due to turbulent bronchiolar flow. Stridor is high pitched and suggests a degree of obstruction at/below the larynx. It can be inspiratory, expiratory, or biphasic.

Periorbital cellulitis

This is an ENT emergency managed jointly with ophthalmology and paediatrics. It is a complication of acute ethmoidal sinusitis and affects young children. It presents with redness, pain, and swelling (Fig. 35.3). It is important to examine for proptosis, a change in visual acuity, colour vision, diplopia, reduced eye movements, and a relative afferent pupil defect (RAPD) as there is a risk of blindness. The condition needs to be managed promptly with IV broad-spectrum antibiotics. A sinus and orbit CT should be performed. If a subperiosteal or intraorbital abscess is present, urgent surgery to decompress the orbit is mandated.

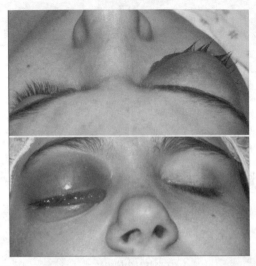

Fig. 35.3 Orbital cellulitis. Reproduced with permission from the *MSD Manual Consumer Version* (Known as the *Merck Manual* in the US and Canada and the MSD Manual in the rest of the world), edited by Robert Porter. Copyright (2018) by Merck Sharp & Dohme Corp., a subsidiary of Merck & Co, Inc, Kenilworth, NJ. Available at http://www.msdmanuals.com/consumer. Accessed (03/01/18).

Ear, nose, and throat surgery: in theatre

Tonsillectomy

You may be asked the reasons for performing this very common operation. There are three main indications: recurrent acute tonsillitis, suspicion of tonsillar malignancy, and obstructive sleep apnoea due to enlarged tonsils. The operation involves bluntly dissecting the tonsil along with its capsule away from the adjacent pharyngeal musculature, working from the upper tonsillar pole, towards the tongue base. The blood supply of the tonsils enters via the lower tonsillar pole, so this is tied to avoid haemorrhage. Many different methods can be used including coblation, electrocautery, and laser but the commonest method which also has the lowest incidence of postoperative haemorrhage is cold steel dissection.

The main complications are infection and haemorrhage which may be primary (occurring in the first 24 hours) or secondary (occurring 5–10 days after surgery). A post-tonsillectomy bleed is an ENT emergency requiring IV resuscitation and antibiotics. A return to theatre may be needed to arrest the bleed.

> ### Honours
> *Indications for tonsillectomy*
> Scottish Intercollegiate Guidelines Network (SIGN) guidelines for tonsillectomy for tonsillitis—patients should meet these criteria:
> - Sore throats are caused by acute tonsillitis.
> - Attacks of sore throat are disabling and prevent normal functioning.
> - Seven or more episodes of sore throat in the past year or five or more episodes in the past 2 years or three or more in the past 3 years.

Grommet insertion

Grommets are tiny tubes inserted into the tympanic membrane in order to drain away fluids and improve ventilation of the middle ear. The procedure is mainly indicated for treating otitis media with effusion (glue ear) lasting >3 months and recurrent acute otitis media. Grommets are inserted using a microscope under either local anaesthetic or GA. A binocular microscope is used for the procedure. A radial cut (myringotomy) is usually made in the inferior-anterior quadrant. Crocodile forceps are used to place the grommet in the incision.

Most microscopes will have a teaching arm allowing you to see what the surgeon is seeing, and this makes it ideal for you ask the surgeon to point out the features of the ear drum. Ask the surgeon before the operation to set up the teaching microscope. Make sure you can identify the different parts of the ear drum, including the umbo, handle of the malleus, incus, and the cone of light. Complications of grommets include otorrhoea which may need antibiotic treatment, scarring, and perforation of the ear drum after the grommet has fallen out.

Thyroidectomy

Performed to treat thyroid carcinoma, a goitre affecting breathing or swallowing, or for hyperthyroidism refractory to medical treatment. Performed increasingly in ENT departments with head and neck units, this is a golden opportunity to assist and to learn about neck anatomy at the same time. Try to see the patient preoperatively to examine their neck. Look out for the important structures as the operation progresses. A good way to remember them is to follow the dissection and work from superficial to deep, starting from the skin, platysma, and the strap muscles which are divided to reveal the trachea, cricoid, and thyroid lobes. The inferior and middle thyroid veins are ligated and divided. The inferior and superior poles are mobilized, and the superior thyroid artery and vein is ligated and divided. You will notice the surgeon concentrating on identifying the recurrent laryngeal nerve which is found in the tracheoesophageal groove. This is essential to prevent iatrogenic damage → vocal cord palsy and hoarse voice. Nerve monitoring devices are increasingly being used to assist with identification. The thyroid is dissected free from the trachea. Complications include recurrent laryngeal or external laryngeal nerve palsy, hypocalcaemia, an airway emergency secondary to haematoma or tracheomalacia, and recurrence.

Neck dissection

Head and neck cancer operations are increasingly being concentrated in regional head and neck centres. If there is limited opportunity for theatre, a neck dissection is a good operation to see in terms of appreciating the anatomy of the neck and the surgical management of head and neck cancer. A neck dissection may be performed: prophylactically for malignancy, therapeutically to treat cancer with lymph node spread, or for obtaining lymph node biopsies (e.g. for lymphoma). The operation involves surgical removal of all or selected lymph nodes on one or both sides of the neck. The sternocleidomastoid, accessory nerve, and internal jugular vein may also be removed.

Surgical tracheostomy

Know the reasons for performing this procedure. They are to secure an obstructed upper airway, to establish an airway in patients with surgery to the head and neck, to facilitate weaning from ventilatory support, to assist removal of respiratory secretions, and to protect the airway from aspiration in patient with a poor cough reflex. It is usually performed under GA and requires excellent teamwork between the surgeon and anaesthetist. A horizontal incision is made midway between the cricoid and sternal notch. Ask your surgeon to demonstrate these landmarks before the operation. The strap muscles are divided in the midline, and the thyroid isthmus is usually divided. A hole is made in the trachea by removing the anterior part of the third and fourth tracheal rings. A tracheostomy tube is inserted, and once the cuff is inflated it is secured. Complications include infection, bleeding, recurrent laryngeal nerve injury, subcutaneous emphysema, pneumothorax, tube displacement, aspiration, and tracheal stenosis.

Ear, nose, and throat surgery: in exams

Your priority during your ENT placement is to practise how to take an ENT history and to perform an ENT examination on real patients. Your GP attachment will also feature a lot of ENT patients.

History station

You will find there is a wide range of different presentations in ENT. As with all histories you start with an open question: 'Can you please start from the beginning and tell me what the problem is?' You can then focus your closed questions based on whether the problem is related to the ear, nose, or throat.

History of presenting complaint

- *Ear review*: ask about which is the affected side, any hearing loss, earache, and ear discharge. Dizziness is a common presentation so differentiate between true vertigo, lightheadedness, and peripheral imbalance.
- *Nose review*: ask about nasal discharge (rhinorrhoea), pain, nosebleeds (epistaxis), obstruction, loss of smell (anosmia), itching, sneezing.
- *Throat and neck review*: inquire about pain in the throat, mouth, neck, ears, change in voice (dysphonia), difficulty in swallowing (dysphagia) or painful swallowing (odynophagia), shortness of breath (dyspnoea), stridor, neck lumps, weight loss, night sweats, and reflux symptoms.
- *Thyroid review*: ascertain the patient's thyroid status. For hyperthyroidism, ask about weight loss, heat intolerance, depression, agitation, anxiety, infrequent menstruation (oligomenorrhoea), weakness, tremor, palpitations, and diarrhoea. For hypothyroidism, ask about weight gain, cold intolerance, depression, memory impairment, heavy menstruation (menorrhagia), constipation, and hoarseness.
- *Systems review*: ask about the relevant ENT area not covered in the PC.

Past medical history

As well as the general enquiry about past medical problems you need to ask specifically about any previous ENT surgery and problems with the ENT.

Family history

Many ENT problems will have a positive FHx. For ear presentations, ask about a FHx of hearing problems. For neck lumps, check if there is a FHx of thyroid disease/surgery.

Drug history

Ask about current medications and allergies. Use of ototoxic drugs (e.g. gentamicin, cisplatin) is important in hearing loss.

Social history

Smoking and alcohol are synergistic risk factors for head and neck malignancy. What is their profession? Anosmia in a chef will have a significant impact on quality of life. Carpenters are exposed to hardwood dust which ↑ the risk of some head and neck cancers.

Examination

Although ENT placements are typically short, ENT cases commonly feature in surgical exams. The good thing is that this is almost always a neck examination, and this may be on an actor with no signs, or on a patient from the head and neck clinic. Therefore, make sure you spend sufficient time in clinic so that you are able to slickly perform a neck examination and to demonstrate any signs.

Neck lump

This is the most likely case to appear in surgical OSCEs. An ENT department will have no shortage in supplying patients with neck lumps to your OSCE.

- Position the patient and expose the neck to the clavicles. The patient's chair is often placed with its back on a wall and the patient may be wearing a scarf. Ensure that you move the chair forwards so you have enough room to examine from behind and ask the patient to remove any clothing that obstructs the view of the neck!
- Ensure hand hygiene, gain consent, and ask the patient if they have any pain in their neck.
- Inspect the neck from front and side. Look for any masses, scars, asymmetry, or skin changes.
- Assess the patient's voice (recurrent laryngeal nerve function) by asking the patient to count from one to ten.
- Ask the patient to take a sip of water, hold, and swallow when asked. Any thyroid mass will move upwards on swallowing.
- Look inside the mouth, then ask the patient to stick out their tongue. Look for any midline masses that move on protrusion such as a thyroglossal cyst.
- Stand behind the patient to palpate their neck using the pulp of your fingers. Work up the midline from the suprasternal notch along the trachea and larynx (level 6 nodes). Palpate the thyroid gland. Palpate the submental and submandibular area (level 1) and then palpate inferiorly along the sternocleidomastoid (levels 2, 3, and 4). Palpate the supraclavicular and infraclavicular area, and then move superiorly along the posterior edge of the sternocleidomastoid and the posterior triangle (level 5). Palpate the occipital, post- and pre-auricular nodes, and the parotid gland. You may be taught to palpate the neck in a different order but the important thing is not to miss out on any areas.
- Use a system to describe any lump you find. Comment on the site, size, shape, surface, consistency, tenderness, transillumination, pulsatility, and attachment to underlying structures.
- For a parotid or submandibular mass, perform bimanual palpation.

Things you should practise beforehand

Thyroid examination

Students are often unsure whether they should perform a full thyroid examination when examining the neck in OSCEs. Usually you will be clearly instructed to examine the thyroid gland. However, if you are only asked to examine a patient's neck, and you suspect a midline lump, then you should suspect a thyroid mass. Ask the examiner if you can proceed to examine the thyroid status.

Neck anatomy

The neck is divided into two triangles which are used to describe the site of a neck lump (see Fig. 35.4):

- *Anterior triangle*: bound anteriorly by the midline of the neck, superiorly by the inferior border of the mandible, and posteriorly by the anterior border of the sternocleidomastoid.
- *Posterior triangle*: formed anteriorly by the posterior edge of the sternocleidomastoid, inferiorly by the clavicle, and posteriorly by the anterior edge of trapezius muscle.

In addition to the full neck examination, the thyroid examination also includes the following points:

- Inspect the patent's skin and look for any restlessness.
- Examine the hands for sweatiness, thyroid acropathy, palmar erythema, and tremor.
- Feel the pulse to look for AF or tachycardia.
- Inspect the eyes for lid retraction, exophthalmos, lid lag, chemosis, and loss of hair from the outer third of the eyebrows.
- Inspect the neck and ask the patient to swallow.
- Ask the patient to cough and count to ten.

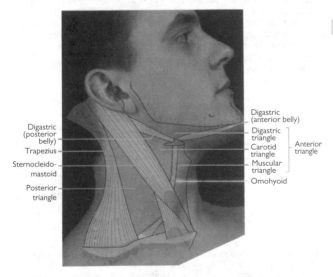

Fig. 35.4 Triangles of the neck. Reproduced with permission from Ellis H. and Mahadevan V., *Clinical Anatomy*, Thirteenth Edition, Wiley-Blackwell, Oxford, UK, Copyright © 2013.

- Palpate the thyroid gland while asking the patient to swallow water and then to protrude their tongue. Feel the thyroid lobes and isthmus gland, and then palpate the neck for any lymphadenopathy.
- Percuss over the upper sternum to detect any retrosternal extension.
- Auscultate over the thyroid to listen for any bruit.
- Ask the patient to stand up with their arms folded (proximal myopathy).
- Look for pretibial myxoedema and assess the ankle reflexes.

Ear examination
This can be practised during both your ENT and GP attachments. The important thing is to become familiar with handling the otoscope. Common pitfalls include holding the otoscope with the wrong hand, or pushing the otoscope too far into the EAC, thereby causing pain. Hold the otoscope with the right hand when examining the right ear and vice versa.
- Ask if there is a better hearing ear and start with that ear.
- Check if there is any pain in the ears.
- Inspect the post- and pre-auricular area, mastoid, pinna, and external auditory meatus. Look for any scars, discharge, sinuses, or inflammation. Scars behind the pinna are particularly hard to miss.
- Use the otoscope to examine the EAC while pulling the pinna upwards and backwards in order to straighten out the EAC. Look for any inflammation, wax, debris, or polyps. It is easy to cause pain by pushing the speculum of the otoscope too far into the ear canal. Prevent this by steadying your hand holding the otoscope with your little finger on the patient's cheek.
- Examine all four quadrants of the tympanic membrane. Look at the ossicles and comment on whether the tympanic membrane is intact, perforated, or retracted. What colour is the drum?
- Repeat this with the worse hearing ear.
- You would then perform tuning fork tests: Rinne and Weber tests (Table 35.1).

Table 35.1 Rinne vs Weber test results

	Weber without lateralization	Weber lateralizes *left*	Weber lateralizes *right*
Rinne both ears AC >BC	Normal	*Right* sensorineural loss	*Left* sensorineural loss
Rinne *left* BC >AC		*Left* conductive hearing loss	Combined loss: *left* conductive and sensorineural loss
Rinne *right* BC >AC		Combined loss: *right* conductive and sensorineural loss	*Right* conductive hearing loss
Rinne both ears BC >AC	Conductive loss in both ears	Combined loss in *right* ear and conductive loss in *left*	Combined loss: *right* conductive and sensorineural loss

AC, air conduction; BC, bone conduction.

Tuning fork tests

Make sure you ask your ENT registrar/consultant to first demonstrate how to perform tuning fork tests, and then practise on patients with both normal and abnormal hearing. Tuning forks are found in the ENT clinic. Always request a 512 Hz tuning fork, and practise striking it on your elbow or knee to make it vibrate.

Weber test

Place the vibrating fork end on the patient's forehead, vertex, or chin. Ask the patient if they can hear it loudest in the right, left, or in the middle. In a person with normal hearing, the sound is loudest in the middle. Sensorineural hearing loss results in the sound lateralizing to the unaffected ear. In conductive hearing loss, the sound lateralizes to the affected ear.

Rinne test

The vibrating fork is first placed behind the ear against the mastoid process to test bone conduction. The fork is then held in front of the ear, in line with the external auditory meatus, to test air conduction. Ask the patient which was the loudest sound. This is repeated for the other ear. The test assesses air conduction against bone conduction. A normal result occurs when air conduction is louder than bone conduction, and unintuitively this is known as a positive Rinne test. An abnormal result is known as a negative Rinne test and occurs when bone conduction is louder than air conduction.

Neurosurgery

Neurosurgery: overview

Neurosurgery is the surgical speciality that deals with disease involving the brain and spinal cord. It is a tertiary centre-based speciality located in large teaching hospitals. Neurosurgery can broadly be subdivided into neurovascular, neuro-oncology, skull base, pituitary, functional, paediatric, and spinal.

Cases to see

Subdural haematoma (SDH)

A bleed within the subdural space as a result of a shearing injury to bridging cortical veins. These occur in the young as a result of severe traumatic brain injury (TBI), are typically acute, and require an emergency craniotomy to evacuate the clot. Elderly patients on anticoagulants may suffer from a chronic collection that presents as a headache or neurological deficit, which is drained with one or two burr holes.

Subarachnoid haemorrhage (SAH)

This type of haemorrhage occurs within the subarachnoid space and most commonly is as a result of trauma. Cases you will encounter on the neuro-surgical ward will be as a result of a ruptured aneurysm.

Traumatic brain injury

TBI remains the commonest cause of death in the under 40s. TBI is a non-specific term describing blunt, penetrating, or blast injuries to the brain. It is further classified into mild, moderate, or severe based on the GCS score. Neurosurgical departments and neurointensive care units look after patients with severe TBI (GCS score <9; mortality is 40%; see Table 36.1).

Brain tumours

There are a variety of tumours observed within the CNS. It is important to appreciate that there are several classification systems to describe brain tumours (i.e. by location or cell type). In the forebrain and cerebellum, tumours can be thought of as within the brain matter (intra-axial) or outside the brain matter (extra-axial). The most common intra-axial tumours are metastases (breast in females and lung in males).

Hydrocephalus

The ventricular system within the brain plays a central role in the production (choroid plexus) and transport of CSF. In adults there is 150 mL of CSF produced at a rate of 20 mL/hour.

Table 36.1 Classification of head injury

Classification	GCS score	Mortality
Mild/minor	13–15	0.1%
Moderate	9–12	10%
Severe	<9	40%

Therefore, any obstruction to flow and/or failure to absorb CSF will result in ↑pressure within the system giving rise to ventriculomegaly and death if not treated.

Cauda equina syndrome (CES)

This is a neurosurgical emergency. It is a clinical syndrome resulting from compression of the spinal roots (cauda equina). It presents with pain (sciatica), paraesthesia/anaesthesia in the sacral distribution (saddle), urinary retention or incontinence, and/or faecal incontinence. The most likely cause of CES is a prolapsed lumbar intervertebral disc. Appreciate that emergency surgery for decompression is required within 24 hours of the onset of urinary or faecal symptoms to preserve some sphincteric function.

Degenerative spinal disease

Refers to any disease of the spinal column that results from the ageing process (i.e. wear and tear) that occurs to the bone and soft tissues of the spine. This is observed in the cervical spine (termed cervical spondylomyelopathy) and most commonly affects levels C5/6, C6/7, and C7/T1 as well as in the lumbar spine affecting levels L4/5 and L5/S1 most frequently. You should develop an understanding of the anatomy of the spine, the relation of the nerves to the surrounding structures, and tie this in with dermatomes/myotomes so that you may correlate clinical signs with anatomy.

Procedures to see

Cranial procedures

Insertion of an intracranial pressure monitor

This is a pressure transducer placed within the subdural space or brain parenchyma to measure ICP (normally 5–15 mmHg) in the unconscious patient with a severe TBI.

Insertion of an external ventricular drain

This is a catheter placed into the frontal horn of the lateral ventricle in the non-dominant hemisphere and is used to divert CSF flow in patients with acute hydrocephalus or a severe TBI in which a rising ICP needs controlling.

Spinal procedures

Lumbar puncture

This is a diagnostic procedure which involves the insertion of a spinal needle into the spinal subdural space both to measure the CSF pressure (in communicating hydrocephalus) and to sample the CSF (diagnosis of SAH and meningitis).

Operations

Burr hole drainage of acute-on-chronic subdural haematoma (ACSDH), image-guided biopsy of tumour, decompressive craniectomy, anterior cervical discectomy, and laminectomy.

Neurosurgery: in clinic

Cranial pathologies

The patients you may see in clinic can be broken down in to either cranial or spinal. The most commonly observed cranial cases in clinic are those that broadly fall into neurovascular conditions, brain tumours, and disorders of CSF flow. Spinal cases are either degenerative or spinal tumours.

Neurovascular conditions

Intracranial vascular disorders can be broadly categorized into (1) cerebral aneurysms, (2) arteriovenous malformations (AVMs), and (3) cavernomas.

Cerebral aneurysms

These are out-pouching of the tunica interna and media through deficient external layers of arterial bifurcations within the circle of Willis. When they rupture they result in bleeding within the subarachnoid space and are classified according to anterior or posterior circulation. Size is observed on digital subtraction angiography (DSA). Incidental unruptured aneurysms are followed up after coiling or clipping.

Arteriovenous malformations

AVMs are congenitally dilated communications between the arterial system and the venous system without intervening capillaries. Present with haemorrhage, seizures, or neurological dysfunction. Around 80% of AVMs will have haemorrhaged by the age of 50 years but the average age of diagnosis is ~33 years with an annual risk of bleeding of 2–4% per year. They can be diagnosed on CT, MRI, and DSA. It must be noted that 10% of AVMs will be associated with a cerebral aneurysm.

Cavernomas

These are bundles of sinusoidal capillaries with no arterial supply or venous drainage. They are low-flow, low-pressure vascular malformations with a propensity to haemorrhage. Present with seizures, progressive neurological deficit, ± haemorrhage. These lesions are not seen on angiography but can be seen on MRI and CT with a popcorn appearance. Depending on their location, these lesions can be resected if they are giving rise to intractable seizures or a neurological deficit secondary to repeated haemorrhage (0.25–0.75% yearly risk).

Brain tumours

The commonest brain tumour is a secondary (i.e. metastasis). The commonest primary brain tumours are of glial origin called gliomas. The WHO grade gliomas as follows:

- 1 = astrocytomas—commonest primary brain tumour occurring between the ages of 40–60 years with 2:1 male:female ratio.
- 2 = diffuse astrocytoma—occurring in younger adults with a mean age of 30 years.
- 3 = anaplastic astrocytoma—mean age of presentation 40–50 years. These lesions have a tendency to progress to grade 4 tumours.

- 4 = astrocytoma—glioblastoma multiforme represents 55% of all astrocytomas in between ages of 50–70 years. They can be primary (i.e. tumours that occur *de novo*) or secondary (i.e. tumours that were initially low grade and progressed).

All cases are discussed in the neuro-oncology MDT. Diagnosis is made by an image-guided biopsy of the lesion. If the lesion is clearly a high-grade lesion then a craniotomy and resection of tumour may be undertaken without prior tissue biopsy. Intraoperative tissue samples are taken and sent to the neuropathology laboratory as a 'frozen section' to confirm the histological diagnosis. Higher grades (rather expectedly) have a poorer prognosis despite complete resection and adjuvant treatment.

Disorders of CSF flow

The disturbance of CSF formation, flow, or absorption → an ↑ in the volume occupied by this fluid in the nervous system is called hydrocephalus. One essential concept that you must appreciate when trying to understand pathologies of CSF flow is the *Monro–Kellie doctrine*. The doctrine states that as the volume of the cranium is fixed, any expansion of either of its constituents (i.e. blood, CSF, and brain tissue) must be compensated for by the remaining constituents to maintain a state of equilibrium. Hence any expansion of either CSF volume (e.g. through failure of absorption or obstruction of flow) or blood (through haemorrhage) will result in compression of the brain parenchyma. After this compensatory mechanism (e.g. reductions in the venous and CSF volumes) is exhausted, brain parenchyma will be compressed from rising ICP → inevitable neurological compromise.

Obstructive hydrocephalus

This is ventriculomegaly secondary to an obstruction of CSF flow between the ventricles, which are characteristically over-expanded on imaging. This is typically caused by compression of the system from the outside (i.e. within the surrounding brain parenchyma) by bleeds, tumours, or by intraventricular lesions. CSF flow diversion can be either through an external ventricular drain, endoscopic third ventriculostomy, or insertion of a ventriculoperitoneal shunt.

Communicating hydrocephalus

This is ventriculomegaly that results from failure of CSF absorption by the arachnoid villi. The absorption process is hindered by CNS infection, during and soon after SAH and high protein states. There is free communication between the different ventricular compartments so use an external ventricular drain, serial LPs, or a ventriculoperitoneal shunt if persistent.

Spinal pathologies

Spinal neurosurgery can be broken down into (1) degenerative disease, (2) tumours, (3) infection, and (4) haemorrhage.

Degenerative spinal disease

The level of the disc protrusion is identified by the myotomes and dermatomes affected.

Cervical disc disease

Typically causes neck pain, radicular symptoms (pain along a dermatomal distribution as a result of compression/irritation of the nerve root), and myelopathy (weakness along a specific myotome secondary to cord compression). A large central disc herniation will compress the cord and → a 'myelopathic picture' such as spasticity and limb weakness. A lateral disc protrusion will compress the exiting nerve root leading to radicular symptoms that are typically pain, numbness, weakness, and paraesthesia. Cervical myelopathy is managed via an anterior (i.e. anterior cervical discectomy and fusion) or a posterior (cervical laminectomy) decompression.

Lumbar degenerative disease

This is characterized either by root compression (i.e. sciatica = radiculopathy) or canal stenosis. Spinal stenosis → neurogenic claudication that occurs during walking and or standing. Flexing the hips, bending forward, or sitting down relieves the pain. Neurogenic claudication is unlike arterial claudication, which can occur at rest. Another distinguishing factor is the presence of arterial pulses in neurogenic claudicants, so remember to examine for peripheral pulses. Treatments are analgesia, nerve root injections, and surgical (i.e. removing the offending disc (discectomies) or decompression (laminectomy)).

Spinal tumours

Tumours affecting the spine are classified by their anatomical location. Extradural tumours are commonly located close to the vertebral bone from which they receive their blood supply. Intradural intramedullary tumours are those arising from the spinal cord parenchyma. (See Fig. 36.1.)

The management of all spinal tumours is centred on three important tenets:
• Decompression
• Stabilization
• Diagnosis.

It is critical to decompress the spinal cord to prevent further neurological deterioration and obtain a tissue diagnosis to determine appropriate postresection therapy. Treatment option for metastasis is radiotherapy, but most intradural extramedullary lesions are benign and do not need more than surgical resection. Intradural intramedullary lesions are surgically resected and patients undergo postoperative radiotherapy.

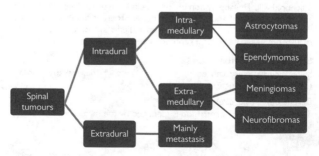

Fig. 36.1 Classification of spinal tumours.

Neurosurgery: in the emergency department

The neurosurgical team are an essential part of the on-call trauma team. After Airway, Breathing, and Circulation have been stabilized, Disability (i.e. level of consciousness) needs to be assessed. This is best done using the universally accepted Glasgow Coma Scale (GCS).

Glasgow Coma Scale

The GCS was developed to facilitate concise and reproducible assessment of the level of consciousness of a patient, which would in turn allow for effective communication regarding that patient between all members of the medical team. The score for the scale is out of 15, with 3 denoting coma or death. It must be remembered that you cannot score <3 (considered a major faux pas). Patients scoring 8 or less are considered at imminent risk of airway compromise and need urgent anaesthetic assessment with a view to being intubated, ventilated, and sedated. Patients with a neurological cause for a low GCS need hourly neuro-observations. (See Table 36.2.)

Traumatic brain injury

There are around 20,000 cases of major trauma in the UK per year, which result in over 5000 deaths. Up to 80% of these patients will have sustained a TBI. These cases will present to the ED where they will be rapidly assessed using the ATLS® protocol. Following stabilization of their airway, breathing, and circulation a CT brain scan will be performed as part of the radiographic trauma series. Neurological signs can be easily documented using the ASIA (American Spinal Injury Association) chart.

Diagnosing traumatic brain injury
- Extradural haematoma.
- Acute subdural haematoma.
- Traumatic SAH.
- Cerebral contusions.
- Skull fracture.

- Pneumocephalus.
- Coning.
- Diffuse axonal injury with loss of grey–white differentiation.

Table 36.2 Glasgow Coma Scale

Eyes (E)	Verbal (V)	Motor (M)
1. No eye opening	1. Makes no sounds	1. No movements
2. Opens eyes to painful stimuli	2. Incomprehensible sounds	2. Extensor posturing
3. Opens eyes to voice	3. Inappropriate words	3. Flexor posturing
4. Opens eyes spontaneously	4. Confused, disorientated	4. Move limb away from pain
	5. Oriented, converses normally	5. Moves limb towards pain
		6. Obeys command
(This reflects the AVPU scale too)	T. If the patient is intubated	

Extradural haematomas

- Arise as a result of an injury to the middle meningeal artery (derived from the external carotid artery) as it courses behind the pterion— the bony junction between the frontal, parietal, temporal, and sphenoid bones.
- Typically, the patient sustains a blow to the side of the head without suffering a deterioration in level of consciousness at the time (defined as the lucid period) and then has a sudden drop in GCS score.
- Depending on the size and degree of mass effect, an urgent surgical evacuation via a craniotomy may be warranted.

Traumatic subarachnoid haemorrhage (tSAH)

- Results from injury to pial bloods vessels.
- It is normally observed over the surface of the brain, (i.e. the convexity), and is managed conservatively, but one must be careful when taking the history from these patients to make sure that an aneurysmal bleed did not give rise to a collapse and a subsequent TBI.
- Find out about any regular anticoagulants/antiplatelet therapy. These only ↑ the risk of bleeding after trauma but not before a traumatic episode. (See Fig. 36.2.)

Associated skull injuries

- In addition to injury to the brain parenchyma, accompanying bony injuries to the calvarium (skull) are also common.
- Skull base fractures are another subset of bony injuries. They can result in a CSF leak (rhinorrhoea and otorrhoea). These patients may have periorbital (panda eyes) and retromastoid (Battle sign) bruising. Samples of fluid leaking from their nose or ears need to be sent for beta-transferrin (biochemical marker specific to CSF) testing in the biochemistry laboratory. Pneumovax is needed as a prophylaxis.
- If the CSF leak does not settle, they may need a surgical repair of the dural defect that has resulted from the skull base fracture.
- Any evidence of air locules within the brain parenchyma (pneumocephalus) on (an ideally fine-cut) CT brain scan should signify that there is likely either a skull base fracture or compromise of an air-containing sinus (i.e. frontal, sphenoid, or ethmoid sinus).

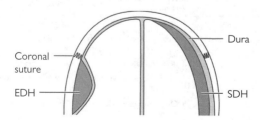

Fig. 36.2 Types of brain haemorrhage. EDH, extradural haematoma; SDH, subdural haematoma. Reproduced with permission from Richard Graham and Ferdia Gallagher, *Emergencies in Clinical Radiology*, 2009, Oxford University Press.

Honours

Cushing response and Cushing's triad

Cushing response refers to the compensatory mechanisms that the brain undertakes to compensate for rising ICP (secondary to a change in one of the components described in the Monro–Kellie doctrine). Early signs of rising ICP are decreased or decreasing GCS, agitation, and confusion. As ICP rises even more, the patient will start to vomit in the absence of nausea secondary to medullary compression. Cardiac monitoring may also demonstrate new-onset arrhythmias. As coma develops, the patient may only have reflexive responses to painful stimuli which may subsequently disappear. Once the brainstem has herniated the patient will have cardiorespiratory arrest.

Cushing's triad is made up of three signs that are observed: *hypertension*, *bradycardia*, and *apnoea*.

Radiology in TBI

- At the most severe end of the TBI spectrum there are two radiographic observations that demonstrate that the injury has been so severe that no neurosurgical intervention would alter the outcome.
- Severe displacement (in relation to the Monro–Kellie doctrine) of the brain parenchyma results in migration of the brainstem through the foramen magnum, better known as 'coning'. This is a terminal event that is characterized by the Cushing response.
- Diffuse axonal injury with loss of grey–white matter differentiation is observed when either the brain has endured a severe acceleration–deceleration injury or when the brain has had a prolonged period of hypoxia due to neurovascular or cardiopulmonary compromise.
- Both these radiological findings are catastrophic and are terminal/unsurvivable.

Aneurysmal subarachnoid haemorrhage (aSAH)

- Annual estimated rate of 6–8 per 100,000 in the Western world.
- Up to 15% of patients die before they reach medical care.
- aSAH has a mortality of 10% in the first few days and almost 50% in the first 2 weeks. The peak age of presentation is between 55–60 years of age and 30% of bleeds occur during sleep.
- Classically patients complain of a sudden-onset, worst-ever headache in 97% of cases ('the worst headache in my life', 'being kicked at the back of the head' or a 'thunderclap headache').
- Up to 60% of patients may have a preceding ('sentinel') headache of lessor severity or shorter duration.
- Patients may complain of symptoms of meningism (i.e. neck stiffness, N&V, photophobia and visual disturbance (double vision ± ptosis)).
- They may be admitted to the ED unconscious or in a coma.
- Following a concise history taking and a thorough neurological examination, a non-contrast CT brain scan is performed urgently.

- If the patient is scanned within 48 hours of the headache the blood appears as an area of high density (like bone-white) within the subarachnoid space. The blood may also extend into the ventricles (intraventricular haemorrhage).
- If the CT brain scan is inconclusive, a LP is performed 12 hours after the onset of the headache. If the red cell count in serial bottles (i.e. xanthochromia) and the bilirubin is above the threshold in these samples then a diagnosis of SAH is made. Xanthochromia, a yellow discolouration of CSF due to breakdown pigment is indicative of SAH.
- Upon diagnosis, THE patient is started on nimodipine (A calcium channel blocker). The patient is then admitted to the neurosurgical ward and will undergo a CT-guided catheter cerebral angiogram to identify and further define an aneurysm.
- A decision is then made whether the aneurysm can be treated endovascularly or neurosurgically via clipping.

Cauda equina syndrome (CES)

The clinical condition arising from dysfunction of multiple lumbar and sacral nerve roots within the spinal canal as a result of compression of the cauda equina (L2 to sacrum and Latin for horse's tail). Compression may occur from disc herniation, spondylosis, trauma, local neoplasm, or abscess. It is a relatively uncommon condition and represents only 0.4% in those presenting with low back pain. Up to 90% of proven cases of CES will have experienced urinary retention at some point along their course, and anal sphincter tone is reduced in 60–80% of cases. Saddle anaesthesia is the most commonly observed sensory disturbance. Weakness along more than one nerve root is also common. Patients will often present with SPINE:

- Saddle anaesthesia
- Pain
- Incontinence
- Numbness
- Emergency.

Patients may complain of longstanding unilateral sciatica that has become bilateral. Male erectile dysfunction is a late feature. Patients with CES have variable time courses that can be broken down into three groups. Take a clear history from all patients with low back pain associated with sphincteric dysfunction in the ED to identify CES:

- First group have sudden-onset symptoms of CES with no previous history of back symptoms.
- Second group have a longstanding history of recurrent low back pain and sciatica.
- Third group present with low back pain and bilateral sciatica.

All cases of suspected CES need an urgent MRI and be booked for surgical decompression on the next-day operative list if confirmed.

Neurosurgery: in theatre

You should develop an understanding of the more commonly performed procedures. These are typically those procedures that are performed in an emergency to prevent further and irreversible neurological deficits. The layers you need to know about are **SCALP**:

- **S**kin
- Subcut **C**onnective tissue
- **A**poneurosis
- **L**oose connective tissue
- **P**ericranium (cranium → brain matter).

Burr hole drainage

- The drainage of acute-on-chronic subdural haematoma (ACSDH) may be achieved by the placement of one or two burr holes through the skull with a dural incision to release the underlying collection.
- Two burr holes are placed either side of the apex of the haematoma.
- Warmed normal saline is then irrigated through both burr holes until the effluent is no longer blood stained.
- The scalp is infiltrated with xylocaine containing adrenaline (epinephrin) (to reduce scalp bleeding).
- Two incisions are placed over the frontal and parietal aspects of the collection.
- Burr holes are fashioned with a handheld electric (if the patient is awake) or a pneumatic drill (if patient is under GA).
- A cruciate incision is then made through the dura.
- If the collection is under high pressure, it will be discharged through the first dural incision.
- Copious wash of the subdural space is performed with normal saline until the effluent is clear.
- A drain is passed from the parietal burr hole into the subdural space.
- This drain is secured and connected to a free drainage bag.
- The scalp is then closed; first the galea with an absorbable suture and then the skin with clips or a non-absorbable suture.
- The patient then returns to the ward and remains on flat bed rest for 24–48 hours.
- The drain is taken out after 24 hours and 4 hours later the patient is started on DVT prophylaxis.

To ask the boss

To leave a subdural catheter or not following burr hole drainage of ACSDH?
Recurrence rates following ACSDH drainage are up to 30%. Santarius et al.[1] demonstrated through a RCT that the use of a subdural drain more than halved the incidence of ACSDH recurrence at 6 months (9.3% vs 24%). There are, of course, risks involved too.

Fronto-temporo-parietal trauma craniotomy

- Acute SDHs overlie the fronto-temporo-parietal cortex.
- The craniotomy also provides access to the middle meningeal artery, which is the commonest cause of an acute extradural haematoma.

- Both these neurosurgical entities require emergency evacuation when the patient is neurologically compromised or if there is significant mass effect.
- Time is of the essence and once the patient is on the operating table decompression should occur within 10 min and in the absence of unforetold complications the whole procedure should not take more than 60 min 'skin to skin'.
- The skin is shaved and a large question mark incision is marked out starting just below the zygomatic arch 1 cm in front of the tragus.
- The scalp is incised to the bone with a scalpel and haemostasis is maintained by the application of Raney clips.
- The temporalis muscle is then cut. The scalp flap is reflected and up to four burr holes are fashioned with a handheld drill.
- The burr holes are connected together using a craniotome.
- Using elevators the bone is lifted off the dura.
- If there is an extradural haematoma it is evacuated with copious wash. Any points of bleeding (i.e. middle meningeal artery) are stopped using bipolar diathermy.
- In the presence of an acute SDH, a C-shaped incision is made through the dura and the underlying haematoma is evacuated.
- Once the clot has been evacuated, the dural defect is closed using continuous sutures and the bone flap is secured to the skull using bioplates and screws.
- The scalp is then closed in a layered manner (galea first with an absorbable suture and subsequently metallic clips to skin).

Cervical and lumbar laminectomy

- Spinal decompression can either be anterior or posterior.
- Anterior approaches are typically performed on the cervical spine, although they can be performed in all other parts of the vertebral column, and involve the removal of one or two discs with implantation of an artificial disc, and are sometimes reinforced by metalwork.
- Posterior approaches can be performed in all segments of the vertebral column. Most commonly a laminectomy is performed.
- A midline incision is made along the avascular aponeurosis.
- Intraoperative radiography is used to accurately locate the correct site.
- Dissection down the midline is performed using monopolar diathermy until the spinous processes are reached.
- The musculature is reflected off the midline laterally until the lateral extent of the laminae is observed bilaterally.
- Using either a drill or a handheld rongeur the lamina is removed.
- The underlying ligament is removed until the spinal theca is observed. Care is taken not to puncture the dura or injure the exiting nerve roots.
- The wound is then closed in layers with placement of a drain depending on the degree of haemostasis achieved.

Reference

1. Santarius T, Kirkpatrick PJ, Ganesan D, et al. (2009). Use of drains versus no drains after burr-hole evacuation of chronic subdural haematoma: a randomised controlled trial. *Lancet* 374(9695):1067–73.

Neurosurgery: in exams

During your time on the neurosurgical firm it is critical you master both the neurological examination and the use of the GCS. Take every opportunity given to you both in clinic and on the admissions ward at taking a focused history. Hold back from finding out what the admitting diagnosis is and try to formulate your own differentials.

History station

The most common neurosurgical stations in examinations are usually aSAH or brain tumours. A patient actor may give a history of a sudden-onset, worst-ever headache associated with nausea, vomiting, photophobia, neck stiffness, and possible neurological deficit. The diagnosis should be obvious to you immediately and once you pick up on the cues you will then have ample opportunity to showboat your knowledge of the field by asking more probing questions.

History of presenting complaint

As with all other histories, feel free to use SOCRATES for pain histories. Once you have exhausted this you need to be able to obtain a concise sequence of events in your head and subsequently formulate a series of focused questions that are tailored according to the pathology being discussed. In the case of the sudden-onset headache you need to know:

- when, where, and how it came on
- what they were doing at the time
- have they had something like it before (sentinel headache or regular migraine?)
- was it relieved by simple analgesia (unlikely in aSAH)
- did they develop a neurological deficit (unlikely in migraine) etc.

PMHx

Ask if your patient suffers from any other medical conditions for which they have seen a doctor. This is a sure-fire way of assuring that you get a comprehensive medical history. Uncontrolled hypertension and the use of anticoagulants for cardiac arrhythmias are of interest to neurosurgeons as they are associated with cerebral haemorrhage.

FHx

Your risk of aSAH ↑ in the presence of polycystic renal and liver disease and first-degree family members who have suffered an aSAH. All oncological history is of interest as it may mean the patient has a genetic predisposition to cancer.

DHx

Is critical as the risk of significant blood loss or uncontrollable haemorrhage is massively ↑ when the patient has recently taken anticoagulants such as warfarin, aspirin, and clopidogrel. The exact dates and times need to be identified.

Recent INR needs to be obtained and normalized prior to surgery. Blood products may minimize the risk of intraoperative haemorrhage.

SHx

Smoking and the use of illicit drugs such as cocaine ↑ your likelihood of suffering a SAH.

Examination

Simple things are common, you are unlikely to be presented with a complex neurosurgical case in your exams. In all probability you may be asked to examine a patient's motor and sensory function. Alternatively, you may be asked to examine a set of cranial nerves looking specifically for a cranial nerve deficit. The eyes are the easiest to examine because ocular deficits are reproducible. The slick use of an ophthalmoscope is essential and you will be expected to be able to identify papilloedema and mention its causes (remember raised ICP links in directly with the Monro–Kellie doctrine so it can only be related to haemorrhage, a space-occupying lesion, and/or a disorder of CSF flow). You need to do this confidently and the only way you can achieve this is to pair up with somebody and pretend to have different scores and assess each other.

Lumbar puncture

- Although you are unlikely to perform a LP during your neurosurgical attachment, you need to make sure you have practised performing a LP in the skills laboratory on a mannequin.
- This needs to be done with a colleague observing and you need to be comfortable talking through the procedure while performing it.
- A central tenet of the procedure is that the spinal cord ends at L1/2 (continuing as the cauda equina below), hence the ideal intervertebral space to aim for is the L3/L4 or L4/5.
- This is easily identified as it is the highest point of the iliac crest and is located on a level with the spinous process of the L4 vertebrae.
- It is important to point your spinal needle rostrally and keep it in the midline.
- The needle will 'give' once the dura is breached.
- You will feel three pops as you penetrate the supraspinous, interspinous, and ligamentum flavum ligaments.
- Always attempt to measure the opening and closing pressure (diagnostic tool for communicating hydrocephalus) or at least say that you would as it is likely to score points in an OSCE station.
- Throughout the procedure always check that the patient is comfortable and on completion of the procedure place a dry dressing over the puncture site and instruct the patient to lay flat for at least an hour to reduce the occurrence of a post-LP headache.
- The severity of headache correlates to the size of the puncture so use a pencil-point, small-gauge spinal needle if possible.

Oral and maxillofacial surgery

Oral and maxillofacial surgery: in clinic

Oral and maxillofacial surgery (OMFS) specializes in the diagnosis and treatment of diseases affecting the mouth, jaws, face, and neck. OMFS requires qualification in both medicine and dentistry, treating conditions that require expertise from both backgrounds.

Background and relevant anatomy

The mouth has over 500–1000 different bacteria orally, particularly anaerobes and Gram-negative bacteria. Therefore broad-spectrum antibiotics are commonly required both as cover for elective procedures and infections. Familiarize yourself with basic dental anatomy and that of the head and neck.

Intra-oral lesions

Abnormal mucosal patches may indicate dysplastic or cancerous change and any suspicious features warrant investigating and biopsy to confirm diagnosis and exclude neoplastic change.

Lichen planus

Affects ~1% of the population worldwide. It is an itchy, non-infectious rash that usually occurs in adults over the age of 40 and is believed to be auto-immune related. An oral component affects the buccal mucosa and gingiva in 50% of people who have cutaneous lesions. Patients complain of burning or stinging in the mouth when eating or drinking spicy foods, citrus fruits, and alcohol. A white, lace-like pattern is often seen on the tongue and buccal mucosa, occasionally with surrounding erythema or ulceration. There is a 0.5–2% risk over a period of 5 years of undergoing cancerous change. *Treatment*: topical or oral corticosteroids, antiseptic and analgesic mouthwash.

Candidiasis

Acute pseudomembranous candidiasis is the oral candidiasis commonly referred to as thrush. It is common in the immunosuppressed or those on antibiotics. Although usually painless, it can cause a burning sensation so should be excluded in patients in whom burning mouth syndrome is being considered. *Treatment*: oral antifungal drops, e.g. nystatin.

Oral submucosal fibrosis

Is a chronic disease of the oral mucosa with inflammation and fibrosis of the submucosal tissues. The main presenting feature is a progressive inability to open the mouth (trismus) due to oral fibrosis and scarring, pain, and burning on consuming spicy food. It has ~8% malignant transformation potential to SCC. The condition is particularly associated with areca nut chewing (prevalent on the Asian subcontinent).

Aphthous ulceration

Is a common condition characterized by recurrent small, round, well-circumscribed ulcers with erythematous margins and yellow or grey slough. There are three subtypes: minor, major, and herpetiform. It is worth noting that they are not infectious and herpetiform implies it has some similarities to HSV infection in appearance only.

Recurrent oral ulcers

Have many potential causes and suspicion for oral carcinoma warrants biopsy (e.g. painless, non-healing ulcers with raised borders, cragginess, surrounding dysplasia, hardness, induration, or persistence >3 weeks). Common sites for oral cancer are the lateral aspect of the tongue, floor of the mouth, and soft palate. Commonest causes of recurrent oral ulceration are local trauma, cessation of smoking, stress, food sensitivities (coffee, nuts, strawberries, tomatoes, etc.), hormones, deficiency (vitamin B12, folate, and iron), infection (HSV type 1) and irradiation.

Salivary gland masses and swellings

Parotid swelling

The commonest neoplastic mass in the parotid is a secondary from a skin cancer within the head/neck. The most common primary tumour is a pleomorphic adenoma whereas the commonest malignant salivary gland tumour is the mucoepidermoid tumour.

Pleomorphic adenoma: 'rule of 80s'

- 80% of salivary gland tumours occur in the parotid gland.
- 80% of parotid tumours are pleomorphic adenomas.
- 80% of parotid pleomorphic adenomas are in the superficial parotid.
- 80% of salivary pleomorphic adenomas are in the parotid.
- 80% are of parotid tumours are benign.
- 80% of untreated pleomorphic adenomas remain benign.

Submandibular glands

Less commonly have malignant masses, the commonest malignant tumour in the submandibular gland is adenoid-cystic carcinoma. Though the submandibular glands are more commonly affected by sialoliths or strictures causing sialadenitis and painful swelling of the gland, either pathology can occur in any gland.

Parotiditis

Tends to occur in elderly patients usually due to a reduction of salivary flow secondary to medical or pharmacological causes. *Treatment:* is rehydration and antibiotics.

Sialoliths (stones)

Can commonly be palpated in a bimanual fashion along the length of the duct. Patients can complain of facial swelling in thinking about or consumption of food (*meal time syndrome*). Subsequent salivary stagnation can predispose to sialadenitis. It is important to consider imaging to help exclude oncological causes as they may cause similar symptoms through duct compression. *Imaging:* this can either be done by indirect visualization through US, sialography, MRI, or by direct visualization via sialendoscopy. *Treatment:* initially, treat by rehydration and antibiotics. Once the infection has settled, options include sialendoscopy, ultrasonic lithotripsy, gland resection, or enucleation of the stone by gland-preserving surgery.

Oral and maxillofacial surgery: in the emergency department

Always exclude head injury, loss of consciousness, and cervical spine (C-spine) injury. Upper facial injury assessment must exclude retrobulbar haemorrhage.

Lip and facial lacerations

Rarely cause tissue loss, but may appear to due to maceration, in folding of skin and swelling. Infiltrate local anaesthetic with a vasopressor (e.g. lidocaine 2% with 1:80,000 adrenaline (epinephrine)) for haemostasis and allow assessment of the wound. If unable to tolerate, use an infra-orbital or mental block. Match the vermillion of the lips (where mucosa meets skin) before closing the skin. Perform a layered closure with absorbable sutures for deeper structures and mucosa, and non-absorbable sutures for superficial closure. Leave sutures in for 7 days.

Facial trauma and fractures

Clinically ask about mechanism of injury to help you rule out other injuries such as head or C-spine injury. Fully assess both intra- and extra-orally and document the cranial nerves examined. If the midface is involved, exclude globe injury, retrobulbar and septal haematoma. Check that damaged teeth have not been aspirated. These fractures are treated with miniplates and screws. Usually they can be placed with all the cuts inside the mouth or hidden in skin creases.

Fractured mandible

This commonly breaks in two places (like a polo mint) so always check for a second fracture. A direct blow to the chin can result in a classic fracture pattern called a *guardsman's fracture* with a symphyseal and bilateral condylar fractures. Patients regularly complain of altered occlusion and numbness. The latter is due to damage to the inferior alveolar nerve, and it is important that you document if sensation is present in the lower lip, as well as the tongue. Look for the standard features of a fracture (pain, swelling, bruising, deformity). Look inside the mouth for haematoma on the floor of the mouth, laceration in the gingiva, step in the line of the teeth, or bleeding from around the teeth. Commonly, teeth around a fracture are mobile, so feel for movement. Imaging usually used to assess a mandible fracture is an orthopantomogram (OPG) and a PA mandible X-ray. Treatment is usually antibiotics, followed by surgery (miniplates) and a soft diet for 6 weeks.

Retrobulbar haemorrhage

Any orbital trauma or surgery can result in bleeding behind the globe, due to the confined space an orbital compartment syndrome can develop. This is an OMFS emergency due to the threat of blindness.

Signs and symptoms
- Pain.
- Proptosis.
- Paralysis of ophthalmic muscles.
- Loss of pupillary responses.
- Blindness (colour vision goes first).
- Tense eye (firmer and painful on ballottement).

Fundoscopy: pale disc and pulseless retinal arteries.

Treatment

Urgent decompression using lateral canthotomy and cantholysis is essential as the window for visual recovery from the onset of ↓visual acuity is ~120 min. Medical management with acetazolamide, mannitol, and hydrocortisone might buy some additional time but the eye will still require urgent surgical decompression.

Orbital floor fracture

It is important to exclude entrapment, retrobulbar haemorrhage and globe injury.

Signs and symptoms

Epistaxis, bony tenderness, step deformity on orbital rim, paraesthesia over maxilla (infraorbital nerve), and subconjunctival haemorrhage are all suggestive of orbital floor fracture. Check for visual acuity, that the pupils are equal and reactive to light, and accommodation, full range of eye movements, and exclude diplopia. Look for hypoglobus (the pupils sit at different vertical heights) and enophthalmos (where the eye sinks back into the socket). Tissues can become entrapped, especially in children due to the greater flexibility in their bone causing the fracture to spring back up like a trap door. This entrapment can cause a 'white eye blowout' where on looking upwards, one eye remains fixed. In paediatric cases it can stimulate the oculocardiac reflex associated with hypotension, N&V. In extremis, it can induce a potentially life-threatening bradycardia or arrhythmia. If tissues are left entrapped this can → muscle necrosis and permanent disturbance in eye movements.

Imaging

Facial view X-ray or CT orbits. Look for the black eyebrow sign of air in the orbit (Fig. 37.1), tear drop sign of entrapped tissue, and fluid level (blood within the maxillary sinus) as suggestive features. If the patient has eye signs and the fracture is minimally displaced, then it can be treated conservatively. Large orbital floor defects are reconstructed using alloplastic (titanium mesh, Medpore®, etc.) or autogenous (bone) materials. Patients must avoid nose blowing, be covered with antibiotics, and reviewed with orthoptics in clinic 7–10 days after the injury/surgery. Numbness is common over the maxilla due to the position of the infraorbital nerve.

Panfacial fractures

Involve trauma to the upper, middle, and lower facial bones. Because of the force necessary to create such severe facial injuries they are commonly associated with multisystem injury as well as head and C-spine trauma. Hence, they're manage initially through standard ATLS® algorithms. Le Fort fracture patterns are worth knowing but it is best to describe the fracture relative to the anatomy. Sometimes no primary repair is done and the bones are allowed to heal in an abnormal position and a corrective osteotomy planned for later.

Ludwig's angina

This is a tracking cellulitis of the floor of the mouth that occurs in association with dental infections. It is *life-threatening* if left untreated as it can cause airway obstruction. Usually there is a history of preceding dental pain or dental work. There is submandibular and submental swelling with

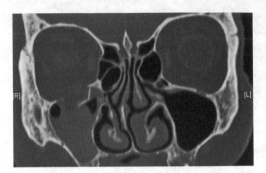

Fig. 37.1 CT right orbital floor fracture. Reproduced with permission from Cyrus Kerawala and Carrie Newlands, *Oral and Maxillofacial Surgery*, 2014, Oxford University Press.

a raised floor of the mouth crossing the midline. The patient has difficulty talking and swallowing their own saliva. They may have a '*hot potato*' like voice. Commonly there is erythema over the anterior neck, which can track all the way down to the sternum. The patient can deteriorate very quickly so early anaesthetic review and OMFS referral is essential. In the intervening period they should be placed in the resuscitation bay, nursed vertically, and placed on monitoring. Treatment is with antibiotics (IV co-amoxiclav) ± steroid (IV dexamethasone) and early surgery to decompress the submandibular and submental spaces. Patients may require a tracheostomy or prolonged intubation depending on severity.

Dental trauma and avulsed teeth

Always exclude head injury and enquire about any loss of consciousness and the mechanism of injury. Ask about disturbance in their bite, as there may be a luxation injury, or an associated dentoalveolar or jaw fracture. Dental injuries are treated conservatively (antibiotics, analgesia, and soft diet for 2 weeks) with early dental review within 24 hours. Very mobile subluxed teeth, extrusions, lateral luxations, and any associated dentoalveolar fractures are treated with reduction, splinting, and a soft diet in addition to this. Ensure you account for the tooth if avulsed.

Types of dental injury

- *Concussed*: injury to the tooth and supporting structures without ↑mobility or displacement. Pain occurs on percussion.
- *Subluxed*: mobility without displacement.
- *Laterally luxated*: displacement of the tooth other than axially.
- *Extruded*: partial displacement of the tooth out of its socket.
- *Intruded*: displacement of the tooth into the alveolar bone.
- *Infraction*: crack in the tooth with no loss of substance.
- *Fractured*: loss of tooth structure. It can be described as being enamel only, dentine and enamel, enamel with dentine and pulp, and root fracture.

Oral and maxillofacial surgery: in theatre

Oral cancer

Oral cancer makes up to 4% of all cancers in the Western world and are on the rise, but can be as high as 40% in the Indian subcontinent. 85% of oral cancers are mucosal SCC. Commonest sites are floor of mouth, tongue, and retromolar trigone (behind the wisdom tooth). *Risk factors:* smoking, drinking alcohol, chewing paan/ghat (can also cause submucosal fibrosis which is pre-cancerous). *Treatment:* resection with or without reconstruction. Adjuvant radiotherapy is occasionally used if margins on the resection are close, as is chemoradiotherapy. Risk of a second head and neck primary is in the region of 35% over a lifetime.

Flaps and grafts

These commonly close surgical and traumatic defects as well as mould and model tissues. A graft draws its blood supply from the recipient area, relying on ingrowth of new vessels whereas a flap arrives in the recipient area with its own blood supply.

Grafts

Full thickness

(Also known as a Wolfe graft.) Commonly used to reconstruct larger skin lesion defects in the head and neck. Usually taken from the supraclavicular area or behind the ear as an ellipse of the full thickness of skin with a small cuff of underling fat, this facilitates primary closure of the donor site. The flap is then thinned with a knife by removing the fat. It is important to note that the recipient area must be covered by soft tissue (and not on bone) as it draws its blood supply locally.

Split thickness

Used for additional cover of muscular flaps or donor site defects unable to be closed primarily. Usually taken from the thigh using a dermatome, a partial thickness of skin to include a partial thickness of dermis. The residual dermis allows the donor site to regenerate epidermis.

Major flaps

Various types of flaps are used, from pedicled, where their own blood supply is not disrupted, to free flaps, where an anastomosis of blood vessels is required. The most common way to describe them is in terms of their composition (e.g. musculocutaneous, composite (mixture of bone, muscle and skin)). The major workhorses of flap reconstruction in the head and neck are the radial forearm, fibula, and deep circumflex iliac artery (DCIA) free flaps, along side pectoralis major and latissimus dorsi pedicled flaps.

Local flaps

These are when you borrow tissue from the adjacent area to fill a defect, such as following the excision of skin cancer. They can be rotational, advancement, or transposition flaps and various designs exist (e.g. rhomboid, bi-lobed, nasolabial, V-Y closure, and O-Z closures). They are relatively robust and do not require rigorous monitoring. They can be done under local anaesthetic, and the patient can go home on the same day.

Oral and maxillofacial surgery: on the ward

Tracheostomy management

Tracheostomies are placed for a number of reasons such as protecting the airway pre-emptively, to secure an airway in an emergency following upper airway obstruction, or to aid ventilation in patients who are intubated for long periods of time. It is important to find out why they have one. They can become blocked through secretions, blood, or displacement into the soft tissues; therefore, they must be secured at all times. Most have an inner tube that slides out to facilitate cleaning. This inner tube can be fenestrated to allow speech, or a complete tube. If a patient loses their airway, then the inner tube should be removed and high-flow oxygen applied over the tracheostomy site. If there is no improvement, consider letting their cuff down on the tracheostomy and giving additional oxygen via the mouth and nose. The UK National Tracheostomy Safety Project has excellent advice on the management of tracheostomies (➲ www.tracheostomy.org.uk).

Flap monitoring

As a flap brings its blood supply with it there is potential for it to be compromised, therefore postoperatively it is important the flap is monitored. No one feature should be taken in isolation but they help build the picture of the health of the flap and patient factors such as whether they are warm and well perfused and inotropes should also be considered. The things commonly looked for in flap observations are as follows:

- *Colour*: a pale flap suggests not enough blood supply, a dark or blue tinted flap implies a compromised venous return.
- *Capillary refill*: a delayed capillary refill means poor arterial supply, a brisk refill can mean poor venous return.
- *Texture*: a boggy flap may be oedema, however it may be an underlying collection; a hard flap may be a large tense haematoma underneath.
- *Temperature*: a cool flap indicates poor perfusion.
- *Doppler signal*: though not always tested, it is useful to test patency of the arterial supply.

The observations should be done regularly and when handing over a patient with a flap it is important for both parties to see the patient together so that they can see and confirm what the flap looks like to establish a baseline. You do not want the first time you see a flap to be at 3 am with the nurse saying 'They think it's a little blue'. It is worth noting that oral flaps have a tendency to be paler than other flaps. When reviewing the flap ensure the patient is optimized; with a sufficient mean arterial pressure (70–80 mmHg), Hb >80, lactate <2 adequate urine output (>0.5ml/kg/hr), that the pedicle is not stretched (e.g through hyper extension), and there is no pressure over the pedicle (such as from tracheostomy straps).

Oral and maxillofacial surgery: in exams

Examination of the head and neck

Tailor your examination to the patient's presentation (e.g. deformity vs oncology vs trauma). Adopt a systematic approach and break it down into extra-oral and intra-oral components of the examination.

Extra-oral

In trauma, always exclude head and C-spine injury first, then break the examination of the face down into thirds, work from upper, to middle, to lower third using the '*look, feel, and move*' approach. Look specifically for signs of base of skull fracture:

- Reduced GCS score.
- Global neurology.
- Battle's sign (bruising of mastoid).
- Panda/raccoon eyes (periorbital bruising).
- Otorrhoea (leaking CSF).
- Rhinorrhoea (leaking CSF).
- New irritant cough (leaking CSF down their throat).

Review C-spine for tenderness on bony prominences and guarded neck movements. Commonly imaging is performed in at-risk cases to aid diagnosis. You should then specifically assess for the following:

- *Facial asymmetry*: examine from above the patient's head, front, side, and below, thinking of the face in 3D assessing in AP, vertical, and horizontal planes. Use your fingers to help you assess the symmetry of bony prominences and their projection.
- *Scars/lacerations/ecchymosis*: should all be looked for, past OMFS scars can be very well hidden, look especially closely around the pre-auricular area and skin creases.
- *Eye*: if there is any possibility of orbital injury look specifically for proptosis, hypoglobus, enophthalmos, limitation in eye movement, acuity, reaction to light, and accommodation. Seek an ophthalmology opinion if any abnormality or globe injury cannot be excluded. Restriction of upward gaze suggests entrapment of soft tissues, such as inferior rectus; if left, this can cause a permanent visual defect as the muscle will become ischaemic and fibrose. This is an emergency in children in whom it is more common due to the orbital floor fracture green-sticking and forming a trap door to spring shut on the muscle.
- *Nose*: deviation in upper, mid, and lower thirds should be documented, with septal deviation and haematoma excluded. The latter is crucial—it can lead to an ischaemic septal cartilage.
- *Mouth opening*: look for deviation to one side, limitation (normal is >4 cm), and check for pain on lateral excursion. Assess for any lock, click, crepitus, and pain on movement.
- *Palpate*: for steps, feel along the bony prominences of the face for step deformities and spot tenderness. Feel for crepitus in the soft tissues, and palpate the lymph nodes systematically.
- *Move the midface*: check for movement at Le Fort 1 (base of the nose), 2 (medial orbit), and 3 (lateral orbit) levels. To do this, place one finger

on the hard palate and pull the mid face in an AP direction while looking and feeling with the other hand over the mid face at the three Le Fort regions.
- *Cranial nerves*: these should be formally assessed and documented, especially cranial nerves V and VII. Classically, malignant parotid tumours affect cranial nerve VII but benign do not. Weakness of the tongue also suggests a malignancy. Altered sensation in lip and chin is regularly seen following a fracture jaw, and numbness over the maxilla common following an orbital floor fracture.

Intra-oral

- *Roof of mouth* (hard and soft palate).
- *Floor of mouth*: if it is raised where infection is suspected then it may be a Ludwig's angina, an OMFS emergency that can compromise the airway. With fractures of the jaw it is common to get bruising, so look specifically for a sublingual haematoma.
- *Buccal aspects*: a dental mirror or tongue depressor and torch are particularly useful here to retract the tissues so you can specifically inspect the sulci.
- *Tongue*: look over lateral, dorsal, and ventral areas. As many cancers occur proximally, ensure the patient sticks out their tongue as far as possible; to aid this, a dry piece of gauze can be used to pull the tongue forwards and at the same time you can feel the tongue for abnormalities. Cancers tend to feel hard and craggy.
- *Oropharynx and tonsils*: these are best viewed by getting the patient to say 'ahhhh'.
- *Gingivae*: commonly lacerated over fracture lines.
- *Teeth*: when reviewing teeth look at them individually (quality, quantity) and how they meet together (occlusion) and establish if this has changed. On individual teeth, check for caries, cavities, and fractures. Feel for sharp or jagged edges that can cause ulcers, then assess mobility and tenderness to percussion. If tapping on a tooth with an instrument causes pain it is suggestive of apical inflammation, likely secondary to trauma or an abscess. Account for any missing teeth in trauma, if any concerns perform CXR to exclude inhalation or lateral facial view to exclude avulsion into soft tissues.
- *Glands*: commonly missed, they are important, as the parotid is the most common site for head and neck skin cancer secondaries. Bimanually palpate the parotids and submandibular glands, try to milk out saliva from ducts (opposite the upper first molars for the parotid and either side of the lingual frenulum for the submandibular gland). Dry the area using a gauze swab, to aid in visualization before milking the gland.
- *Muscles of mastication*: palpate for tenderness, common with bruxists (excessive teeth grinding or jaw clenching).
- *Lumps and bumps*: if you do find any masses, or lesions in glands or intra-orally, describe them in the usual fashion such as site, size, shape, symmetry, surface, scars, colour, consistency, compressibility, temperature, tenderness, transillumination, fixation, etc.

Paediatric surgery

Paediatric surgery: overview

Imagine operating on a 450 g baby with necrotizing enterocolitis. The name tells you what it is. She would sit comfortably in the palm of your hand if she were not ventilated on inotropes, fighting for her life. Deciding when to operate on these delicate babies is tough. While most surgical specialties are defined by an organ system, we are defined only by age, from fetal surgery to 16 years. *Why can't adult surgeons operate on children, aren't they just little adults?* No, their physiology, pharmacology, anatomy, and psychology are different.

Honours

Top tips

If the child is old enough, first you will need to earn their trust. When they are scared this is even more difficult, and the ability to play with a child, distract them, and make them laugh is a skill you should enjoy practising. So spend time with the play therapists and clown doctors (you may learn some child development in the process) ... and carry a bottle of bubbles.

Oncology

Adjunctive treatments

The most common malignancies in childhood are the leukaemias, followed by brain tumours, and then solid organ tumours. Paediatric surgeons offer a range of adjunctive procedures to assist paediatric oncologists in managing these conditions, which have seen great improvements in their survival rate:

- Core needle (Tru-cut), incision/excisional biopsies.
- Long-term venous access is required for frequent blood tests and chemotherapy.
- Gastrostomy insertion to aid in feeding.
- Ovarian preservation surgery when chemotherapy and radiotherapy threaten fertility.

Solid organ tumours

If slow growing, benign, or localized complete excision alone may be curative. In other cases, surgery is part of a multimodal treatment regimen aimed at curing the patient. This may include adjuvant and neoadjuvant chemotherapy and radiotherapy. In more aggressive tumours, 'debulking' surgery may → symptomatic relief or prolonged survival. Common solid organ tumours amenable to surgery are:

- Wilms tumour (nephroblastoma)
- neuroblastomas
- germ cell tumours
- sarcomas.

General surgical conditions

Inguinal hernias

In children these are usually indirect, transmitting bowel through the deep inguinal ring. This is a congenital failure of closure of the processus vaginalis. Herniorrhaphy (repair usually with mesh) in adults, herniotomy (division and closure of the patent processus vaginalis) in children. A thickened cord ('*silk glove sign*') may be palpable. An irreducible hernia is a surgical emergency, reducible ones may be repaired electively. Complications of hernia include:

- incarceration = irreducible
- obstruction = blockage to lumen
- strangulation = compromised blood supply → infarction.

Umbilical hernia

Unlike inguinal hernias these are less likely to complicate, and may close spontaneously.

Undescended testicles

Occurs in 5% at birth but in 1% by age 1 year. Orchidopexy (offered from 6-12 months age), improves cosmesis, prevents torsion and may improve malignancy and fertility rates, both of which are adversely affected in undescended testes.

The paediatric foreskin

It is normal for the newborn foreskin to be adherent to the glans and not retract. This is not a pathological phimosis, and resolves naturally with growth. By 3 years of age, 90% of foreskins will retract. Non-retractile foreskins may cause ballooning, which on its own is of little consequence and will subside once the foreskin is retractile. Definite indication for circumcision is balanitis xerotica obliterans, where there is whitish scarring; rare before 5 years of age.

Abdominal pain

Is a common occurrence in childhood and usually transient, self-limiting, and dealt with at home or in the community. When persistent, severe, associated with other symptoms (e.g. vomiting, diarrhoea) or a systemically unwell child, accurate assessment requires a detailed history and experienced examination. Causes include:

- UTI
- mesenteric adenitis
- pneumonia
- DKA
- IBD
- sickle cell disease
- gall stone disease
- congenital cysts
- intussusception
- malrotation
- gastroenteritis
- appendicitis.

Appendicitis

Is difficult to diagnose in children. If in doubt, US scanning can be very useful. As children are less able to localize their pain, perforation and its complications are more common.

Neonates

The neonatal period is defined as the first 28 days of life, although some 'neonatal' babies will spend many months on the unit.

Many congenital abnormalities are today diagnosed antenatally which can → ethically and emotionally difficult decisions about whether to continue or to terminate the pregnancy.

Necrotizing enterocolitis (NEC)

Is bowel inflammation that → necrosis prior to severe sepsis ± perforation. Ninety percent of cases occur in premature babies after introduction of feeds. In the early stages there will be signs of systemic sepsis (brady- or tachycardia/desaturation/blood glucose instability/pyrexia/poor handling). There should also be some sign of bowel dysfunction (↑/green aspirates, bloody stools, distension) and abdominal wall discoloration. AXR may show an ileus (suspected NEC), or intramural gas (proven NEC). NEC can → perforation. Early NEC can be managed with bowel rest, antibiotics, and organ support. Failure of medical management and perforation → laparotomy.

Gastrointestinal atresia

Oesophageal atresia (OA) is a discontinuity in the oesophagus, and usually a fistula with the respiratory tract. The most common configuration is OA with distal tracheo-oesophageal fistula. The baby is unable to swallow secretions and feed and so froths at the mouth and vomits. Aspiration → respiratory symptoms. If there is clinical suspicion, a NG tube should be passed and will get stuck at about 10 cm from the lips and not go into the stomach. This should be confirmed on an X-ray. This tube should be kept on regular suction to prevent further aspiration. In theatre after a right thoracotomy, the lung is retracted forwards, the fistula is identified as it enters the trachea and divided and closed, and an anastomosis performed between the two ends of the oesophagus (less than half the diameter of your little finger). Small bowel atresias present with bilious vomiting and are usually easy to diagnose with an AXR. The number of gas bubbles seen on the X-ray will give you some idea of the level of the obstruction. A single gastric bubble suggests pyloric atresia (very rare), a 'double-bubble' sign is seen in duodenal atresia (larger stomach bubble and smaller duodenal bubble), a 'few' bubbles suggest jejunal atresia, more bubbles suggest ileal atresia. Large bowel atresia is less common. The more distal the atresia, the more the number of bubbles, but the more difficult to diagnose on a plain X-ray, in which a contrast study may help.

Anorectal malformations

Are easy to diagnose as usually the anus is not where it should be. Some have no opening, but most have a fistulous tract opening into the perineum or genitourinary tract. A few can be corrected in the first few days of life with a primary anoplasty (repair), most require a stoma to allow the child to defecate and feed while awaiting definitive repair when older.

Neonatal biliary abnormalities

Biliary atresia is a cause of prolonged jaundice in neonates. It remains the most common indication for liver transplantation in children. Choledochal cysts do not usually present until infancy, childhood, or even later, with either obstructive jaundice, abdominal pain, ± mass.

Spina bifida

Is failure of fusion of the posterior column of the spine. It ranges from occulta (hidden) with no neurological defect to various types of spina bifida aperta (open) where the meninges (meningocele) or meninges and spinal cord (myelomeningocele) are exposed → neurological damage. Most commonly the lumbosacral spine is affected. These nerves supply the lower limbs, bowel, and bladder, all of which can be variously affected. The defect is usually repaired in the first few days. In utero surgery before birth is also possible. Many patients subsequently develop hydrocephalus, which requires surgical drainage. A MDT approach to management of limb, bowel, and bladder dysfunction is the mainstay of treatment. In the UK with (1) folate supplementation, (2) antenatal diagnosis, and an (3) increasing decision for termination, this condition is less commonly seen in the newborn period.

Abdominal wall defects

In gastroschisis, the baby is born with bowels protruding through a defect usually to the right of the umbilicus. The bowels have been exposed to amniotic fluid *in utero* and hence are thickened and often matted together. Sometimes they can be returned into the abdomen and the defect closed at one operation but if there is too much bowel, a plastic silo is attached to the umbilical defect (there are both operative and non-operative methods) to contain the bowel as it is gently squeezed into the abdomen over the course of a few days. The abnormal bowel takes some weeks to start working during which time nutrition is maintained with total parenteral nutrition. In high-income countries, survival is >90%, but in developing countries survival is probably <10%. In exomphalos the bowels ± the liver are outside the abdomen, but contained within a membrane. As such, the bowel is usually healthy and feeding can be commenced at birth. However, exomphalos can be associated with other serious abnormalities so while the bowel may be healthy, survival can be worse than for gastroschisis.

Congenital diaphragmatic hernia

Usually diagnosed antenatally in high-income countries, congenital diaphragmatic hernia is less commonly seen in low-income countries, probably because newborns with severe respiratory distress don't make it to central hospitals. The underlying lung has various degrees of pulmonary hypertension, so these children may be born in severe respiratory distress, or in some cases present as older children with mild, recurrent chest symptoms or GI symptoms. Intensive care management of those born with severe pulmonary hypoplasia is complex. Pulmonary hypertension not only → respiratory failure but also right heart failure. Deciding the best time to operate can be challenging, and there is still significant mortality from this condition.

Gastrointestinal surgery

Pyloric stenosis

Typically presents with projectile, non-bilious vomiting in a hungry child from 3 weeks to 3 months. Blood gas analysis reveals a hypochloraemic, hypokalaemic metabolic alkalosis. A test feed in patient, experienced hands reveals a palpable a palpable 'olive' in the RUQ. If in doubt, US scanning usually confirms the diagnosis. Treatment is by pyloromyotomy after correction of dehydration and acid–base imbalance.

Voluvulus

Bilious (green) vomiting is a child must make you consider malrotation. Normally the duodenojejunal flexure (DJF) is high on the left, and the caecum low on the right. This produces a broad, stable mesentery. Failure of normal rotation results in a low DJF on the right, a high caecum, and a narrow mesentery, which is prone to twisting. This twist may be intermittent but can progress → ischaemia and infarction of the entire small bowel and catastrophe. *Therefore, green vomiting should be investigated with an urgent contrast follow through to exclude malrotation.*

Intussusception

During neonatal laparotomies for other indications one may see a transient intussusception, when the proximal bowel (intussusceptum) is propulsed into the distal bowel (intussuscipiens). These are self-resolving. If, however, there is a lead point (e.g. lymph nodes, Meckel's diverticulum, polyps/tumours), this may progress to obstruction and ischaemia. The classical clinical triad is intermittent inconsolable crying, redcurrant jelly stool (sloughed, bloody, ischaemic mucosa), and bilious vomiting (obstruction). The priority is vigorous fluid resuscitation and NG drainage. Abdominal X-ray may show obstruction and a meniscus sign but US scanning is more specific and sensitive. If caught early, air enema reduction is successful in up to 90% of cases. Bowel resection may be avoided if the intussusception is manually reduced (squeezed out).

Hirschsprung's disease

Is congenital aganglionosis of the distal bowel. This causes a tonic contraction with subsequent massive proximal dilatation (many years ago it was the dilated bowel that was thought to be abnormal, it is actually the collapsed distal aganglionic bowel that needs to be resected). There is usually a history of delayed passage of meconium and constipation and this may be associated with distension and vomiting, especially during an episode of Hirschsprung's-associated enterocolitis which is potentially fatal. The initial management is bowel rest, antibiotics if enterocolitis is expected, and decompression of the distal bowel. This may be achieved with rectal washouts but if unsuccessful, a stoma is required. The diagnosis is confirmed with a rectal biopsy.

Urology

Upper tract dilatation

In high-income countries is today mostly diagnosed on routine antenatal scanning. While many resolve *in utero*, of those that persist at birth some require urgent action (posterior urethral valves), others careful follow-up (pelviureteric junction (PUJ) obstruction, vesicoureteric junction (VUJ) obstruction, and vesicoureteric reflux (VUR). Follow-up may involve biochemical tests of renal function (U&E or glomerular filtration rate) or radiological studies looking at anatomy (degree and site of dilation, e.g. US) or function (percentage function of each kidney and/or clearance, e.g. nuclear medicine scans). If symptomatic, increasing dilatation or decreasing function surgery may be indicated. PUJO is treated with open or laparoscopic pyeloplasty, VUJO by ureteric reimplantation, and sever VUR by narrowing the ureteric orifice with endoscopic submucosal injection or by reimplanting the refluxing ureter.

Hypospadias

It is a triad of defects all due to deficient tissue on the ventral aspect of the penis: proximally sited meatus, chordee, and hooded foreskin. Surgery can repair the defect but most involve using the foreskin, so parents should be advised not to circumcise children with hypospadias.

Disorders of sexual differentiation

An embryo with two X chromosomes will become female, the gonads develop as ovaries. The Y chromosome contains the *SRY* gene. This codes for TDF (testis-determining factor), which causes the gonads to become testicles and produce testosterone (which causes development of male external genitalia and has an effect on the brain) and Mullerian inhibiting substance (which causes regression of the female internal genitalia, uterus, and fallopian tubes). Disruption in any of these pathways → a plethora of abnormalities in which the sex of the child may not be clear and cause life-threatening biochemical abnormalities. These children will be cared for by an MDT in partnership with the parents to decide the sex of rearing. At some point, surgery may be required to make the external genitalia look more normal.

Plastic surgery

Plastic surgery: overview

Plastic surgery is a broad surgical speciality which encompasses the management of a wide range of elective and acute pathologies. Its spectrum includes skin and soft tissue oncology, microvascular reconstruction, hand and upper limb, oncoplastic breast, aesthetics, head and neck, burns, lower limb trauma, and paediatric/cleft/craniofacial surgery. Plastic surgeons are heavily involved in cancer and trauma reconstruction of all parts of the body that require surgery following tissue loss, or for specialist functional and aesthetic considerations. Plastic surgery aims to restore optimal 'form and function' for patients.

> **Trivia**
> Originally derived from the Greek '*plastikos*' (which means to mould or reshape), plastic surgery is a surgical specialty which encompasses both reconstructive and aesthetic surgery.

Cases to see

Lumps and bumps

These patients usually undergo day case surgery under local anaesthetic (for smaller lesions). These are excellent cases to practise basic lump examinations and to assess important characteristics such as the depth, mobility, and attachments of the lesion to the surrounding structures. Understanding these relationships early will help you develop a solid foundation for future examinations (including lymph nodes and malignancies).

Hand trauma

Injuries range from soft tissue lacerations, to bony fractures and complex injuries involving both hands. Follow the on-call surgeon, assess these acute injuries, learn how to interpret radiographs, and present your findings; these activities provide powerful learning experiences.

Skin cancer

These can typically be seen at dedicated skin oncology clinics and operating lists (smaller lesions will likely be on day case local anaesthetic lists; larger lesions requiring major reconstruction will tend to be performed under GA). Learn to comment on skin lesion appearances (including the size, shape, symmetry, attachment and surface of the lesion) and to examine the local and regional lymph node basins.

Cleft lip and palate

Seen in specialist cleft centres due to the specialist MDT input required (e.g. surgeons, psychologists, geneticists, speech therapists, and specialist nurses). Attend outpatient clinics, sessions with the speech therapists, and other specialists to gain a broader understanding of the patient journey from birth, through surgery, to speech therapy and later development.

Burns

Patients usually present to the ED but are only managed definitively in specialist burns centres or units. Make yourself available to join the burns team on-call. The resuscitation and multifaceted management of major burns is highly specialized, exciting, and can be very satisfying.

Lower limb trauma

Lower limb trauma such as open tibial fractures are one of the most common injuries referred by orthopaedic surgeons. These injuries are typically high-energy polytraumas and can be extremely gory! Get involved with every aspect of care in these patients, from the initial assessment and resuscitation to the surgical debridement and reconstruction.

Things to do

Plastic surgery is an ideal rotation to master the techniques of delicate tissue handling, meticulous suturing, and to gain an appreciation for aesthetic refinements (e.g. when repairing facial wounds). You can learn to use a hand-held Doppler (also used by vascular surgeons) for finding the tiny blood vessels (perforators) in the skin and when assessing certain flaps in the postoperative period.

Investigations

FNAC

Uses a thin, hollow needle to aspirate samples of tissue or fluid from an organ of the body or a lump (e.g. lymph node). It can identify the type of cells within a mass, or provide information on the treatment progress of a previously known lump. It is commonly used to investigate lumps found in the breast or thyroid, but it can also be used in other palpable lymph nodes, and is a useful way of detecting cancer (e.g. melanoma metastases to the groin).

Sentinel lymph node biopsy

A diagnostic procedure that identifies and removes the sentinel lymph node (the first node to be involved in lymphatic spread from a particular area of the body). This is an excellent modality to identify if a cancer has spread to the lymph nodes. There are two important technical aspects that aid the procedure: (1) preoperative injection of radioactive tracer into the lymphatics of the primary lesion, which highlights the location of the node in the associated lymph node basin. This can then be detected intraoperatively on table by a gamma probe; (2) the surgeon may inject blue dye in the same area; this stains the lymphatics and involved lymph node(s) draining this site.

CT angiogram

Used in the planning phase for free flap reconstruction of the lower limb (to assess availability and patency of vessels) or breast (to identify appropriate perforators in DIEP (deep inferior epigastric artery perforator flap) autologous reconstruction). It enables the visualization of the vascular supply and also the position and size of arterial perforators and veins which can influence the design and choice of free flaps.

Plastic surgery: in clinic

Skin oncology

Skin cancer is a broad subspecialty which encompasses BCC, SCC, malignant melanoma (see ⮕ p. 217), adnexal, rare skin and other soft tissue cancers.

Risk factors

Sun exposure (UV radiation), pale skin (lower Fitzpatrick types), radiation or chemical exposure (tar/soot), age, immunosuppression, PMHx, FHx, and dysplastic naevi (for malignant melanoma).

Excision margins

British Association of Dermatologists (BAD) guidelines recommend specific excision margins for skin carcinomas. These currently guide treatment approaches in the UK, with continued research taking place.

BCC

Small BCCs <2 cm = 3–5 mm margin (a 3 mm margin will clear tumour in 85% of cases; a 4–5 mm margin will ↑ the peripheral clearance rate to 95%). Larger lesions will require larger excisions. Also, note that lesions are classified into low risk and high risk. Morphoeic subtype lesions require 13–15 mm margins to achieve 95% peripheral clearance.

SCC

Treated by wide local excision with 4 mm margins in low-risk tumours (<2 cm, well defined) and ≥6 mm in higher-risk cases which gives a 95% confidence of complete excision. Tumours classified as higher risk (e.g. >2 cm wide, >4 mm thick, ear/lip/nose, moderately/poorly/undifferentiated, extending into the subcutaneous tissue) are removed with a wider excision margin. Deep margin clearance is also important in skin cancer excisions.

Malignant melanoma

Excisional biopsy confirms subtype and Breslow thickness among numerous microscopic characteristics. This subsequently guides excision margins of the residual scar (e.g. <1 mm thickness on excision biopsy requires 1 cm wide local excision, 1.01–2 mm thickness requires 1–2 mm excision). Patients who have had non-melanoma skin cancer have a tenfold higher risk of a second non-melanomatous skin cancer. Melanoma patients have a threefold higher risk than the average risk of getting a non-melanomatous skin cancer. These patients require regular follow-up for monitoring—for local recurrence, satellite lesions, and distant metastases.

Mohs micrographic surgery

Involves progressive circumferential (peripheral and deep) layered excision of tumour; each layer is analysed under the microscope in frozen sections in real time until clearance is achieved, to avoid extensive tissue resection. Recommended technique for certain anatomical or cosmetically sensitive areas (e.g. nose, eyelids) and tumour types (e.g. morphoeic BCC) to optimize treatment and reconstruction.

Honours

Clinical manifestation of melanomas

The ABCDE rule is an easy guide or recognition tool for melanoma: A—asymmetry, B—border, C—colour, D—diameter, E—evolving. Other general warning signs

- A sore that does not heal.
- A new growth.
- A new itch within a mole.
- Change in the surface like scaling, oozing, bleeding, nodule, etc.
- Spread of pigment (colour) from the border of a spot.
- Redness or a new swelling beyond the border.

Pressure sores (pressure ulcers/decubitus ulcers)

An area of skin and underlying subcutaneous tissue damaged as a result of sufficient and persistent pressure that impairs the blood supply. They can develop at any site; however, certain pressure area points such as the *occiput, sacrum, ischium,* and *heels* are at higher risk. Locally they can be worsened by moisture, infection, and shear forces, and systemically by poor wound healing (e.g. in diabetics and PVD). All patients are at risk of developing pressure sores although particularly susceptible groups include the elderly, malnourished, acutely ill, quadriplegic, and bed-bound patients. It must be noted that pressure sores are preventable, and NICE has published guidelines for the prevention and management of these sores. 10% of patients in acute care facilities develop pressure sores. Pressure sores are graded 1–4, depending on how deep the tissue damage extends (in grade 4, tissue necrosis extends down to muscle or bone). Management always begins with optimizing the local and systemic factors that contributed to the pressure sore in the first place (i.e. pressure relief, wound toilet and appropriate dressings, adequate nutrition, etc.) Surgery may be required in complex pressure sores for debridement and reconstruction.

Honours

Waterlow risk assessment

This is a method of assessing patients for the risk of developing pressure sores, based on their comorbidities and other factors: BMI, skin changes, age, sex, adverse healing, continence, neurological deficit, mobility, surgical intervention, nutrition, and drugs (steroids).

Cleft lip and palate

The face and upper lip develop between weeks 5–9 of pregnancy. Most clefts are identified either at the time of the routine 20-week scan, or soon after birth. The cleft can affect the lip, palate (roof mouth), or both. The cleft can involve a part or the whole area (i.e. partial or complete) and may be one-sided (unilateral) or affect both sides (bilateral). The management of cleft patients begins in the neonatal period and continues until their teenage years and adulthood. A cleft lip and palate is the most common facial birth defect in the UK (1 in 700). The most common finding is a cleft palate, found in ~ 50% of all cases; ~25% of affected children have a cleft lip and ~25% have both a cleft lip and palate.

A cleft palate is repaired because it can affect hearing, feeding, and, later, speech. A cleft lip (particularly if it extends from the lip to involve the alveola) may affect the growth of teeth. Repairing a cleft lip is important to restore the normal function of the mouth as well as to improve the cosmetic appearance, which is extremely important. Surgery is the usual treatment for cleft lip and palate. Other interventions consist of speech and language therapy and orthodontics. Most tend to have a normal appearance with minimal scarring and good speech postoperatively.

Craniosynostosis

A rare condition (1 in 2000 births) involving the premature fusion of one or more of the fibrous sutures of the infant's skull, causing the baby to be born with or develop an abnormally shaped head. 75% of cases affect boys. The skull compensates by growing in the direction parallel to the fused suture. If, however, the compensatory growth is insufficient to allow for normal brain growth, ↑ICP → persistent headaches, learning difficulties, and visual impairment (all in later childhood). Treatment is surgical, involving remodelling of the cranium. 80–95% of cases are isolated (non-syndromic) but may be associated with >150 syndromes.

Plastic surgery: in the emergency department

As for all surgical patients, remember your ATLS® approach: ABCDE.

ABCD plus ...

Exposure: open fractures, degloving injuries, skin loss, extravasation injury, burns.

Hand trauma

Make sure you take a detailed history and perform a meticulous examination every time. Remember that what may appear to be innocuous injuries on the surface, can be extensive and in actual fact be extremely disabling for the patient. There are some crucial aspects to the hand history: *age, hand dominance, occupation, smoking status, and specific hobbies (e.g. musical instruments)* are the first five details that should be elucidated. Ask about the exact circumstances that led to the injury including the timing (particularly important for amputations and open injuries) and the mechanism of injury (e.g. power tools, broken glass, and slamming doors).

Honours

Managing traumatic wounds

Irrigate the wound thoroughly with saline or warm running tap water to remove debris. Local anaesthesia may need to be infiltrated to avoid pain, but try to assess nerve function prior to this. Give a tetanus booster if the primary vaccination course is incomplete or boosters are not up to date. Consider human tetanus immunoglobulin in high-risk wounds (e.g. in soil/manure contamination).

Glass injuries will never fail to surprise you by the severity of internal damage to tendons, nerves, and vessels; power tools and DIY injuries tend to be bloody and involve extensive bone and soft tissue damage. Explore the patient's social circumstances, as these may prompt you to think about home help and community therapy upon hospital discharge. Assessment is based on *look, feel, move, plus special tests*. In summary, assess for skin, soft tissue, bone, and joint injuries systematically. Soft tissue in the hand includes tendons (flexors and extensors), nerves (motor and sensory), and blood vessels (arteries and veins). Dirty or contaminated wounds (e.g. animal bites, human bites, and work-related, dirty machinery-induced injuries) need to go to theatre as soon as possible (ideally within 24 hours for a washout), but clean cuts (including tendon and nerve injuries) can safely be done on the next available operating list as long as the wound has been irrigated and there is no joint exposure. Some patients may require antibiotics.

Closed fractures that require an operation may best be fixed a few days after the original injury, particularly if there is significant swelling which would first benefit from elevation (e.g. in a Bradford sling) to reduce oedema.

Amputation and ischaemic limbs

If a traumatic episode results in complete amputation whereby the body part is totally severed (e.g. a finger that has been sliced off and is brought in separately by the patient/family), this can sometimes be replanted (re-attached), especially when proper care is taken of the severed part and stump. Smoking → unfavourable outcomes. In a partial amputation, some soft tissue connection remains. A partially severed extremity may or may not be able to be reattached in which case a '*terminalization*' (down to the next proximal joint) is advised.

Lower limb trauma

Plastic surgeons are frequently involved in the management of open fractures, working closely with the orthopaedic surgeons. Polytrauma patients need thorough assessment and resuscitation. It is important to consider the mechanics of the injury (i.e. low- vs high-energy impact). Plastic surgery involvement is mainly for soft tissue reconstruction (skin, muscle, nerve, and vessels) but bone injury must be documented (fracture site, size, shape, comminution, contamination, loss). The Gustillo–Anderson classification for open fractures is used to describe these injuries. Reconstruction in theatres involves repair of soft tissues plus providing adequate bone cover (if exposed). National lower limb trauma guidelines have been established, and can be found online (⌗ www.bapras.org.uk) and are a British Orthopaedic Association/British Association of Plastic, Reconstructive and Aesthetic Surgeons collective endeavour. A thorough neurovascular examination should be performed of the limb involved. There should be a high suspicion of compartment syndrome if there is severe pain or swelling peri-injury and perioperatively.

Burns

Can be caused by thermal (hot and cold), chemical (acid or alkali), or electrical injuries. Most burn accidents occur at home and in the workplace. About 75% of all burn injuries in children are preventable. Flame burns are the leading causes of burn injury in adults, while scalding is the leading cause of burn injury in children. Infants and the elderly are at the greatest risk for burn injury. Burns are classified by the *mode of injury* (e.g. scald/flame/chemical/electrical), their *depth* (e.g. superficial partial thickness/deep partial thickness/full thickness), and also the *extent* (e.g. dependent on total body surface area (TBSA) involved). Major burns are those covering >15% of the TBSA in adults and 10% in children. If major burns are taken to theatre, due to skin damage (what would have been their main barrier for thermoregulation), theatre temperatures are usually turned up to very warm levels.

Assessment

The depth of the burn will depend on the temperature of the heat and how long it is applied for:

- *Superficial erythema*: involves the dermis only, skin is dry and intact, bright red, usually no/small blisters, very painful. This does not contribute towards TBSA calculation in a burn (e.g. sunburn).

- *Superficial/partial thickness*: the skin is pink/red and blistered, blanches on pressure application, and is very painful. This should heal spontaneously within 10–14 days.
- *Deep dermal/deep partial thickness*: the skin is pinky red or white, feels thickened, no blisters, does not blanch on pressure application, and has reduced sensation. This should heal in 3 weeks if left to heal alone and will likely leave a scar. Such burns may require debridement and grafting to heal more quickly.
- *Full thickness*: the skin is white, brown, or black, leathery, dry and painless. May need debridement ± skin grafting. There are indications for hydrosurgery, enzymatic debridement, or maggot therapy.

Fluid resuscitation

IV fluid resuscitation is required in burns of 15% in an adult, and 10% in a child or the elderly, and inhalation injuries, so these patients require admission. People who have lesser burns but in special areas such as the face or perineum usually also require admission, and suspected NAI must be seen by the paediatric on-call team. Refer obviously large full-thickness burns, or hand burns, and those requiring surgery.

The Parkland formula = 4 mL/% body surface area burned/kg

The original formula noted a volume of 3.7–4.3 mL but has since been modified. It is currently one of the most popular formulas used (4 mL/%TBSA/kg). This calculates the total millilitres of crystalloid (e.g. Hartmann's or Ringer's lactate) required for the first 24 hours after the time of the burn. Give half of this volume in the first 8 hours, the remainder over the next 16 hours. Children additionally require maintenance fluid (dextrose saline) calculated based on their weight. The aim is to achieve adequate urine output and avoid fluid overload. Fluid resuscitation is a dynamic process and with regular assessments, fluid volumes can be titrated as necessary. Other formulas have been described; e.g. Mount Vernon, Brooke, Shriner's (paediatric), and Galveston's (paediatric).

Honours

Referral criteria for burns centre
- Consider if >3% TBSA, partial thickness burns (2% TBSA in children).
- All deep dermal and full-thickness burns.
- All burns associated with electrical shock, chemical agents, NAI, relevant anatomy (face, hands, perineum, feet), circumferential to limbs/trunk/neck, and inhalation injury.
- All burns not healed within 2 weeks.

Plastic surgery: in theatre

Survival tips

Plastic surgery should be considered a collection of specialized surgical techniques that once mastered (some with steep learning curves), can be utilized to solve difficult reconstructive challenges in most areas of the body.

Debridement and reconstruction

Plastic surgeons are often required to deal with complex wounds following trauma, infection, or cancer. A vital skill that you can learn is how to assess a wound, debride it effectively, and decide on the type of procedure that is required to reconstruct it. When assessing a wound in theatre, it is imperative to identify and differentiate viable vs non-viable tissue. In the context of necrotic and infected wounds or heavy contamination, this can be more challenging.

> **Tips and tricks**
>
> *Wound assessment*
>
> There are a few assessment tools to keep in mind which will help you identify non-viable from viable tissue (dead from the living):
> - *Colour*: of the tissue compared with surrounding similar tissue. Dermis which is black or is a fixed, non-blanching red is probably non-viable. When assessing fat, a bright, shiny yellow is healthy, whereas pale, cream-coloured or red fat is probably not.
> - *Temperature*: changes in the skin can be very useful in determining if tissue is alive and hence well perfused or not.
> - *Bleeding*: if in doubt, you can check for bleeding using a needle or by scoring with a knife.
> - *Tug test*: when assessing a complex wound with fracture fragments and contamination, any tissue that is easy to pull away with a pair of forceps with minimal little resistance is unlikely to survive and should be removed.

The next task is to debride the wound. Effective debridement involves removing all non-viable tissue and contaminants and irrigating the wound with copious volumes of saline. Wounds should be debrided to remove all dead and contaminated tissue, exposing healthy, bleeding edges. Any devitalized tissue left *in situ* may become necrotic and liquefy → collections, infections, and delays in wound healing. Reconstruction of a wound is the next step along this pathway. Achieving tissue healing in the quickest time, when possible, is the best way to prevent infections and complications. A plastic surgeon will always aim to reconstruct a wound with three factors in mind: *form, function*, and *safety*. Re-establishing form and function can get the patient back on the path of recovery and rehabilitation.

An example is the reconstruction of a burn scar contracture above a joint. By releasing the scar and reconstructing with a skin graft (with or without a dermal substitute) or flap, function is restored to what could otherwise become a stiff and immobile joint. Arguably the most important consideration is safety. The plastic surgeon must choose the most appropriate reconstruction to achieve the best form and functional result; however, it must be appropriate and safe for the individual patient. For example, it would be considered inappropriate to perform a highly technical reconstruction on a frail patient who may suffer if a prolonged GA is required, especially when there is an easier, shorter, and safer option available.

Honours

Reconstructive ladder

This model was originally devised to help plan appropriate management. It includes a number of reconstructive options, which are progressively more complex:
1. Healing by secondary intention (allow to heal by granulation).
2. Healing by primary intention (suture).
3. Skin grafting (split thickness and full thickness).
4. Local flap (transposition, advancement, rotation).
5. Regional flap.
6. Distant flap (pedicled or free).

When faced with a reconstructive challenge, choose the simplest option first and consider if it will give the best outcome in terms of form and function and if it is safe for the patient before moving up. This concept has been superseded by the *reconstructive elevator*—signifying the importance of selecting the most appropriate level of reconstruction as opposed to defaulting to the least complex; sometimes one may have to jump several options, or start immediately with a free flap as best management. We also now have other options to consider: topical negative pressure dressings (e.g. vacuum assisted closure) and dermal substitute matrices, in addition to tissue expansion.

Graft

A graft is a unit of tissue that is harvested from a donor area and transferred to another area of the body. The crucial factor is that the graft does not carry with it its blood supply; instead, in order to survive, it must get its blood supply from its new tissue bed. It is a reliable and repeatable procedure that reconstructs tissues with like-tissues using relatively simple techniques. Skin grafts are the commonest grafts performed. Skin grafts are used when a wound is too large to close directly, such as following a large skin cancer excision or an extensive defect following a large burn or necrotizing fasciitis.

Skin can be harvested as a shaving of the epidermis and part of the dermis (termed split-thickness skin graft) vs excised as full thickness of the skin (termed full-thickness skin graft). When a large amount of graft is required at several sites, split-thickness skin grafts are preferentially harvested. Meshing is a process of cutting the split-thickness skin graft in a criss-cross pattern making numerous small holes in the skin (using a mesher). This is performed to allow the graft to drape more easily in an uneven wound and to allow any fluid or blood to escape from underneath the graft (which may otherwise have lifted off the graft). Furthermore, when massive wound areas are encountered, such as in the case of large burns, then a skin graft can be meshed and expanded up to nine times its original size!

Skin grafts initially stick to the wound bed by fibrin adhesion. They are nourished directly by the plasma in the wound (*plasma imbibition*) for 48 hours. It is followed by a process of *inosculation*, which involves cut ends of arteries in the skin graft lining up and 'kissing' with ends of arteries in the wound bed. The graft is dependent on these processes for its survival over the first 4–5 days, after which *revascularization* of the graft occurs and it can then survive by itself.

Honours

Blood supply of the skin
The skin receives its blood supply through a series of deep and superficial plexuses (networks): *subepidermal, dermal, subdermal, subcutaneous,* and *prefascial*.

Cartilage grafts are sometimes needed to reconstruct a defect of the nose or ear. These defects may be congenital, traumatic, or following cancer excisions. Cartilage is needed to provide shape and can be harvested from the ears, nasal septum, and ribs (costal cartilage). Bone grafts are used to fill gaps in the bone since skeletal continuity is vital for support and movement. Defects in the bone can result from trauma, infection (osteomyelitis), and congenital defects. Cancellous bone is typically harvested from the pelvic bone (e.g. iliac crest). Other forms of tissue grafting include, muscle, nerve, vein, and fat, which have specific indications.

Honours

Split- vs full-thickness skin grafts
Split
- *Advantages*: large grafts can be harvested, meshed to expand coverage, rapid healing, donor sites heal spontaneously with minimal scarring.
- *Disadvantages*: easily sheared and traumatized, less natural colour and texture, meshing pattern remains visible, significant contracture.

Full
- *Advantages*: better match for normal skin colour and texture, less contracture, less contour deformity, remains soft and pliable, better over joints.
- *Disadvantages*: limited size of graft as donor site should be amenable to direct closure, higher risk of graft failure, scar at site.

Flaps

A flap is a unit of tissue which is transferred from one part of the body to another, but at all times retains its blood supply. This enables surgeons to transfer much larger, more bulky tissues to fill deep defects and also transfer them to areas that may not be suitable for grafting, such as directly onto bone and over tendons. Remember, however, that attention must be paid to the resultant donor site, minimizing deformity and disability. Flaps can be classified according to their *contents, circulation, contour*, and *contiguity*.

Circulation

Flaps can get their blood supply through a named artery that runs within that flap (axial flaps) or through a random network of small blood vessels that supply blood through the base of the flap (random pattern flaps). Random pattern flaps are relatively easy to raise, however they have a limited length:width ratio (up to 2:1 on the body, and 4:1 on the face possible due to its excellent blood supply). Axial pattern flaps receive their blood supply directly from a named artery and accompanying vein. They allow for a much greater length of flap to be raised and are generally more reliable. Axial flaps are subdivided into fasciocutaneous and musculocutaneous depending on the course that the blood vessels take before reaching and supplying the skin. Perforator flaps are now popular and have their own evolving nomenclature; they are generally named with a focus on the perforating vessel that the flap contains (e.g. ALT (anterolateral thigh flap), based on a perforator from the descending branch of lateral circumflex femoral artery).

Contents

A flap may be composed of any layer of soft tissue including skin, fat, fascia, muscle, or bone. The most common flaps that you will encounter in plastic surgery are fasciocutaneous flaps (containing skin and fascia) and muscle flaps (gracilis, latissimus dorsi, etc.).

Contiguity

Flaps can be described as local, regional, or distant depending on their origin. Local flaps are composed of tissue adjacent to the defect; regional flaps are composed of tissue from the same region (e.g. upper limb, head and neck or trunk); and distant flaps are composed of tissue from another part of the body and can be transferred whilst pedicled (still attached) or free (completely detached) flap, the latter requiring microsurgical anastomoses.

Contour

The contour of a flap describes the movement that a flap makes in order to reach its destination. These can be described as advancement, rotation, transposition, and interpolation. This refers mainly to local flaps (e.g. performed on the face: bilobed, V-Y advancement, cheek rotation). If a perforator vessel is identified (e.g. on Doppler or imaging), where a local flap can be designed, then a local perforator flap can be used for reconstruction of the defect (e.g. a lumbar artery perforator flap to reconstruct a defect on the back).

Microsurgery

In trauma, microsurgery is often required for the anastomosis of tiny arteries and veins in amputated limbs, digits, and appendages. In breast cancer reconstruction, free flaps are usually harvested from the abdomen, e.g. DIEP flaps (and in certain cases from the medial thigh or buttocks) and transferred to reconstruct the breast. The arteries and veins of the abdominal tissue are anastomosed to recipient vessels in the chest or axilla. Nerves in the brachial plexus or peripherally in the arms or hands often need reconstruction. It is important to align the nerve axons accurately under a microscope to achieve the best re-innervation and functional outcomes from the nerve repair.

Aesthetic surgery

Aesthetic principles pervade all aspects of plastic surgery, including trauma, cancer reconstruction, burns, and, of course, aesthetic surgery.

The plastic surgeon will use the principles of aesthetic/cosmetic surgery, such as skin tension lines, natural creases, and ideal proportions in order to achieve the best aesthetic outcome in any scenario, wherever possible. Aesthetic surgery is a branch of plastic surgery which is concerned with providing an enhancement of shape and form of the body. History and examination must still be thorough, e.g. when taking a history for a breast reduction patient, you should ask about risk factors for malignancy and when examining you must also examine the breast and axillae for lumps; when taking a history for a blepharoplasty (eyelid rejuvenation) you must ask about vision/glasses/contact lenses/dry eyes, etc.

Aesthetic surgery is performed on all parts of the body including the face, breasts, trunk, and limbs.

Trivia

Breast enlargement remains the most popular procedure, with 11,135 augmentations performed in 2013, up 13% year-on-year, according to figures collected by the British Association of Aesthetic Plastic Surgeons.

There are numerous types of implants. For example, in very basic terms these can be described by their shape (rounded vs. anatomical), or surface (textured vs. smooth). Breast implant associated anaplastic large cell lymphoma (BIA-ALCL) is topical. It is a rare and highly treatable type of lymphoma that can develop around breast implants, mainly certain textures. The ABS (Association of Breast Surgery), BAAPS, BAPRAS and MHRA have recently issued a joint UK update; it is important that you remain aware of this discussion for the future.

Autologous fat grafting for breast enlargement is also commonly performed, in both aesthetic and reconstructive cases.

Trauma and orthopaedic surgery

Trauma and orthopaedic surgery: overview

Trauma and orthopaedic (T&O) surgery is the branch of surgery concerned with the musculoskeletal (MSk) system. Orthopaedic surgeons treat MSk trauma, sports injuries, infections, tumours, and congenital and degenerative diseases. In some hospitals, they may also be involved in spine surgery (alt. neurosurgeons) and hand surgery (alt. plastics).

Most consultants are involved in trauma (injuries and fractures), however they also have one or two subspeciality interests:
- Wrist and hand
- Shoulder and elbow
- Hip and knee
- Foot and ankle
- Spinal surgery
- Pelvic surgery
- MSk oncology
- Sports medicine
- Paediatric orthopaedics
- Arthroplasty (joint reconstruction).

Cases to see
- Trauma/emergency:
  - Polytrauma
  - Cauda equina
  - Neck of femur (NOF) fracture: intra/extracapsular
  - Ankle fracture
  - Wrist (distal radius) fracture
  - Limping child
  - Hot, swollen joint
- Elective:
  - Osteoarthritis (OA e.g. hip ± knee)
  - Carpal/cubital tunnel syndrome
  - Rotator cuff pathology
  - Soft tissue knee injury (e.g. meniscal tear)
  - Arthroscopy (mainly knee + shoulder)
  - Bunions
  - Removal of metalwork
  - Arthroplasty (joint replacement).

Investigations/procedures to see
- Joint reduction
- Manipulation under anaesthesia
- Fracture repair
- K-wire
- Plate (ankle, wrist)
- Screws (e.g. hip fracture)
- Intramedullary nailing (e.g. long bone fractures)
- External fixator ('ExFix').

Things to do

- Go to the plaster room,
- Joint injection/aspiration.

Factoid

Orthopaedic surgeons sometimes have the negative reputation of being simple minded, bone-centric, and interested only in private practice. You will hear it said that orthopods are strong as an ox and half as clever, however a multicentre prospective study found that orthopaedic surgeons were both stronger and more intelligent than their anaesthetic colleagues.[1] In reality, most orthopods are enthusiastic, energetic, and approachable.

Reference

1. Subramanian P, Kantharuban S, Subramanian V, et al. (2011). Orthopaedic surgeons: as strong as an ox and almost twice as clever? Multicentre prospective comparative study. *BMJ* 343:d7506.

Trauma and orthopaedic surgery: in clinic

Not surprisingly, the T&O clinic is divided into trauma (fractures and injuries) and orthopaedic (elective conditions) clinics. Try to sit in on both types. This is an opportunity to practise your focused orthopaedic history and examinations. (See Table 40.1.)

The most common presenting complaint to an orthopaedic clinic is pain—either following an injury or through a degenerative process. If from an injury, what is the mechanism? The impact on quality of life and the level of disability caused must be established and therefore it is important to ask about hand dominance and occupation. Focus on conditions that may affect potential surgery in the PMHx. For instance, establish whether the patient has risk factors for undergoing anaesthesia. Diabetes, long-term steroid use, immunosuppression, and smoking are important as these are risk factors for poor wound healing. Any anticoagulant use should also be noted as this will need to be withheld prior to surgery. Finally, it is equally important to establish the patient's goals and expectations. What activities would they like to return to? The treatment for a premiership footballer with an ACL rupture will be different to an elderly patient with a sedentary lifestyle with the same condition. The following cases are likely to form the mainstay of your clinic caseload.

Orthopaedic/elective clinic

Osteoarthritis (OA) is defined as degenerative arthritis (joint inflammation) predominantly affecting articular cartilage and subchondral bone. The overwhelming majority of arthritides are degenerative (OA).

Predisposing factors are age, weight-bearing (e.g. obesity and knee OA), and previous injury to the joint (e.g. infection/trauma/malalignment/damage to articular cartilage). Symptoms are predominantly pain and stiffness. The key to OA management is to understand this is not a life-threatening condition, and focus on improving quality of life. Initial treatment is lifestyle changes (weight loss, exercise) and analgesia. Later treatments include joint injections (steroid and local anaesthetic/hyaluronan), joint reconstruction (resurfacing/replacement), or fusion (arthrodesis). (See Fig. 40.1.)

- *Rheumatoid arthritis (RA)*: a chronic multisystem disease with predominant MSk manifestations. It attacks synovial tissues, i.e. synovial joints, tendons and bursae, and → deformities. Use of DMARDs has significantly reduced this.

Table 40.1 A favourite question is features of OA vs RA on X-ray

Cardinal signs of OA (LOSS)	Cardinal signs of RA (LESS)
Loss of joint space	Joint space narrowing
Osteophytes	Erosions
Subchondral cysts	Soft bones (osteopenia)
Subchondral sclerosis	Soft tissue swelling

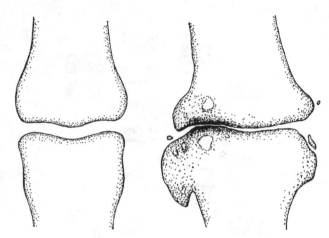

Fig. 40.1 X-ray features of osteoarthritis. Reproduced with permission from Wilkinson, Ian, et al, *Oxford Handbook of Clinical Medicine* 10e, 2016, Oxford University Press. Courtesy of Dr DC Howlett.

- *Carpal tunnel syndrome*: entrapment of the median nerve at the wrist causing pain, paraesthesia, and numbness in the distribution of median nerve. Risk factors include pregnancy, diabetes, RA, hypothyroid, acromegaly. It is a matter of debate whether repetitive injury is associated with carpal tunnel syndrome. Treatment involves splinting, steroid injection, and surgical decompression.
- *Rotator cuff (RC) pathology*: affects the group of muscles that stabilizes the shoulder (supraspinatus, infraspinatus, subscapularis, teres minor). Common problems include RC tear, impingement, and RC arthropathy. Most are managed conservatively (e.g. physiotherapy, steroid injections). Refractory cases require surgery, usually arthroscopic.
- *Bunions*: hallux valgus (big toe) deviating laterally at metatarsophalangeal joint; associated with biomechanical forces typically related to wearing tight shoes or high-heels. Treatment involves pads, splints, wedges between toes, realignment surgery (e.g. scarf/Akin osteotomy), or arthrodesis in advanced cases.

Trauma/fracture clinic

- *Soft tissue injury*: tendon/ligament injuries and meniscal tears are common. Meniscal tears can be treated with physiotherapy and/or arthroscopy. Tendon ruptures can often be treated conservatively or with repair/reconstruction. Many soft tissue injuries can be treated with RICE (Rest, Ice, Elevation, and Compression).
- *Fracture (fx or #)*: discontinuity in the cortex of a bone *with an associated soft tissue injury* (do not forget this important point).

See Fig. 40.2.

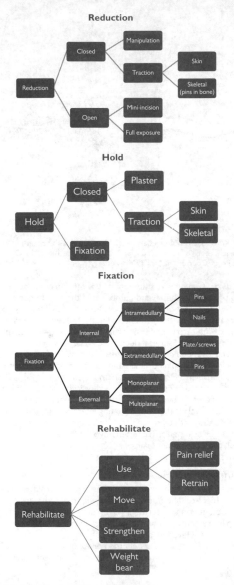

Fig. 40.2 Principles of orthopaedic management.

The management of any fracture follows the 4R algorithm
1. *Resuscitate*: ATLS® algorithm.
2. *Reduce* (hold): closed (in ED) or open (in theatre) reduction.
3. *Restrict* (fixation): external (cast, splint, traction, brace, ExFix) vs internal (plate, screw, nail).
4. *Rehabilitate*: physiotherapy, occupational therapy.

There are two main types of types of fracture fixation: fixation with *absolute stability* and *relative stability* (see Table 40.2).

Relative stability

This is the 'classic' four-stage method you will have read about:
1. Bleeding from bone ends creates a haematoma, generating an *inflammatory* reaction. Haematoma is gradually replaced by granulation tissue. Necrotic bone is removed.
2. Periosteal cells develop into *chondroblasts* and fibroblasts which form hyaline cartilage and woven bone. This culminates in a new mass of tissue known as *soft callus*.
3. The soft callus is converted into stronger *hard callus*.
4. The bone then *remodels* to the normal stresses it is placed under and returns to its normal shape over months to years.

Absolute stability

Fixation by *absolute stability* 'fools' the body into thinking no fracture has occurred by obliterating the fracture gap. New bone is laid down without callus. These methods are used in different scenarios depending on the fracture pattern.

> **Top tips**
> - Attend the trauma meetings in the morning to learn how to present. *It is not an X-ray, it is a plain radiograph!*
> - X-rays are like ECGs in the sense that you need (1) your own system, and (2) to see lots of normal to recognize abnormal. As an undergraduate it is usually enough to name the bones (common question), and recognize simple fracture patterns.
> Never comment on a fracture based on one view, *always ask for two orthogonal views* (e.g. AP and lateral views); and remember the joint above and below may also need imaging.

The rate of bone healing is multifactorial, including which bone is affected, fracture pattern, blood supply, age and general health of the patient, and type of fixation (plaster vs plate etc.). Children heal much faster than adults.

Table 40.2 Difference between absolute vs relative stability

Stability	Absolute	Relative
Movement	No movement at fracture gap	Limited movement, resulting in callus formation
Fracture gap	No gap	Small fracture gap
Bone healing	No callus (direct, hence primary)	Callus (indirect, hence secondary)
Examples	Lag screws, plate-and-screws (some)	Intramedullary nailing, plate-and-screws (some)

Terminology: importance of describing X-rays systemically

Imagine you are on the phone describing the radiograph to your consultant who cannot see it:
- Site:
  - Bone (e.g. femur).
  - Distal vs proximal.
  - Intra-/extra-articular.
- Pattern: spiral/oblique/transverse/impacted/avulsion/incomplete.
- Simple/comminuted (number of fragments).
- Displacement:
  - Minimal vs complete.
  - % change.
  - Shortened.
- Angulation:
  - Varus vs valgus.
  - Dorsal vs volar.
- Rotation.
- *Dislocation*: complete loss of congruity between the articular surfaces of a joint. *Subluxation* is *partial* loss of congruity between the articular surfaces of a joint. Both can be associated with fractures ('fracture-dislocation' and 'fracture-subluxation').

See Fig. 40.3 for an example.

Ask the boss ...

When to remove metalwork?
- Infection.
- Wound dehiscence.
- Pain.
- Restricted range of movement.
- Healed fracture.
- Overlying skin/soft tissue irritation.
- Kirschner wires (K-wires).

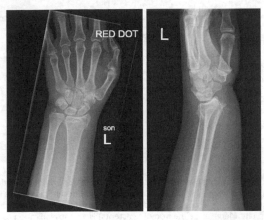

Fig. 40.3 This is a plain radiograph of a 45-year old right hand dominant carpenter taken this morning, who fell onto his outstretched right hand today. He sustained a closed wrist fracture and is neurovascularly intact. This is a simple transverse fracture of the distal radius, which is extra-articular. There is 50% displacement, 1 cm shortening with dorsal angulation. There is also an associated ulna styloid fracture.

What are the possible complications in fracture healing?

When fractures heal, the fragments unite. However, this also depends on optimal conditions (see Table 40.3).

- *Union*: bone healing within an expected time frame (generally 6 weeks for children and 12 weeks for adults for long bones).
- *Delayed union*: failure to reach union in 6 months after fracture and fractures that take longer to heal.
- *Non-union*: an arrest in fracture repair due to infection, biomechanical instability, or poor vascularity (avascular necrosis/PVD). It is usually divided into atrophic vs hypertrophic.
- *Malunion*: fracture healing in a suboptimal and non-anatomic (abnormal) position.

Common orthopaedic imaging modalities

- *X-ray*: uses a beam of electrons to pass through the body to generate an image on a photographic film. The vast majority of UK hospitals use an electronic version without need for films (e.g. picture archiving and communication system (PACS)).
- *Ultrasound*: uses high-frequency sound waves to visualize soft tissues (e.g. tendons). No ionizing radiation is used, but it is very operator dependent. It is faster, cheaper, and generally more readily available in hospitals than the following listed modalities.
- *CT*: takes X-rays of bones in 3D. It is mostly used to image complex fractures, but can also assess the degree of fracture healing.

Table 40.3 Complications of orthopaedic surgery, fracture, and trauma

Timeframe	
Short term	Medium to long term
Infection	Delayed/mal-/non-union
VTE and fat embolus	Joint stiffness
Compartment syndrome	Osteoarthritis
Haemorrhage	Avascular necrosis
Fracture blisters	Complex regional pain syndrome
Neurovascular and visceral injury	Myositis ossificans

- *MRI*: uses a strong magnetic field to generate images without radiation. It is used to image soft tissues but may also spot occult fractures. It is expensive, takes a long time, and can be difficult to get in district general hospitals. Metal inside the body (e.g. stents) is a contraindication to its use.
- *Dual-energy X-ray absorptiometry (DXA)*: uses two beams of different densities to estimate bone mineral density. Used mostly in the context of fractured hips.
- *Nuclear medicine scans* (bone scan/scintigraphy): used to detect occult tumours, metastases, and stress fractures using radioisotopes such as technetium-99m.

Trauma and orthopaedic surgery: in theatre

'The bone is a plant, with its roots in the soft tissue, and when its vascular connections are damaged, it often requires not techniques of a cabinet maker, but the patient care and understanding of a gardener.' (Gathorne Robert Girdlestone, 1932)

You will see various methods of fracture fixation in theatre. Remember to (1) always wear a face mask according to the adage 'you can sneeze into an abdomen but you cannot cough into a joint' to minimize risk of infection, and (2) wear a lead gown when a C-arm is present to protect yourself from radiation.

Trauma surgery

K-wires

These are thin, smooth wires driven into bone using a driver which pin fragments together. They act as blocking wires to stop further displacement of fracture fragments until healing begins. They are usually left protruding from the skin and need to be removed at a later date, usually in clinic.

Plate and screws

Widely used for absolute stability but requires enough bone at either end of the plate to ensure screw fixation. It often requires a large incision and soft tissue stripping (risks compromising the periosteal blood supply to the bone) because the plate must be applied directly to the bone (e.g. ankle, wrist) through open reduction and internal fixation (ORIF).

Screws alone

For example, cannulated screws are used to fix the femoral head *in situ* in an undisplaced intracapsular fracture or in slipped upper femoral epiphysis (SUFE), or for fixing the medial malleolus. This is a minimally invasive technique that requires only a small incision.

Intramedullary nailing (IMN)

IMN is essentially a rod placed through the centre of the bone (the medullary canal), usually for fractures of the diaphysis of long bones (humerus, tibia, and femur) through closed reduction and internal fixation (CRIF).

C-arm

K-wires, screws, and IMN are inserted using small incisions using an image intensifier machine (called a C-arm) in theatre that provides fluoroscopic imaging, while plates require wide-open incisions allowing the entire plate to be visualized with the naked eye. Often a C-arm is used to confirm restoration of length, alignment, and rotation. The X-ray images can be stored for evidence of surgical outcomes and comparisons to preoperative planning in revision surgery.

External fixator
This is an external device which acts as a scaffold to hold fractures from the outside of limbs. Protruding pins are driven into bone and connected by external bars. This has a wide range of indications:
- Heavily comminuted fracture.
- Deep contamination.
- Non-unions.
- Polytrauma/temporary stability.
- Heavy soft tissue disruption.
- Limb-lengthening.

Neck of femur fractures
Hip hemiarthroplasty is replacement of the fractured femoral head only, leaving the native acetabulum untouched (compare with total hip replacement (THR) where both are replaced). The usual indication is a displaced intracapsular fractured NOF where there is presumed disruption to the blood supply of the femoral head which will likely undergo osteonecrosis. Extracapsular fractures require a *dynamic hip screw* (DHS), which fixes the fractured femoral head onto the femoral shaft using a special plate-and-screws design such that weight-bearing compresses the fracture. Both options fulfil the goals of treatment which are to allow mobilization without restriction, preventing mortality and morbidity associated with being bed-bound.

Elective surgery

Arthroscopy
This is minimally invasive surgery of a joint, typically knee and shoulder, and can be diagnostic or therapeutic (washout, reconstruction, repair, e.g. torn ligaments and menisci). Scars are 1–2 cm long, and usually two to four in number.

Honours

Arthroscopic meniscal knee surgery
- Menisci are C-shaped discs of cartilage in the knee. They ↑ the congruency of the knee joint and act as shock absorbers.
- Tears are common in young, sporty patients who forcefully twist the knee on weight-bearing.
- Patients report 'mechanical symptoms' of pain, locking, and giving way of the knee.
- Examination may reveal joint line tenderness, reduced range of movement, and positive McMurray's test (do with caution as this can be very painful!).
- Tears give characteristic MRI appearances.
- Physiotherapy is the mainstay of treatment but if it fails, patients undergo arthroscopy. Tears in the outer third where there is a blood supply are usually repaired with sutures; tears in the inner third have to be trimmed as they are not repairable. Menisci must be preserved as much as possible.

Arthroplasty

Almost every joint can be reconstructed or replaced; however, hip and knee are the most common, typically required for OA. These can be partial or total, and with or without bone cement. Research shows reduced pain, and improved quality of life and lifespan. The aim is to delay surgery until the last resort since every implant has a shelf life (~10–20 years on average) before it is inevitable to do revision surgery which becomes more complex and risky every time. Cement and implant loosening may be septic or aseptic.

Carpal tunnel decompression

Division of the skin → fat → superficial palmar fascia → transverse carpal ligament (flexor retinaculum) in order to decompress the underlying median nerve. The flexor retinaculum contains four flexor digitorum profundus (FDP), four flexor digitorum superficialis (FDS) tendons, flexor pollicis longus (FPL), and median nerve. This is usually a day case procedure performed under local anaesthetic.

Anatomy

There are three main nerves supplying motor and sensory innervation to the upper limb: (1) median, (2) ulnar, and (3) radial nerves. The flexor retinaculum has four bony attachments: laterally, scaphoid tubercle and ridge of trapezium; medially, pisiform and hook of hamate. Guyon's (ulnar) canal runs superficial and ulnar to the flexor retinaculum (outside the carpal tunnel) and contains the ulnar nerve and artery (hence 'ulnar sparing' in carpal tunnel syndrome). (See Fig. 40.4.)

Pathology

These nerves can become compressed at various sites along their course, especially where they travel between muscles and within tight tunnels. The most common is carpal tunnel syndrome, which constitutes compression of the median nerve as it travels through the carpal tunnel in the volar aspect of the wrist.

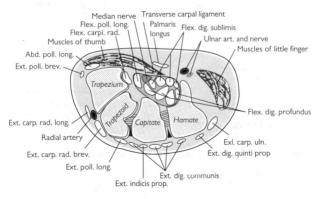

Fig. 40.4 Cross-section of the carpal tunnel. Reproduced from https://commons.wikimedia.org/wiki/File:Carpal-Tunnel.svg, licensed under the Creative Commons Attribution-Share Alike 3.0 Unported license.

Presentation

Compressive neuropathy produces typical symptoms:
• Pain.
• Numbness.
• Pins and needles (paraesthesia).
• Reduced grip strength.
• Thenar wasting.

Symptoms characteristically worsen at night and are relieved by shaking the hand or dangling it off the edge of the bed.

Risk factors

Most cases of carpal tunnel syndrome are idiopathic, however it can be caused by pregnancy, hypothyroidism, diabetes, and rarely by tumours within the carpal tunnel.

Special examinations

Can provoke the symptoms and add to the weight of clinical evidence:
• Durkan's (pressure over tunnel).
• Tinel's (tapping over the tunnel).
• Phalen's tests (flat palms together in wrist hyper-flexion/extension).

Investigations

Nerve conduction studies are useful to correlate with clinical findings but this is essentially a clinical diagnosis. MRI excludes space-occupying lesions within the carpal tunnel, which is rare.

Management

Non-surgical management can be attempted with night splints and steroid injections around the median nerve. Definitive treatment is carpal tunnel decompression (via open vs endoscopic).

Complications

Sparing of sensation of the thenar eminence is due to its supply by the palmar cutaneous branch of the median nerve, which comes off the main nerve 5 cm proximal to the carpal tunnel. Symptomatic persistence ± recurrence can take 3 months to resolve. The commonest complication is scar sensitivity (pillar pain).

Trivia

What is bone cement?

It is a synthetic material which fills the free space between bone and implant. It is composed of a powder and a liquid which is mixed together. This generates an exothermic polymerization reaction to form polymethyl methacrylate (PMMA), commonly known as Plexiglas®.

Why is it green?

Cement contains extract of chlorophyll to enable it to be seen easily.

How is it visible on X-ray?

Barium or zirconium is added to make cement radio-opaque.

Trauma and orthopaedic surgery: in the emergency department

Polytrauma

Multiply injured patients in England are now triaged to major trauma centres, where they are looked after by a trauma team trained to deal with these complex injuries on a daily basis. The team includes ED, general surgery, vascular surgery, anaesthetics. and orthopaedics. It may also include neurosurgery and plastic surgery. Assessment and management of polytrauma patients are performed according to the ATLS® algorithm:

- *A*: airway with C-spine protection.
- *B*: breathing and ventilation control.
- *C*: circulation and haemorrhage control.
- *D*: disability/neurological assessment.
- *E*: exposure and environmental control.

Borrow a copy of the latest ATLS® manual; it is easy to read and will cover the whole scope of managing major trauma. It is beyond the scope of medical school but may be interesting/useful. *Make sure you see a trauma call with primary and secondary surveys.*

See Fig. 40.5 for types of hip fracture.

Open (compound) fracture

This is a fracture communicating with an overlying skin wound. A fracture where the skin remains intact is a closed fracture. You cannot tell from an X-ray if the fracture is open or closed.

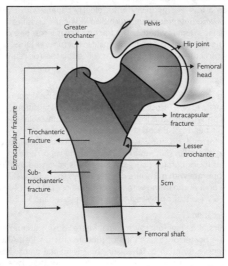

Fig. 40.5 Types of hip fractures. Reproduced with permission from Parker, M., Johansen, A., Hip Fracture, *BMJ*. 2006 Jul 1; 333(7557): 27–30.

Use the six As to guide open fracture management:
- *Assessment*: ATLS® plus assessment of the neurovascular status of the limb, viability of soft tissues, photograph the wound.
- *Antisepsis*: remove gross contaminants, and seal with saline-soaked gauze and impermeable dressing.
- *Alignment*: align fracture and splint (for immobilization, analgesia, and haemorrhage control).
- *Anti-tetanus*: check status and immunize appropriately.
- *Antibiotics*: e.g. IV co-amoxiclav.
- *Analgesia*: e.g. opioids.

Compartment syndrome

Tissue (osseo-fascial) pressure in a closed compartment exceeds the perfusion pressure resulting in ischaemia due to microvascular compromise and congested venous return. It is a clinical diagnosis and must be diagnosed promptly as the only treatment is immediate fasciotomy (in theatre) to save the limb. Complications include ischaemia/rhabdomyolysis → necrosis → contracture, chronic pain, dry and wet gangrene → amputation.

> **Top tip**
>
> You will often hear and read that compartment syndrome is characterized by the six Ps which are actually signs of *acute limb ischaemia*. It is typified by pain out of proportionate to the underlying injury, especially on passive stretch of a tense compartment. Opioids have no effect!

Neck of femur (NOF) fracture (Fig 40.5)

This is often a low-energy injury in an elderly patient with osteoporosis. There are a number of fracture patterns; however, the classification that determines management is whether the fracture line is intra- or extracapsular. In general, the rule is fix/repair extracapsular fractures → DHS, and replace intracapsular fractures → hemiarthroplasty if displaced (or repair with cannulated screws/DHS if undisplaced).

Ankle fracture

Can involve medial, lateral, or posterior malleolar fractures. Lateral malleolar fractures are most common (Weber classification). Treatment will depend on whether the fracture is 'stable' or 'unstable' (displacement on full weight-bearing). Be on the lookout for (1) fracture dislocation (if obviously deformed, do not waste time waiting for an X-ray, just reduce it immediately), (2) talar shift, and (3) syndesmotic rupture which all add to instability and more complex surgery. Surgery is governed by Muller's rule of 6: either operate within 6 hours or after 6 days to avoid swelling, in which case elevate on a Braun frame with ice compression and wait. Ankle ORIF is followed by 6 weeks of non-weight-bearing in plaster and VTE prophylaxis.

Shoulder dislocation

Usually occurs after high-energy trauma where most are anterior dislocation (>90%) > posterior (5%) > inferior (luxatio erecta <1%). Always check for axillary nerve function by checking the regimental patch. Reduce and re-X-ray. Patients aged <30 years have >90% dislocation rate and those aged >30 years have <10%. Initial management requires rest (polysling), physiotherapy, and ruling out rotator cuff injury. Recurrent dislocation requires arthroscopic stabilization.

Hot, swollen joint

This is septic arthritis until proven otherwise, as if missed will → avoidable problems including septicaemia and hastened OA. Septic arthritis (pus in the joint due to infection) rapidly → destruction of the articular cartilage and the joint itself. Causes are numerous, including:

- exacerbation of gout
- pseudogout
- OA
- RA
- psoriatic arthritis.

Must exclude infection and gout using blood markers including WCC, ESR, CRP, and urate. Do a joint aspirate (arthrocentesis) for urgent MC&S and crystallography (gout/pseudogout). Always X-ray to look for erosive changes in septic, autoimmune, and gouty changes. Treat according to cause (proven septic arthritis requires antibiotics and washout in theatre). Do not start antibiotics blindly without sampling synovial fluid and blood cultures for MC&S for Gram-staining (only takes hours and can better guide specific antibiotic therapy).

Limping child

This is a worrying presentation. Causes depend to some extent on age and include trauma, infection (septic arthritis, osteomyelitis), Perthes disease (idiopathic osteonecrosis of the femoral head, 5–10 years), SUFE (epiphysis slips through the growth plate in 10–15 years, half of which are obese), and transient synovitis.

Wrist (distal radius) fracture

This is usually a low-energy injury in an osteoporotic, elderly patient. They are also very common in children. Some eponymous names you may hear include:

- Colles' fracture
- Smith's fracture
- Barton's fracture.

Intra-articular fractures have a greater risk of being unstable, thus are likelier to require surgery. But there terms are fortunately largely obsolete. They can be immobilized in a cast, but unstable fractures require surgery (manipulation under anaesthesia → K-wires → ORIF with plates and screws).

Honours

- Gout and pseudogout crystals look different under polarized light: gout is needle-shaped and strongly negative birefringent; pseudogout is rhomboid-shaped and weakly positive birefringent.
- Damage control surgery (DTS) works on the principle that the primary insult (the injury) exerts metabolic damage which is worsened by prolonged complex surgery (secondary insult), → death (via (1) coagulopathy, (2) hypothermia and (3) metabolic acidosis). DTS aims to stabilize the patient quickly with minimal additional insult, with the plan for further surgery when the patient is systemically stable. The alternative is early total care (ETC) where definitive surgery (often taking significant time) has become obsolete.

Trauma and orthopaedic surgery: in exams

Clinical orthopaedic examinations are more difficult than those of other specialties as there is no single routine and lots of body parts! We urge you to ask a friendly registrar/consultant to show you how to examine a hip, knee, hand, shoulder, spine, and ankle/foot.

The good news is that all orthopaedic exams are a variation on *look, feel, move, special tests*, and *imaging* (see ➔ 'Orthopaedic examinations: general' pp. 941–3). Remember, you have two limbs so you should always examine the normal side before the abnormal/painful side. You should also always offer to examine the joint above and below.

Like other specialties, you are unlikely to see emergency cases (e.g. fractured NOF, dislocations, septic arthritis). The most common cases are:
- knee/hip OA or arthroplasty postoperatively
- joint arthroscopy postoperatively
- arthritic hand
- shoulder impingement (in an actor).

Beware postoperative patients (of which there are many) with minimal scarring. It is common for candidates to be presented with a 'normal' knee; the majority will miss small arthroscopic port scars on the sides. When you look this is not just for show, it is important that you really look!

Also remember to look around the room for sticks, crutches, braces, etc. Ask the patient to remove their shoes and look at the soles for abnormal wear, and inside the shoes for insoles. These adjuncts will give you a clue as to what is wrong with the patient! Also remember that for lower limb joint examinations, stand the patient up and observe their stance and gait. This will allow you to thoroughly inspect all around and the back of the limb for any muscle wasting, scars, or deformities.

It is likely that you will be asked to comment on radiographs after the examination. Commonly this will be knee or hip OA (so know your radiographic features). Occasionally it may be a fracture (practise describing a fracture). Learn what THR, total knee replacement, DHS, hip hemiarthroplasty, plate-and-screws, and K-wires look like on X-ray.

Top tips

Orthopaedic jargon
- *Arthro*: joint.
- *Arthrocentesis*: joint aspiration.
- *Arthroscopy*: looking into the joint.
- *Arthroplasty*: joint reconstruction/replacement (± implant/cement).
- *Arthrodesis*: surgical fusion of the joint to immobilize.
- *Arthrography*: joint imaging ± contrast (usually radiological).

Vascular surgery

Vascular surgery: overview

Vascular surgery is the surgical specialty that deals with diseases of the arterial, venous, and lymphatic systems.

Cases to see

Critical limb ischaemia

Most patients on the vascular ward will have peripheral vascular disease with rest pain and/or tissue loss (ulceration, toe gangrene, etc.).

Intermittent claudication

You might catch these patients in hospital having investigations (e.g. angiography) but will have to work around lots of other processes (consent, blood tests, etc.)

Varicose veins

Ligation, sclerotherapy, and ablation usually performed as day cases so you could need to catch these patients in clinic or at day surgery unit.

Foot ulcers

Spend a day in the diabetic foot clinic if you want to see many in one place. Try to see examples of arterial, venous, and neuropathic ulcers as well as clean, healing, and infected cases.

Abdominal aortic aneurysms (AAAs)

Large palpable AAAs are likely to be fixed quickly and ruptured aneurysms are few and far between. You must use your vascular rotation to feel AAAs as students often struggle to distinguish 'pulsatile' from 'expansile'.

Acute limb ischaemia

Unpredictable and requiring swift intervention so may be missed during a short placement.

Procedures to see

Duplex ultrasound scanning

Look for the vascular lab or radiology department to observe duplex US scan of the lower limb arterial, venous, and carotid systems.

Angiography and angioplasty

Operations

Lower limb arterial bypass, AAA repair (open and endovascular), major lower limb amputation (e.g. below-knee amputation), carotid endarterectomy, and operative management of varicose veins (e.g. sclerotherapy, laser ablation). Carotid endarterectomy provides a rare opportunity to appreciate neck anatomy.

Things to do

Master the use of a hand-held Doppler and perform an ankle–brachial pressure index (ABPI).

Vascular surgery: in clinic

Abdominal aortic aneurysm

An aneurysm is an abnormal permanent dilatation of a blood vessel by >50% of its normal diameter. The most common aneurysm is of the infra-renal (below the renal arteries) abdominal aorta. Aortas are considered aneurysmal once they reach a diameter of 3 cm and most are detected by the NHS AAA Screening Programme (single US scan for all males from age 65). They may also be found incidentally, e.g. on clinical examination or when patients are scanned for other conditions. Mortality associated with ruptured AAA is >50%. Aetiology is poorly understood but may be related to atherosclerotic disease so risk factors are cardiovascular (e.g. hypertension, diabetes, male, age, smoking). Small aneurysms (<5.5 cm) are followed up by annual US surveillance. Large aneurysms are repaired electively as the risk of operation usually outweighs rupture at 5.5 cm. Repair is by open or endovascular techniques. Associated with this are femoral and popliteal aneurysms.

Honours

UK Small Aneurysms Trial (UKSAT)

The UKSAT was a multicentre, randomized controlled trial of two management strategies for AAAs: 'early elective open surgery' and 'regular US surveillance'. The study included 1100 patients and showed that small AAAs (<5.5 cm) can be monitored safely with US scanning without any ↑ in mortality. Indications for electively repairing AAAs are now often stated as >5.5 cm, growing >1 cm/year, or becoming tender.

Intermittent claudication

Is a cramping pain in the muscle that occurs during exercise and is relieved by rest. Smoking is the biggest modifiable risk factor, claudication distance and rest period correlate with degree of arterial insufficiency and collateral supply respectively. The differential is spinal claudication (associated back pain, claudication relieved on leaning forward). Also needs distinguishing from critical limb ischaemia—arterial insufficiency with rest pain (e.g. at night when legs elevated) and/or tissue loss (e.g. ulceration) which needs prompt intervention. Most patients are managed conservatively: stop smoking, control modifiable CVD risk factors, walk through claudication distance, and primary prevention for CVD (aspirin and statin). Other interventions are to improve quality of life or for critical limb ischaemia (e.g. angioplasty, bypass, amputation).

Honours

Classification of arterial disease

One traditional method for classifying PVD was proposed in 1954 by Rene Fontaine. The key thing is that PVD is a spectrum of disease severity which may be progressive, hence 'staging'. Fontaine's classification:

- Stage I: asymptomatic, incomplete blood vessel obstruction.
- Stage II: mild claudication pain in limb.
- Stage III: rest pain, mostly in the feet.
- Stage IV: necrosis and/or gangrene of the limb.

Varicose veins

Are dilated and tortuous veins of the superficial venous system (e.g. great and lesser saphenous veins). Secondary varicose veins may be caused by DVT and the three Ps (pelvic mass, pregnancy, previous history). These are unsightly but symptoms include **AEIOU**:

- Aching
- Eczema
- Itching
- Oedema
- Ulceration/ugly.

Compression stockings followed by invasive options if unsuccessful: ligation/stripping, sclerotherapy, radiofrequency, or laser ablations.

Lower limb ulceration

An ulcer is a break in the skin or mucous membrane that fails to heal. The textbooks tell us these are arterial, venous, or neuropathic, although in practice most are mixed.

Venous ulcers

Caused by venous insufficiency (haemosiderin deposition → skin breakdown and eczema → chronic ulceration) and managed by elevation and four-layer compression bandages. Venous ulcers often have an arterial component in which case four-layer bandaging may be contraindicated as risks worsening arterial disease.

Arterial ulcers

Caused by chronically inadequate blood supply (e.g. PVD → skin breakdown without healing → ulcer. Treatment to optimize blood flow (e.g. angioplasty, bypass).

Neuropathic ulcers

Caused by loss of peripheral sensation and microtrauma. The most common type is the diabetic ulcer, which also frequently has an arterial component of poorly understood aetiology. Other causes are those of peripheral neuropathy. These are managed by a MDT (e.g. tight glycaemic control, chiropody, orthotic devices).

Carotid artery stenosis

Is caused by atherosclerosis. The problem is plaque embolization (e.g. causing TIA and/or stroke) rather than occlusion of the vessel itself as there is usually an adequate collateral supply through the circle of Willis. Patients at high risk of CVA (e.g. significant stenosis and evidence of embolization) may benefit from carotid endarterectomy.

> ### Honours
> *Primary prevention of cardiovascular disease*
> Primary prevention describes measures to avoid disease in patients thought to be at ↑risk. This is different to secondary prevention, e.g. treatment to avoid recurring coronary disease in a patient following acute MI. Patients with PVD (e.g. intermittent claudication) also probably have coronary and/or cerebrovascular disease. They may therefore be treated with strict risk factor management (smoking cessation and BP/glucose/cholesterol control). Most benefit from a statin and aspirin.

Critical limb ischaemia

Lies on a spectrum of intermittent claudication. It is defined as inadequate arterial supply that threatens limb viability. Key red flags are rest pain, night pain, and tissue loss (e.g. ulceration, gangrene). These patients require urgent investigation and/or revascularization. It is distinct from acute limb ischaemia in that it often represents the slow deterioration of PVD rather than an acute event disrupting arterial supply (e.g. thrombosis, embolus).

Investigations

Duplex US scanning
Allows simultaneous visualization of tissue architecture and flow which are overlaid onto a single image. It is non-invasive, safe, and relatively cheap but operator dependent, not therapeutic and can be limited by bowel gas, calcifications, and body habitus.

Angiogram
Imaging technique using injected radio-opaque contrast agent (e.g. femoral artery) and X-ray imaging techniques such as fluoroscopy. The words angiogram and arteriogram are often used interchangeably, but technically refer to arterial imaging as opposed to the venous system (venogram). It can be therapeutic (e.g. angioplasty, stenting) as well as diagnostic. Disadvantages includes contrast allergy, nephrotoxicity, and complications of arterial puncture (e.g. bleeding, pseudo-aneurysm, limb loss).

CT and MR angiography
Non-invasive angiograms providing detailed imaging of the arterial system, although it is not possible to intervene and risks of contrast remain.

Vascular surgery: in the emergency department

Leaking AAA

Present as abdominal/back/loin–groin pain. Patient may be very well/ stable initially. Requires high index of suspicion; often misdiagnosed as renal colic. All older (>55 years old) patients with pain should have active consideration of AAA ± US scan. The commonest presentation is collapse with hypovolaemic shock, and massive transfusion requirements. US can measure the aortic diameter (is there an aneurysm?) but bleeding is better identified by CT angiogram. CT should not delay transfer of an unstable patient to theatre, as only definitive haemorrhage control will save the patient (giving blood is supportive but ultimately need to turn off the tap). Management is as per elective aneurysms (open or endovascular aneurysm repair (EVAR)) or palliation may be appropriate.

Honours

IV resuscitation

One approach to the bleeding and compromised patient is fluid resuscitation. This is a matter for discussion, however most leaking aneurysms cause bleeding into the retroperitoneum which tamponades the haematoma. Raising the systolic BP with excessive fluid resuscitation could rupture this haematoma and cause intra-abdominal bleeding with consequent circulatory collapse. Hence, maintain the systolic BP ≤100 mmHg but ensure the patient remains conscious—a concept known as '*permissive hypotension*'.

Acute limb ischaemia

Main causes are thrombosis (e.g. of a popliteal aneurysm), (embolism, e.g. commonly intracardiac due to AF), and trauma (e.g. arterial transection). Presents as 6 'P's:

- Pain
- Paraesthesia
- Paralysis (late sign)
- Pallor
- Pulseless
- Perishingly cold (poikilothermia)

Investigations include duplex US and angiography to identify the lesion site. An acutely ischaemic limb needs to be revascularized within 4–6 hours to avoid amputation. Possible interventions include thrombolysis through an indwelling arterial catheter as an infusion, embolectomy, and bypass. An insensate, paralysed limb with fixed mottling is very unlikely to be rescued and probably requires amputation. Revascularization of a necrotic limb releases a deadly concoction of metabolites into the systemic circulation (SIRS, myoglobinuric AKI, death).

Vascular surgery: in theatre

The principles of operative vascular surgery are to gain proximal and distal control of the relevant vessel (e.g. using clamps or small rubber bands called 'sloops') before investigating the site of injury.

Open AAA repair

Most AAAs are infrarenal (70%) which means they lie entirely below the origin of the renal arteries. Supra- and juxtarenal aneurysms are more complicated. The procedure involves laparotomy, clamping the aorta proximally, excision of the diseased vessel, and suturing in a graft (usually made of a polyester called Dacron®) prior to removing the clamp. As with any laparotomy, recall layers of the abdominal wall before you are asked. You may be asked to identify a large vessel running anterior to the aorta—this is probably the renal vein, which is sometimes sacrificed to gain better access. (See Fig. 41.1 for anatomy.) Mortality rate of elective open AAA repair is 5%. Risks of cross-clamping above the renal arteries include renal and gut underperfusion so try not to disturb the surgeon once the clamp is applied as they will want to proceed swiftly with minimal interruptions. Other complications are those of any laparotomy. Open repair of a ruptured AAA is more urgent and it is best not to interrupt the surgeon at any time if you happen to encounter one of these. It is often impossible to close the abdomen without risk of abdominal compartment syndrome and the abdomen may therefore be left 'open'. A potential long-term complication of any open AAA repair is an aorto-enteric fistula (→ small 'herald' rectal bleed preceding massive GI haemorrhage), which is rare in practice but common in exams.

Honours

Physiology of cross-clamping the aorta
You will hopefully notice the surgeon warning the anaesthetist before placing a cross-clamp across the aorta. This is because the clamp leads to ↑afterload to raise arterial pressure with consequent potential for heart failure and myocardial ischaemia.

Endovascular aneurysm repair

EVAR may be performed by an interventional radiologist, specially trained vascular surgeon, or both. A guide wire is passed (usually through the femoral artery) under fluoroscopic (X-ray) guidance, and placed above the aneurysm in the aorta. A stent is deployed over the guide wire to exclude the aneurysm sac from the circulation. Juxtarenal aneurysms are often repaired using a fenestrated stent, i.e. with holes to accommodate branches of the aorta. Fluoroscopic images 'light up' the aorta and its branches. Unsuspecting students may well be asked at this point to identify major branches so learn them (plus vertebral levels at which they emerge from the aorta) beforehand. Specific complications are related to contrast (e.g. nephrotoxicity), the stent itself (e.g. infection, migration), occlusion of aortic branches (gut, kidneys, and spinal cord at risk), and groin puncture. An endoleak describes blood refilling the aneurysm sac due to a 'leak' around the stent—there are multiple types (e.g. depending on whether the leak is proximal, distal, or due to back-filling from small vessels). This can be an early or a late complication. Elective mortality of EVAR is around 1%, although the scale of long-term complications (e.g. stent migration) is not yet known and these patients require regular imaging surveillance. Some patients are technically unsuitable for EVAR, e.g. small tortuous iliac artery.

Carotid endarterectomy

The neck is dissected (you might be asked about platysma—a large superficial subcutaneous muscle) and the arteries exposed. Know the contents of the carotid sheath (common carotid, internal jugular, vagus) and relative location of key structures before getting too close to a surgeon performing this operation. The external carotid is identified by its first branch (superior thyroid artery), the internal carotid having no branches outside the skull. The artery is controlled proximally and distally (e.g. with clamps or sloops), opened, and the intimal layer with associated atherosclerotic plaque removed. The artery is then repaired, e.g. with a vein patch which prevents stricture formation if the artery was closed primarily. Sometimes a shunt (temporary tube) is used to temporarily bypass the operative site. Complications include cranial nerve damage (VII, XII, and X at risk), stroke, haematoma, and hyper-perfusion syndrome.

Honours
Indications for carotid endarterectomy
Carotid endarterectomy (surgical excision of plaque from the carotid artery) is performed to prevent embolization cranially which can cause disabling stroke. There is a <5% risk of death or disabling stroke perioperatively and so the procedure must be balanced carefully against its potential benefits. Commonly accepted indications include:
- symptomatic patients with >70% stenosis
- symptomatic patients with 50–69% stenosis—marginal benefit
- asymptomatic patients with >60% stenosis—marginal benefit.

Arterial bypass

'Bypass' is a method of re-plumbing vessels so blood proceeds past an obstruction. Every bypass requires an inflow, conduit, and an outflow. Inflow describes adequate blood supply proximally, the conduit may be vein (e.g. great saphenous vein) or synthetic (e.g. PTFE), and the outflow describes distal '*run-off*': vessel patency distal to the occlusion. Bypasses are described by their origin (anatomical vs extra-anatomical) and insertion (e.g. femoral–popliteal, axillary–femoral). Complications are of the graft (e.g. thrombosis, infection) and '*steal*' phenomenon in which a limb is deprived of blood which has been diverted elsewhere (e.g. to the other leg).

To ask the boss
Choice of vein or prosthetic graft
Possible factors might include the presence of a suitable vein, projected bypass length, infection risk, and likelihood of thrombosis/reocclusion). In some patients, the decision might be obvious (e.g. great saphenous vein previously harvested for CABG) but in others less so.

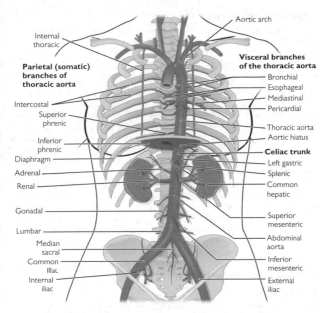

Fig. 41.1 Abdominal aorta anatomy. Reproduced from *Anatomy & Physiology*, Connexions Web site. http://cnx.org/content/col11496/1.6/, Jun 19, 2013. under the Creative Commons Attribution 3.0 Unported license.

Embolectomy

The artery (e.g. brachial or femoral) is dissected, the surgeon gains proximal and distal control, a small cut is made in the artery, and a Fogarty catheter is passed along the vessel. A small balloon at the end of the catheter is inflated with water and withdrawn to remove the embolus. Complications include intimal lesions (causing thrombosis), cholesterol emboli, and those related to arterial puncture.

Trivia

The Fogarty catheter

Dr Thomas J. Fogarty (b. 1934) watched lots of operations before going to medical school and was concerned that the amputation rate for patients with acutely ischaemic limbs due to embolus was >50%. At this time, a large part of the artery had to be cut out and the embolus removed with forceps. Fogarty tied a piece of glove to the end of a urethral catheter and proposed that it could be used to scoop out the embolus. No one accepted this idea until he went to medical school, trained as a cardiovascular surgeon, and proved the concept on his own patients. The Fogarty catheter is now used worldwide 300,000 times per year and is thought to have saved 15 million patients from death and/or amputation.

Major limb amputation

Amputation describes removal of a body extremity. Its indications are sometimes described as either:

• 'dead limb' (e.g. ischaemic necrosis)
• 'deadly limb' (e.g. malignancy, life-threatening infection)
• 'dead loss' (e.g. paralysed limb hampering function).

Major lower limb amputations are described anatomically (e.g. below knee, through knee, above knee, hindquarter). The knee is preserved if possible as it functions as a useful lever even when little is left distally. Prosthetic fitting is also something to consider. However, this must be balanced against the need for adequate stump healing (significant proximal vascular lesion → unlikely adequate supply to heal below-knee amputation stump).

Significant complications include those related to the wound (e.g. infection, dehiscence) and stump (e.g. phantom pain, need for revision). Most patients require prolonged rehabilitation and are assessed for suitability to receive a prosthetic limb. Try to see a major amputation if possible—it is an important operation and a great opportunity to revise lower limb anatomy. Although they may be performed by other specialties (e.g. orthopaedic surgery), the vascular surgeons do more than anyone else. You are likely to be asked about the four compartments of the lower limb (anterior, lateral, posterior superficial, posterior deep) and their contents so look these up beforehand. When asked to identify structures, start by recalling the level of the amputation (e.g. no popliteal artery in a below-knee amputation).

Angiography

This term describes injection of dye into an artery (e.g. coronary angiography). In the vascular setting, angiography is often of arteries in the lower limb. A radio-opaque dye is injected through a catheter in the femoral artery and X-ray technology used to visualize arterial flow. It can be diagnostic (e.g. showing occlusions) and/or therapeutic (e.g. stent insertion) in which case it may be called angioplasty. Complications are due to the dye (e.g. nephrotoxicity, anaphylaxis), arterial puncture (e.g. arterial rupture, pseudoaneurysm), and distal embolization of thrombus.

Angiography is usually performed in a specialist angiography suite, possibly signposted as 'fluoroscopy', rather than in theatres. It is usually performed by an interventional radiologist rather than a surgeon. Interventional radiologists are usually approachable and enthusiastic about teaching as they are rarely assigned their own medical students. The best place to find them is at the end of the vascular MDT meeting—going direct to fluoroscopy risks catching them mid procedure.

Vascular surgery: in exams

During your vascular placement, ensure that you can perform and elicit the procedures and signs in this section.

History station

The most common vascular history will be intermittent claudication because this beautifully tests all elements of the standard history structure. A patient or actor will give a history of leg pain on exercise and you will doubtless draw out the following features within a few minutes of effective history taking. Practise this history on real patients before the exam—vascular wards are full of cheerful older men awaiting angioplasty/bypass/amputation who are otherwise bored and keen to aid learning.

History of presenting complaint (HPC)

SOCRATES pain history. In 'site', which leg is worst? In 'onset', ask about claudication distance (short distance claudicants, e.g. 10 m, have worse arterial disease). In 'symptoms', ask about vascular red flags: rest pain, night pain, and tissue loss. Although tissue loss is usually something you would find on examination, play safe in a history station and ask 'Have you noticed any breaks in the skin of your feet?' Do not leave the exam room without asking explicitly about these features.

Past medical history (PMHx)

Ask generally, 'Do you have any medical conditions?', then demonstrate your understanding of PVD by asking specifically about risk factors (hypertension, high cholesterol), consequences (MI, stroke), and complicating factors (diabetes).

Family history (FHx)

Assessment of risk so specifically MI and stroke with ages (first-degree relative MI at 40 years is a greater risk than at 90 years).

Drug history (DHx)

Ask generally, 'Do you take any medications, and have any allergies?', then ask specifically: statin, aspirin, clopidogrel?

Social history (SHx)

Smoking (including pack-years and 'Have you ever smoked?'), alcohol, and impact on life ('How do you get around normally? What stops you from walking further? What do these symptoms stop you doing?'). These last questions are not tick-box exercises in PVD: revascularization will not cure chronic heart failure or if SOB on exertion/painful knees are the main restrictions to mobility. Disabling PVD warrants aggressive intervention. One other possibility (although less likely) is a history of TIAs in a patient with carotid disease. Ask about amaurosis fugax, limb weakness, and time to resolution of symptoms. Ask about AF (and any associated treatment) in PMHx.

Examination

Vascular cases are common in surgical exams because they are chronic, often stable, and effectively test your ability to elicit clinical signs. The most common cases are:

Peripheral vascular disease

Many patients with PVD will have a full constellation of vascular signs (e.g. cool foot with prolonged capillary refill and absent pulses) so the best students will trot out a full list (assuming all signs are present!) when summarizing their findings.

Chronic venous disease

There are many patients with chronic venous disease and they can be recognized by their legs which are said to be shaped like an 'inverted champagne bottle'. Create a script for describing these characteristic legs as above for chronic arterial disease, e.g. 'both legs exhibit thickened shiny skin with brown discoloration which is consistent with long-standing chronic venous insufficiency. There is no evidence of cellulitis, ulceration, or varicose eczema'. If asked to examine such a patient, do not be fooled into thinking that there is a separate venous disease exam. Carefully inspect and assess the arterial system (including sensation etc.) as well as noting features of chronic venous disease.

Varicose veins

This case tends to make students uncomfortable as there is a huge 'inspection' element which students often race through so they have time for the complex (but probably less important) clinical tests. It is nothing more than gambling to go into a surgical exam without having performed the tourniquet test on a real patient with varicose veins. Although this is not commonly used in practice, ask a doctor in the veins clinic to show you if textbook descriptions are unhelpful. YouTube and online videos may also be instructive.

Things you should practise beforehand

Feeling peripheral pulses

These are palpable when a good arterial supply crosses an underlying non-compressible structure, e.g. pressing the radial artery against the radius. It should not take >20 sec to grip both hands (temperature), inspect them carefully (colour, ulceration), then palpate the distal pulses:

- *Radial*: lateral aspect of the distal wrist on the volar aspect.
- *Ulnar*: medial aspect of the distal wrist on the volar aspect.
- *Brachial*: medial to the biceps tendon in the antecubital fossa. Ask the patient to flex their elbow while feeling in the antecubital fossa for the biceps tendon which becomes taut.
- *Carotid pulse*: is palpated between the trachea and sternocleidomastoid. It is a vital landmark in cardiac arrests and you will need to be fairly confident about its presence (to certify death).
- *Abdominal aorta*: ends at L4 which is identified by palpating the iliac crests and is approximately at the umbilicus in slim people. An aneurysm should feel like an expansile mass on the abdomen.
- *Femoral*: mid-inguinal point—halfway between ASIS and pubic symphysis (not to be confused with midpoint of the inguinal ligament).
- *Popliteal*: flex knee to 90° and feel behind deeply with your finger pulps. It is often impalpable so do not be surprised if it is absent.

- *Posterior tibial*: Pimenta's point—halfway between medial malleolus and insertion of Achilles tendon. Alternatively 2 cm 'below and behind' the medial malleolus.
- *Dorsalis pedis*: lateral to extensor hallucis longus (EHL). Ask the patient to point their toe towards their head in dorsiflexion to bowstring the tendon. Follow on the lateral side of EHL until you find bone where the pulse should be present. Absent in 2–3%!

Use the hand-held Doppler US probe

Common pitfalls include insufficient gel but there is a definite technique to angling the probe appropriately to detect flow. Three waveforms (triphasic) relate to arterial wall expansion/contraction: three 'whooshes' = normal, two = stenosed, and monophasic = severe stenosis. You are more likely to have to use this as part of measuring ABPI.

Ankle–brachial pressure index

ABPI is a ratio calculated by systolic BP leg/systolic BP in arm. A BP cuff is applied to the arm, Doppler probe applied to the brachial artery, and the cuff inflated until the signal disappears, which signifies the systolic BP. The same process is repeated at the ankle with the cuff around the calf, measuring both the anterior tibial and posterior tibial. The best score at the leg is used. Beware diabetics with calcified arteries who may have abnormally high ABPIs.
- 0.9–1.2: normal
- 0.5–0.9: claudicant
- ≤0.4: critical ischaemia.

Berger's test

This is a test/sign seen in patients with severe lower limb arterial disease. The patient lies supine and one leg is raised. In the presence of arterial insufficiency, the leg may become white at an angle known as 'Berger's angle'. The white leg is then swung over the side of the bed in which case it may become dark red/purple (anaerobic metabolites → vasodilatation → hyperperfusion)—a positive 'Berger's sign'.

Tourniquet/Trendelenburg test

These are two very similar tests, both of which are used to determine the level of venous incompetence. With the patient supine, lift the leg and milk the varicose vein proximally—back hand along the path of the vein. Once the leg is raised and the vein 'milked', place two fingers over the saphenofemoral junction (SFJ) in the Trendelenburg test or apply a tourniquet at this level in the tourniquet test. The SFJ lies 4 cm lateral and inferior to the pubic tubercle. Once the SFJ is occluded, ask the patient to stand and observe for refilling of the varicose vein. If the incompetence is limited to the SFJ, varicosities will not reappear. If they return, then repositioning the tourniquet sequentially along the lower limb (mid thigh, above knee, and below knee) will help identify the level of the incompetence.

Upper gastrointestinal and hepatopancreatobiliary surgery

Upper gastrointestinal (UGI) surgery: overview

UGI surgery specializes in conditions of the oesophagus, stomach, gall bladder, biliary system, and duodenum. Surgical management of splenic conditions often falls within the remit of a UGI surgeon. UGI surgical oncology, bariatric surgery, and some oesophagogastric surgery are centralized to specialist hospitals. There is some overlap with hepatopancreatobiliary (HPB) surgery.

Places to be

Emergency department

Many conditions associated with UGI will present via the ED. Take initiative and clerk patients and present them to the on-call SHO/specialist registrar.

Radiology

This is a high-yield activity, particularly in consolidating your anatomy learning with diagnostic radiology. As with HPB surgery, interventional radiology plays a role in managing patients including procedures such as percutaneous transhepatic cholangiography (PTC), image-guided aspiration/drain insertion, oesophageal stenting, radiologically inserted gastrostomy insertion, and fluoroscopy studies.

Wards

There are lots of drains and tubes—observe where they placed on the patient and look at what they are producing and how much. You will also learn about perioperative care and complications that can arise from surgery.

Endoscopy

This is performed by gastroenterologists and some general surgeons. They have both diagnostic and therapeutic value and many UGI patients will have these procedures performed on them.

Theatre

This is an exciting and often very rewarding place to spend time. Theatre activity includes emergency cases (CEPOD theatre, named after the Confidential Enquiry into Perioperative Deaths), day surgery, and elective operating lists. Be enthusiastic and you will be able to scrub and assist in cases. Read up on the patients prior to the operation and anticipate questions the seniors may ask you about the case (e.g. essential anatomical questions).

ITU

Surgical patients constitute some of the sickest patients in the hospital and often need to be managed in critical care. This is a great place to relearn your physiology and link it to clinical care.

UGI surgery: multidisciplinary teams

UGI cancer MDTs will be useful in gaining exposure to cases of oesophageal and gastric malignancy. It is also a useful place to bring together your basic science (anatomy, pathology, tumour biology) and clinical science (GI, radiology, oncology, surgery).

Procedures to see

Radiology

Transabdominal ultrasound

Non-invasive, safe, and is particularly useful for evaluating liver, gall bladder, and biliary pathology.

Fluoroscopic contrast studies

This is a form of continuous X-ray imaging method to produce a live and dynamic study. Combined with an oral contrast agent such as barium, this can be used to investigate (1) oesophageal motility disorders (e.g. 'birds beak' sign in achalasia), (2) anatomical disorders (e.g. pharyngeal pouch), (3) hiatus hernia, (4) if a surgical anastomosis is leaking, or (5) where OGD is contraindicated.

Endoscopy

Oesophagogastroduodenoscopy

OGD allows direct luminal visualization of the oesophagus, stomach, and duodenum. This confers great diagnostic value and can also be used to provide biopsies and minor interventions. This is a great learning opportunity to build your anatomical understanding of the UGI tract and observe pathologies.

Endoscopic retrograde cholangiopancreatography (ERCP)

(See ⊃ p. 330.)

Endoscopic ultrasound (EUS)

GI physiology

Oesophageal manometry

This involves a transnasal insertion of a manometric catheter into the oesophagus to detect pressures within the lumen. This is the gold standard test in detecting motility disorders of the oesophagus including achalasia and oesophageal spasm. Occasionally used in assessing GORD.

pH monitoring

This is usually performed in patients being considered for antireflux surgery, confirming the presence of GORD and avoiding operations on patients with functional heartburn. A transnasal catheter with a pH sensor is inserted above the lower oesophageal sphincter (5 cm above, position confirmed with manometric measurements).

UGI surgery: oesophageal disease

Key anatomy: oesophagus
- Upper oesophageal sphincter: cricopharyngeus.
- Lower oesophageal sphincter: functional zone of higher pressure above gastro-oesophageal sphincter.
- Upper two-thirds: stratified squamous epithelium. Striated muscle fibres.
- Lower one-third: transition to columnar epithelium.

Oesophageal dysmotility
Pathological contraction or malcoordination of the oesophagus can result in conditions such as achalasia or oesophageal spasm.

Achalasia
Results in loss of inhibitory neurons required for lower oesophageal sphincter (LOS) relaxation and peristalsis of the oesophagus. The LOS fails to relax and the peristalsis of the oesophagus becomes disorganized.

Symptoms
Usually include gradual-onset dysphagia which initially is worse for fluids than solids. Regurgitation, chest pain, heartburn, and weight loss can occur.

Investigations
Manometry is the gold standard for diagnosis and will demonstrate lack of coordination of peristalsis and a high integrated relaxation pressure. Barium swallow fluoroscopy classically shows smooth distal tapering with the 'bird's beak' sign.

Management
Can be treated endoscopically with balloon dilatation. Botulinum toxin injections have also been used in selected patients. Myotomy is the most definitive procedure with a success rate of 95%, and 85% of patients remaining symptom free at 5 years. Heller's procedure is a type of myotomy, and may be combined with antireflux procedures to prevent reflux post myotomy.

Honours
Chicago classification of achalasia
- Type 1 (classic): minimal oesophageal pressurization.
- Type 2: achalasia with oesophageal compression, pan-oesophageal pressurization.
- Type 3: premature spastic contractions or preserved fragments of distal peristalsis.

Oesophageal cancer

New onset of dysphagia must prompt you to think of a tumour as an important differential diagnosis, particularly in those patients aged >45 years. Can present with dysphagia to solids followed by liquids. Presentations with true dysphagia, ~25% have oesophageal cancer.

Presentations

Dysphagia, ongoing reflux, regurgitation, odynophagia (painful swallowing), hoarse voice from recurrent laryngeal nerve invasion, cervical lymphadenopathy, cough, and haemoptysis and other systemic features such as weight loss, anorexia, and anaemia.

Types and risk factors

Adenocarcinoma and squamous carcinoma. Adenocarcinomas are increasing in the Western population and may be associated with GORD, Barrett's oesophagus, and obesity. Most commonly affects the lower third of the oesophagus. Squamous carcinoma has a higher incidence in Japan and northern China. This can occur throughout the oesophagus and is associated with smoking, high alcohol intake, and diet low in fruit and vegetables.

Diagnosis

OGD and biopsy with histopathological examination.

Management

Most patients at time of presentation have incurable disease and treatment will be focused on palliative measures. Dysphagia from structuring or obstruction of the oesophagus may be treated with endoscopic luminal stents. Surgery with curative intent may involve neoadjuvant chemoradiotherapy and radical resection. Surgical approaches to removing oesophageal tumour include laparotomy plus right lateral thoracotomy (Ivor Lewis oesophagectomy), left thoracoabdominal oesophagectomy, and the transhiatal approach.

Key revision: Barrett's oesophagus

- Oesophageal metaplasia: normal squamous epithelium in oesophageal mucosa replaced with columnar epithelium.
- Pre-cursor to oesophageal adenocarcinoma.

Pharyngeal pouch

Also known as a Zenker's diverticulum, this is an acquired diverticulum between the inferior constrictor and cricopharyngeus muscle (known as '*Killians dehiscence*'). This mostly occurs in the elderly and can present with an intermittent lump appearing in the neck on swallowing (usually deviated to one side), regurgitation of undigested food, halitosis, cervical dysphagia, chronic cough, and aspiration. Diagnosis can be made clinically or with barium swallow fluoroscopy, which will show contrast filling in the pouch. Treatment can include an endoscopic or external open approach.

UGI surgery: gastric

Hiatus hernia

The presence of hiatus hernia is common and is usually asymptomatic. It affects females proportionally more than males. By definition, this involves protrusion of the stomach into the thoracic cavity and is associated with a widening or weakness of the diaphragmatic crura. It can be classified as (1) *sliding* (commonest), (2) *rolling* (aka paraoesophageal), or (3) *mixed* (when both coexist).

Symptoms

Reflux, dysphagia, vomiting, post-prandial fullness, substernal pain, and dyspnoea if a large hernia is present.

Diagnosis

Plain X-ray, OGD, barium swallow tests, or on CT imaging.

Management

Reducing precipitating factors (smoking, obesity, alcohol, caffeine) and reducing acid secretion with PPIs. Indications for surgical treatment include failure of symptom control with maximal medical therapy, complications associated with hiatus hernia (e.g. gastric volvulus), and GORD associated with hiatus hernia. Surgical management reduces the herniating stomach/contents back through the hiatus and fixing the stomach to prevent migration (gastropexy). Hiatus hernia surgery is usually combined with antireflux procedures.

Gastro-oesophageal reflux disease

Affects up to 40% of the population.

Presentation

Heartburn (retrosternal burning), regurgitation, waterbrash, or dyspepsia. May also present as chest pain, epigastric pain, cough, odynophagia, and a hoarse voice. Symptoms are often worse after eating or when lying down. It is important to learn how GORD presents, not just because it is very common but there are a wide range of differential diagnoses (including ones never to be missed—cancer, MI, aortic aneurysm). Pathological consequences include oesophagitis (inflammatory changes in squamous lines oesophageal lumen), stricturing, and Barrett's oesophagus.

Pathology

When protective mechanisms are lost, GORD can develop consequently. The mechanisms that normally prevent acid reflux are:
- the LOS
- the flap valve—formed by a fold of gastric mucosa that serves to occlude the oesophageal lumen
- the angle of His (acute angle between cardia at entrance of stomach and oesophagus)
- an intra-abdominal length of oesophagus
- relatively elevated intra-abdominal pressure surrounding the abdominal segment of oesophagus.

Investigations

Further investigations may be performed if there are concerns around complications, non-response to treatment, diagnostic uncertainty, or if the patient is being considered for antireflux surgery. Reflux can be confirmed by continuous 24-hour pH monitoring. Changes in pH need to correspond to symptom episodes. An OGD may be performed to exclude malignancy.

> ### Ask the boss: antireflux surgery
> *Further reading and discussion to have while on UGI firm*
> - Indications for antireflux surgery, medical vs surgical therapy (LOTUS trial).
> - Antireflux surgery for Barrett's oesophagus and reducing cancer risk.

Management

GORD is normally treated in the community with proton pump inhibitors (PPI). Symptomatic response usually confirms the diagnosis.

PPI therapy can be effective (70–80%) and lifestyle modifications (smoking/ETOH/weight reduction, avoid eating 2–3 hours prior to bedtime, and eating small meals) can help in managing symptoms. Other medications that may be used include H_2 receptor antagonists, antacids, sucralfate, and prokinetics. Only a few patients will need surgery, the commonest being the laparoscopic antireflux procedure (e.g. wrapping of the fundus around the oesophagus—Nissen fundoplication is a 360^n wrap).

> ### Honours
> *NICE criteria for urgent OGD for dyspepsia*
> Urgent '2-week wait' referral for OGD in patients with dyspepsia with:
> - weight loss
> - iron deficiency anaemia
> - persistent vomiting
> - palpable mass
> - chronic GI bleeding
> - >55 years, new or unexplained case.

Gastric cancer

Most common form of gastric cancer is adenocarcinoma (from mucosal tissue). Other forms include gastrointestinal stromal tumours (GIST) arising from the connective tissue of stomach wall, neuroendocrine tumours, or lymphomas.

Presentation

Upper abdominal pain, dyspepsia, weight loss, UGI bleed, and mass. Many gastric cancers are not amenable to surgical resection due to the local extent of metastatic disease.

Management

Treatment goals in this setting are symptomatic and palliative. In potentially curative cases, surgical management includes either distal gastrectomy or total gastrectomy depending on the anatomical location with the aim of removing all neoplastic tissue with adequate margins. (See Fig 42.1.) (Neo-) Adjuvant chemotherapy is combined with surgery.

UGI perforation

Acute UGI perforation can be caused by a duodenal ulcer, gastric ulcer, tumours, and traumatic origin (e.g. fishbone). Rarely, ischaemia can precipitate a perforation. Remember, the oesophagus can perforate too (e.g. Boerhaave syndrome).

Presentation

Patient will be acutely unwell and present with acute-onset upper abdominal pain and peritonism. Erect CXR gives the diagnosis by free air under the diaphragm (pneumoperitoneum); however, beware that the absence of free air on CXR does not exclude a UGI perforation!

Management

Immediate resuscitation (following acute life support principles). The definitive treatment is urgent operative intervention. This usually is a laparotomy; however, laparoscopy is sometimes favoured by some surgeons. A perforated duodenal ulcer is treated with an omental patch as is a prepyloric gastric ulcer. Ulcers on body of the stomach should be biopsied and closed. Patients will also be commenced on PPI therapy and receive empirical *Helicobacter pylori* eradication therapy.

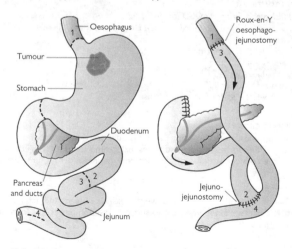

Fig. 42.1 Operative diagram of a total gastrectomy with a Roux-en-Y reconstruction. Reproduced with permission from Chris Callaghan et al, *Emergencies in Clinical Surgery*, 2008, Oxford University press

Upper GI surgery: bariatric surgery

Obesity represents one of the biggest public health challenges faced by developed countries. At present, the only effective treatment proven to achieve substantial weight loss is surgery. This surgical specialist interest is termed 'bariatric surgery'; it is typically performed by UGI surgeons and is rapidly expanding as access to these services is being made more widely available.

Operations

Although many there are a multitude of different operations used for weight loss, the most commonly performed operations in the UK are (1) sleeve gastrectomy, (2) gastric bypass and (3) gastric band. (See Fig. 42.2.)

1. Sleeve gastrectomy

Was initially designed as the first stage of a more complex duodenal switch procedure but was found to be effective in its own right as a weight loss procedure. It is technically straightforward relative to the other operations and involves the removal of the greater curve of the stomach.

2. Gastric bypass

This is the most commonly performed (and perhaps the most effective) weight loss procedure globally. It involves the creation of a small 30 mL pouch of stomach using a linear stapler and then dividing the small bowel distally and bringing up the distal end to anastomose with the small pouch of stomach (gastrojejunostomy). This leaves the pancreatobiliary limb (proximal end of divided small bowel), which is anastomosed to the small bowel distal to the gastrojejunostomy completing the Roux-en-Y reconstruction.

3. Gastric band

Involves the creation of a small (~30 mL) proximal pouch of stomach by applying an inflatable silicone band around the stomach. The band is connected to a subcutaneous port, allowing inflation and release of the band to adjust for the patient.

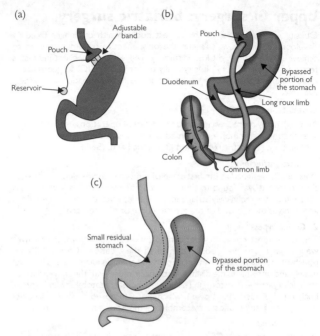

Fig. 42.2 Types of bariatric surgery. (a) Adjustable gastric band—a small bracelet-like band is placed around the top of the stomach to create a small pouch, thereby limiting food intake; the outlet size can be varied by injecting/removing saline from a small reservoir connected to the band. (b) Roux-en-Y—works by restricting food intake and by ↓ the absorption of food; a small pouch (similar in size to the adjustable gastric band) is created; in addition, absorption is reduced by 'excluding' most of the stomach, duodenum, and upper small intestine and routing food directly from the pouch into more distal small bowel. (c) Vertical sleeve gastrectomy—works by reducing the capacity of the stomach and altering gastric emptying. Reproduced from Jolly, E., et al, *Training in Medicine* 2016, OUP, Fig 7.62.

Hepatopancreatobiliary (HPB) surgery: overview

HPB surgery is the surgical subspecialty concerned with diseases of the liver, pancreas, and biliary tree. It has become increasingly centralized to major centres, especially for major resections and complex cases (including liver transplant). That said, a great deal of the bread-and-butter surgical take is concerned with the more common HPB conditions.

Procedures to see

Radiology
Percutaneous intervention: this may be diagnostic (obtaining a biopsy of a liver lesion of liver parenchyma to establish a histological diagnosis or therapeutic such as a PTC to decompress the biliary system or an image-guided aspiration/drain insertion. Liver abscesses and peripancreatic collections can be drained with image guidance by the interventional radiology team.

Endoscopy
ERCP: this is performed in endoscopy, often by the gastroenterologists, and is a key part of the investigation and management of patients with obstructive jaundice. Although performed at most acute hospitals, access is often limited in a district general hospital.

  EUS: this is a combination of endoscopy and US scanning used in specialist centres to assess the UGI tract including pancreas and distal common bile duct (CBD), as well as being a method of radiologically guiding biopsies/FNAs (e.g. for pancreatic cyst lesions).

Theatre/operations
Cholecystectomy: laparoscopic or open, typically the former ± intraoperative cholangiogram. One of the most commonly performed elective and emergency general surgical procedures—this is a must-see! Make sure you have revised your biliary anatomy read the patient's notes for indication, and LFTs, and reviewed the US report/images.

  Liver resections: these are specialist procedures done laparoscopically or as open procedures. Typically carried out in major centres so it may be difficult to see much of this without going to a teaching hospital. If going to theatre—make sure you ask a specialist registrar to go over the scans and surgical anatomy with you before surgery.

Things to do

Within HPB surgery there is a huge variety of activities and lots of opportunities for you to get involved—just turn up early and introduce yourself! These patients are also some of the sickest surgical patients you may encounter, often presenting with classic signs—so make sure you take the opportunity to examine these patients in ED or on the ward.

HPB surgery: biliary diseases

Gallstone disease

Common conditions with 100,000 gallstone-related admissions per year in the UK. Affects 10–20% of the population with majority asymptomatic. 1–4% of patients with gallstone per year will develop symptoms. Female >male incidence (2:1) and ↑ with age.

Biliary colic

Clinical syndrome characterized by severe RUQ pain, typically colicky (usually constant in cholecystitis), radiating to the back or shoulder, which is for a short duration. Symptoms are related to the impaction of a gallstone in Hartmann's pouch, cystic duct, or CBD. Diagnosis is made by a typical history of episodic RUQ pain after eating fatty meals combined with gallstones seen on USS/magnetic resonance cholangiopancreatography (MRCP). 10% seen on plain X-ray.

Biliary colic must be distinguished from other gallstone-related presentations and are associated with:
- acute calculous cholecystitis
- choledocholithiasis
- ascending cholangitis
- acute pancreatitis.

> #### Differential diagnosis
> Ruptured AAA, perforated peptic ulcer disease, acute pancreatitis.

Signs

Absence of jaundice and fever with Murphy's sign negative in RUQ (this Charcot triad usually present in acute cholangitis).

Bloods

Normal inflammatory markers, amylase and LFTs.

Treatment

Initially conservative with analgesia and a low-fat diet, occasionally requiring admission for symptom control. Definitive management is elective laparoscopic cholecystectomy.

Acute calculous cholecystitis

Occurs due to impaction of a gallstone in Hartmann's pouch resulting in chemical cholecystitis which progresses to bacterial cholecystitis. This may progress to necrosis, perforation, or empyema. Acalculous cholecystitis may occur secondary to systemic sepsis, long-term total parenteral nutrition, DM, and hepatitis A.

Presentation

RUQ pain (constant) for >24 hours, N&V, associated systemic upset (tachycardia and pyrexia), and a positive Murphy's sign.

Honours

Organisms associated with biliary tract infections are typically Gram-negative organisms:

- *Escherichia coli*
- *Klebsiella* spp.
- *Streptococcus. faecalis.*

Investigations

Bloods

Elevated inflammatory markers (WCC—leucocytosis, CRP) but usually *normal* LFTs.

US

Gallstones and sludge present in the gall bladder plus thickening of gall bladder wall plus pericholecystic fluid/oedema.

Treatment

Nil by mouth, IV fluids, IV antibiotics (with Gram-negative cover), analgesia (NSAIDs).

Ask the boss

Emergency 'hot' vs delayed laparoscopic cholecystectomy for acute cholecystitis

Traditionally, patients were managed conservatively in the acute phase and offered delayed cholecystectomy 6 weeks later. However, latest guidelines and evidence now recommend early laparoscopic cholecystectomy (within 72 hours of onset or during the index admission); variation in practice still exists though—ask your boss about the pros/cons.

Obstructive jaundice

Any interruption in the flow of bile from liver to GI tract (ultimately, via the CBD) can be a cause of obstructive jaundice. A thorough history and examination coupled with basic blood tests will provide useful clues as to where the obstruction is likely to be and the underlying pathology.

Choledocholithiasis (CBD stones)

These patients may be asymptomatic but often present with jaundice plus RUQ pain ± fever. These patients need to be monitored closely as they can quickly deteriorate, especially if elderly. An obstructed and infected biliary tree is a surgical emergency and needs urgent attention.

Honours

Signs of ascending cholangitis

- *Charcot's triad*: fever + RUQ pain + jaundice.
- *Reynolds' pentad*: Charcot's triad + septic shock + confusion.

Investigations

US

Always check the calibre of the CBD (<9 mm is normal), also look for evidence of intrahepatic duct dilation.

MRCP

Should be performed if stones are suspected and then proceed to ERCP decompression.

Treatment

ERCP plus stone retrieval ± stent and sphincterotomy. Essentially the duct needs to be cleared prior to laparoscopic cholecystectomy.

Head of pancreas (HOP) mass (pancreatic cancer) and cholangiocarcinoma

It is important to be aware that obstructive jaundice may be the presentation of something more sinister! Always do your systemic enquiry and look for signs and symptoms of malignancy (weight loss, malaise, fatigue).

Ask the boss

ERCP vs intraoperative cholangiogram (IOC) and laparoscopic CBD exploration at time of surgery

Surgical CBD exploration is usually reserved for cases where ERCP is unavailable, contraindicated, or unsuccessful. However, some units routinely perform IOC and may go straight to surgery without ERCP. Ask your consultant about the pros/cons.

Laparoscopic cholecystectomy

Common procedure. 50,000 cholecystectomies are performed every year in the UK so it is definitely worth getting to theatre and seeing this procedure.

Honours

Courvoisier's law

'If a patient presents with painless mild obstructive jaundice and a palpable gall bladder, the cause is not gall stones!' → the implication is that this is a *malignant* process. Therefore, the patient will need a CT chest/abdomen/pelvis and tumour markers checked (carcinoembryonic antigen plus CA 19-9).

Surgical anatomy

Calot's triangle

This is the anatomical location where the surgeon should reliably find the cystic artery (branch of the right hepatic artery) (Fig. 42.3). Boundaries are:
- liver (superior)
- cystic duct (lateral)
- common hepatic duct (medial).

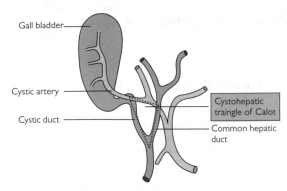

Fig. 42.3 Calot's triangle. Reproduced from Agarwal, Anil, et al, *Oxford Handbook of Operative Surgery* 3e, 2017, Oxford University Press.

Operation

Cholecystectomy (surgical removal of the gall bladder) can be performed laparoscopically or open, but the vast majority are now done laparoscopically (or at least start that way!). Once the surgeon has carefully dissected Calot's triangle, exposing the anatomy of the key structures, they have established the '*critical view of safety*' so that clips can be applied to the cystic duct and artery and these structures divided safely. The gall bladder is then carefully dissected off the liver bed (using an electrocauterizing hook—remember to '*look, hook, cook*') and extracted from the abdominal cavity via an umbilical port.

Honours

Complications of laparoscopic cholecystectomy
- Bile leak associated with an accessory cystic duct of Luschka.
- Iatrogenic CBD injury (Bismuth and Strasberg classification).
- Bleeding.
- Visceral injury.
- Conversion to open (if gall bladder is 'stuck' down).

Cholangiocarcinoma

This is an uncommon malignancy that affects males more than females and has a peak incidence in the 70s. Most are adenocarcinomas with 90% being extrahepatic. Risk factors are PSC and congenital anomalies, with PSC having a 5–15% lifetime risk. Few cases are resectable with poor outcomes. Palliative stenting (via ERCP/PTC) relieves jaundice for symptom control, but can also present its own complications.

HPB surgery: pancreatic disease

Acute pancreatitis

(See ➜ pp. 325–6.)

> ### Rule number 1: 'Don't mess with the pancreas!'
>
> This group of patients represents some of the sickest patients you will see and they can often end up on ITU requiring support for multiple organ systems.

Local complications: acute fluid collections

Peripancreatic fluid collection

This occurs within or around the pancreas early in acute, severe pancreatitis; it lacks an enclosing wall and will often resolve spontaneously without intervention. However, this can become infected creating an *infected* peripancreatic collection which can cause rapid deterioration and may require percutaneous US/CT-guided drainage (or another form of minimally invasive intervention).

Acute pancreatic pseudocyst

This is a collection of pancreatic juice within or adjacent to the pancreas enclosed by a wall of fibrous or granulation tissue. This often succeeds a peripancreatic fluid collection and forms over 4–6 weeks. It should also be treated conservatively so long as it remains sterile. Once infected and the patient is unstable, intervention is necessary (US/CT/endoscopic drainage).

Peripancreatic abscess

This is a well-circumscribed collection of pus in close proximity to the pancreas within the abdomen; it is usually the result of an infected peripancreatic collection or acute pancreatic pseudocyst. This needs to be drained.

Pancreatic necrosis

This is an area of non-viable pancreatic parenchyma that may be focal or diffuse and associated with peripancreatic fat necrosis. This is a dangerous condition with a high mortality. If this previously sterile condition becomes infected it is (surprisingly) called '*infected* pancreatic necrosis' and these patients can deteriorate rapidly needing aggressive resuscitation and management with IV antibiotics ± drainage where possible. Outcomes of intervention are poor and the traditional approach of open surgical necrosectomy (removal of necrotic pancreatic tissue) is increasingly controversial and less frequently performed, in favour of minimally invasive strategies. *This is largely because it breaks rule number 1!*

HPB surgery: pancreatic operations

Whipple's procedure or pancreaticoduodenectomy (PD)

This a major operation performed in highly specialized units for patients with cancers affecting the head of the pancreas or invading duodenum.

Resection

It involves en block resection of the head of the pancreas, distal stomach, duodenum, CBD, and gall bladder.

Reconstruction

Pancreaticojejunostomy (duct to mucosa), hepaticojejunostomy, gastrojejunostomy, jejunojejunostomy, and feeding jejunostomy. This 4–7-hour process of replumbing the flow of bile, pancreatic juices, and food into the small intestine is pretty physically demanding, so if you decide to go to theatre, make sure you have your Weetabix!

Pylorus-preserving pancreaticoduodenectomy (PPPD)

This is a variation of the classic Whipple's procedure and was designed to avoid two of the challenging complications: *postoperative dumping syndrome* and *bile reflux*. In this procedure, the pylorus is preserved to maintain the physiological valve effect of the distal stomach.

Distal pancreatectomy ± splenectomy

For lesions of the tail of the pancreas (benign and malignant), a distal pancreatectomy may be recommended. This may also involve splenectomy. This procedure is increasingly done laparoscopically.

If the patient has a splenectomy they will require *lifelong prophylactic antibiotics, usually penicillin (V)*, and they need to have vaccinations against:

* *Streptococcus pneumoniae*,
* *Haemophilus influenza* type B
* *Neisseria meningitides*
* Annual flu vaccine.

Honours

PD (traditional Whipple's) vs PPPD (modified)

Meta-analysis and randomized controlled trials have shown no difference in cancer survival, morbidity, or mortality between these two procedures.

Ask the boss

Controversies in acute pancreatitis management

1. Nutrition: early enteral nutrition vs parenteral nutrition.
2. Prophylactic antibiotics: is there a role?
3. Surgery for pancreatitis (necrosectomy): what (if any) are the indications? What is the optimal approach?
4. Timing for laparoscopic cholecystectomy for gallstone-related acute pancreatitis: when is it safe to operate?

Urology

Urology: overview

Urology deals with surgical and medical diseases of the male and female urinary tract system and the male reproductive organs. The surgical procedures involved can be classified into those of the upper and lower urinary tract respectively. The majority of urological procedures are performed electively (e.g. as day-case procedures).

Subspecialties include
- endo-urology
- onco-urology
- urogynaecology
- paediatric urology
- trauma and reconstructive urology
- andrology
- neuro-urology.

Cases to see
- Transurethral resections (e.g. transurethral resection of the prostate (TURP) for prostate; transurethral resection of bladder tumour (TURBT) for bladder tumours).
- Surgery for renal stones (e.g. lithotripsy in theatre, and extracorporeal shockwave lithotripsy (ESWL) in the clinic).
- Nephrectomy.
- Circumcision.
- Paediatric urology (e.g. hypospadias, orchidopexy).
- Urethroplasty.
- Orchidectomy.

Investigations/procedures to see
- X-ray (plain/contrast)/CT KUB/CT urography.
- US renal tract.
- Isotope renography.
- Cystoscopy (i.e. flexible in clinic, rigid in theatre).
- Urethral/suprapubic catheterization (ward/ED).
- Bladder irrigation (specialist nurse clinic or on ward/ED).
- Urodynamics (often by specialist nurses in clinic).

Things to do
- Digital rectal examination of prostate
- Testicular exam.
- Urine dipstick.
- Urethral catheterization and attending trial without catheter (TWOC) clinic.
- Flexible cystoscopy on a model (ask the doctor whether you can navigate a cystoscope inside an upturned plastic cup with lesions drawn inside).

Urology: in clinic

Haematuria

This is strictly the presence of RBCs in the urine. It can be classified into microscopic (i.e. normal urine colour) and macroscopic (i.e. looks red). Classify the causes *anatomically* (i.e. upper tract—kidney; middle tract—ureter; lower tract—bladder/prostate/urethra). The commonest causes are infection (e.g. cystitis, pyelonephritis), stones (anywhere along the urinary tract!), tumours (prostate, bladder, and kidney), autoimmune disease (rarer, e.g. glomerulonephritis), and postoperative (more common, e.g. after TURP).

Renal stones

Typically cause renal colic (a rapid, severe, sharp, and colicky loin-to-groin pain). You might often see dipstick haematuria, and if not, you would definitely need to think about the most common alternative causes (appendicitis, gallstones, (gynae) cyst rupture, bowel obstruction, gastroenteritis, etc.). Commonest sites of stone formation are at the narrowest sites: pelviureteric junction (PUJ), mid ureter, and vesicoureteric junction (VUJ). Predisposing factors include dehydration (think lorry drivers), infection (*Proteus* infections associated with large staghorn calculi), metabolic abnormalities (rare but exam favourites, e.g. hyperparathyroidism), congenital deformities (rare, e.g. horseshoe kidney), and familial. 80% of stones are radio-opaque (e.g. oxalate/phosphate) due to calcification (the other 20% include struvite, urate, and cysteine stones). Management depends on size of stone: stones <5 mm are likely to pass spontaneously where medication may offer symptomatic relief (alpha blockers); those >5 mm may require lithotripsy (in clinic) or extraction (in theatre).

Benign prostatic hyperplasia (BPH)

This is the most common cause of bladder outlet obstruction, and often presents in elderly males with symptoms such as hesitancy, poor stream, frequency, and terminal dribbling. After the classical history, this diagnosis is assisted by DRE which identifies a smooth, symmetrically enlarged prostate. You should know how alpha-adrenergic antagonists (tamsulosin) or 5-alpha reductase (finasteride) work to alleviate symptoms. TURP may be necessary if the bladder is still functional and therefore will not → incontinence. (See Fig 43.1.)

Phimosis

This is a condition defined as the inability to retract the foreskin (over the glans). It is normal in <6-year-olds, but when (1) it persists, (2) it is associated with pain, or (3) there is swelling on urination, it can precipitate underlying infection (balanitis). It can be associated in adults with infections, as well as various skin conditions, in particular lichen sclerosis, and this can be an indication for circumcision. Remember, paraphimosis, is when the foreskin cannot be returned to its original position after retraction. This can occur if you forget to return the foreskin after urinary catheterization. The glans swells and becomes painful (due to restricted penile blood flow) and should be manually reduced (or rarely warrants emergent circumcision).

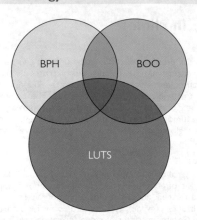

Fig. 43.1 The relationship between BPH, LUTS (lower urinary tract symptoms), and BOO (bladder outflow obstruction). The cause of LUTS is multifactorial; however, they remain the usual trigger for men to seek medical attention and may → a diagnosis of BPH, with or without evidence of BOO. Reproduced with permission from William E. G. Thomas et al, *Oxford Textbook of Fundamentals of Surgery*, 2016, Oxford University Press.

Urinary incontinence

This is defined as the leakage of urine after ↑intra-abdominal pressure and is due to a weak urethral sphincter. This can be classified most commonly into stress, urge, overflow, and mixed. There are several causes, the commonest being pelvic floor weakness from childbirth and exacerbated by age in females, and BPH in males. Other causes include diabetes, stimulants (e.g. caffeine), and neuro-degeneration (e.g. multiple sclerosis, spinal cord injury, etc.). Try to understand abdominal vs bladder pressure traces during urodynamic testing, and how these can differentiate between the causes. Patient management begins with physiotherapy (i.e. pelvic floor exercises for stress incontinence) and medications (oxybutynin for urge incontinence), but surgery may be required (e.g. tension-free transvaginal tape).

Paediatric urology

Consists of a vast range of conditions. Common ones include cryptorchidism (undescended testis associated with subfertility and malignancy), hypospadias, and vesicoureteral reflux (a common renal disease due to abnormal backflow of urine).

Uro-oncology

Involves cancer anywhere along the urogenital tract but commonly in the prostate (adenocarcinoma), bladder (transitional cell carcinomas), and kidneys (various types including clear cell tumours). Testicular tumours include germ and stromal tumours, teratomas in second decade (*Troops*) and seminomas in third decade (*Sergeants*). These are all incredibly variable, as are their investigations and the chemotherapeutic, radiation, and surgical management that may be used.

Testicular lumps

Commonly seen in clinic (and finals), including hydrocoeles (fluid within the tunica vaginalis, typically transilluminating), varicocoeles (dilated veins of the pampiniform plexus, typically feeling like a 'bag of worms'), and testicular tumours. A good mantra is to consider a scrotal lump a cancer until proven otherwise, while an acute, painful testicular swelling is a testicular torsion until proven otherwise.

Investigations

- Intravenous urography (IVU) was traditionally the investigation of choice for suspected abnormalities of the renal tract (especially the ureter) but has now been replaced by CT imaging (e.g. non-contrast CT KUB for renal stones, or CT urography for other renal tract abnormalities). Plain film KUB often accompanies a CT KUB to establish whether they can be identified so they can be used for follow-up. Always ask for a 15–30 min interval film in IVU, looking for a standing column to confirm a calculus. (See Fig 43.2.)
- US scans of the kidneys may demonstrate structural abnormalities (e.g. hydronephrosis, cysts). Transrectal US scanning is used for biopsy of suspected prostate cancer, and scrotal US scanning is used for suspected testicular cancer.
- MRI rather than CT can be useful in the assessment of the prostate gland (and seminal vesicles).
- Isotope renography provides anatomical and functional information about the renal tract. DMSA (dimercaptosuccinic acid) provides a functional image of the renal parenchyma, while MAG3 (mercaptoacetyltriglycine) renography provides dynamic assessment of renal excretion, and excludes the presence of obstruction.

Honours

Testicular tumours may present atypically (e.g. as testicular torsion or scrotal haematomas) but offer good prognosis if managed early. Teratomas are associated with raised serum alpha-fetoprotein and beta-human chorionic gonadotropin (hCG), and are usually managed with orchidectomy and chemotherapy, while seminomas are associated with raised serum beta-hCG and are very sensitive to radiotherapy.

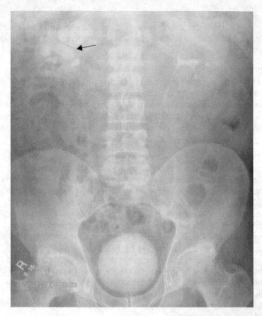

Fig. 43.2 An intravenous urogram demonstrating excretion of contrast material by the left kidney into the bladder. There is some excretion of contrast from the right kidney along with multiple, large, round radio-opaque lesions in the kidney consistent with multiple renal calculi (arrow). Reproduced with permission from Jolly, E. et al, *Training in Medicine*, 2016, OUP.

Urology: in theatre

Cystoscopy

This is a central endoscopic procedure for urologists. Flexible cystoscopy is performed under local anaesthetic to examine the urethra and bladder, while rigid cystoscopy is performed under GA and allows for a greater degree of instrumentation. Cystoscopy (and ureterorenoscopy) can be used for insertion of retrograde ureteric stents, stone fragmentation/extraction, as well as tissue resection and biopsy.

Circumcision

This is a common procedure and may be performed under GA or local anaesthesia. Alongside hydrocele repair and other 'lumps', it can often be found on a theatre list of day cases and make for excellent cases to scrub in with and assist (make sure you know your relevant inguinal and scrotal anatomy beforehand).

Hydrocoele

This may resolve spontaneously or is amenable to drainage (often associated with recurrence): Lord's repair (plication of the tunica vaginalis), Jaboulay's repair (inversion of the hydrocele sac).

Varicocoele

This may rarely be repaired by embolization.

Orchidectomy

This may be performed for certain advanced testicular tumours, or upon finding a non-viable testis during scrotal exploration for testicular torsion (find out whether the surgical access is via inguinal vs scrotal skin). If a testis is deemed viable during exploration, orchidopexy is commonly performed on both the affected and normal testes.

TURP

This is performed via rigid scopes and involves circumferential excision of the inner transitional zone of the prostate. It can be performed with traditional diathermy or more modern laser-based tools to excise/vaporize the prostatic tissue. Complications of TURP include haematuria (requiring bladder irrigation), retrograde ejaculation, incontinence, erectile dysfunction, and TURP syndrome. This procedure is not used for prostate cancer, which may require radical prostatectomy (via an open or laparoscopic approach) for curative intent.

TURBT

This removes bladder tumours (together with intravesical BCG or mitomycin C). More advanced bladder tumours may be amenable to radical cystectomy (± chemotherapy or radiotherapy), but often begin with a TURBT for the purpose of obtaining histological information.

Nephrectomy

This is for (1) removing tumours of the proximal renal tract, (2) extraction from donor patients, and (3) cystic renal disease. Indication for benign or malignant disease determines the ancillary procedure (e.g. lymph node, vascular and ureteric excision).

Nephrostomy

This is performed by interventional radiologists, usually percutaneously, to decompress an obstructed (± infected) kidney.

Anatomy

Simple anatomies of the male and female reproductive systems are found in Fig. 43.3. Learn the basics which will be asked in theatre.

Honours

- The irrigation fluid used for TURP and endoscopic procedures involving diathermy is usually glycine (instead of normal saline), due to its electrical non-conductivity and relative hypotonicity.
- *TURP syndrome* may occur after transurethral surgery, due to excessive absorption of irrigation fluid perioperatively → *hyponatraemia* (confusion, hypotension, bradycardia, vomiting, and collapse). The patient may need ITU support alongside 'slow' restoration of Na^+.

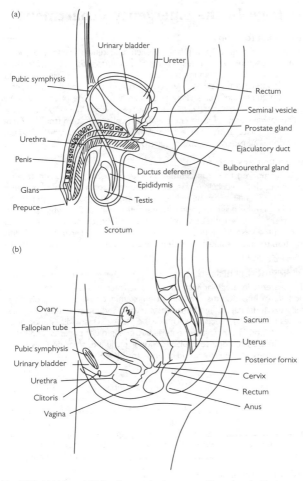

Fig. 43.3 (a) Male and (b) female reproductive systems. Reproduced with permission from Glasper, A. et al, *Oxford Handbook of Children's and Young People's Nursing* 2e, 2015, Oxford University Press.

Urology: in the emergency department

Testicular torsion

Presents as sudden pain in a hot, swollen, and tender testicle, occurring spontaneously in young males. This is a clinical diagnosis for which there should be a low threshold for suspicion. There is a 6-hour window to untwist the affected testicle after which the risk of testicular death (necrosis and subsequent subfertility likely due to an autoimmune phenomenon) is significant. Because it is a clinical diagnosis (Doppler), US is only supportive and not always done. Treatment is with surgical exploration (midline raphe incision or bilateral transverse scrotal incisions) for detorsion ± fixation (orchidopexy). Necrotic testes require orchidectomy.

Acute urinary retention

Painful compared to chronic retention. May be secondary to prostate enlargement, clot, calculi, infection, and strictures. Confirmation of retention by bladder scanning may be helpful, but history and palpation/percussion should clinch the diagnosis, and catheterization will confirm while providing swift relief. Coude catheters, introducers, and cystoscopes aid in difficult cases. In the case of clot retention, a three-way catheter permits bladder irrigation to clear residual clots. Suprapubic cystostomy is reserved in case of contraindications.

Epididymo-orchitis

This presents in a similar way to testicular torsion but is often subacute, and signs of infection may be evident on examination (e.g. penile discharge or pyrexia), urinalysis, and blood tests (e.g. raised inflammatory markers). Causes include (1) infections such as TB, STIs (e.g. chlamydia/gonorrhoea) in younger and Gram-negative enteric bacteria in older patients; and (2) recent catheter. Provided testicular torsion is excluded, treatment with antibiotics is commenced after sending urine for MC&S.

Renal colic

This is due to urinary calculi. Dipstick haematuria is highly sensitive for this pathology, and CT KUB is commonly used to confirm the diagnosis, establish the size/location, and guide treatment. It will be prudent to remember other differential diagnoses (especially ruptured AAA) when high-risk cardiopathy patients present with similar symptoms. Renal colic rarely occurs in the elderly, so always rule out AAA first with a history, examination, and imaging (e.g. bedside US scan in the ED or formal CT angiogram).

Frank haematuria

This is usually secondary to bladder or prostate pathology. Admission is warranted if blood loss is significant, if there is evidence of haemodynamic instability, and more typically for three-way catheterization and irrigation. The patient must be stabilized and able to urinate freely or via an unblocked catheter before being discharged. Most importantly, exclude malignancy with outpatient investigations.

Urology: in exams

Any examination of the urological system should be accompanied by an examination of the abdomen, hernia orifices, and include a DRE (i.e. for examination of the prostate).

Imaging—interpretation of plain film KUB or contrast IVU (i.e. to recognize renal tract abnormalities, calculi (e.g. staghorn), horseshoe kidney, or a duplex collecting system). Try to navigate CT urography on your urology attachment so you are used to tracing the renal system from kidneys down to bladders.

Urine dipstick testing is a common and simple procedure, and students should be familiar with the equipment involved and interpretations. Catheterization is a core skill which you should be able to talk through and demonstrate on female and male models including the reasons for each step.

Examining a testicular mass is a basic requirement, and you should be asking the following questions relating to the mass:
- Can you get above it?
- Is it separate from the testis?
- Does it have a cough impulse?
  - Consider indirect inguinoscrotal hernia.
- Is it cystic/solid (and does it transilluminate)?
  - Cannot get above: inguinoscrotal hernia or hydrocele extending proximally
  - Separate and cystic: epididymal cyst.
  - Separate and solid: epididymitis/varicocele.
  - Testicular and cystic: hydrocele.
  - Testicular and solid—tumour, orchitis, haematocele, granuloma, gumma.
- Signs pointing towards *torsion*:
  - Prehn's sign: lifting up the testicles relieves the pain of epididymitis (positive) but not the pain caused by testicular torsion (negative).
  - Blue dot sign: tender and blue discoloured nodule on the upper pole of the testis (appendix testis or hydatid of Morgagni).

Honours

Foley catheters are made of dark yellow latex (*beware allergies*), are more flexible, and are for shorter-term usage than silicone catheters, which are clear in colour. Long-term catheters need to be changed every few months, and the formation of microbacterial biofilms is common; prophylactic 'pre-change' antibiotics may reduce the risk of infection at catheterization. If the patient is symptomatic of an infection they may require antibiotics but bacteriuria in asymptomatic catheterized patients is typical and should not be treated.

Part 4

Clinical skills

Chapter 44

Radiology

Radiology: in the radiology department

Plain radiographic film

Uses X-rays to image the skeleton and soft tissues.

Physics

Metal filament in X-ray tube heated causing emission of electrons. Electrons are accelerated and focused onto a metal target. Collision of electrons with nuclei of metallic atoms causes emission of X-rays. X-rays pass through body and hit X-ray plate detector which goes black. The more X-rays that hit the detector, the more black the target gets. Higher-density tissue absorbs and deflects more X-rays so less X-rays reach detector. Six main densities seen on X-ray image: air (black), fat, soft tissue, fluid, bone, and metal (white).

Indications

- *Chest*: useful in primary workup to assess heart and lungs. Also useful in follow-up to monitor progression of disease and/or resolution.
- *Abdomen*: limited use with the ↑availability of CT but still used to look for bowel obstruction or perforation or to see radio-opaque kidney stones.
- *ED trauma*: used following trauma (trauma series including cervical spine, chest, pelvis, likely fracture sites) to identify fractures and in follow-up to assess response to treatment/complications.
- *Orthopaedics*: used to assess joint destruction to decide on management or to follow-up joint replacements or metalwork placement. Also used for follow-up on conservative and operative management (e.g. non-union, malunion, etc.).
- *Rheumatology*: used to assess arthritic distribution, changes over time, and response to treatment.
- *Mammography*: exclusive breast X-rays to look for soft tissue lumps and calcifications as part of the national screening programme for breast cancer.

Drawbacks

- 2D representation of 3D structures.
- Does not image soft tissues well.
- Radiation exposure.
- Limited views obtainable.

Ultrasound

Uses sound waves to image internal tissues.

Physics

Current passed through piezoelectric crystal causes it to resonate and produce sound waves. Sound waves pass through body and reflect off different density interfaces.

Echoes are detected by crystal which allows formation of image showing interfaces. Sound waves pass easily through fluid due to low echogenicity and appear black on image. Sound waves cannot pass through air or bone due to high echogenicity and reflect off showing no image beyond.

Different soft tissues have different echogenicities and the interface between the densities can be differentiated and displayed as an image.

Indications

Abdomen

- *Liver*: focal lesions, cirrhosis, biliary duct dilatation, portal or hepatic vein occlusion.
- *Spleen*: focal lesions, infarcts, haemorrhage.
- *Pancreas*: tumours, cysts, pancreatitis.
- *Gallbladder*: gallstones, cholecystitis, cholangiocarcinoma.
- *Bowel*: can also see and assess free fluid. Often bowel can be seen (if fluid filled) however, air-filled bowel will obscure underling structures as US unable to pass through air.
- *Kidneys*: stones, hydronephrosis, renal artery/vein occlusion. (See Fig. 44.1.)

Pelvis

- *Bladder*: tumours, calcification, stones.
- *Uterus*: endometrium, fibroids.
- *Ovaries*: cysts, torsion.
- *Prostate*: size, focal lesions including transvaginal or transrectal US.

Chest

Can be used to assess size of pleural effusion and to characterize the fluid contents including the presence of septations ± loculations (can be hard to detect on CT). Drains can be inserted under US guidance.

Breast

Can give excellent views of lumps which are not seen on mammography or find lesions to biopsy. Also used to assess or biopsy axillary lymph nodes.

Testes

Excellent views looking for focal lesions, microlithiasis, torsion, hydroceles, or varicoceles.

Thyroid

Assess goitres, nodular thyroid, and to guide FNA sampling.

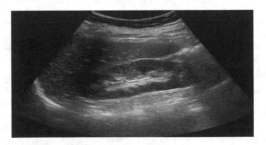

Fig. 44.1 Renal ultrasound.

Vascular

Almost any vessel can be imaged including arteries (carotids to assess in patients at risk of TIA, aorta looking for AAA, iliacs, femorals, arm and leg arteries looking for atherosclerotic disease) and veins (jugulars and subclavians to assess for central line placements, arm and leg veins looking for DVT or thrombophlebitis).

Musculoskeletal

Most peripheral joints can be imaged to assess the tendons, bursae, and capsules having the benefit of dynamic imaging unlike CT and MRI.

Transcranial

Used in neonates with patent fontanelles to give intracranial views in preference to CT due to ionizing radiation.

Superficial tissues

Any superficial tissue can be imaged (lipoma, seroma, superficial collections, pseudoaneurysms, etc.).

Drawbacks

- User dependent.
- Cannot travel through air so cannot image aerated lung or air-filled bowel.
- Time-consuming.
- Difficult to replicate images for follow-up.

Computed tomography

Uses X-rays to build up an internal view of the body and can formulate 3D models of patients. Any part of the body can be imaged.

Physics

X-rays pass through body from 360° around patient. Depending on different absorptions of intervening tissues, different amounts will pass through to other side, which are detected. By adding all the different images from 360° a 3D image is formed of all internal structures. Each pixel is given a number (Hounsfield unit (HU)) which denotes its density or attenuation. Each tissue type has a particular HU which aids in differentiating pathology. Contrast agents can be given via various routes and at different stages in the scan process to help improve image quality. Oral or rectal contrast can be given to help identify a leak in the GI tract or to simply opacify the bowel so it is easier to differentiate it from the other structures. Contrast can also be injected into the bladder for similar reasons.

IV contrast can be given to help identify various structures (see Fig. 44.2). The length of time following administration and image acquisition will determine what type of scan is performed:

- At 15–25 sec the contrast will be in the pulmonary arteries, as in CTPA to diagnose PE.
- At 30–40 sec the main systemic arteries will opacify which would help to look for aneurysms or acute bleeding.
- At 70–90 sec the abdominal organs will begin to take up contrast and this helps to identify focal lesions or delayed bleeding.

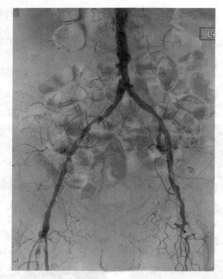

Fig. 44.2 CT contrast angiogram showing the abdominal aortic bifurcation.

- After 2 3 min the contrast would start to be excreted by the kidneys and therefore the ureters and bladder would begin to fill with contrast helping to identify obstruction or tumours in the renal tract.

Drawbacks
- Radiation.
- Requires patient to lie flat and completely still.
- Can induce contrast-induced nephropathy in patients with renal impairment.
- Anaphylaxis seen in patients with contrast allergy.

Magnetic resonance imaging

MRI uses magnets and radiofrequency pulses to build up an internal view of the body. It is particularly useful for soft tissue characterization and musculoskeletal imaging to view tendons and ligaments which cannot be identified on CT. This modality is also useful for identifying different tissue types within lesions. Any part of the body can be imaged (see Fig. 44.3).

Physics
Hydrogen nuclei are aligned in a strong magnetic field. Radiofrequency pulses cause hydrogen nuclei to flip by varying degrees.

Nuclei spin back to their original alignment and give out varying signals dependent on what type of tissue they are located in. A computer detects signals returned from nuclei and displays them as an image. Different

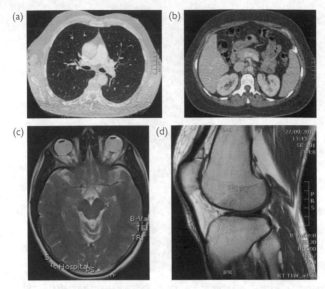

Fig. 44.3 MRI of various body parts. (a) MRI chest; (b) MRI abdomen; (c) MRI brain; (d) MRI knee.

sequences can be performed by altering degrees of spin and by repeating radiofrequency pulses which help differentiate different tissue types.

Drawbacks
- Takes very long time to scan a patient.
- Small tube and so cannot scan large or claustrophobic patients.
- Cannot scan patients with ferromagnetic implants.

Fluoroscopy

Real-time sequential X-ray pictures can be acquired of any region of the body

Contrast studies: administration of contrast via any cavity in the body and fluoroscopy performed to monitor the passage of that contrast through the body.

Oral or rectal administration of contrast enables opacification of the GI tract to demonstrate luminal pathology such as polyps, strictures, diverticula, or tumours (see Fig. 44.4).

Injection of contrast via a catheter into the uterus is used to opacify the uterus and fallopian tubes to identify patency in patients with subfertility (see Fig. 44.5).

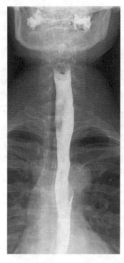

Fig 44.4 Barium swallow/meal/follow through/enema.

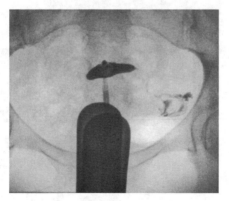

Fig. 44.5 Hysterosalpingogram.

Nephrostogram/cystogram

Injection of contrast into a nephrostomy or urinary bladder catheter or opacify the renal tract or identify a bladder leak or urethral injury.

Tubogram/linogram

Injection of contrast into any drain, line, or indwelling tube to ascertain its position and/or patency such as blocked venous lines or abdominal drains.

Nuclear imaging

Radio-labelled pharmaceuticals are injected into patients which migrate to various tissues and emit gamma rays. These are then picked up by a gamma camera and show where the pharmaceutical has migrated to. This enables physiological activity within various cells in the body to be determined. There are numerous pharmaceutical agents which can be radiolabelled depending on where you want the tracer to be absorbed such as thyroid, kidney, bone (Fig. 44.6), heart, lung, white cells, etc.

PET-CT: this is a fusion of PET (a cross-sectional version of nuclear imaging) and CT to produce images with anatomical data from CT with overlayed physiological data from PET. This shows the exact sites of ↑physiological activity such as small metastatic deposits.

Drawbacks
- High-dose radiation.
- Image acquisition takes a long time requiring the patient to remain still.
- Patient remains radioactive for some time following procedure.

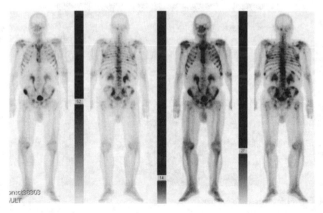

Fig. 44.6 Bone scan.

In the interventional radiology suite

This is a vastly expanding subspeciality field of radiology. Procedures range from simple US-guided biopsies to fluoroscopy-guided complex EVARs. Interventional radiology is divided into two further fields of vascular and non-vascular. Common procedures can be divided into vascular and non-vascular cases which include:

Vascular interventional radiology

- Angioplasty/venoplasty and stenting of atherosclerotic or aneurysmal vessels.
- Endovenous laser treatment of varicose veins.
- Thrombolysis for acute clot and emergency embolization in acute haemorrhage, including postpartum haemorrhage.
- Inferior vena cava filter placement and retrieval.
- Embolization of arteriovenous malformations.
- Tunnelled central line insertion.
- Transjugular intrahepatic portosystemic shunt (TIPS) for portal hypertension.

Non-vascular interventional radiology

- Nephrostomy tube insertion for hydronephrosis.
- Radiologically inserted gastrostomy (RIG).
- Cholecystotomy.
- Radiofrequency ablation of tumours (liver, kidney, lung, bone).
- Vertebroplasty.
- US/CT-guided biopsies and drains.

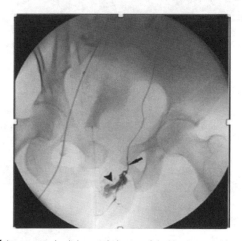

Fig. 44.7 Interventional radiology: embolization of the bleeding vessel by microcatheterization. Reproduced with permission from McCormack and Keith Kelly, *Oxford Case Histories in Anaesthesia*, 2014, Oxford University Press.

Practical procedures

Introduction to practical procedures

Successfully placing your first cannula, relieving a patient in urinary retention—these are often the highs of medical school when you feel that you have actually done something helpful. Each medical school will have its own list of competencies and rules around how these are supervised and achieved but you should aim to start as soon as you can on your clinical rotations so that you are not overwhelmed when you hit the wards as a junior doctor.

'*See one, do one, teach one*' has worked pretty well over the decades as a teaching philosophy but the key is to find a senior you feel comfortable with who has time to oversee your first attempts at procedures. Also, pick your patients—you are far more likely to succeed with a relaxed patient who tells you before you even declare yourself that it is fine to fail than an anxious and needle-phobic one. Also, practise really does make perfect. While putting needles into plastic arms is useful hands-on experience, and there are excellent teaching videos on YouTube and that now form part of some textbooks, these cannot replace the experience of setting up beforehand, winning the trust of your patient, and getting a feel of how a procedure is done.

Gain consent and explain what you plan to do. Defer to your seniors in a situation where you are unable to obtain consent (e.g. patient in a coma, an adult with learning difficulties). Wash your hands.

Hand hygiene and asepsis

Hand hygiene is a vital public health intervention to help prevent the spread of hospital-acquired infection from drug-resistant microbes such as meticillin-resistant *Staphylococcus aureus* (MRSA). But despite the near miraculous reduction in maternal deaths in 1847 at the Vienna General Hospital's obstetrics unit, after Dr Ignaz Semmelweis insisted doctors washed their hands before seeing patients, we are still not very good at washing our hands.[1]

Remember handwashing in OSCEs, even if the arm you have been asked to draw blood from is a plastic one. Like giving your name, it is easy marks and you are unlikely to pass the station if you have not done so. And patients have been rightly empowered to ask if you *have* washed your hands!

Most hospitals are only allowed to declare up to three iatrogenic MRSA incidents before being heavily fined and assessed for quality of care. It is your responsibility to prioritize personal hygiene to uphold patient safety for a vulnerable population.

Asepsis and aseptic non-touch technique (ANTT)

The best place to learn to scrub for surgery is in theatre and you will get faster in time! However, even if you are not going to be a surgeon, you will be doing basic procedures as a junior doctor and you must know how to do these aseptically (and document that the technique was aseptic). The premise of ANTT is basic—if you do not touch something, you will not infect it. The following is generic for any ward-based procedure where there is a chance of introducing infection (e.g. urethral catheterization). It also helps to have someone else available to open and hand things to you if you are scrubbed.

Prepare a trolley (clean surface with antiseptic wipes). Put trolley next to patient and then wash your hands and prepare kit (e.g. opening out a wound dressing pack using the edge of the packaging, putting antiseptic solution into gallipots, dropping sterile items into middle of sterile field, half opening sterile gloves ready to put on, etc.)

For the procedure, wash your hands, double-glove if cleaning an area first (you can then carefully discard the top pair of gloves without having to re-scrub) and carry out the procedure, making sure you have a sterile drape over the surrounding area while doing so. Afterwards, ensure all sharps are safely discarded in a sharps bin (it is good practice to always identify and discard your own sharps) and that any clinical waste is removed. Clean your trolley!

Reference

1. Gawande A (2008). *Better: A Surgeon's Notes on Performance*. London: Profile Books.

Measuring blood pressure

BP is the force exerted by the heart on the blood vessel wall as blood is pumped round the body. Measuring BP is a basic skill on which you will be examined at OSCEs. As the examiner listens in with a dual earpiece stethoscope, you will not be able to fake it. You might think with automated BP machines that this is a pointless skill—you would be wrong. Many automated machines are badly calibrated so if you really want to know what someone's BP is, measure it manually. (See Table 45.1.)

Indications

BP is a part of standard observations and is also used for screening for hypertension, risk stratification for cardiovascular disease, and suitability for procedures (e.g. preoperative optimization).

Contraindications

There are no absolute contraindications but relative ones do exist. Do not take BP from an arm with an arteriovenous fistula (e.g. used for haemodialysis), lymphoedema, and burns on the arms or legs.

Procedure

- The bladder (cuff) should cover approximately two-thirds of the upper arm (or cuff width should be >40% of upper arm circumference).
  NB: the cuff can also be placed around the calf if the arms are not accessible (e.g. burns patient).
- A cuff that is too small will give an erroneously high BP, and a cuff that is too big will underestimate BP.
- Ensure the patient is relaxed as can be—pain, anxiety, and fear of healthcare staff (white coat hypertension) will cause a high BP reading. Get the patient to relax the arm on a desk/table/bedside at the level of the heart.
- Place stethoscope over the brachial artery and inflate the cuff to 30 mmHg above the disappearance of pulse sounds, then slowly release until you can 'hear' the pulse—this is systolic BP, or Korotkoff 1 sounds.
- Continue lowering the cuff pressure until the sounds disappear (Korotkoff V)—this is diastolic BP. Choose the muffling of sounds in individuals whose diastolic goes down to zero (e.g. pregnant women).
- You cannot diagnose hypertension from one BP measurement—repeated measurements are needed. Note down the best of three.

Hypertension

This is a 'silent' but major risk factor for stroke and MI. Systolic BP is most strongly associated with risk of CVS disease (see Fig 45.1).[1]

Do not forget the importance of BP in:

Pregnant women

Hypertension (with proteinuria, oedema, upper abdominal pain, and headache) can mean pre-eclampsia, an obstetric emergency.

Table 45.1 Blood pressure monitoring: some definitions (adult, in mmHg))

Optimal adult BP	Systolic <120 and diastolic <75
Borderline	>140/90
Requiring treatment	>160/100
Malignant hypertension	>200/130

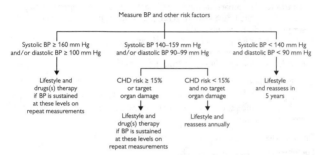

Fig. 45.1 Managing adult hypertension. Reproduced from British Cardiac Society, et al, Joint British recommendations on prevention of coronary heart disease in clinical practice, *Heart* 1998;80(supplement 2):S1–S29.

Children

BP should be a routine observation for children as well as adults. There are normal values based on a child's age and height. A quick formula for children >1 year: median systolic BP = 90 mmHg + (2 × age in years). Remember the 6-year-old who made repeated presentations with non-specific abdominal pain and was found to have a BP of 203/157 mmHg, secondary to a phaeochromocytoma.[2]

References

1. Tin LL, Beevers DG, Lip GY (2002). Systolic vs diastolic blood pressure and the burden of hypertension. *J Human Hypertens* 16:147–50.
2. Corcoran J, Bird C, Side L, et al. (2008). Diagnosis at dusk: malignant hypertension and phaeochromocytoma in a 6-year-old girl. *Emerg Med Australas* 20:66–9.

Inserting a nasogastric tube

There are generally two types of NG tubes. Wide bore (Ryles) tubes are used for drainage of the stomach and UGI tract in bowel obstruction or postoperatively. Fine-bore (8–12 Fr) tubes are used for feeding and administering drugs if a patient does not have a safe swallow, is delirious and so not regularly eating, or is sedated in ITU. Feeding via an NG tube is not a permanent feeding system as the risk of tube displacement is too high.[1]

Indications

Inserted into the stomach via the nose (if via the mouth, an orogastric tube) for:
- *surgical*: intestinal obstruction, acute pancreatitis, post-abdominal surgery (wide-bore tube)
- *medical*: risk of aspiration (and therefore also used to empty the stomach prior to emergency anaesthesia), dysphagia
- *nutrition*: for feeding (fine-bore tube).

Contraindications

Possibility of facial fracture or recent UGI or ENT surgery (especially with delicate anastomosis, talk to the patient's surgical team); be cautious if concurrent rhinitis/pharyngitis/oesophagitis present.

Procedure

Equipment

Non-sterile procedure (but wear gloves and prepare clean tray): NG tube, water-based lubricant, syringe, bile bag, securing tape, and pH indicator.

Sizes

16 Fr (large), 12 Fr (medium), 10 Fr (small)—smaller sizes available for children. The tube should be able to fit comfortably in the nostril (right often easier than left). Measure the length to be inserted by placing the end of the tube at the nares, passed back round the ear and then down to the xiphisternum.

Complete the following steps:
- Lubricate tip of tube. Ask the patient to touch their chest with their chin.
- Use curvature of the tube to pass it back and downwards through the nostril (do not force the tube—if resistance felt, try other nostril and if still not working, find your senior).
- When the tube passes into the throat (patient will gag), twist tube 180° to prevent tube curving back out through the mouth.
- When inserted to the measured length, tape in place to nose.
- Do not use until pH tested (aspirate >0.5 mL stomach contents and test on pH paper—must be 1–5.5).
- If no fluid can be aspirated initially, the patient should be turned (onto the left side) and aspiration tried again in 20 min.
- As incorrect siting of an NG tube is a 'never event', many hospitals now insist on a CXR to ensure the tip is in the stomach.
- Look for correct positioning on CXR (see Fig 45.2).
- If struggling, you can refrigerate the tube for 15–30 min to make it more rigid or use a smaller size NGT.
- If wide-bore tube used, options are to allow free flow of gastric contents into a bag, aspirate the NGT every 2–4 hours, or to spigot (i.e. place a cap) to allow absorption of medication.

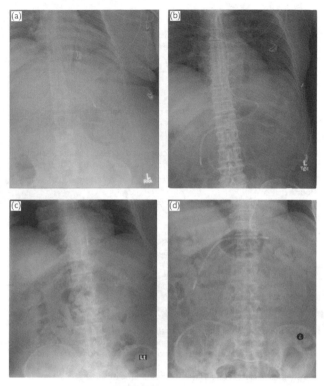

Fig. 45.2 Common positions of nasogastric tube (upper row (correct): mid gastric, postpyloric; lower row (incorrect): oesophageal, and descending duodenum. Reproduced with permission from Wijdicks, Eelco F.M. *Providing Acute Care*, 2014, Oxford University Press.

NG tube placement pointers
- Does the tube path follow the oesophagus?
- Can you see the tube bisect the carina?
- Can you see the tube cross the diaphragm in the midline?
- Does the tube then deviate immediately to the left?
- Can you see the tip of the tube clearly below the left hemidiaphragm?

Reference

1. Lamont T, Beaumont C, Fayaz A, et al. (2011). Checking placement of nasogastric feeding tubes in adults (interpretation of x ray images): summary of a safety report from the National Patient Safety Agency *BMJ* 342:d2586.

Bladder/urethral catheterization

A catheter is placed into the bladder via the urethra. You should know how to do both male and female catheterizations and make sure you have a chaperone (and know your anatomy; see Fig. 45.3). You should practise on plastic models in the clinical skills lab before attempting it on patients on the ward/theatre.

Indications

Main indications are to treat urinary retention and monitor urine output. Other indications include immobility and intravesical chemotherapy.

Contraindications

Possible urethral injury (e.g. pelvic fracture) and acute prostatitis. Ask about *latex allergy*. When explaining the procedure, also advise about the risk of infection and false passage.

Procedure

This is a *sterile* procedure (poor technique can introduce infection). You will need a catheterization pack (with sterile drape, kidney dish, gauze swabs, forceps, drainage bag, a size 12–16 Fr catheter), sterile gloves, apron, and local anaesthetic (e.g. lidocaine) gel (see Fig. 45.4). Your non-dominant hand will be 'dirty' and your dominant hand, the one inserting the catheter, will be 'sterile'. The steps are as follows:

• Explain procedure and gain consent.
• Prepare trolley and kit (aseptic technique), and expose patient from umbilicus to above knees.
• Wash hands and put on sterile gloves.
• Tear a small hole in middle of sterile drape and place over genitals.
• With the non-dominant hand hold the penis upright, retract foreskin, and clean around urethral meatus and outwards (use plastic tongs to hold antiseptic-soaked swabs). In women, the non-dominant hand is used to part the labia.
• Instil local anaesthetic gel into the urethral meatus and give it a minute to take effect.
• Place kidney dish just below ready to catch urine.
• Tear off the top of the catheter's inner plastic wrapping, without touching the catheter, and introduce the tip into the urethra.
• Gently feed the catheter, peeling back the wrapper as you go, into the bladder up to the hilt—urine will begin to drain.
• *Do not force the catheter*—you could create a false passage.
• Then inflate the catheter balloon with sterile water (the volume required will be marked on the catheter) to secure it in place, watching all the while that inflating it does not cause the patient pain (indicating that it could be in the wrong place).
• *NB*: beware of excruciating pain and frank traumatic haematuria if the balloon is inflated within the urethra as opposed within the base of the bladder.
• Attach the catheter to a urine bag (urinometer if monitoring hourly output) and ensure that in a male patient that you draw the foreskin back down—*otherwise the patient is at risk of paraphimosis → possible gangrene or necrosis of the glans penis*.

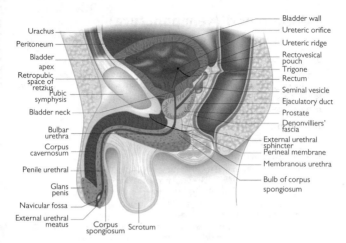

Fig. 45.3 Sagittal section of the male bladder and urethra. Reproduced with permission from Hamdy, F.C., and Eardley, I., *Oxford Textbook of Urological Surgery*, 2017, Oxford University Press.

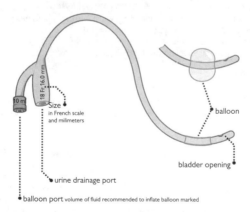

Fig. 45.4 Anatomy of a urinary catheter. Reproduced from https://commons. wikimedia.org/wiki/File:Foley_catheter_inflated_and_deflated_EN.svg, licensed under the Creative Commons Attribution-Share Alike 3.0 Unported license.

In male patients, if there is some initial resistance when passing the catheter, try moving the angle of the penis down to overcome resistance at the prostate. There are two bends but the membranous urethra has more resistance. Remember that the urethra forms an angle of roughly 45° (range 0–90°) at the midpoint of the prostatic urethra.

Taking blood (venepuncture)

There are several different systems for taking blood samples (from central lines on the ICU to heel pricks in infants). Remember that if you are siting an IV line, ensure you take blood samples from the back of the cannula if required. Also, beware taking samples from areas that will give you false results (e.g. above an IV infusion). Practise with a plastic arm—the feeling is not the same but it is useful to rehearse the steps before trying on a real patient. See Table 45.2 for common blood tests.

Indications

Blood sampling and infusion.

Contraindications

Leave patients with bleeding or clotting problems to your seniors (e.g. the patient with haemophilia). Likewise, if you are inexperienced, do not learn on patients with known HIV, hepatitis infection, or the combative patient. Remember that any patient might have a blood-borne infection and that you must take precautions to avoid a *needle-stick injury*. If you do accidentally stick yourself, tell your seniors immediately, make sure a risk assessment is made, and that your local hospital needle-stick policy is followed.

NB: never re-sheathe a needle!

First aid for needle-stick injury

- Splash to mouth/eyes—wash thoroughly with water.
- Skin puncture—encourage bleeding, wash with soap and water/ chlorhexidine—do not scrub or suck wound.
- HIV exposure possible—urgent clinical review for PEP.
- Follow hospital guideline on sharps injury.

Procedure

Kit

Trolley/tray, sterile wipe, gloves, tourniquet, tape/cotton/plaster, needle (green, 21 G, less likely to haemolyse sample), syringe (or vacutainer), sample bottles, and sharps bin.

Choosing your vein

(See Fig. 45.5.) *Do not* use arteriovenous fistulas, damaged areas of skin (e.g. burns or dermatitis due to risk of infection), thrombosed or recently used veins, and be careful when trying for a vein near an artery such as the median cubital vein that runs over the brachial artery in the antecubital fossa, protected by the bicipital aponeurosis which lies between them (known as the 'grace a Dieu', or 'by the grace of God' fascia in the barber surgeon days). The best place to start is either the top of the hands or in the antecubital fossae.

- Gain verbal consent.
- Consider anaesthetic gel, which takes about 45 min to work, especially in needle-phobic or young patients.
- Wash your hands and wear non-sterile gloves.
- Once you have identified a suitable vein, place tourniquet (but not so tight that you stop arterial flow) and *never* walk away from a patient with a tourniquet in place.

Table 45.2 Common blood tests

Usual bottle colour type)	Test name	Testing for
Lavender/purple (EDTA)	Full blood count (FBC)	Hb, WCC (and subtypes), platelets, MCV, haematocrit
	Erythrocyte sedimentation rate (ESR)	ESR
	Glycated haemoglobin	HbA1c
Yellow/gold (SST II)	U&E/renal profile	Urea, creatinine, sodium, potassium, bicarbonate
	Bone profile	Adjusted calcium, phosphate
	Creatine kinase	CK
	LFT	Bilirubin, AST, ALT, ALP, albumin, gamma-glutamyl transpeptidase (GGT)
	TFT	TSH, T4, T3
	Complement-reactive protein	CRP
	Lipid profile	Low-/high-density lipoprotein/triglycerides
	Iron studies	Serum iron, ferritin, transferrin saturation, and total iron-binding capacity (TIBC)
	Others	Magnesium
		Troponin
		Drug concentrations
		Urate
		Tumour markers
		Toxicology
		Autoantibodies
Light blue (sodium citrate)	Clotting screen (CS)	Prothrombin time (PT), APTT, INR, thrombin time (TT), fibrinogen, factor assays
	International normalized ratio	INR
	D-dimer	D-dimer
Grey (fluoride oxalate)		Blood glucose
		Lactate
Pink	Group and save	G&S
	Cross-match	XM
Green (heparin & PST II)		Vitamins, insulin, ammonia, aldosterone
Dark blue	Trace element	Zinc, copper, selenium
Blood cultures		Blue—aerobic
		Purple—anaerobic

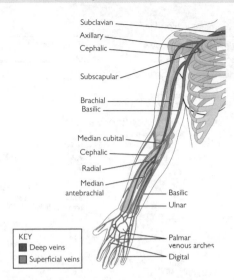

Fig. 45.5 Upper limb venous system. Reproduced from https://commons.
wikimedia.org/wiki/File:2134_Thoracic_Upper_Limb_Veins.jpg, licensed under the
Creative Commons Attribution-Share Alike 3.0 Unported license.

- Gently tap or rub the vein if it is still hiding.
- Clean the area with antiseptic wipe.
- Pull the skin down below the vein to stabilize and straighten it.
- Insert needle at angle of 20° (go through the skin quickly, and then slow down), until you have a flashback.
- If using a syringe, withdraw required amount.
- If using a Vacutainer® system (double-ended needle), you will not have a flashback—you know you are in the right place if the collection bottle on the rubber-coated needle fills with blood.
- *Release* tourniquet, *then* remove needle from vein.
- Apply gentle but firm pressure with cotton/gauze until bleeding stops and cover with a plaster.
- If you have used a syringe, do not use the needle to fill the bottles (risk of sharps injury)—take the needle off, and syringe the blood into the bottles (with their caps removed).
- Fill lithium heparin bottles (U&E) *before* EDTA and clotting bottles so that samples are not inadvertently contaminated. Ensure samples are correctly labelled.
- Dispose of your sharps carefully in a sharps bin.

Butterfly needles with clear tubing to attach to a syringe, allow you to see a flashback and their wings help you to guide the needle in. Some have a rubber-coated safety needle at the other end of the tubing to attach to a Vacutainer® system.

Arterial blood gas

Indications

Assess gas exchange (respiratory component) and acid–base status (metabolic component), and immediate information on electrolytes.

It is also useful to monitor the patient after comparing to previous results. This is particularly important if your patient is known to have chronic respiratory disease with existing chronic ABG changes.

Normal values (for arterial blood; lower pO_2 and higher pCO_2 in venous sampling):

- pH: 7.35–7.45.
- pO_2: 10–14 kPa.
- pCO_2: 4.5–6 kPa.
- Base excess (BE): −2 to 2.
- HCO_3: 22–26 mmol/L.
- Lactate: <2 mmol/L.

Contraindications

Include arteriovenous fistulae, abnormal Allen test, local infection, or severe PVD.

Equipment

Trolley/tray, sterile wipe, gloves, tourniquet, tape/cotton/plaster, ABG needle plus syringe, and sharps bin.

Procedure

- Choosing your artery: common arteries sampled from include radial > femoral > posterior tibialis. If sampling from the radial artery, perform the Allen test which measures arterial competency to the hand (arterial supply: radial = 30–40% vs ulnar = 60–70%):
- Instruct the patient to clench the fist → occlude both ulnar and radial arteries → check that the palm has blanched → release pressure on the ulnar artery only:
  - *Positive test*: if the hand flushes within 15 sec it indicates that the ulnar artery has good blood flow.
  - *Negative test*: if the hand does *not* flush within 15 sec, it indicates that ulnar circulation is insufficient or non-existent → do not sample from radial artery.
- Place your index and middle finger tips over the radial artery.
- In between your two finger tips, slowly aim the needle either at 90° (perpendicular) or angle at 45°.
- If the artery is punctured, then there will be a flush of flashback as the syringe fills up with bright red blood.
- Beware, if the blood is dark red and fills the syringe slowly you may have likely sampled venous blood instead. This may not be an issue if you are mainly after electrolyte and Hb results quickly.
- Once completed, remove the needle and replace with a bung.
- Remember to sample a sufficient volume. The ABG machine will not be able analyse insufficient amounts.
- You have ~10–15 min to get your sample to the ABG machine for analysis or the sample may clot. The ABG syringes are pre-filled with an anticoagulant additive to reduce the risk of this. Yet, ABG sample clotting happens all the time!
- Make a note of the details and FiO_2 for the ABG machine.

Intravenous and intraosseous cannula insertion ('line', 'drip')

Intravenous access

Get good at this early. It can save a life. And as with other procedures, do not lose heart when you are struggling to get a line in—everyone, however senior, still has their bad cannula days. Much of the advice for venepuncture applies here (and read the venepuncture pages first, to ensure you are aware of what to do in the event of a *needle-stick injury*). Make sure you are supervised and ensure you follow your medical school guidelines on what you can and cannot do, especially the injection of fluids through the cannula (e.g. a 0.9% saline flush to keep the line open). Again, practising on a plastic arm in the clinical skills lab is helpful.

Indications

This is a standard hospital procedure for repeated blood sampling, resuscitation, administration of IV medications (including fluids, antibiotics, chemotherapy, nutrition, anaesthesia, blood transfusions and contrast for imaging (e.g. CT and MRI)).

Thomas Latta, cholera, and the invention of IV fluid therapy

The 1831 cholera pandemic came by sea from India and spread across Europe, reaching the UK that winter. *The Lancet* contained several conflicting articles, extolling either venesection or oxygen gas but a Scottish physician, Dr Thomas Latta, published a letter which recommended injecting large quantities of salty, distilled water through the basilic vein, via a silver syringe, being careful to avoid air embolism. His first patient, after initial recovery, relapsed and died.

His second patient, after receiving ~9 L of fluid in 12 hours, recovered after 48 hours.[1] Timely fluid treatment using oral rehydration salts and, if the patient is shocked, IV fluids saves tens of thousands of lives each year from cholera outbreaks in poor-country settings.

Contraindications

As in the venepuncture guidance, be wary of placing cannulas in patients with bleeding or infection problems.

Procedure

Kit

Trolley/tray, sterile wipe, gloves, tourniquet, tape/cotton/plaster, IV cannula, syringe (to flush line with 0.9% saline, another to take blood samples from back of cannula), cannula dressing and tapes, and sharps bin.

Size of cannula

- 14 G (orange), 16 G (grey): wide-bore cannulas used in large veins to help resuscitate a patient (e.g. haemorrhage in trauma/*per vaginam* (PV) blood loss). Remember Poiseuille's law: if you double the diameter of a catheter, you ↑ the flow by 16 times (i.e. r^4).
- 18 G (green), 20 G (pink): adults.
- 22 G (blue), 24 G (yellow): children/neonates.

Choosing your vein

Do *not* use arteriovenous fistulas, damaged areas of skin (e.g. burns, dermatitis and previous sites of phlebitis), or thrombosed or recently used veins, and be careful when trying for a vein near an artery.

- Gain verbal consent.
- Consider anaesthetic gel, which takes about 45 min to work, especially in needle-phobic or young patients.
- Wash your hands and wear non-sterile gloves.
- Once you have identified a suitable vein, place tourniquet (but not so tight that you stop arterial flow) and *never* walk away from a patient with a tourniquet in place.
- Gently tap or rub the vein if it is still hiding. Choose a vein that is straight.
- Clean the area with antiseptic wipe.
- Pull the skin down lightly below the vein to stabilize and straighten it.
- Insert needle at angle of 10–20° (go through the skin quickly, and then 'low and slow'), until you have a flashback. It is sometimes worth puncturing the skin just before the vein—do not jump onto it half-way up.
- When you have flashback, withdraw ever so slightly and then gently flick/slide the cannula into the vein over the stationary needle.
- *Release* tourniquet, *then* remove needle from vein.
- Place a small tape across the cannula to keep it stable while you take bloods (if needed, using a syringe) and flush the line with 0.9% saline to make sure the line is patent. You know you are in if the cannula bleeds back well and flushes easily. You might have to reapply the tourniquet to take blood.
- Ensure a sterile bung is placed over the end.
- Dispose of your sharps carefully in a sharps bin.

Intraosseous (IO) access

Trying to get IV access in a sick patient who is peripherally shut down can take time, especially in young children—with devastating consequences. In the resuscitation scenario, standard guidance now teaches that clinicians should not take more than 60–90 sec trying to obtain emergency IV access and that after this, they should use the IO route. Originally a tough, wide-bore cannula (Cook's needle) was hand-screwed into the bone (most often within distal femur, proximal tibia, or proximal humerus), but most resuscitation trolleys now carry a battery powered drill, with which access takes seconds. The commonest insertion site in children is ~2 cm below and medial to the tibial tuberosity. Ask the ED or ward staff to show you the kit and you can practise on plastic limbs. All resuscitation fluids, drugs, and blood products can be put through an IO needle. (See Fig 45.6.)

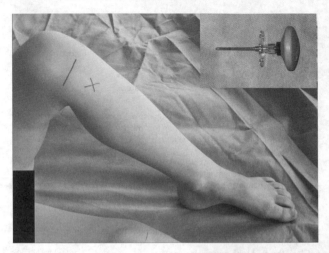

Fig. 45.6 Insertion sites for intraosseous needle in children <6 years, with intraosseous needle (inset). The line indicates the level of the tibial tuberosity; X indicates the insertion point 2–3 cm below on the anteromedial surface of the tibia. Reproduced with permission from Jackson, Guy, et al., *Practical Procedures in Anaesthesia and Critical Care*, 2010, Oxford University Press.

Reference

1. Foëx BA (2003). How the cholera epidemic of 1831 resulted in a new technique for fluid resuscitation. *Emerg Med J* 20:316–18.

Ankle–brachial pressure index

Indication

Quantifying the severity of chronic peripheral arterial disease (PAD) in the lower limb.

Contraindications

- DVT
- Intractable pain
- Open wounds.

Kit

- Sphygmomanometer
- US Doppler probe and gel.

Procedure

See Fig 45.7.

Interpretation

See Table 45.3.

Table 45.3 ABPI = ankle systolic BP/brachial systolic BP

ABPI ratio	Interpretation	Action/follow-up
>1.2	Incompressible/calcified arteries (DM, CKD)	Refer to specialist, control chronic disease
0.9–1.2	Normal	N/A
0.8–0.9	Mild PAD	Modify lifestyle and risk factors
0.5–0.8	Moderate PAD	Routine vascular referral
0.3–0.5	Severe PAD—rest pain	Urgent vascular referral/ED
<0.3	Gangrene/ulceration	

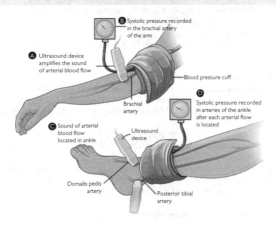

Fig. 45.7 Measuring ABPI. Reproduced from wikimedia under the Creative Commons Attribution-Share Alike 3.0 Unported license.

Basic plastering

Indications
- Splinting/immobilizing for comfort.
- Moulding/maintaining fractures.
- Localized infection.
- Postoperative protection of metalwork.
- Protecting bony and soft tissue injuries.
- Holding joint dislocations.

Contraindications
- Open wounds
- Allergies
- Non-compliance.

Kit
- Plaster of Paris (POP) or fibrecast
- Water in a bowl
- Gloves
- Wool
- Crepe dressing
- Tape
- Gloves and apron
- Stockinette
- Scissors.

Procedure
- Place the stockinette or layer of wool over limb.
- Measure length of limb and cut POP accordingly.
- Place POP/fibrecast in lukewarm water and drain excess water.
- Place POP/fibrecast onto limb and do three-point moulding.
- Ensure there are no cracks in POP.
- Wrap crepe dressing and apply tape.
- Take plain radiograph to ensure no further displacement post plastering.

Notes
- POP is made out of calcium sulphate (gypsum).
- POP can be half (backslabs) to allow for swelling in the acute setting or full casts (e.g. paediatric fractures). Disadvantage is that POP feels heavy.
- Fibrecasts are circumferential full casts and have the advantage of being lightweight.
- Full casts can be removed by being split with an electric oscillating saw.
- The balance is between optimal moulding (difficult with too many layers) and optimal protection (appropriate amount of layers).
- Prolonged immobilization with casting leads to muscle atrophy, joint stiffness, and disuse osteopaenia.
- Split plaster if any danger of swelling.
- Elevate limb.
- Monitor neurovascular observations.

Basic investigations

Urine tests

Urine dipsticks, microscopy, and biochemistry have replaced taste to help screen for infection, renal disorders, pregnancy, and pregnancy-related disorders but inspection (haematuria) and smell (smell of burnt sugar in maple syrup urine disease, an autosomal recessive metabolic disorder) are still useful!

Urine dipstick

Dip the test strip in the sample for 1–2 sec, then wait for 30 sec before reading the different tabs against the dipstick container. (See Fig. 46.1.) Most wards have automatic readers which give a printout of the urinalysis.

Ketones

Are a product of incomplete fat metabolism and a measure of starvation. Used to help diagnose and monitor treatment response to DKA but this has been replaced by measuring blood ketones (beta-hydroxybutyrate) which is a more accurate measurement of ketosis.

Glucose

Normally absent in urine. Can be caused by drugs (some antibiotics, steroids). If positive, requires a blood glucose (see ➜ p. 847).

Specific gravity

Measures the amount of solute in urine compared to water (1.0) and so the kidney's ability to concentrate urine. If <1.005, excessive hydration or inability to concentrate urine (glomerulonephritis, pyelonephritis, diabetes insipidus, AKI). If >1.035, indicates dehydration (diarrhoea/vomiting), SIADH, heart failure, proteinuria, or glucose.

pH

The kidneys help regulate acid–base balance, with normal range anywhere between 4.5 and 8.0 (but usually 5–7).

Blood

Must rule out malignancy! Otherwise indicative of trauma, infection (if tropical travel, think of schistosomiasis), stones, clotting disorder, or a tumour (Wilms' tumour). Also, haemolysis (e.g. sickle cell crisis, toxins). Ask if a female patient is currently menstruating.

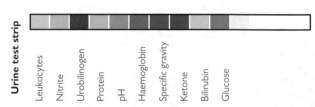

Fig. 46.1 Urine test strip. Reproduced from https://en.wikipedia.org/wiki/Urine_test_strip.

Leucocytes
White cells indicate infection (but also trauma, stones, tumour) so is a non-specific marker of inflammation.

Protein
Normally <150 mg/day excreted. Fever, exercise, hypertension, CCF, infection, nephrotic syndrome, pregnancy (think of pre-eclampsia if hypertensive), and multiple myeloma (although urine dipstick detects albumin and not Bence Jones proteins. Urine is collected over a 24-hour period for more accurate assessment of proteins and solutes).

Nitrites
More sensitive marker for infection (vs leucocytes) as urinary nitrates converted to nitrites by Gram-negative bacteria such as *Escherichia coli*. However, not all bacteria do this (e.g. enterococci) and so test is not very sensitive in infants who pass urine more often than adults.

Microscopy
Some hospitals still count microscopy as a bedside test but most samples are likely sent to the microbiology lab before culturing:
- *RBCs*: >2/mm^3, abnormal (haematuria).
- *Leucocytes* >10 mm^3, pyuria.
- *Organisms*: >50,000 colony-forming units, likely infection (although lower thresholds to treat in patients symptomatic of UTI).
- *Crystals*: may be normal but precursor to calculi (stones).
- *Epithelial cells*: marker for possible contamination with skin flora.
- *Casts*: hyaline—clear, colourless, normal in concentrated urine; granular—breakdown of plasma proteins, indicate CKD; tubular—indicates AKI; waxy—longstanding renal disease.
- *Yeast cells*: most commonly *Candida*.

Urine collection

Important to consider how urine was collected to know likelihood of contamination. A '*clean catch*' is where the patient, after wiping the area around the urethral meatus, voids half the contents of the bladder (to flush off contaminants) and then collects the urine sample—easier said than done, especially in children. You should be alert to the possibility of contamination or colonization of indwelling catheter specimens. Use of in-out catheters, especially in infants, or suprapubic aspiration, reduces likelihood of contamination (but with pain/discomfort and possible complications). Do not use urine bags to obtain urine samples for ?UTI—they will likely be contaminated.

Pregnancy

Urine strips can be bought over the counter for self-testing at home, which detects beta-hCG after the egg implants. Essential test to rule out *ectopic pregnancy* in women of child-bearing age who present with PV bleeding/acute abdominal pain.

Toxicology

For drugs of abuse (but beware over-the-counter medications, e.g. codeine tests positive for opiates).

Urine osmolality

A measure of solute concentration in the urine (more accurate than specific gravity), normally 400–800 mOsm/kg of water but dependent on hydration status. *Low* (<100 mOsm/kg): excessive fluid intake and with AKI (where kidneys unable to concentrate urine). *High* (>1100 mOsm/kg): in dehydration.

Serum osmolality

(Normal = 280–300 mOsm/kg.) When paired with urine osmolality can be used to diagnose SIADH (serum osmolality <270 mOsm/kg and a urine osmolality > than serum level). But this is the other way round in diabetes insipidus, with serum osmolality >320 mOsm/kg and urine osmolality <100 mOsm/kg.

Full blood count

The most commonly ordered blood test in rich country settings, the FBC (or complete blood count, CBC, in North America), has a wealth of information that is often overlooked. Be systematic. Remember, a recent transfusion will affect the results.

Haemoglobin

Amount of oxygen-carrying protein in the blood. A low Hb is <11.5 g/dL for women and <13.5 g/dL for men at sea level. Hb normal ranges vary for children. Anaemia, a low concentration of Hb, has many causes, the main clue being MCV.

Mean cell volume

Normal MCV is 76–96 femtolitres (fL). The MCV is used to classify the three main types of anaemia (see Table 46.1).

Platelets

Normal value 150–400 × 10^9/L. Involved in *primary haemostasis*, triggered by injury to vessel wall, forming a platelet plug. Reduced in bleeding disorders, autoimmune diseases (e.g. idiopathic thrombocytopenic purpura), marrow infiltration (e.g. leukaemia) and marrow suppression (e.g. chemotherapy). ↑After blood loss, surgery, inflammation, and infection.

Haematocrit

The space taken up by RBCs in blood as a %.

Table 46.1 Narrowing your differential for anaemia

Anaemia type	Associated disease
Microcytic anaemia (low MCV)	• Iron deficiency (also, look for raised red cell distribution width) • Thalassaemia (suspect if MCV abnormally low for Hb level and if raised RBC count) • Sideroblastic anaemia (ineffective erythropoiesis secondary to myeloproliferative, congenital, and toxic causes, e.g. lead poisoning)
Normocytic anaemia (normal MCV)	• Acute blood loss • Haemolysis • Anaemia of chronic disease • Pregnancy • Bone marrow (look at WCC and platelets) • Renal failure
Macrocytic anaemia (raised MCV)	• Alcohol excess • Vitamin B12 or folate deficiency • Drugs (cytotoxics)

Red cell distribution width

An ↑ in variation in RBC size (anisocytosis) is suggestive of iron deficiency.

White cell count

WCC is the total number of white blood cells (WBCs) in a given volume of blood (normal range for adults 4–11 × 10^9/L), with the differential breaking down the number of five different types of infection (see Table 46.2).

Mean cell haemoglobin (MCH)

Mass of Hb in RBCs, read alongside mean cell haemoglobin concentration (MCHC): concentration of haemoglobin inside RBCs, low in hypochromic anaemias (e.g. iron deficiency), high in hyperchromic anaemias (e.g. hereditary spherocytosis).

> **Top tip**
>
> *Common pitfalls with bloods*
> - Filling plain blood tubes *after* those with anticoagulant (EDTA, clotting), which can affect results.
> - Ensure clotting bottles are full (or lab will reject sample).
> - Taking blood from an arm with an IV line (false electrolyte results).
> - Squeezed/old samples can falsely raise potassium level.
> - *Be obsessive about labelling samples.*

Table 46.2 The differential white cell count

Type of WBC	↑WCC	↓WCC
Neutrophils (2–7.5 × 10^9/L)	• Bacterial infection • Inflammation (e.g. MI) • Malignancy	• Viral infection • Chemotherapy • Severe sepsis • Bone marrow failure
Lymphocytes (1.5–4.5 × 10^9/L)	• Viral infection • Chronic infection (TB, syphilis) • Leukaemias, lymphomas	• HIV • Steroid treatment
Eosinophils (0.04–0.4 × 10^9/L)	• Allergy (asthma, eczema) • Parasites (e.g. helminths)	
Monocytes (0.2–0.8 × 10^9/L)	• Chemo/radiotherapy • Chronic infection (TB) • Malignancy	
Basophils (0–0.1 × 10^9/L)	• Viral infection • Myeloproliferative disorders • IgE-mediated hypersensitivity reactions (e.g. urticaria) • Inflammatory disorders (e.g. rheumatoid arthritis, UC)	

Other haematology tests

Iron studies

Not part of the FBC but iron, total iron binding capacity (TIBC), and ferritin are looked at to interpret a low Hb level. Ferritin is also an acute phase reactant so can be raised in infection. (See Table 46.3.)

Reticulocyte count

This is a measure of new red cell production (new RBCs contain RNA while mature RBCs do not—normal range 0.8–2%) as a percentage of total RBCs and can further help determine the cause of anaemia: raised in haemolytic anaemias (along with ↑bilirubin); ↓ in bone marrow failure from cancer, infection, iron deficiency anaemia, and aplastic anaemia.

Blood film

A haematological diagnosis can be made with careful examination of a peripheral blood film, including *malaria*. Some common blood film terms:
- Anisocytosis: varying RBC size (iron deficiency anaemia).
- Basophilic stippling: denatured RNA seen in RBCs secondary to haemoglobinopathy, lead poisoning, and megaloblastic anaemia.
- Blast cells: abnormal, nucleated precursor cells, diagnosis of leukaemia.
- Heinz bodies: denatured haemoglobin seen in oxidative haemolysis (e.g. G6PD deficiency).
- Howell–Jolly bodies: remnants of DNA usually removed from RBCs by the spleen, so seen post splenectomy or in hyposplenism (e.g. sickle cell disease).
- Hypochromia: pale staining of RBCs secondary to ↓Hb.
- Left shift: immature neutrophils, seen in infection.
- Right shift: hypermature white cells seen in megaloblastic anaemia (e.g. vitamin B12 deficiency), liver disease.
- Rouleaux formation: RBCs stack up together (like rolls of new coins), seen in chronic inflammation (see ➲ 'Erythrocyte sedimentation rate' p. 847).
- Toxic granulation: ↑granulation in neutrophils, from infection.

Table 46.3 Interpreting plasma iron studies

	Iron	TIBC	Ferritin
Iron deficiency	↓	↑	↓
Anaemia of chronic disease	↓	↓	↑
Chronic haemolysis	↑	↓	↑
Haemochromatosis	↑	↓	↑
Pregnancy	↑	↑/n	n
Sideroblastic anaemia	↑	n	↑

Reproduced with permission from Wilkinson, Ian, et al., *Oxford Handbook of Clinical Medicine* 10th ed, Oxford University Press 2017, p327.

Clotting/coagulation studies

Clotting studies look at secondary haemostasis, the fibrin clot formation that occurs after primary haemostasis (platelet plug formation and vasoconstriction). This is made to happen via the coagulation cascade, which follows either the intrinsic or extrinsic pathways, joining in a final common pathway and fibrin clot formation (see Fig. 46.2). Knowing which part of the clotting profile tests which part of the cascade will help you to a diagnosis.

Prothrombin time (PT)

Tests the *extrinsic system* but is more often expressed as an *INR* to aid the monitoring of warfarin therapy (*normal* = 0.9–1.2). The PT/INR is prolonged (abnormal) by warfarin, liver disease (e.g. paracetamol overdose), vitamin K deficiency, or DIC.

Activated partial thromboplastin time (APTT)

Normal: 35–45 sec. Tests the *intrinsic pathway* and is prolonged by heparin, DIC, liver disease, and haemophilia (Factor VIII or IX deficiencies).

Thrombin time (TT)

Normal: 10–15 sec. Used to assess function of fibrinogen. Prolonged by heparin and DIC.

Fibrinogen

Normal: 1.5–4 g/L. Tests fibrinogen activity. Reduced by consumption of fibrinogen from bleeding/trauma, liver disease, and DIC.

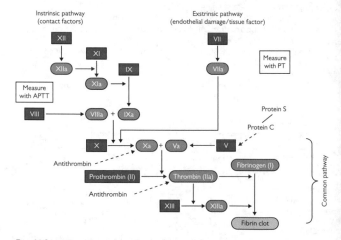

Fig. 46.2 Coagulation cascade. Reproduced from Marco Tubaro et al. (eds.), *ESC Textbook of Intensive and Acute Cardiac Care*, Oxford University Press, Oxford, UK, Copyright © European Society of Cardiology 2011, by permission of Oxford University Press.

Clinical chemistry

Blood glucose

The quickest way to measure blood glucose is with a bedside blood glucose test strip (often called a 'BM' which actually stands for a company that made them) but their accuracy is limited with either very low (important in hypoglycaemic neonates) or very high readings. Get someone to show you how to use one. A venous blood glucose level should be sent for either abnormally high or low readings. Remember the fitting or unconscious patient, ABC and DEFG ('don't ever forget glucose').

Normal fasting blood glucose
- Adults: 3.5–5.5 mmol/L.
- Children: 3–5.3 mmol/L.

Diabetes (WHO)
Fasting venous glucose >7 mmol/L on two separate occasions or random level >11.1 mmol/L. Oral glucose tolerance test (OGTT), 2-hour value >11.1 mmol/L.

C-reactive protein

CRP is a marker of inflammation but one which must be taken in clinical context. A protein produced by the liver, it was first identified in patients in the 1930s with pneumococcal infection, where the protein reacted with a 'C' antigen of the pneumococcal bacterium. It rises quickly in infection and other inflammatory disorders but also goes down quickly with either resolution or the right treatment. However, a low CRP does not rule out a serious bacterial infection (could this level be an early rise?) so is of less use if thinking about discharging a patient from the ED. Also, highly sensitive CRP (hs-CRP) has begun to have a role in predicting cardiovascular disease outcomes in adults. (see Table 46.4).

Erythrocyte sedimentation rate

An alternative marker of inflammation is the ESR ('sed' rate) but this goes up and down more slowly and takes longer to process in the lab. However, it is still used to screen for joint infections and inflammation (e.g. IBD). Upper limit of normal: men = age/2; women = age + 10/2.

Table 46.4 CRP levels: a rough guide

Condition (adults)	CRP level (mg/L)
Normal	<10
Mild inflammation (viral illness, steroids, obesity, ulcerative colitis)	10–40
Bacterial infection, Crohn's	40–200
Sepsis, severe trauma	>200

Urea and electrolytes

The kidneys are vital to homeostasis in several areas:
- Acid–base balance, electrolyte levels (Na^+, K^+, Ca^{2+}, and PO_4^{3-}).
- Removing waste products (including urea).
- RBC production (erythropoietin).
- BP (renin).
- Vitamin D (hydroxylating 25-hydroxyvitamin D → 1,25 hydroxyvitamin D).

Know the differentials for *pre-renal* (poor blood supply, e.g. blood loss, heart failure, renal artery stenosis), *renal* (toxins, sepsis, cancer, trauma), and *post-renal failure* (preventing urinary flow and so backing up to the kidneys, e.g. bladder/prostate cancer, urinary retention, posterior urethral valves in male newborns).

U&E is a commonly ordered panel, especially for patients on fluid therapy or where fluid balance is an issue. In the 2009 National Confidential Enquiry into Patient Outcome and Death (NCEPOD), it was found that 43% of patients with post-admission *AKI* (see ➔ p. 420) were diagnosed late, and it recommended U&E for all emergency admissions.[1] U&E are used as a simplified marker for disease and, hopefully, disease resolution in this highly complex organ. *Always take a drug history* to look for drug-induced causes of impaired renal function.

Sodium (Na)

Normal: 135–145 mmol/L. Risk of seizures, arrhythmias if *sodium <120 mmol/L* (severe hyponatraemia, e.g. Addison's, diuretics, DKA, D&V, nephrotic syndrome, cardiac failure, SIADH, iatrogenic) *or >155 mmol/L* (hypernatraemia, e.g. fluid deficit from D&V, burns, osmotic diuresis secondary to DKA, diabetes insipidus, iatrogenic). Serum sodium needs to be corrected in the presence of hyperglycaemia, i.e. in DKA. Corrected (i.e. actual) Na = measured Na + 0.3 (glucose − 5.5) mmol/L.

Potassium (K⁺)

Normal: 3.5–5 mmol/L. A high potassium (severe *hyperkalaemia, >6.5 mmol/L*) is an emergency. Remember, presumed artefactual results should be repeated. Causes include metabolic acidosis (e.g. DKA), renal failure, Addison's, massive blood transfusion, burns, and drugs.

A low potassium (severe *hypokalaemia, <2.5 mmol/L*) can present with cramping pain, palpitations, muscle weakness, and ↓muscle tone and can cause arrhythmias (ECG: prolonged PR interval, ST depression, small/inverted T waves, U waves). Causes include severe gastroenteritis, pyloric stenosis in infants, diuretics, intestinal fistula, Cushing's (glucocorticoid excess), and Conn's (aldosterone producing adenoma) syndromes.

Urea

Normal: 2.5–6.7 mmol/L (blood urea nitrogen, or BUN in North America). A waste product from protein metabolism produced by the liver (converted from toxic ammonia) that is excreted by the kidneys in urine. A raised serum urea points to renal failure, acute or chronic. Remember that urea can also be raised by dehydration and blood loss (e.g. a marker for upper GI bleeding). It is used alongside creatinine (see next paragraph) to monitor kidney function.

Creatinine

Normal: 70–150 μmol/L. The most common measure of renal function, 'creatinine' is derived from the Greek 'κρέας', or 'flesh', as it is derived from creatine phosphate, a waste product from muscle that is excreted by the kidneys. However, a 'normal' creatinine level depends on an individual's muscle mass (see Fig. 46.2).

Estimated glomerular filtration rate (eGFR)

Normal: >90 mL/min. A more accurate way to test renal function than serum creatinine is an estimate of the glomerular filtration rate, i.e. how much the kidney is filtering, normally around 100 mL/min. An example of its importance is prescribing nephrotoxic drugs—an elderly patient's creatinine may be 'normal' but his low muscle mass might be masking poor renal function, which would more likely to be picked up by eGFR.

There are logistical difficulties in finding out accurate creatinine clearance from both *24-hour urine collection* and *inulin clearance* (requires IV inulin infusion) so most labs use the *MDRD equation* (Modification of Diet in Renal Disease Study Group), which calculates eGFR based on serum creatinine, sex, age, and ethnicity (African-Caribbean/non-African-Caribbean).

However, the MDRD's accuracy is debated alongside that of the CKD-EPI and Cockcroft–Gault equations.[2] You should be aware of the *Cockcroft–Gault equation*, which takes into account the patient's serum creatinine, age, sex, and weight:

Creatinine clearance = (140 − age in years) × (weight in kg) × 1.23 (for males, 0.85 for women)/serum creatinine μmol/L

References

1. National Confidential Enquiry into Patient Outcomes and Death. Acute Kidney Injury (2009). *Adding Insult to Injury*. ℰ www.ncepod.org.uk/2009report1/Downloads/AKI_summary.pdf

2. Willems JM, Vlasveld T, den Elzen WP, et al. (2013). Performance of Cockcroft-Gault, MDRD, and CKD-EPI in estimating prevalence of renal function and predicting survival in the oldest old. *BMC Geriatr* 13:113.

Liver function tests

Remember, *clotting studies* are also an important marker of the liver's synthetic function, e.g. production of proteins (and the liver team will groan if a clotting has not been taken alongside LFTs in assessing a patient with suspected liver disease). There are some common patterns to liver disease but there are important caveats (e.g. other systems can upset the results). As with the kidney, look at the *drug chart* for potential culprits in liver disease.

Albumin

Normal: 35–50 g/L. Alongside clotting, another marker of the liver's synthetic function. It *decreases* when abnormal and is a marker for more chronic liver disease. It is also reduced in malnutrition, sepsis (leaky capillaries), and malabsorption. Albumin can also be a marker for protein loss, e.g. peeing out proteins in nephrotic syndrome or loss from burns. *Oedema* is the clinical sign of a low albumin.

Alkaline phosphatase (ALP)

Normal: 30–150 IU/L. Raised ALP is a marker for liver disease, primarily cholestasis but also in cirrhosis and malignancy. A high ALP is seen in bone metastases, healing fractures, and other bone disease but is normal during the growth spurt in children and in pregnant women (produced by the placenta).

Alanine and aspartate aminotransferase (ALT, AST)

Normal: both 5–35 IU/L. Raised with damage to hepatocytes (viral or drug-induced hepatitis). ALT is specific to the liver while AST is also raised with damage to cardiac and skeletal muscle. Can be normal in end-stage liver cirrhosis. An AST:ALT ratio of >2:1 is suggestive of alcoholic liver disease.

Gamma-glutamyl transferase (GGT)

Normal: 0–45 IU/L. Raised in alcoholic liver damage, cholestasis, and secondary to drugs.

Total bilirubin

Normal: 3–17 μmol/L. *Jaundice*, the yellowing of skin and sclerae, is visible when the bilirubin level is 35–40 μmol/L. Bilirubin is formed by the breakdown of haemoglobin; unconjugated bilirubin is (1) taken up by the liver; (2) conjugated by hepatocytes with glucuronic acid, making it water soluble; then (3) excreted in bile, some of which is changed either to urobilinogen by gut bacteria (and then excreted by the kidneys) or stercobilinogen which makes stool brown.

A *split bilirubin* can point to whether the problem is:
- *pre-hepatic* (unconjugated): haemolysis from haemoglobinopathies, physiological jaundice in neonates, drugs (e.g. antimalarials)
- *intra-hepatic* (mixed picture): viral hepatitis, cirrhosis, drugs
- *post-hepatic* (conjugated): obstructive, e.g. gallstone obstructing biliary duct or carcinoma of the pancreas obstructing the CBD (NB: pale chalky stools and dark urine are signs of a conjugated hyperbilirubinaemia as bilirubin is concentrated in the urine but not making it to the stools—a crucial bit of information not to miss in a neonate who might have biliary atresia). (See Table 46.5.)

Table 46.5 Some common patterns in liver disease

Type of liver disease	LFTs
Acute hepatitis (e.g. viral, drug-induced)	↑↑ALT/AST (>1000 μmol/L), ALP and bilirubin slightly raised, clotting abnormalities
Alcoholic liver disease	AST:ALT ratio of >2:1, ↑GGT, ↑MCV (macrocytosis), ↓albumin
Obstructive jaundice (e.g. cholestasis)	↑↑ALP, ↑GGT, ↑bilirubin (conjugated)
End-stage liver disease	↓Albumin, ↑AST (ALT often normal)

Remember to include *viral hepatitis* in your differential in travellers, health workers, those at risk of STI, IV drug users, and patients with tattoos/body piercing. Hepatitis B and C are spread through exposure to infected body fluids (hepatitis D infections occur only in those already infected with hepatitis B). Hepatitis A and E are spread through the faecal-oral route—usually a self-limiting illness, although hepatitis E has a high mortality in pregnant women. Hepatitis A and B are vaccine preventable (also hepatitis D via hepatitis B vaccine).

Amylase: normal <100 IU/L (up to 180 IU/L in Asians, West Indians, and Chinese). Not a LFT but a marker for *pancreatitis* (if result >1000 IU/L or three times the upper limit of normal). Often ordered as part of the workup for an acute abdomen. It can also be raised in DKA, parotitis (salivary glands produce amylase), and severe gastroenteritis. Not useful for chronic pancreatitis as amylase levels drop after 48–72 hours.

Bone profile

The interplay of parathyroid hormone (PTH), calcium, phosphate, and Vitamin D is complex. When interpreting the bone profile, remember that PTH regulates the level of ionized calcium in the bloodstream (important for cardiac and muscle function and blood clotting). High *phosphate* levels are seen in chronic renal failure and can → calciphylaxis, the deposition of calcium and phosphate in tissues other than bone.

Calcium (Ca^{2+})

Normal: 2.12–2.65 mmol/L. A corrected calcium is usually reported to account for calcium bound by the protein albumin. It is unbound, ionized calcium that is active.

If calcium is low (*hypocalcaemia*), PTH is released to grab stores from bone (↑osteoclast activity)—a problem in patients with kidney failure who can't replace calcium stores as the kidney is unable to process vitamin D, or for those who've had their parathyroid glands removed. Signs and symptoms, 'SPASMODIC':

- Spasms (e.g. Trousseau's sign—carpopedal spasm on inflating BP cuff)
- Prolonged corrected QT interval (QTc) on ECG
- Anxious
- Seizures
- Muscle tone↑
- Orientation impaired
- Dermatitis
- Impetigo herpetiformis
- Chvostek's sign (twitching of face when facial nerve tapped over parotid gland).

For *hypercalcaemia*, remember '*bones, stones, groans, and moans*'—bone pain, renal stones, depression, abdominal pain, lethargy, confusion; bony metastases, primary and tertiary hyperparathyroidism, TB, sarcoidosis, vitamin D overdose, and lithium are some of the causes. Also, can → cardiac arrest (shortened QT on ECG).

Blood gases

Blood gas analysis is straightforward—honest!—if you look at the result in a systematic way. But also look at *all* the results—remember some gas machines will give blood glucose (*DEFG*—'*don't ever forget glucose*'), Hb, bilirubin, lactate, and carbon monoxide levels, any of which might need treating. Remember, you can get most of the information you need from a venous sample (or capillary sample in infants), thus avoiding a painful arterial stab, but venous gases are not as accurate for CO_2 and O_2 measurement.[1]

The numbers

- *pH: normal* = 7.35–7.45. Below 7.35 and your patient is acidotic, above 7.45 and she is alkalotic.
- *CO_2: normal* 4.7–6.0 kPa. Acidic, so if raised, e.g. with a respiratory problem, and the pH is <7.35, you have a *respiratory acidosis*. If the CO_2 is down and the pH is >7.45, you have a respiratory alkalosis (from hyperventilation). If the pH is <7.35 but the CO_2 is also low (e.g. 3.0 kPa), your patient is compensating for acidosis.
- *HCO_3^- (bicarbonate): normal* = 22–28 mmol/L. Alkaline, low in acidosis and raised in alkalosis. A change to HCO_3^- → *metabolic* problem.
- *Anion gap: normal* = 10–18 mmol/L. An indirect measure of anions in plasma, e.g. ketones. Anion gap = cations (Na^+ and K^+) – anions (Cl^- and HCO_3^-). Helpful to pin down cause of a metabolic acidosis. ↑*Anion gap*: DKA (ketones), shock (lactic acidosis), drugs/toxins (e.g. salicylates) (see ➲ metabolic acidosis later in this topic for more detail).

Some examples:

- ↓*pH*, ↑*pCO₂*: *respiratory acidosis*, e.g. a problem with alveolar ventilation (e.g. asthma, COPD), a neuromuscular problem, foreign body in airway, or depressed respiratory drive (e.g. opiate overdose)—this hypercapnia (raised pCO₂) is *type 2 respiratory failure*. Type 1 respiratory failure is hypoxaemia with a normal CO_2, where the problem is either a low ambient oxygen level (e.g. altitude) or V/Q mismatch (e.g. PE, acute pulmonary oedema) where oxygen is not getting into the blood.
- ↑*pH*, ↓*pCO₂*: *respiratory alkalosis*, from hyperventilation (e.g. stroke, and other central causes, anxiety, pregnancy).
- ↓*pH*, ↓*HCO₃⁻*: *metabolic acidosis*. If you have this picture, work out the *anion gap* (see earlier in topic) to help determine the underlying cause—'MUDPILES':
  - **M**ethanol
  - **U**raemia
  - **D**iabetic ketoacidosis
  - **P**araldehyde
  - **I**soniazid/Iron overdose
  - **L**actic acidosis
  - **E**thylene glycol intoxication
  - **S**alicylate intoxication.

  A normal anion gap—renal tubular acidosis, diarrhoea, GI fistula.
- ↑*pH*, ↑*HCO₃⁻*: *metabolic alkalosis*, e.g. vomiting, burns, ingestion of alkali/base.

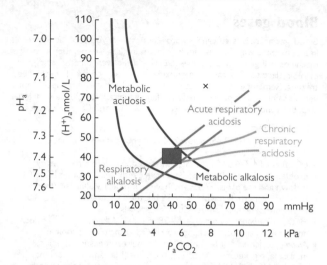

Fig. 46.3 Blood gas analysis. Reproduced with permission from Wilkinson, Ian, et al., *Oxford Handbook of Clinical Medicine* 10th ed, Oxford University Press 2017, Fig 14.2.

Honours

The above, standard approach to blood gas analysis is what we tend to use in everyday clinical practice but be aware that this is based mainly on the carbonic acid reaction, using pH, PCO_2, HCO_3/base excess to work out the respiratory and/or metabolic causes underlying a patient's presentation. There is now growing interest in Canadian physiologist Peter Stewart's *strong ion theory* which, alongside the carbonic reaction, shows the following also affect pH:

- strong ion difference (SID)—difference between positively charged ions (cations, e.g. sodium) and negatively charged ions (anions, e.g. chloride)
- the action of non-volatile weak acids, e.g. plasma proteins, mainly albumin

Standard blood gas analysis is a simplification![2]

References

1. Byrne AL, Bennett M, Chatterji R, et al. (2014). Peripheral venous and arterial blood gas analysis in adults: are they comparable? A systematic review and meta-analysis. *Respirology* 19(2):168–75.
2. Samuels M, Wieteska S (Eds) (2016). *Advanced Paediatric Life Support: A Practical Approach to Emergencies*. Oxford: Wiley.

Electrocardiogram

The electrocardiogram, or electrocardiograph (ECG or EKG in the US), provides a snapshot of the heart's electrical activity, the patterns of which change with various disease processes. This summary cannot possibly teach all the normal variants and caveats that come with looking at ECGs on the wards and reading elsewhere in greater depth on how to interpret them is recommended. The following basics apply to adults (there are several important age-dependent variants in children).

Top reference for ECG interpretation

Hampton JR (2013). *The ECG Made Easy*. 8th ed. Edinburgh: Churchill Livingstone.

Be systematic in your approach and you will not miss important pathology—it is worth checking:
- it is the right patient!
- Rate and rhythm
- axis
- P-wave morphology, PR interval
- QRS complexes (description)
- ST segments
- T waves
- QTc.

Quick revision of what the ECG is looking at

- *P wave*: depolarization of atria (remember, repolarization is hidden behind the QRS complex) → atrial contraction.
- *QRS complex*: depolarization of ventricles → ventricular contraction.
- *T wave*: repolarization of the ventricles.
- *Limb leads*: I, II, aVL—left cardiac lateral surface; aVR—the right atrium; III and aVF—the inferior surface of the heart.
- *Chest leads*: V1, V2—right ventricle; V3, V4—ventricular septum; V5, V6—left ventricle.

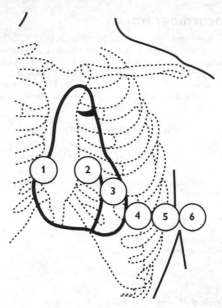

Fig. 46.4 Placement of ECG leads. 1, right sternal edge, 4th intercostal space. 2, left sternal edge, 4th intercostal space. v3, between 2 and 4; 4, 5th intercostal space, mid-clavicular line. 5, anterior axillary line. 6, mid-axillary line. (7, posterior axillary line.) Reproduced with permission from Wilkinson, Ian, et al., *Oxford Handbook of Clinical Medicine* 10th ed, Oxford University Press 2017, Fig 3.6.

Electrocardiogram assessment

Rate/rhythm

Normal heart rate in adults = 60–100 bpm (sinus tachycardia >100 bpm, sinus bradycardia <60 bpm). Normal sinus rhythm means that a P wave always precedes a QRS complex (i.e. the atria contract before the ventricles). Atrial fibrillation will have no easily identifiable P waves and the QRS complexes will be 'irregularly irregular'—like the patient's pulse (you can prove this to yourself by placing a piece of paper over the top of three successive R waves, marking them and then moving the paper along to the next set of R waves on the rhythm strip—they will not line up). Remember that in children and young people, the heartbeat can vary with respiration and so the irregularly spaced QRS complexes—which are all preceded by a P wave—are normal (sinus arrhythmia).

Axis

The sum of all the competing electrical forces during depolarization of the ventricles. If you imagine a clock over the front of the heart, the normal path of depolarization runs from 11 o'clock to 5 o'clock. As this spreads towards leads I, II, and III, the QRS complexes are predominantly positive (i.e. the R wave is greater than the S wave).

- If the right ventricle enlarges (hypertrophies)—e.g. due to conditions that put a strain on the right side of the heart—the depolarization wave spreads towards the right (or 7–8 o'clock), causing lead I to be negative (downward deflection) while III is positive. This is *right axis deviation* (RAD).
- If depolarization spreads towards the left (2 o'clock), there will be a negative deflection in lead III (and more pronounced if also in lead II). This is *left axis deviation* (LAD), a sign of left ventricular hypertrophy. RAD can be normal in tall, thin patients and LAD normal in short patients with a raised BMI but look for pathology with either, especially LAD.

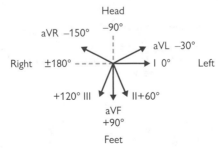

Fig. 46.5 Planes represented by the limb 'leads'. Reproduced with permission from Wilkinson, Ian, et al., *Oxford Handbook of Clinical Medicine* 10th ed, Oxford University Press, 2017, Fig 3.4.

P wave

Must be present before each QRS complex for sinus rhythm. Normal PR interval = 0.12–0.2 sec (3–5 small squares). If >0.2 sec, it signifies first-degree heart block (prolonged conduction time between atria and ventricles).

Peaked P wave

Right atrial hypertrophy (*P pulmonale*).

Bifid P wave

Left atrial hypertrophy (*P mitrale*). A shortened PR interval suggests faster atrioventricular conduction, e.g. *Wolff–Parkinson–White syndrome* (which also has a 'slurred upstroke' known as a delta wave at the start of the QRS complex).

QRS complex

Normal is <0.12 sec duration (3 small squares), i.e. narrow complexes. Broad complexes (i.e. >0.12 sec) associated with bundle branch block (conduction problem) and left ventricular hypertrophy. Q waves >0.04 sec wide (1 small square) or >2 mm deep indicate myocardial infarction, with the lead indicating where the ischaemic damage has occurred. Normal Q waves can be seen in leads V6, I, and aVL, mirroring septal depolarization.

ST segment

Should be at the same level as the line of the PR interval, i.e. isoelectric. ST elevation (the ST segment moves to a level >1 mm higher than the line of the PR interval) indicates acute myocardial infarction (death of cardiac muscle) or, if across most leads, pericarditis. ST depression indicates myocardial ischaemia (lack of blood supply and therefore oxygen to the heart).

T waves

Normally upright except in aVR, V1, and up to V3 in children. An inverted or 'flipped' T wave can be a sign of bundle branch block, myocardial ischaemia, treatment with digoxin, or ventricular hypertrophy. Peaked T waves in hyperkalaemia, flattened T waves in hypokalaemia.

QTc

Calculated to look for a prolonged QT interval (measured from start of QRS to end of T wave). Calculated as follows: $QTc = QT / \sqrt{RR}$. Causes of prolongation include congenital, certain drugs (e.g. tricyclics, macrolides), electrolyte abnormalities (hypokalaemia/hypocalcaemia/hypomagnesaemia), and myocardial ischaemia.

Ethics and law

The basics

Although medical schools take different approaches to ethics, in the UK the starting point will usually be the consensus statement. It lists the areas every medical student should learn during their training and also describes competencies that students should develop. The consensus statement in medical ethics is summarized in the following section with some examples. The full version is available on the Institute of Medical Ethics website (℗ www.instituteofmedicalethics.org). The eagle-eyed will notice that even the summary includes areas in which few, if any, medical students, will be directly involved. Medicine is a mixture of the applied and the arcane. However, it is helpful to think about the relationship between what you are learning and your practice.

For example, in sessions on genome editing or cloning, you can relish (really) the intellectual gymnastics of debates about personhood and identity. In contrast, when you are learning about consent, it is important to think of it both in terms of its conceptual elements and its practical application. What are the basics of ethics? One way to answer that question is to think about the transition from the lecture theatre to the clinical environment. The ways in which you experience consent, confidentiality, questions of dignity (sometimes yours as well as the patient's), capacity (ditto), and decision-making are fundamental. These areas have both conceptual and practical meaning. For that reason and given that our time together is limited, let us focus on those.

Consensus statement in medical ethics

- Patients: their values, narratives, rights, and responsibilities.
- Consent and refusal in medical decision-making: e.g. the constituent elements of valid consent, proxy consent.
- Capacity: e.g. the Mental Capacity Act, Deprivation of Liberty Safeguards, best interests.
- Confidentiality: e.g. the limits to confidentiality, the role of trust in therapeutic relationships.
- Justice and public health ethics: e.g. resource allocation.
- Ethico-legal aspects of working with children and young people: e.g. the Children Act, Gillick competence, the concept of assent.
- Mental health ethics and the legal framework: e.g. the Mental Health Act.
- Ethics at the beginning of life: e.g. reproductive ethics, neonatal ethics.
- Towards the end of life: e.g. assisted dying, resuscitation decision-making, death certification.
- Medical research and audit: e.g. research governance, research with people who lack capacity, global considerations in research.
- Generic competencies: e.g. awareness of ethical questions or considerations, analytic and reasoning skills, reflective practice.

Capacity and consent

As a medical student, you will seek consent hundreds, possibly thousands, of times. It is a familiar task, yet it is also the way in which you demonstrate a fundamental ethical commitment, namely your respect for self-determination. For students, consent is particularly important—no one has to talk to a student or let someone who is not qualified examine them—you always have to ask permission. For a patient to make an informed choice, you must explain your student status. The four elements of consent are each experienced differently as a student. First, there is the question of capacity, i.e. can this person understand, remember, and weigh up what is happening or being proposed? If a patient does not have capacity, they cannot agree or disagree to you doing anything. Anything that happens to a patient without capacity should be either on the basis of proxy consent (if there is a valid lasting power of attorney) or best interests. It is difficult to argue that it is in best interests of a person who lacks capacity to have a student, rather than a qualified doctor, perform an examination or provide treatment, although in some settings you may be invited to contribute under close supervision.

Assuming the patient has capacity, he/she has to give consent voluntarily. You need to be clear that it is a choice whether a student is involved. Next, is the question of information: the patient needs enough to make a decision with the emphasis being on what the patient wants to know rather than what the professionals want to tell. Relevant information includes that you are a student and your stage of training. Occasionally, you may be introduced misleadingly (e.g. as a 'colleague' or a 'doctor in training'). It is your job to ensure that the patient understands that you are a student and not yet qualified. Finally, consent has to be continuing which means the patient can change his or her mind.

The excitement of clinical placements can mean that even the best students forget the basics of consent. However fascinating the learning opportunity, the essence of your privileged status as a medical student is trust. And trust depends on your honesty and sensitivity in seeking consent, always. Whatever the pressures, you obtain permission. No exceptions.

Confidentiality and dignity

There is a tension between what you learn about confidentiality and dignity and the realities of clinical practice. Attending to the dignity and privacy of a patient is essential. People reveal themselves at their most vulnerable and they do it because they assume you will respect their dignity and protect their privacy. Yet, there is much about healthcare that can compromise privacy and dignity. Many of these things are systemic. Curtains round the bed can (usually) be pulled to protect others seeing what is happening, but sound travels easily whether the curtains are closed or not. Ward rounds share personal information within a group that continues its conversations as it moves through the hospital. Teams meet in the canteen partly because everyone is craving coffee and partly because there is no spare room. Whiteboards, visible to all, aid clinical care, but are less effective at protecting confidentiality. You cannot be an ethical superhero and defend against all these systemic failures, but you can think about your own behaviour. Beware of lunchtime conversations with friends in public spaces. Think about ways you can protect a patient's dignity. For example, you can cover them up after an examination, check that they are comfortable, and give them quiet space to talk through the implications of their diagnosis with their family. Students often describe feeling powerless as if there is 'nothing they can do'. Yet, sensitivity to privacy and dignity can be transformative and these small ethical acts are valuable.

Decision-making in the clinical setting

People often assume that students do not make any decisions, ethical or otherwise, until they qualify. In fact, students make ethical choices every day: how to introduce themselves, whether to put their own learning before the patient's comfort, and what to do when they are concerned about a peer or a superior. Nonetheless, it is true that students are rarely the ones making decisions about clinical care. However, you can learn much from watching the ways in which decisions are being made, particularly ethical decisions. Sometimes they will be implicit—you observe no discussion, yet everyone appears agreed on the next steps. Other times, you will see explicit decision-making both with patients and their families and within clinical teams. Whatever the subject, from safeguarding to resuscitation and from the determination of best interests to information sharing, you have a unique opportunity as a student to observe decision-making. Try to make your observations count. Does it reflect what you have learnt? Why has this decision been taken? Do you agree with it? Who was involved in making the decision? Will it be reviewed? If so, how, when, and by whom? What was written in the notes about the decision? How is it going to be communicated both to the patient and his or her family and to other professionals? These are not just prompts for the incurious—they are the basis of ethical practice both as a medical student and a doctor.

Do not be afraid to ask politely about why and how decisions have been reached. These conversations provide the foundations for the day when you are the one making the decisions.

Role models and cautionary tales

You will meet a range of people in your training. Some will inspire you and become role models. Others will be more cautionary tales than role models. There is something to learn from everyone you meet, although it may not always be what they claim to be teaching. Role models are essential, especially when times get tough. Everyone has moments of doubt in medical school, particularly after bruising days. Role models are invaluable for helping you get through those moments. Find people who remind you why you want to do medicine and what kind of a doctor you want to become. Notice what it is about them that inspires you and hang on to it in your own practice. They have; you can too.

What of the cautionary tales? Those whom you would dread becoming or even simply just dread? They are important too. They represent your ethical boundaries and identity. You respond to them negatively because something is at odds with what you believe or know to be right. That is the hidden gem in these horrid encounters. In rejecting their approach, you affirm your own commitment to ethical practice and maintaining your integrity. Now, that is all well and good, but how does that get you through the day when you are working with someone who is causing you distress? You do not need to struggle on alone. All medical schools will have members of staff who will support students who have concerns about the practice they encounter in the clinical setting and most will also have systems to allow for confidential feedback about student experiences. I know that the perceived 'risk' of confiding in someone about a senior is significant, but there are safe ways of speaking out and getting some support. Please find and use them.

'Be kind, no exceptions'

Whether it is in a lecture theatre, an OSCE, or a real clinical setting, you will encounter ethics in many ways. Sometimes, you will need to hit the books and get to grips with specific knowledge. Sometimes, you will practise how to apply conceptual learning to clinical situations. Sometimes, you will experience ethics in ways that seem far removed from what you have encountered in the classroom or examination room. Whether you love or loathe the subject, it is inescapable and how you respond is often, in itself, a moral choice. As you shift between types of learning in different places, perhaps the most important thing is to remember what brought you to medicine in the first place. Although motivation will vary, you will never meet anyone who entered medicine wanting to do a poor job.

Part 5

Assessments and examinations

Clinical assessments

Clinical assessments: overview

What are they for?

A number of different assessments will occur during clinical school, which may be *formative* (i.e. largely for the student's benefit in terms of learning and reflection), *summative* (a minimum mark is required to progress through the course, and could count towards your final grade), or may even contribute to job applications. The purpose of this section is to outline the different *clinical* assessments you may face during your clinical attachments and at the end of clinical school.

Case presentations

It is common at the end of a clinical attachment to be asked to present a patient you have encountered. You should expect to spend ~5 min presenting and perhaps 10 min discussing the issues raised. Your examiner is likely to be a consultant or registrar.

Some important tips include the following:

- Keep it brief! Imagine you are on a post-take ward round where there are 20 patients to be seen in a morning. Include pertinent information only (including important negatives) and state it succinctly.
- Start with some medical background if it is immediately relevant to the current admission; breathlessness 4 weeks after a CABG raises a very particular list of differential diagnoses to be considered compared to breathlessness in someone with no PMHx.
- Also add some social detail early on if this is likely to have a major impact on the patient's management: 'This is a 92-year-old lady from a nursing home with end-stage dementia ...'
- After describing the patient's history and your examination findings, list the differential diagnoses, perhaps with a brief comment about which are the likeliest, or the most important to exclude.
- You should then propose a management plan (remember that management includes investigations and treatment). Include some detail about which would be the most discriminating tests, or what you would be looking for in each case.
- Summarize the case with one or two sentences: 'To conclude, this is a 64-year-old man who presents with right upper quadrant pain and fever. The most likely cause is gallstones and I would investigate him further with an ultrasound of the biliary tree.'
- Be prepared for questions about the differential diagnoses, the value of different investigations (e.g. V/Q scan vs CTPA in possible PE), and risks/benefits of different treatments.
- What learning points or issues has this case raised?

You may also be asked to compile a portfolio of written case presentations, in which case you should use the same format as in medical note keeping with a brief section at the end discussing relevant issues.

Objective structured clinical examinations

OSCEs test clinical examination, practical skills, and communication skills, usually in 10 min 'stations' around which you rotate in turn. You could be asked to dipstick urine, perform a cognitive assessment, or certify death in the same sitting. Although a somewhat artificial environment, the OSCE reflects the multitasking and varied nature of life as a junior doctor.

Some important points to remember include the following:

- Behave as you would in real life, by washing your hands, introducing yourself to the patient, and asking permission before acting.
- Ensure patient dignity, only exposing them after seeking permission and checking with the examiner that it is necessary. Be mindful that the patient may see 20 medical students that morning and may be fatigued.
- Time keeping is also very important. If you have only 7 min to perform a neurological examination of the lower limbs, you need to be mindful of this and ensure you cover all aspects in this time. This will require practice!
- Do not be disheartened by a bad station. As soon as the bell rings, you should move on to the next task and forget what has passed. The next examiner will not know what has just happened and you can start afresh and make a good impression.
- A critical point to remember is that OSCEs are scored using a very prescriptive mark sheet. There is little allowance for the examiner's subjective impression of performance (as there would be in real life). If you are not seen to wash your hands or to state that you are looking for scleral jaundice, then the mark will not be awarded. State the obvious!
- The mark sheets may well be based on whatever learning materials have been made available to you. If you have been given a suggested routine for BP taking, it would be unwise to do much differently in the exam. Read and learn the routines!
- Remember the most vital traits in a new doctor are patient safety and appropriate respect/concern for the patient. These values are likely to be reflected in mark schemes.
- OSCEs provide a robust (and quantitative) assessment of all-round performance in clinical school. As a result, they often contribute significantly to the final mark. It is well worth putting in the time to practise these routines in advance.

Some examples of OSCE stations include:

- handwashing/scrubbing up
- venepuncture
- systems exam (e.g. CVS/GI)
- consenting for procedures
- counselling/break bad news
- urinary catheterization
- urine dip/DRE
- focused history taking.

Learning portfolios

Some medical schools use learning portfolios as a method of gathering evidence about your performance at medical school through work-based assessments (WBAs) or supervised learning events (SLEs). The assessments are often based on those that will be used in your graduate training and beyond, e.g. mini-clinical evaluation exercises (Mini-CEX), case-based discussions (CBDs), direct observation of procedural skills (DOPS), and multisource feedback (MSF). The assessor will usually be a doctor in the team to which you are currently attached.

Mini-CEX

A focused encounter such as assessing a patient's airway or performing an abdominal examination.

CBD

The student chooses a case for discussion, starts with a brief presentation, and then explores the issues raised.

MSF

Sometimes known as a 360° appraisal or mini-peer assessment tool (mini-PAT). The student selects a number of colleagues (doctors, nurses, healthcare assistants, physiotherapists, and administrative staff) to complete a form describing their performance, attitude, team work, and professionalism.

DOPS

There are a set of procedures where you need to demonstrate competency under supervision (cannulation, catheterization, peak flow, etc.)

Developing the clinical teacher

Assessment of teaching and/or making a presentation, and to develop skills in preparation and scene-setting, delivery of material, subject knowledge, and ability to answer questions.

All assessments are done electronically through an e-learning website. If the assessor is not there in person to sign you off, you can generate an e-ticket to be sent to the assessor's email address to be signed off later. This is an opportunity for both of you to highlight your strengths and weaknesses as well as an action plan to continue your professional development.

Situational judgement test

The SJT is an essential requirement in the final year of clinical schools nationwide, and the score is considered in ranking Foundation Year applications. It is worth getting right! Further information can be found at ℬ http://sjt.foundationprogramme.nhs.uk.

The SJT tests attitudes, priorities, and professional behaviour, replicating as best it can the nuances and thought processes involved in making clinical decisions. You are asked to rank answers, e.g. in order of the most to least appropriate, or to select three appropriate responses from a list of eight.

Example questions are shown in Box 48.1.

Top tip

There are plenty of examples and a rich question bank available from Metcalfe D, Dev H (2018). *Situational Judgement Test*, 3rd ed. Oxford: Oxford University Press.

Box 48.1 Example situational judgement tests

Example 1

You are just finishing a busy shift on the Acute Assessment Unit (AAU). Your FY1 colleague who is due to replace you for the evening shift leaves a message with the nurse in charge that she will be 15–30 min late. There is only a 30-min overlap between your timetables to handover to your colleague. You need to leave on time as you have a social engagement to attend with your partner.

Rank in order the following actions in response to this situation:
(1= most appropriate; 5= least appropriate.)

A. Make a list of the patients under your care on the AAU, detailing their outstanding issues, and leave this on the doctor's office noticeboard when your shift ends and then leave at the end of your shift.

B. Quickly go around each of the patients on the AAU, leaving an entry in the notes highlighting the major outstanding issues relating to each patient and then leave at the end of your shift.

C. Make a list of patients and outstanding investigations to give to your colleague as soon as she arrives.

D. Ask your registrar if you can leave a list of your patients and their outstanding issues with him to give to your colleague when she arrives and then leave at the end of your shift.

E. Leave a message for your partner explaining that you will be 30 min late.

Answer: ECDBA

Clearly this question is assessing professionalism and prioritizing clinical responsibilities over social concerns. It emphasizes the importance of face-to-face verbal handover rather than written notes. Although handing over jobs to your registrar may seem inappropriate, in the interest of patient safety it is preferable to leaving notes in this instance.

(Continued)

Box 48.1 (Contd.)

Example 2

You review a patient on the surgical ward who has had an appendicectomy done earlier on the day. You write a prescription for strong painkillers. The staff nurse challenges your decision and refuses to give the medication to the patient.

Choose the THREE most appropriate actions to take in this situation:

A. Instruct the nurse to give the medication to the patient.

B. Discuss with the nurse why she disagrees with the prescription.

C. Ask a senior colleague for advice.

D. Complete a clinical incident form.

E. Cancel the prescription on the nurse's advice.

F. Arrange to speak to the nurse later to discuss your working relationship.

G. Write in the medical notes that the nurse has declined to give the medication.

H. Review the case again.

Answer: BCH

The aim here is to assess your ability to interact effectively with colleagues in challenging situations, and also to recognize your limitations and accept your decisions being questioned.

Reproduced from ♒ http://sjt.foundationprogramme.nhs.uk/sample.

Preparing for clinical examinations

Introducing clinical examinations

Clinical examinations will test your ability to perform effective history taking, communication, physical examinations, and procedural skills. The method employed by most medical schools is the OSCE which consists of a series of short and highly focused 'stations'. The exact format of clinical examinations is often subtly different between medical schools and even between year groups within the same medical school, and it is important you establish the nature of your clinical examinations. They may utilize actors particularly in history taking stations where the examiners can ensure identical patient responses to each candidate's questions, in order to ensure an objective and reproducible assessment. While they are often focused on a specific system (see ⊃ Chapter 50) it is important to behave authentically as you would in a clinical setting.

What are they testing?

OSCEs were first introduced to medical schools in 1975 to assess skills not measured by written assessments. These include:

- observational skills
- ability to build rapport
- communication skills
- problem-solving ability
- clinical knowledge
- practical skills.

You will note that some of these skills are generic (i.e. they will apply across all specialties) while others can be specific (i.e. clinical knowledge) (see Table 49.1). The balance of emphasis on these skills will be different in different specialties. For example, communication skills may make up a very small proportion (or may not be marked at all) at an advanced life support station when you are performing CPR on a dummy, while active listening and good communication may be the main component of a psychiatry station. However, both of those are extreme examples and you will find that almost all OSCEs assess manner, communication, and the ubiquitous hand hygiene (communication skills and respect for patient dignity are still marked if you are performing a pelvic exam on a plastic model, for example.)

Table 49.1 Examples of skills

Examples of specific skills	Examples of generic skills
• Recognition of T-wave inversion on ECG	• Explains procedure to patient and gains consent
• Elicits dull percussion note on chest examination	• Good hand hygiene
• Able to describe maculopapular rash	• Presents examination findings succinctly
• Identification of effusion on chest X-ray	• Able to form differential diagnoses

You will find it very difficult to pass your OSCEs if you emphasize speedy diagnosis and fact-reciting at the expense of politeness, consideration, and kindness. Ignore these 'soft skills' at your peril. They are at the heart of good medical practice.

How do they work?

A typical OSCE consists of a number of stations (usually around 10–15), each comprising a clinical scenario—taking blood, for example, or breaking bad news. Each station typically has one or two examiners. Sometimes there is another person in the room acting as an independent examiner, who will be assessing the way the OSCE is taking place, and not you. Sometimes a layperson is brought in to give a 'person on the street' opinion of your manner and communication skills. This is more common in stations where communication is the main skill being assessed, such as a breaking bad news station, or an alcohol counselling station in psychiatry or general practice.

OSCE stations use a variety of methods to illustrate clinical scenarios. These include:

- models (e.g. a plastic arm for venepuncture, or a torso for CPR)
- actors (e.g. playing a bereaved partner or angry family member)
- multimedia (e.g. a photo of a rash or a radiograph)
- real patient (e.g. with rheumatoid arthritis or a heart murmur).

Most OSCEs will have a mix of these components, but the balance will be different depending on the specialty.

Taking a history

You will be asked to take either a formal history (e.g. for 10–15 min) or a focused history (e.g. for 5–10 min). Even a formal history requires constant refinement of a differential diagnosis throughout the process, asking closed questions to exclude or highlight possible diagnoses. This will take time to develop, but is essential to score well in clinical examinations. One way of achieving this will be to ask about specific risk factors for common presentations (e.g. jaundice, haemoptysis, and melaena).

Focused history of risk factors for jaundice

Ask about:

- blood transfusions, unprotected intercourse, IV drug usage and sharing needles (hepatitis B and C)
- recent travel (e.g. hepatitis A)
- medicine (e.g. co-amoxiclav causing cholestasis 6 weeks later)
- alcohol (e.g. cirrhosis, hepatocellular carcinoma)
- constitutional symptoms—anorexia, weight loss (cachexia), night sweats (e.g. hepatic/pancreatic malignancy)
- FHx (e.g. Gilbert's syndrome)
- recent HPB surgery (e.g. postoperative complication, retained biliary stone post cholecystectomy).

Examinations

You may have up to 10 min to complete an examination of one particular system (cardiovascular, respiratory, endocrine, etc.) You will be expected to follow the standard procedure of inspection, palpation, percussion, and auscultation (IPPA). In joint exams, you may present your findings as look, feel, and move.

Some students prefer speaking through the examination to report the presence or absence of pertinent clinical signs, while others report their findings at the end.

Practical procedures

You will be given 5–15 min to perform a task in which you will not only be assessed on your practical skills but also how you communicate with the patient through the procedure. Set aside time every week to practise basic practical skills in the skills laboratory. Some common procedures include venesection, ABG, blood cultures, IV cannulation, urinary catheterization, suturing, DRE, vaginal examination, measuring BP, urine dipstick, performing an ECG, measuring peak expiratory flow, and prescribing and administering IV fluids.

Explaining a procedure and gaining consent

You are usually given 10 min to explain a procedure (breast biopsy, colonoscopy, etc.) or gain informed consent. While you will need to have an understanding of the procedure, your assessment will be weighted towards your communication skills. Your task is to explain an invasive procedure, without using medical jargon or complicated terminology. This may also involve explaining the risks of a procedure— knowing the rates of perforation, haemorrhage, infection, failure of procedure, and mortality can be helpful, although precise figures need to be used cautiously if at all. You will need to be able to provide the patient with all the information they require in a way they understand it, and respond to any concerns they may have.

Breaking bad news

This is an important skill to learn but should ideally be done by a senior doctor with a nurse at a scheduled meeting, in an appropriate environment with the patient and their relatives. In the exam situation, you will not be afforded such a luxury, and it will be your task to break bad news alone (e.g. you are on call and have to explain the death of a patient to visiting relatives at night). The following points may be of help:

• *Prior preparation*: this is essential for both you and the patient/relatives. Read the patient's notes beforehand including all the latest results (e.g. blood tests and scans). Mentally rehearse the consultation and the questions you might be asked. Be ready to discuss the significance of results from investigations, and opinions from other specialities and your seniors.

• *Consent*: this must be sought from the patient, where possible, in order to divulge information in front of anyone else, including family members. Patients still have the right to their autonomy and you must respect their wishes, even if they prefer not to know about their diagnosis.

- *Introductions*: these are necessary so that you know who you are addressing. Also make a note of all those present in the patient's notes.
- *Establish pre-existing knowledge*: this should be asked about at the beginning of the meeting to establish what is already known, and what the patient/family would like to know.
- *Signposting and warning shots*: these are effective in psychologically preparing patients to receive some bad news; cryptic and ambiguous language will not help. It is acceptable to say 'Unfortunately, I have some bad news to share with you'.
- *Time*: this is a powerful component in such consultations. After breaking bad news to the patient sensibly, allow adequate time for the information to sink in and do expect emotional reactions such as denial, crying, anger, and shock.
- *Amount of information*: this should be given at the patient's pace, and will need to be judged individually. Everyone can process bad news better if given in manageable chunks. Keep monitoring their responses to the information given, and move forward with the consultation while reconfirming their understanding.
- *Empathy*: this will avoid the patient feeling isolated. You may not fully understand what they are feeling but demonstrate that you can relate to them by imagining being in their position. Offer hope but not at the expense of being honest and realistic about treatment and prognosis. Do not commit to a time-frame or make any false promises.
- *Language*: must be simple, understandable, and without jargon.
- *ICE*: this is a mnemonic (Ideas, Concerns, and Expectations) for you to address the patient's ideas and concerns about the bad news given and expectations from your team.
- *Summarize*: do this at the end because the patient may still be processing the bad news as opposed to all the other matters discussed including management options and counselling. Make sure that the patient is able to understand and repeat the information given back to you at the end of the consultation.
- *Follow-up*: by arranging another time to meet with the patient and family members which will give them more time to process the bad news, and provide them with contact details to get in touch if any further questions arise in the meantime.

Use one of the items in Box 49.1 as a model to guide your consultation.

Box 49.1 Items to guide your consultation

Setting	Advanced preparation	Background
Communicate	Build a therapeutic environment	Rapport
Perception	Exploring	Announce
Invitation	Deal with reactions	
Knowledge	Follow-up plan	
Empathy	Kindling	
Summarize.		

How marks are awarded

OSCE scoring systems differ between medical schools. The two main systems are 'tick-box' or 'global impressions.' Their main points are summarized in Table 49.2.

There are plenty of example OSCE mark sheets for each system in Chapter 51.

Table 49.2 OSCE scoring systems

OSCE type	'Tick-box'	'Global impressions'
How it is marked	1 point scored for each action performed. Examples: • Handwashing • Introduction and consent • Ensures patient dignity during examination • Palpate for thrill or heave • Describes systolic murmur over the mitral area • Mentions mitral valve regurgitation in list of differentials • Able to describe other pathological findings in association with mitral valve regurgitation, e.g. pulmonary oedema, signs of heart failure (1 point for each)	General impression of student's approach, courtesy, communication, knowledge of subject, technical skills, and presentation.
Pass mark	Individual stations marked and results totalled Global pass mark for all stations (i.e. total of 160/200 to be achieved overall), or minimal mark for each station to be attained determined by examiners	Each station judged 'fail', 'borderline', or 'pass' Overall 'fail', 'borderline', or 'pass' given based on analysis of performance in all stations
Pros	• Good for point-by-point feedback • Objective	• Evidence shows highly correlated with 'real-life' clinical performance • Used in professional exams
Cons	• Not how many professional exams are marked • Assesses actions but not necessarily quality or confidence—difficult to distinguish between excellent and average candidates	• More subjective • Lacks specific feedback—difficult for student to target areas needing improvement

How examination results are used

Generally speaking, clinical examinations are used in assessment with a written component, but both will have a minimum mark that needs to be exceeded to pass—you cannot fail your OSCE completely then pull yourself up by the written component, or vice versa.

While medical school OSCEs can be left behind you when you graduate, it is worthwhile honing your performance while you can, because OSCEs are here to stay for the rest of your medical training. The GMC is currently running a pilot scheme to incorporate standard OSCEs into specialty interviews from 2017. As well as this official move towards a more standardized grading system, an ↑number of specialties are now using OSCE-style stations for interviews, where applicants analyse a paper, break bad news, or describe clinical imaging, in a break from the increasingly old-fashioned 'Tell me about your greatest achievement' style of interview. PACES (Practical Assessment of Clinical Examination Skills) and MRCS (Member, Royal College of Anaesthetists) may seem a million years off, but the same skills you are developing as a first-year medical student will pay dividends when you become a registrar.

Finally, and most importantly, think about how you will use your exam results to improve your own practice. Remember that the skills you use to pass OSCEs are those you use every day to communicate to your colleagues, assess patients, and formulate a management plan. They are all part of what will make you an excellent doctor.

Will a bad mark affect my future?

We have all had that sinking feeling when opening the results envelope. Perhaps the realization hit early—as you frantically tried to elicit a sign—any sign—from the patient in the 'murmurs' station as the seconds ticked away, or perhaps the mark on the paper came as an unwelcome surprise. Either way, it is not a pleasant feeling.

The good news is that your medical school OSCEs are meant to be formative—to mould you into a better doctor and to teach you about your own weaknesses. A bad mark is not a millstone around your neck—use it as a launching pad to improve your practice. When you are a cardiology registrar, no one will remember that time you listened for the heart on the wrong side in your fourth-year OSCE.

Formative vs summative exams

Formative exams are mock exams to prepare you for finals at the end of the academic year. The exam mark may not count towards your degree but it is a strong indication of your progression in medical studies and may be a warning sign for you, your tutor, and the medical school that you are lagging behind. Summative exams are your final exams of an academic year which count towards completing your degree.

Disabilities/extenuating circumstances

Extra time is given to those with a disability in the form of a physical or mental impairment which has a long-term adverse effect on the person's ability to carry out normal activities according to the Office of

Qualifications and Examinations Regulation (Ofqual). Students with dyslexia or other learning difficulties qualify for extra time in exams as well as governmental support to purchase learning aids. If you are experiencing personal difficulties that may affect your ability to perform in exams, it is crucial that you put this in writing after discussing it with your personal tutor, the welfare officer, and the Dean. No one can help you if you report any issues after you have sat exams.

Intercalated degrees

These are marked by weighted averages according to classes as seen in Table 49.3. A degree may be awarded with or without honours. It is worth noting that most institutions expect those pursuing a higher degree afterwards (e.g. a Master's or PhD) often require at least an upper second in their bachelor's degree. Percentages traditionally correlate with classes (see Table 49.3).

Merits and distinctions

These count on your CV, for your portfolio, and job applications. Less than a quarter of your year will graduate with a distinction in a subject which will appear on their degree certificate. Some universities, like the ones in London, hold an annual Gold Medal competition for only the best.

Awards and scholarships

These are awarded to students scoring the highest marks in both written and clinical examinations. These awards tend to be internal and offered by the board of examiners. Prizes vary but usually consist of several hundred pounds as well as formal recognition on your degree.

Curriculum vitae

This will feature any significant grades such as your merits, distinctions, and intercalated degree award classification. Demonstrating a consistent track record of academic achievement is very important to obtain the jobs you want to progress in your career.

Job applications and interviews

Your employers will look for a strong sense of academic merit. Your accolades demonstrate your knowledge, skill, and attitude. You can discuss these in depth at your job interviews which sets you apart from other candidates.

Table 49.3 Classes of awards for degrees

Class	Average weighted %
First	>70
Upper second	60–69
Lower second	50–59
Third	45–49
Ordinary pass	40–44

Revision strategies

'He who studies medicine without books sails an uncharted sea, but he who studies medicine without patients does not go to sea at all.'

William Osler.

To succeed at clinical examinations, you need clinical experience. No amount of reading will replace hours spent on the wards, which will consolidate your reading, enhance your practical skills, teach you examination tricks not mentioned in books, and show you how doctors communicate with patients, interpret results, and decide on management plans. Never lose sight of the fact that while the immediate and all-consuming concern may be the looming exam and the need to pass, the ultimate goal is to achieve your full potential as an excellent clinician and to pave the way for a lifetime of learning. See your exams as a tool to hone your clinical skills, to alert you to areas of weakness, and to push you to be the best possible doctor you can be to your patients.

1. Know the curriculum

Dull but true. Start by going through the curriculum. You may find surprising areas of weakness that seems to have been missed out in lectures or by yourself. Start by making a list. These will help direct your clinical learning. A word of warning—while it is important to be familiar with the whole curriculum, in case there are any nasty surprises, do not forget the old medical truism: *common things are common*. Examiners like horses, not zebras, and their favourite topics will tend to coincide with the important, bread-and butter sections of clinical medicine. You are very likely to get shown a picture of a fundus with diabetic retinopathy and laser scars—you are unlikely to get a picture with neurosarcoidosis and granulomatous papillitis. Indeed, part of learning to be an excellent doctor is being excellent at recognizing common things, and being excellent at treating them—as well as knowing when to be suspicious that something is out of the ordinary.

2. Develop a system

Tempting as it is to simply open a book and hope the entire contents make their way into your brain so you can repeat it verbatim on demand, it is far better to develop a system for dealing with each condition you come across. Exams are not presented like a textbook, nor will examiners take kindly to you regurgitating a long, meandering list of causes and effects when what they want is a succinct diagnosis, followed by a few pertinent differentials. A system also helps you react to unexpected situations, think through what a surprising examination finding might mean, and try and put the whole thing together into a coherent clinical picture—essential in the stressful environs of an OSCE. Learning in the way exams are presented can be helpful.

For example, you might wish to start learning about lung cancer by beginning with a list of differentials for a radiopaque mass, and go on by considering other ways lung cancer can present, rather than reading through the different types of lung cancer. In terms of presentation, the surgical sieve is a useful start and absolutely priceless if stuck in an OSCE with an examiner demanding to know what could cause this patient to have that weak left arm you have nicely demonstrated. The surgical sieve consists of **VITAMIN ABCDEFG**:

- Vascular
- Infection/inflammatory
- Trauma
- Autoimmune
- Metabolic
- Idiopathic/iatrogenic
- Neoplasia
- Acquired
- Blood
- Congenital
- Drugs/degenerative/developmental
- Endocrine/environmental
- Functional
- Genetic.

There are other systems of presenting and thinking about conditions:
- *Acute vs chronic* (e.g. skin changes in allergic eczema, symptoms of heart failure, causes of a pleural effusion).
- *Immediate vs late* (e.g. side effects of radiotherapy, complications of surgery, symptoms of organ rejection).
- *Local vs systemic* (e.g. symptoms of renal cancer, pulmonary TB).

3. Walk the wards

Armed with a system and a list of target areas, you are ready to hit the wards. Remember, there is no replacement for practical experience. Books are important, and of course there is a balance to be had. However, successful students are overwhelmingly those who have spent more time on the wards. You may know that you have to send off a serum ACTH to diagnose an Addisonian crisis, but only someone who has been on the wards knows the results do not come back for 2 weeks—and that an Addisonian crisis is an urgent clinical diagnosis that needs to be treated without waiting for that blood test. In an OSCE, a few questions can quickly reveal who has put in the time and who has not. More pertinently, that lack of clinical experience will really show when it comes to your first weeks as a nervous doctor. Nevertheless, there are times on the wards when your heart sinks because there is 'nothing to see and nothing's happening'. The key is to bring plenty of reading material and other things to do while you wait for an interesting case—and have faith, because there will be one, sooner or later.

4. Attend clinics

Clinics are an excellent way to spend focused clinical time. They play second fiddle to wards in these revision tips, because too much focus on clinics risks missing out a good deal of general inpatient medicine, which will form the bulk of your medical and surgical exam topics. Having said that, clinics can be extremely useful to swot up on areas of weakness, get exposure to rarer conditions, spend a whole morning just looking at knobbly, arthritic joints, identify suspect skin lesions, or peer into ears—many of which are likely to have actual signs. Do your research before going to a clinic.

5. Tutorials

You can learn from anyone more senior than you—whether it is the students in the year above or the consultant about to retire. You just have to ask. If this seems unbearably impertinent, remember that many students and junior doctors are interested in teaching qualifications, CV points, or need teaching feedback for their ARCP (Annual Review of Competence Progression)—so they may be as keen to teach as you are to be taught. The longer you spend on the wards, the more likely you are to get taught. A spare 10 min may crop up unexpectedly and you may get an impromptu bedside tutorial. Also, the longer you spend getting to know a particular team, the more likely it is they will offer to teach you, or respond well to a request for a tutorial. All levels of seniority will be helpful in teaching. Older students will have just been through the process and may have good tips on good consultants to shadow, common exam topics, or good clinics to attend. Junior doctors also remember what it is like to revise for exams. They will have a huge list of patients with good signs and will grill you on your examination technique. Consultants are, of course, the ultimate authority. They may well be setting your exam, and they will be able to clarify any particularly tricky areas you have been wrestling with. Use them all wisely.

6. Multimedia

There are a wide variety of websites out there to help you revise, with useful videos and pictures. These are particularly useful for learning anatomy, practical techniques, and rare and interesting signs, but can be used to complement any facet of your learning, if you find you are a very visual learner. Podcasts are an excellent way to learn while on the move, and for those with short attention spans or who learn particularly well by listening. There are a number of free podcasts available online, and any medical student forum will come up with a long list of possibilities. There are a number of case-based books. These provide easy bite-sized chunks of revision and are a good way of cramming a little bit of revision into a spare 5 min.

7. Practical labs

Your medical school may organize practical labs as catch-up sessions before OSCEs for stations such as cannula insertion, NG tube placement, suturing, and so on. Take advantage of these. You may be able to organize informal sessions by contacting the practical coordinator in your medical school and arranging access out of hours.

8. Mock exams

- *Practise with your medical friends*. The first time will be excruciating—the second time will be just a bit awkward—and the next time you will be just eager to tell them exactly what they did wrong. Students are the harshest critics—and it is fairly easy to get a group together, pool your knowledge, and share tips.
- *Practise with your non-medical friends*. They will give you hints on communication, manner, and whether you are slipping into medical jargon. They will tell you if your examination leaves them feeling undignified, and if you look convincing when you present, even if they cannot fault you on your knowledge.
- *Practise with doctors*. Junior doctors may be willing to run a 'mock' OSCE in return for teaching feedback—try suggesting it to some you have been shadowing and see if they are open to taking a 30 min session if you can find a small group.

- *Practise in mock exams.* There may be free courses—or very cheap ones—run by other medical students or junior doctors keen for teaching practice. Use these as much as you can—even if they are very informal or not realistic, they are a great way of getting generic feedback and finding your weaknesses.

9. Feedback from previous exams

Feedback from previous OSCEs is an extremely valuable way to inform your exam technique. If you do not automatically get this, try contacting your medical school tutors, who may be able to make this available to you. A helpful way to look at this information is to go through it with a trusted friend or tutor and see if they particularly agree with or can expand on any points made (e.g. if your presentation skills are criticized, might they have noticed you have poor eye contact, or that you tend to repeat yourself?).

10. Take a break!

You cannot study forever. Everyone works more efficiently when they are well rested and energized. So remember to take care of your body as well as your mind. Get enough sleep. Do not burn out just before the exam—an exhausted, demoralized student gives a bad global impression and generally gives a poor performance.

Sources

Clinical examination and skills textbooks

Learn systemic examinations by heart and recognize what signs to look out for in a logical order so that you can perform the examination competently in a timely fashion. Practise your basic clinical skills in the skills laboratory with your colleagues performing the role of the patient. Some popular texts include the following:

- Thomas J, Monaghan T (2014). *Oxford Handbook of Clinical Examination and Practical Skills*, 2nd ed. Oxford University Press.
- Wilkinson IB, Raine T, Wiles K, et al. (2017). *Oxford Handbook of Clinical Medicine*. Oxford University Press.
- Roper TA (2014). *Clinical Skills: Oxford Core Text*, 2nd ed. Oxford University Press.
- Alastair Innes J, Dover AR, Fairhurst K (2018). *Macleod's Clinical Examination*, 14th ed. Churchill Livingstone.

Clinical cases books

Many common clinical scenarios have been compiled in books with recommendations on what to specifically look for and how to present these findings to your examiner in order to gain the highest marks. Some popular texts include the following:

- Farne H, Norris-Cervetto E, Warbrick-Smith J (2015). *Oxford Cases in Medicine and Surgery*, 2nd ed. Oxford University Press.
- Hampton JR (2013). *The ECG Made Easy*, 8th ed. Churchill Livingstone.
- Liakos A, Hill M (2014). *Oxford Assess and Progress: Clinical Medicine*, 2nd ed. Oxford University Press.
- Bain S, Gupta J (2012). *Core Clinical Cases in Medicine and Medical Specialties*, 2nd ed. Hodder Arnold.
- Hall T (2013). *PACES for the MRCP: With 250 Clinical Cases*, 3rd ed. Churchill Livingstone.

Examination videos

Ask your medical school library for any available examination videos. It may be worth watching these videos and then practising each sequential step of the examination with your colleagues. Beware of 'variations' or false advice, particularly online; you will need to develop your own examination style which incorporates the techniques needed to elicit important and relevant signs. Some online references:

- St George's University London: ℘ www.elu.sgul.ac.uk
- Learners TV: ℘ www.learnerstv.com/Free-Medical-video-lecture-courses.htm
- University of Virginia: ℘ www.med-ed.virginia.edu/courses/pom1/videos/index.cfm
- University of Wisconsin: ℘ www.videos.med.wisc.edu
- Ace Medicine: www.acemedicine.com (£59.99/year)
- YouTube.com: examples of most common examinations ℘ www.youtube.com.

Group
Revising with your colleagues allows you to assess each other's performance while gaining the confidence to perform examinations confidently in front of an audience. You can learn from the strengths and weaknesses of others.

Tutor
Request a doctor to act as your group's tutor so that after practising your clinical examinations and skills for a week, you can then be assessed by your seniors for more guidance and tips to polish off your skills. It is worth obtaining a tutor in general medicine and in general surgery and one tutor within each of the clinical specialties (orthopaedics, rheumatology, obstetrics and gynaecology, neurology, etc.) It is important that you learn from your mistakes during practice sessions as opposed to in the exam.

Speak to senior students
Ask for advice from your predecessors who will have recently passed the clinical examinations. They may be able to offer some helpful tips on effective revision strategies, good revision references, personal insights, and may even offer to tutor you for a few sessions.

Observing doctors
While on clinical placements, ask your doctors if they can demonstrate a model example of examining a patient while talking you through each step and justifying their actions. Doctors will also highlight clinical signs on patients during the ward round. They may also offer to observe your examination technique and give some feedback. Bear in mind that there will be some variation in examination technique between doctors but appreciate that everyone has a fixed system of thoroughly examining which is all that matters. Based on a universally accepted method of *inspection, palpation, percussion*, and *auscultation* (or *look, feel*, and *move* in joint examinations).

Wards
These are the most valuable sources of real patients with authentic clinical signs. The more time you spend on the ward clerking and examining patients, the more confident and competent you will become. It is only through repetition you will develop clinical judgement, which will be the product of all your previous knowledge and experiences of different signs and clinical presentations.

Courses
There are an abundant number of courses offered by both medical schools and private groups throughout the year. Although not compulsory, some students feel that they benefit from attending courses near exam time. These courses are usually delivered by registrars and consultants who give brief lectures, demonstrate examinations or skills, and observe you practising your technique on volunteer students/patients under exam conditions. Some of the courses may be of use (see Table 49.4).

Previous mark sheets
Your tutor may have access to some mark sheets used in previous years which give you a template of what is expected of you during clinical examinations. Generic marks are always given for the following actions:

Beginning
- Introduction.
- Hand-washing.
- Explaining the examination/procedure and gaining patient consent.

Middle
- Professionalism and attitude towards patient.
- Fluidity of taking history, clinical examination, or performing clinical skills.
- Being thorough in IPPA or look, feel, and move.
- Clinical knowledge and identifying signs correctly.

End
- Covering and thanking the patient.
- Presenting a concise summary of history/examination and relevant clinical findings/negatives.
- Offering differentials.
- Proposing a sensible management plan.

Table 49.4 Examples of courses

Course	Website	Fee	Days	Location
Q Courses	᧛ www.qcourses.org	£125	2	London
PME	᧛ www.professional medicaleducation.co.uk	£110	2	Nottingham
Ask Dr Clarke	᧛ www.askdoctorclarke.com	£69	1	Nationwide
Hammersmith	᧛ www.hammersmith medicine.com	£75	2	London
Mentor OSCE	᧛ www.mentorosce.com	£140	2	London
Doctors Academy	᧛ www.doctorsacademy.org	£55	1	Manchester
Finalmed	᧛ www.finalmed.com	£167	2	London

15 tips for success in clinical examinations

1. Practice, practice, practice …

… makes perfect. Practise with colleagues everyday on and off the wards. It is often helpful to identify good technique while observing others examining and reflecting. Moreover, if you are able to teach a skill, then you are likely to be competent to perform it yourself since it will force you to simplify and justify the relevant steps. If you are having to think hard about the next item on the agenda, you will not have time to put it together. Practice makes you slick, it helps you recognize patterns, and it will make you outstanding.

2. Preparation

This is the best-kept secret for passing clinical examinations. You cannot rely on last-minute cramming since you need to spend a substantial amount of time applying your clinical skills to real patients.

3. Beginning and end matters

Introduce yourself to the examiner and the patient with your name, grade, consent, and duration of exam so that you put the patient and yourself at ease. Be sure to thank the patient at the end of the clinical encounter.

4. Confidence

This is key to convince both examiner and patient that you are reliable and know what you are doing. Project your voice when speaking and presenting. Do not panic if you get stuck since you will be prompted. In examinations, state whether a sign is present or absent but do not use vague words such as '*I think, it appears, it looks like, it is likely, there could be* …'.

5. Non-verbal communication

This is vital in comforting the patient and empowering them to give you the information you seek and demonstrating your competence to the patient and examiner. Focus on keeping your body language, maintain eye contact, nod to empathize with the patient, and do not forget to smile when re-assuring the patient.

6. Verbal communication

This is one of the most crucial attributes of a good clinician. Engage with the patient's ideas, concerns, and expectations while establishing clinical details. Offer signposts to guide the patient when taking a history. Always summarize at the end to make sure no important information has been over-looked. Avoid medical jargon with the patient at all costs; you may use the correct terminology when presenting your findings to the examiner. Present your key findings first, and tell them the story of your diagnosis. Listen to how junior doctors present to their consultants, and use that as a model.

7. Behave professionally

It is important that you adopt a mindset of a doctor and present yourself appropriately, remembering that your attitude and behaviour will also be assessed. Wear a shirt or blouse, tie, and formal trousers or skirt in neutral colours; dress like a doctor. Be mature and respectful towards the patient and address their concerns to the best of your abilities.

8. Think out loud and putting it all together

Doing this during examinations can minimize the risk of missing out significant clinical signs. Otherwise, you may pick up on something significant which you may forget to mention at the end due to stress and time restraints. If someone has a thyroid mass, look at their legs for pretibial myxoedema, and their hands for thyroid acropachy. If someone has a scar on their chest, look at their legs for vein grafts. This shows everyone you are putting everything together and seeing the bigger picture (look for associations, causes, and complications relevant to the signs you identify). If you do not have time to examine for all those things, mention them in your presentation so the examiner knows you have thought about them.

9. Be systematic

And stick to a format you are used to and have practised over and over again. Always go back to basics if you find yourself struggling: *IPPA* (or *look, feel, and move* in joint examinations).

10. Courtesy

Be courteous to your patient. They are bored and tired and they have had to sit through the same scenario many times already this morning. Remember to help keep their dignity, to ask for consent, and to make sure they are comfortable before you start presenting. If you do this, your examiners will mark you up, and your patients will like you and help you out—they may give you extra clues in the history, or offer up extra information without you explicitly asking for it. This reflects real life, where putting a patient at their ease is likely to result in better communication all round. Be sure to thank the patient at the end of the clinical encounter. Some OSCEs also leave a few marks to be decided by the patient/actor on how they comfortable they felt to have you as their doctor.

11. The little details count

Make sure everything is right. If you are examining confrontational visual fields, make sure you and the patient are on the same level. If you are looking at the JVP and then palpating the abdomen, make sure the patient really is at 45° to start with, and then take the time to lie them completely flat. These are small details but sloppiness here gives a bad impression. More importantly, failing to get the setting right means you may miss key findings. A sloppy clinician is an unobservant clinician.

12. Think laterally

Contrary to popular expectation, OSCEs are not designed by fiends in human form, itching to catch you out on a technicality. However, bear in mind that a 'hand examination' does not always mean musculoskeletal—and can be a catapult to other parts of the examination (e.g. clubbing and yellow nails to the respiratory exam), especially in the 'endocrine' or 'general' station. Remember that certain things can present in the hands—wasting (so think about a lung apex tumour—and exclude a subtle ptosis), or pigmented palmar creases (so look for signs of Addison's).

13. Do not see what you expect to see (or hear)

Develop your skills of really looking and really listening. You might be expecting to hear a murmur in the cardiology station, but if the station is all about identifying the central sternotomy scar and talking about cardiovascular risk factors, then presenting a fictional aortic regurgitation is quite frankly embarrassing. Be confident and back yourself if you think you have found something—but do not go convincing yourself you have found something because you think it should be there.

14. Time yourself

Once you have your routine down in memory, it is time to practise to a strict time limit. Find out what the timings are likely to be in the OSCE, and strictly time yourself. There is nothing worse than running out of time in the exam—you are flustered, worried you have missed something, have not put it together, and now you have to present. If you are not disciplined enough, get a friend or a sibling to do it.

15. Let it go

Do not let failure at one station help you fail the next. Just as with a written exam, do not get hung up on a difficult question. This can be hard, as a bad OSCE station has more psychological impact than turning over an exam page, and is harder to forget. But do it. Turn over that blank page in your mind. The next station is a whole new opportunity. The same goes for the next part in the same OSCE. The examiner may not have noticed you started listening to the heart on the wrong side. Carrying on smoothly and correcting your mistakes mean they may never notice. Drawing attention to it or becoming frustrated and letting it affect the rest of your examination means they definitely will.

Medical history

(See ➲ Chapter 6.)

Presenting complaint

- In the patient's own words, why have they come to see you (what changes (symptoms) have they noticed)?
- Patient's *ideas* about the cause of PC.
- Patient's *concerns*.
- Patient's *expectations* of the consultation.
- Effect/impact of the PC on patient's life (home and work).

History of presenting complaint

- When did symptoms start?
- When were the first changes noticed?
- What has happened since then?
- What has the patient done about it?
- Any over-the-counter medication for PC?
- Previous episodes and what happened last time.
- Characterize pain/symptoms (SOCRATES).
- Investigations and tests.
- Treatment.

Past medical history

- Previous illnesses.
- Previous operations.
- Previous hospitalizations.
- Screening questions: *MJ THREADS*.

Medication/allergies

- Medication for treatment.
- *DRUGS* mnemonic.
- Allergies.

Family history

- Parents, siblings, children, partner—quality of relationships with patient.

Social history

- Age.
- Place of origin.
- Marital status/children.
- Who lives at home?
- Occupation—nature and satisfaction.
- Housing—location and type (e.g. house or flat).

Lifestyle

- Smoking/tobacco:
  - Smoking: 1 pack-year = 20/day/year.
- Alcohol (*CAGE*):
  - 1 unit = ½ pint of beer or 1 glass of wine.
- Recreational drugs.
- Exercise.
- Diet.

Additional lifestyle issues

- Quality of life—effect of illness on daily routine.
  - Activities of daily living: shower, dress, house choirs, shopping.
- Mobility:
  - Independent, needing assistance, walking aids (stick, crutch, Zimmer frame), wheelchair or bed-bound.
- Quality of sleep.
- Sexual history.
- Recent travel.
- Significant life events.

Functional enquiry/systems review

- Systemic/constitutional symptoms:
  - Fever, weight loss, night sweats, lumps, fatigue, loss of appetite.
- Cardiorespiratory:
  - Palpitations, chest pain, breathlessness, wheezing, cough, sputum, haemoptysis, orthopnoea, peripheral oedema.
- Gastrointestinal:
  - Abdominal pain, nausea, vomiting, constipation, diarrhoea, weight change, constipation, PR bleed, mucus discharge.
- Genitourinary:
  - Irritative symptoms (↑frequency, haematuria, dysuria, urgency), obstructive symptoms (hesitancy, intermittent stream, straining, terminal dribbling, incomplete bladder emptying), incontinence, discharge, urinary retention; sexual history.
- Gynaecological:
  - Menstruation, dysmenorrhoea/haemorrhagia; pregnancies.
- Neurological:
  - Headaches, unilateral weakness, neck stiffness, photophobia, seizures, ataxic, falls, dizziness, vertigo, changes in vision/hearing/balance/speech/taste.
- Musculoskeletal:
  - Joint/bone pains, joint stiffness, skin changes, deformed joint, fluid, swelling.
- Psychiatric:
  - Depression, hallucinations, thought (insertion, withdrawal, control), mood.
- Endocrine/thyroid:
  - Thyrotoxicosis (diarrhoea, weight loss, Grave's eye signs, insomnia, tachycardia, palpitations, tremor, acropachy, heat intolerance), hypothyroidism (weight gain, proximal myopathy, alopecia, bradycardia, cold intolerance, constipation), goitre.

Communication tips

- Clarify patient's terms and understanding.
- Make transition statements and signposts.
- Clarify ICE from the patient.
- Empower patients to ask questions.
- Provide a summary at the end.

Useful mnemonics in history taking

Screening for PMHx: MJTHREADS
Malignancy, Jaundice, Tuberculosis, Hypertension/Heart disease, Rheumatic fever, Epilepsy, Asthma, Diabetes, Stroke.

Pain history: SOCRATES

Site	Where exactly is the pain?
Onset	When did pain start, was it gradual or sudden?
Character	Describe pain: sharp, burning, crushing?
Radiation	Pain spreading elsewhere.
Associations	Pain accompanied by other symptoms.
Timing	Pain varying in intensity during the day.
Exacerbating	What makes pain worse or better?
Severity	Score from 0 (no pain) to 10 (maximum).

Medication history (DRUGS)

Doctor	Prescriptions.
Recreational	Non-medicinal drugs (e.g. cannabis, heroin).
User	Pharmacy, over-the-counter, alternative/herbal remedies.
Gynaecological	Contraception.
Sensitivities	Reactions to anaesthetics.

Alcohol overuse screening: CAGE

C	Want to *Cut* down your drinking?
A	*Annoyed* by criticism of your drinking?
G	*Guilty* about drinking?
E	*Eye-opener* in the morning: drinking in the morning to overcome a hangover?

ICE questionnaire—useful phrases
- *Ideas*: what do you know/think/understand about this matter?
- *Concerns*: are you concerned or worried about something?
- *Expectations*: what do you hope for/expect/anticipate from this?

Clinical examinations

Clinical examination: overview

Clinical examination is the art of eliciting physical signs in order to diagnose conditions without recourse to laboratory or radiological investigations. Historically, physical examination was a physician's main diagnostic tool. The advent of technology (e.g. CT scanning) should complement this modality rather than replace it.

Why is it important?

A picture paints a thousand words

A quick glance at a patient can often provide you with more information than a 10 min phone call or two pages of writing. Is the hypotensive patient sitting up drinking tea or unresponsive and in peri-arrest? Is this 80-year-old man sufficiently robust to survive an emergency AAA repair, or frail, malnourished, and better suited for conservative management? Other important skills such as fluid assessments and psychiatric evaluation can only be done well face to face.

'On-the-spot' answers

A number of clinical signs are constant and reliable enough to convey a diagnosis, long before radiological or histological evidence is available. For example, if you see a patient in the ED with spider naevi, gynaecomastia, and palmar erythema, you can be reasonably confident he has chronic liver disease, even if his transaminases are unremarkable and it is days before he has a US showing a cirrhotic liver. In addition, clinical examination can provide answers that other diagnostic modalities can only hint at or infer. A CTPA showing a large PE may also raise the possibility of right heart strain (if paradoxical interventricular septal bowing or reflux into the inferior vena cava is present). However, this information is superseded by your clinical examination of the patient: what is their BP? Is their JVP dilated and raised? Is there a right heart heave? You are unlikely to make the decision to thrombolyse a patient on the basis of CT findings, but clinical signs might change your management.

Targeting investigations

A major part of clinical medicine is knowing what investigations to request in order to reach a diagnosis, while using them responsibly in a targeted fashion. If someone is admitted with breathlessness and your clinical examination finds a gallop rhythm or a heart murmur, you are much more likely to pursue a cardiological approach rather than a respiratory one.

What makes a good clinical examination?

During your first few months of clinical training, the greatest difficulty you will have is remembering which part of the examination comes next, and trying not to forget vital elements of it.

The next challenge will be trying to interpret clinical signs correctly and ultimately synthesize these findings into a coherent list of differential diagnoses ('A systolic murmur could be caused by aortic stenosis or mitral regurgitation').

You then need to use your clinical examination findings to formulate a management plan (e.g. 'In light of these signs, I would like to perform an

ECG, and a lying and standing BP'). In the setting of medical school exams, it is also helpful to be able to pre-empt examiners' questions ('What are the causes of mitral regurgitation?')

This is a lot to ask! Nobody learns how to examine a patient in the space of a week. There is no substitute to repetition; you need to examine patients week in, week out for the duration of your clinical training so that you can perform the examination on autopilot and concentrate on finding the clinical signs. It is clear to examiners which candidates are not comfortable with clinical examinations. Also, you will only learn to recognize 'normal' by seeing as many patients as possible.

Do not invent things. You may think you *should* be hearing a systolic murmur because it would fit in with other findings, but if you do not hear one, then do not report one. It is a greater sin to invent something than to miss it. Be honest. 'I could not see the JVP' or 'I was unable to palpate the carotid pulse' are signs of an honest and trustworthy individual who does not confabulate.

Finally, keep an open mind. In the pursuit of passing finals, it is tempting to think in terms of classical patterns and syndromes. In reality, you will often be surprised by unrelated or unexpected findings which are just as important.

Important *do's* and *don'ts* in clinical examinations

- *Introduce yourself.* Explain that as a medical student, the examination is for your own benefit and will not alter their current management but will help your training. If the patient is obviously distressed or tired, come back another time.
- *Timing.* Medical students should not try to see patients during meal times or any designated rest period. Similarly, try to work around any visitors they may have; seeing family and friends is very important for patient morale.
- *'Popularity'.* Be mindful of the fact that someone with rare but classic signs such as congenital heart disease or polycystic kidneys may have seen scores of students before you.
- *Communication limitations.* Establish early on if the patient has any communication difficulties (e.g. blind or hard of hearing).
- *Ensure patient comfort.* Making sure that they are not in pain or breathless is more important than slavish attention to lying the patient flat or asking them to sit at 45°.
- *Appearance and personal hygiene.* You will be close enough to the patient for them to notice and be affected by your personal hygiene. *Always* wash your hands (soap and water or alcohol gel) in front of the patient. Ensure that you are appropriately dressed in clean clothes and that if you have cycled 5 miles to the hospital that you do not smell as such. If you smoke, you should take measures to disguise the smell. If you openly smell of alcohol from the night before, give patients a miss that day.
- *Dignity and privacy.* You should draw the curtains around the bed for any patient interaction. Ensure you have either a blanket or dressing gown to keep the patient covered if you need to expose any part of them during the examination.

- *Explain what you plan to do.* A patient may agree to you performing a heart examination and then wonder why you spend so long looking at their hands and their neck. Similarly, it may seem obvious to you that you will palpate for the apex beat after inspecting the chest. All the patient will see is you diving towards her left breast. Pre-empt any such difficulties!
- *Reassure.* Explain that most of the signs you are examining for, and indeed are openly discussing, are not specifically relevant to them. Make sure that the patient is not left anxious or bemused by what you have been doing.

Important 'end-of-the-bed' observations

You will learn to pick up on a number of subtle clues to patients' conditions just from inspecting their bed space and looking at the patient from several metres away.

Bed space
- Are you in a high dependency bay? Is the patient on oxygen or a cardiac monitor? Are there infusion pumps running and if so what drug is being administered?
- Are you in a side room? If so, why? (Think MRSA, *Clostridium difficile*, and take appropriate infection control measures.)
- Is the patient on a special air mattress? (Think diabetes, pressure ulcers, immobility, vulnerable skin.)
- Are there walking aids nearby such as a stick, a frame, or even a wheelchair? This gives you a good idea of patient mobility
- Signs above the bed often describe dietary measures (diabetic, low potassium, soft consistency), nursing instructions (e.g. 'red-tray'), or fluid restriction (cardiac or renal failure).
- Patient's effects: magnifying glass or spectacles on the table (visually impaired), hearing aids (hard of hearing), sugar-free drinks (diabetes), sputum pot, inhalers (brown = steroids, blue = salbutamol), glyceryl trinitrate (GTN) spray (red). Cards and gifts may suggest strong family and social support.

The patient
- It is best to start off with obvious but important statements. Let the examiner know that you can spot an acutely ill patient. Confirm the '*three Cs*'; is the patient calm, comfortable, and conscious?
- General appearance. Do they look well or unwell? This is a simple but vital observation that will stand you in good stead in your career. Are they sitting in their chair doing the crossword or lying in bed looking grey?
- Are they overweight or malnourished? Well-kempt or evidence of neglect (prior to admission)? In pain or comfortable?
- Is there evidence of gross abnormality (e.g. amputation, severe peripheral oedema, distended abdomen, facial injuries), surgical scar visible despite clothing (e.g. sternotomy wound), medical devices (e.g. IV cannula, PICC line, central line or urinary catheter), paralysis, hair loss (cytotoxic chemotherapy).

- Patient's affect. Does the patient respond and interact appropriately on your arrival? Could the patient have dementia or be depressed? Is their GCS score clearly compromised?
- Respiratory effort. Is the patient sitting up struggling for breath, using accessory muscles of respiration? Or are they comfortably asleep on their back on your arrival?
- After an overview, you can state more confidently whether the patient initially does or does not present as a medical emergency.
- That is a lot of things to look for in 10 sec, but you will be amazed what you begin to notice.

The following sections are intended as an introduction to clinical examination but are necessarily brief. You should consult monographs for more detail. The following are recommended:

- Thomas J, Monaghan T (2014). *Oxford Handbook of Clinical Examination and Practical Skills*, 2nd ed. Oxford University Press.
- Talley NJ, O'Connor S (2017). *Clinical Examination*, 8th ed. Elsevier.
- Alastair Innes J, Dover AR, Fairhurst K (2018). *Macleod's Clinical Examination*, 14th ed. Churchill Livingstone.
- University of California. *Practical Guide to Clinical Medicine*. ℘ www. meded.ucsd.edu/clinicalmed/breast.htm.
- OSCE Skills: ℘ www.osceskills.com.
- Geeky Medics: ℘ www.geekymedics.com.

Top tip

OSCE mark schemes

Ask your tutor or senior peers about previous mark schemes for your medical school, although most should contain mostly the same criteria. For a comprehensive list of example OSCE mark schemes, visit Mock Marking Schemes for OSCEs (℘ www.scionpublishing.com/resources/osce/OSCEs%20Marking.pdf).

Cardiovascular examination

Heart sounds

The key to a successful cardiovascular examination is being familiar with the heart sounds, and identifying abnormal or additional sounds. As well as spending a number of minutes listening to your own heart sounds, YouTube and recordings on websites are a good place to start.

Normal heart sounds

- S1: 'lub'. Closure of the mitral valve (MV) and tricuspid valve (TV). Think M1.
- S2: 'dub'. Closure of the aortic valve (AV) and pulmonary valve (PV).

Abnormal added heart sounds

Both cause a 'gallop' rhythm:
- S3: 'Kentucky'. Can be normal in young people. In older patients a sign of ventricular dysfunction or volume overload.
- S4: 'Tennessee'. Sign of ventricular stiffness, e.g. LV hypertrophy.
- 'Friction rub': due to serosal inflammation, e.g. viral pericarditis or post MI.

Murmurs

Caused by turbulent blood flow. May be physiological (e.g. in pregnancy) or pathological. Often described numerically to denote intensity (grade 1 = only audible with accentuation, grade 6 = audible with stethoscope just removed from chest wall). Murmurs are also described by their timing in the cardiac cycle:

Systolic murmurs begin at or after the first heart sound and are usually caused by stenosed AV/PV or regurgitant MV/TV. Common examples include:
- ejection: aortic stenosis (AS)
- pan-systolic: mitral regurgitation (MR) (or rarely ventricular septal defect)
- others: MV prolapse, atrial septal defect, hypertrophic obstructive cardiomyopathy.

Diastolic murmurs being at or after the second heart sound and are caused by stenosed MV/tricuspid stenosis or regurgitant AV/PV. These are difficult to identify and rarer than lesions causing systolic murmurs:
- Early: usually aortic regurgitation (rarely pulmonary).
- Mid: mitral/tricuspid stenosis (both rare).

Accentuating manoeuvres

There are a number of techniques to distinguish murmurs which involve manoeuvres to alter the volume/speed of turbulent flow and therefore the intensity of the murmur. The most important are:

Right vs left heart

Right-sided murmurs are louder in inspiration due to ↑venous return and right heart filling. As a result, right sided murmurs are quieter in expiration while left-sided murmurs sound louder (and vice versa). Think *Right Inspiration (RIght)* and *left expiration (LEft)*.

Radiation
The murmur of MR radiates to axilla, AS radiates to the carotid.

Patient position
Sitting forwards in expiration makes aortic murmurs louder as the left side of the heart is closer to the chest wall. Mitral murmurs are accentuated when patients are lying on their left side (lateral decubitus).

Valsalva manoeuvres: accentuates the murmurs of both hypertrophic obstructive cardiomyopathy and MV prolapse due to reduced LV volume and closer apposition of septum and MV. All other murmurs are quieter.

Where to listen for cardiac sounds
See Fig. 50.1.

Jugular venous pressure (JVP)
Another important element of the cardiovascular examination is to understand and identify the position and waveform of the internal jugular vein (IJV). The IJV is found medial to the sternocleidomastoid and can be distinguished from the carotid artery by being impalpable and compressible, having a bifid waveform and changing with respiration. Its position can be accentuated by gentle pressure in the RUQ (hepatojugular reflux or abdominojugular test). Remember, this is not an automatic reflex but a

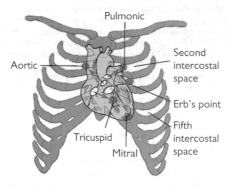

Fig. 50.1 Precordial locations for cardiac palpation and auscultation of heart sounds. Closure of the mitral and tricuspid valves produces the S1 heart sound; closure of the pulmonic and aortic (semilunar) valves produces the S2 sound. Reproduced from Polanski, A, and Tatro, S., *Luckmann's Core Principles and Practice of Medical-surgical Nursing*, 1996, WB Saunders.

Aortic: 2nd intercostal space on right, right sternal edge.

Pulmonary: 2nd intercostal space on left, left sternal edge.

Mitral: 5th left intercostal space, left mid-clavicular line.

Tricuspid: 4th left intercostal space, left sternal edge.

Erb's point: third left intercostal space/left lower sternal border (where S2 is best heard).

pressured reflUx. There are lengthy academic descriptions of the JVP waveform but in practical terms, the following are most important:

- Identify if it is elevated (heart failure or fluid overload, right heart strain, e.g. PE).
- Large 'v wave' (tricuspid regurgitation).
- Cannon or 'a wave' (AF and heart block).

Fluid assessment

Fluid overload is a cardinal sign of heart failure and you should become familiar with looking for signs of intra- and extravascular fluid status:

- *Intravascular*: HR, BP (postural), capillary refill, JVP, urine output.
- *Extravascular*: peripheral/pulmonary oedema, ascites, tissue turgor.

Around the bed space

Look for

Fluid restriction or daily weights sign, GTN spray, infusions such as furosemide, cardiac monitor, oxygen.

Observation of the patient

Breathless at rest? Cardiac cachexia? Gross oedema visible from end of bed, urinary catheter? Consider patient's age (if young, think of congenital cardiac disease). Evidence of systemic disease (ankylosing spondylitis, RA) or syndrome (Marfan's, trisomy 21)? Listen for audible click of metallic valve.

Examination

- *Hands*: capillary refill (<2 sec), clubbing (congenital heart disease), long fingers (Marfan's), tendon xanthelasma, warm and well perfused vs cold and shut down, peripheral cyanosis, peripheral stigmata of infective endocarditis (>three splinter haemorrhages, Osler's nodes, Janeway lesions), tar (*not nicotine*) stains from smoking, palmar erythema (SLE, hyperthyroid, RA).
- *Radial pulse*: regular vs irregularly irregular (AF) vs regularly irregular (sinus arrhythmia). Rate, volume, and character (best assessed from a central artery such as the carotid and femoral). Radio-radial delay (coarctation/aortic dissection) and radio-femoral delay. Recent scar/cannulation in forearm (or groin) from angiogram.
- *Brachial pulse*: collapsing/water hammer (aortic regurgitation). Assess quality of pulse especially if the radial pulse is impalpable.

Ask for patient's BP and calculate the pulse pressure (systolic BP − diastolic BP). Narrow pulse pressure (e.g. 100/80 mmHg) occurs in severe AS whereas wide pulse pressure (e.g. 180/70 mmHg) occurs in aortic regurgitation. A low BP may occur in cardiac failure or if compromised by fast AF.

Eyes

Subconjunctival haemorrhage (infective endocarditis), conjunctival pallor in anaemia, jaundiced sclera, xanthomata (lipid), corneal arcus (pathological if <50 years old) vs corneal senilis (physiological).

Mouth

Central cyanosis (congenital heart disease), high-arched palate (Marfan's), poor dentition (risk factor for infective endocarditis).

Carotid

Slow rising pulse (anacrotic in severe aortic stenosis), scar from endarterectomy, listen for bruit or radiation of AS murmur.

Praecordium

- *Inspection*: midline sternotomy scar, indwelling devices, e.g. permanent pacemaker or implantable cardioverter defibrillator, apical valvotomy scar (unusual).
- *Palpation*: apex beat (fifth intercostal space in midclavicular line), palpate for thrills (i.e. palpable murmurs) at apex and over sternum with hand *lightly* on chest wall. Feel for heaves (ventricular hypertrophy) with the heel of your hand.
- *Auscultation*: listen in the five areas, initially to assess S1 and S2 and then to identify added sounds such as S3/4 or murmur. Perform accentuating manoeuvres to distinguish murmurs while holding their radial pulse to distinguish systolic from diastolic. Take your time and listen carefully. Some even close their eyes to focus.
- *Lungs*: percuss at bases for effusions and listen for pulmonary oedema.

While the patient is sitting forward

- *Sacrum*: assess for sacral oedema. Remember in bed-bound patients that the sacrum/hips are often the lowest part of the body.
- *Abdomen*: assess for AAA. If patient has signs of tricuspid regurgitation, palpate for a pulsatile liver. Look for ascites in heart failure.
- *Lower limb*: palpate for (and auscultate) femoral pulses, and also check for popliteal/dorsalis pedis pulses. Check feet for evidence of emboli/'trash foot'/splinter haemorrhages, and lower limb oedema. Is there evidence of saphenous vein harvest (CABG)?
- *Offer to check*: dipstick urine (microscopic haematuria in infective endocarditis), lying and standing BP, resting ECG, pulse oximetry.

Report your findings

'This is a 69-year-old man who presented with shortness of breath. He is comfortable at rest. Clinical signs include irregularly irregular pulse, displaced apex beat, a pansystolic murmur that radiates to the apex, bibasal crepitations and peripheral oedema. In summary these signs are consistent with mitral regurgitation, atrial fibrillation, and congestive cardiac failure. To investigate further I would like to perform an ECG, an echocardiogram and a plain chest radiograph.'

Anticipate the following questions

- Causes of AF.
- How to distinguish MR/AS.
- Causes of MR.
- Management of MR (medical and surgical).
- CXR signs of heart failure.

If you are doing really well

- Indications for surgery.
- Pros and cons between tissue and metallic valves.
- Management of AF and risk score to guide anticoagulation.

Patterns of findings

It is useful to think of cardiac conditions in terms of patterns or syndromes so that you remember to look for additional signs during the course of your examination. (See Table 50.1.)

Other

- *Tricuspid regurgitation*: PSM at lower left sternal edge louder in inspiration (often absent). Raised JVP with large v waves. Pulsatile liver. Usually functional (dilated RV with normal valves).
- *Prosthetic valves*: midline sternotomy scar, metallic valves audible without stethoscope (think ticking clock).

Table 50.1 Patterns of findings

Common		
Aortic stenosis (AS)	ESM radiating to carotids	Slow rising pulse
	Quiet/normal S1, absent S2	LV heave/hypertrophy
	Presence of S4 (late)	Congestive cardiac failure (late)
	Narrow pulse pressure	(Check for coexisting AR)
Mitral regurgitation (MR)	PSM radiating to axilla	AF
	Quiet/absent S1	Congestive cardiac failure
	Presence of S3	Hyperdynamic circulation
	Displaced apex beat	
Rare		
Aortic regurgitation (AR)	Early diastolic murmur	'Water hammer' pulse
	Usually coexisting ESM	Eponymous signs: Quincke, Corrigan, De Musset, Duroziez
	Austin Flint murmur	
	Wide pulse pressure	Cause: Marfan's, ankylosing spondylitis
Mitral stenosis (MS)	Mitral facies	AF
	Low diastolic murmur at apex	Main cause rheumatic heart disease which is rare now
	Loud S1	

ESM, ejection-systolic murmur; PSM, pansystolic murmur.

Respiratory examination

Breath sounds

Learn to recognize the different breath sounds associated with normal and pathological ventilation. Listen to your own breathing; start with the stethoscope over your lungs to identify vesicular breath sounds. Then move the stethoscope to your sternum to hear bronchial breath sounds. Breathe through your mouth to exclude any nasopharyngeal noise.

Types of breath sounds
- *Vesicular*: this is the sound of normal air transit through the large airways, heard transmitted through normal lung tissue and the chest wall. The inspiratory phase is typically about two to three times longer than expiratory. The volume/intensity is reduced with poor respiratory effort, ↑muscle mass or obesity.
- *Bronchial*: this is the sound of air moving through large airways without being filtered by normal (gas filled) lung tissue. It is normal to hear bronchial breath sounds when listening over the large airways but abnormal when listening over lung tissue. Bronchial breath sounds are heard over consolidated lung and in some cases adjacent to effusion or collapse.

Added sounds
- *Wheeze*: implies airways obstruction, usually expiratory but also present in inspiration. Obstruction of multiple smaller airways (e.g. asthma) causes polyphonic wheeze; beware that severe airways obstruction limits even the airflow required to make wheeze and a 'silent chest' is an emergency. Obstruction of single calibre airways (e.g. bronchial carcinoma) causes monophonic wheeze which does not clear with coughing.
- *Inspiratory crackles* (also referred to as crepitations/creps/rhonchi/rales): crackles are caused by the rapid re-expansion of collapsed airspaces during inspiration. The timing in the respiratory cycle is an important clue to the size of airspace involved. Early inspiratory crackles usually originate in smaller airways as in chronic bronchitis.
- Late inspiratory crackles are due to alveolar re-expansion and are further described by their nature:
  • Fine: like Velcro as in pulmonary fibrosis.
  • Coarse: bronchiectasis/pneumonia.
  • Medium: pulmonary oedema.
- *Pleural rub*: caused by inflammation of the pleural surfaces and seen in response to infection, infarction (PE) or systemic inflammatory disease (e.g. SLE). Described as the crunching of fresh snow. Distinguish from pericardial rub by asking patient to hold their breath (pleural rub disappears).

Percussion

In addition to auscultation, percussion is another very important modality of respiratory examination. Practise tapping one (usually left) middle finger with your other (right) middle finger so that you can do it without looking or concentrating. It is common at early stages to miss and instead strike the patient; this is best avoided.

Percussion utilizes the difference in conduction between air- and liquid-filled tissues. Practise percussing your own chest wall to identify the normal sound over air-filled lung. This sound becomes dull/reduced over consolidated lung or pleural effusions while it becomes hyper-resonant over hyperinflated lung or pneumothorax.

Tactile vocal fremitus (TVF)

Ask the patient to repeat a number while resting the ulnar aspects of both hands over the lung fields. Normally, the air-filled lung tissue greatly attenuates the conduction of sound waves. When the lung is consolidated, the thrill is more obviously palpable through the chest wall. TVF is reduced in effusion and pneumothorax.

Vocal resonance and whispering pectoriloquy

This is the auditory correlate of TVF. Auscultate and ask the patient to say 99. Higher-frequency speech is rapidly transmitted through consolidated lung and sounds louder than over normal lung.

Lung expansion

More helpful in comparing left to right than in absolute terms. Assess upper lobe expansion by resting hands over clavicles or observing clavicle movement with respiration from behind. Lower lobe expansion seen by movement of examiner's hands on rib cage expansion.
- *Unilateral reduction*: pneumonia, collapse, effusion, pneumothorax.
- *Bilateral*: diffuse lung disease, e.g. fibrosis, emphysema.

Tracheal/mediastinal displacement

Tracheal deviation is
- *towards* side of lesion: collapse, lung resection
- *away* from lesion: effusion, pneumothorax.

Significant volume expansion can cause mediastinal shift (e.g. tension pneumothorax). This is life-threatening. Clinical signs include circulatory collapse, tracheal deviation, displaced apex beat, absent breath sounds, and hyper-resonance (see Table 50.2). This is a clinical diagnosis so *do not* wait for the CXR!

Table 50.2 Summary of clinical findings

Condition	Breath sounds	Percussion	TVF/VR	Expansion
Consolidation	Bronchial or ↓	Dull	↑	↓
Effusion	↓	Dull	↓	↓
Emphysema	↓, creps	Hyper-resonant	↓	Bilateral ↓
Collapse	Absent or ↓	Dull		↓
Pneumothorax	Absent	Hyper-resonant	↓	↓
TVF, tactile vocal fremitus; VR, vocal resonance.				

Other aspects of respiratory examination

Signs of pulmonary hypertension/right heart failure

Chronic hypoxia and pulmonary hypertension can → right heart failure (cor pulmonale) and a number of clinical signs which are useful clues to the severity/longevity of the patient's condition:

- Loud P2.
- Right ventricular heave (sternal edge).
- Raised JVP (large a wave).
- Palpable liver.
- Ascites/peripheral oedema.

Specific signs in lung cancer

Lung cancer can give rise to a number of specific signs. These can be caused by the following:

1. Airway obstruction from tumour (cough, monophonic wheeze, distal collapse/consolidation).
2. Local invasion by tumour (brachial plexus, SVC obstruction, Horner's syndrome).
3. Metastatic spread (jaundice, palpable liver, bone pain).
4. Paraneoplasia (Eaton–Lambert, gynaecomastia).
5. Systemic: cachexia, lymphadenopathy, clubbing.
6. Previous surgical scars (thoracoscopy, lobectomy, pneumonectomy) which are usually on the back—so ensure you inspect both front and back.

Suggested routine for respiratory examination

Around the bed space

Look for:

Fluid restriction sign, inhalers (brown = steroid, blue = salbutamol, nebulizers), oxygen therapy (flow rate, nasal specula, or face mask), sputum pot (colour, consistency, viscosity, blood?). Is the patient isolated (TB?)

Observation of the patient

Breathless at rest? ↑Respiratory work (tachypnoea, pursed-mouth breathing, use of accessory muscles, 'tripod' position), added respiratory noises (cough, wheeze, stridor), cachexia, obesity (think sleep apnoea/ventilatory failure), peripheral oedema, age of patient (if young, think cystic fibrosis, alpha-1 antitrypsin deficiency, asthma, neuromuscular disorder).

Examination

- CO_2 *retention flap*: ask patient to stretch out arms/hands and observe for coarse myoclonic jerks. Salbutamol-induced fine tremor will also be evident.
- *Hands*: clubbing (cancer, suppurative lung disease), wasting of small muscles (brachial plexopathy in cancer), palmar erythema (SLE, RA), tar staining (smoking).
- *Wrists*: hypertrophic pulmonary osteoarthropathy (extreme form of clubbing). Peripheral cyanosis.
- *Radial pulse*: tachycardia/AF. Bounding pulse in CO_2 retention. Count respiration rate at this point.

- *Face*: anaemia, central cyanosis, ptosis (Horner's).
- *JVP*: raised in pulmonary hypertension.
- *Trachea*: (warn the patient). Deviated? Palpate sternotracheal distance (reduced in hyperinflated lungs).
- Cervical lymph nodes.
- *The chest*: remember to examine both front and back, especially for hidden surgical scars!
- *Inspection*: pectus carinatum or excavatum, congenital anomaly (e.g. Klippel–Feil syndrome), thoracotomy scar, Hickman line for antibiotics.
- *Palpation*: assess for chest expansion in upper and lower zones.
- *Percussion*: compare like with like (i.e. left upper zone with right). Right axilla identifies right middle lobe. Cardiac dullness attenuated in asthma/COPD.
- *Auscultate*: front and back comparing left with right as you go. Ask patient to breathe through mouth to eliminate nasopharyngeal noise. Remember to auscultate over supraclavicular fossae and axillae. Ask patient to cough to see if crackles clear. TVF/vocal resonance. Listen in the pulmonary valve area for loud P2 (pulmonary hypertension).
- *Lower limbs*: peripheral oedema.
- *Other*: look for evidence of long-term steroid use (skin thinning, central obesity, finger pricks from diabetes).
- *Offer to*: check pulse oximetry, examine the sputum, and perform bedside spirometry.

Report your findings

'This is an 71-year-old woman who presents with breathlessness and cough. She is tachypnoeic and tachycardic at rest. On examination I found tar-stained fingers, reduced sternotracheal distance, bilaterally reduced chest expansion, quiet breath sounds, and expiratory wheeze throughout with a hyper-resonant percussion note. She also has a loud P2, elevated JVP, and pitting oedema of the lower limbs. Finally, she has a number of bruises and thin skin. Taken together, I think this lady has evidence of a smoking history, emphysema treated with corticosteroids, and cor pulmonale. To investigate further, I would perform a plain chest radiograph and pulmonary function test'. (See Table 50.3.)

Anticipate the following questions

- What would you expect to find on pulmonary function testing?
- What are the characteristic radiological findings in emphysema?
- How is COPD managed?
- What are the complications of COPD?
- What are the risks of uncontrolled oxygen therapy?
- What are the other causes of small airways obstruction?

If you are doing really well

- What is the pathophysiology of emphysema?
- What are the criteria for long-term home oxygen therapy?
- What are the indications for surgery in COPD?

Table 50.3 Patterns of findings

Obstructive airways disease	Hyperexpansion, quiet BS, hyper-resonance
	Prolonged expiratory phase
	Steroid use
	Salbutamol tremor
	COPD only: CO_2 retention, smoking, pulmonary HTN, cor pulmonale
Lobar pneumonia	Fever/tachycardia
	Oxygen therapy
	Focal consolidation: dull percussion, bronchial BS, inspiratory creps and/or rub, ↑TVF/VR
Pulmonary fibrosis	Clubbing
	Fine bilateral late inspiratory crackles
	Pulmonary HTN/cor pulmonale
	Systemic disease: SLE, RA, ankylosing spondylitis
	Steroid use
Bronchiectasis/CF	Clubbing
	Sputum pot, haemoptysis
	Coarse bilateral late inspiratory crackles
	Hickman line
	(CF: cachexia, diabetes, Creon)
Pleural effusions	Dull lung base (s), reduced expansion, quiet/absent BS, reduced TVF/VR
	Bilateral: heart/renal failure
	Unilateral: cancer/pneumonia
	Evidence of pleurocentesis
Lung cancer	Clubbing
	Smoking
	Cachexia/wasting
	Lymph nodes
	Monophonic wheeze
	Focal consolidation/effusion
	Specific signs

BS, breath sounds; HTN, hypertension.

Others

- *TB*: ethnicity, cachexia, fever, lymphadenopathy, usually few lung signs. Old TB: pneumonectomy, 'plombage' on CXR, phrenic nerve crush scar above clavicle.
- *Sarcoidosis*: ethnicity, uveitis, lymphadenopathy, visceral involvement (liver, spleen, renal), erythema nodosum, usually few lung signs.

Gastrointestinal examination

The abdominal examination takes in a number of different organ systems, and you need to be able to detect signs of liver disease, IBD, palpable kidneys or renal transplant, stomas, and splenomegaly.

Causes of abdominal distension or masses

Often the principal challenge is to detect organomegaly, and establish which organ it is you are palpating. In many cases, there is no organomegaly, and the diagnosis will be deduced from surgical scars or peripheral stigmata of systemic disease. The abdomen is usually divided into four or nine but remember that there is no such thing as nine quadrants.

Abdominal distension

Is classically described by the 'five Fs': fat, flatus, faeces, fluid, and fetus. Typically there will be generalized and often symmetrical distension. The causes can be identified on percussion (ascites dull, gaseous distension resonant), the presence of shifting dullness (ascites), auscultation (high-pitched bowel sounds in obstruction, absent in paralytic ileus).

Abdominal masses

Can be described as you would any other lump: location, size, shape, appearance, pain, fluctuance, consistency, percussion note, etc. This is a good place to start if you are completely lost and need some structure to gather your thoughts. However, it is more useful to learn the specific features of the intra-abdominal organs on examination so that you can rapidly decide what you are palpating.

Liver

RUQ, descends 1–2 cm in inspiration, upper border ~sixth intercostal space and expands distally. Usually smooth (if craggy, think metastatic disease). Tender if capsule stretched like in rapid expansion (acute hepatitis). Percussion note dull. Bruit present in hepatocellular carcinoma and acute alcoholic hepatitis. Remember that the liver is often impalpable in cirrhosis (small, scarred liver).

Spleen

LUQ, expands inferomedially towards the RIF but often only detectable with patient in right lateral position. Start palpating from the umbilicus, diagonally upwards towards the left hypochondrium in order to detect splenomegaly. Inferior border is notched, though this is rarely discernible. Cannot palpate upper border which is above costal margin. Spleen moves with respiration. Dull percussion note. Splenic friction rub rarely present in acute splenomegaly or capsular inflammation (viral infection, infarction).

Kidneys

Enlarged kidneys are usually bilateral (e.g. ADPKD) but may be unilateral (renal cell carcinoma, hydronephrosis, ADPKD with nephrectomy—look for scar). Main distinction is between spleen and left kidney: kidney moves inferiorly with inspiration but not medially and has no notch. You should be able to palpate the upper aspect beneath the costal margin.

The term *balloting* is often used to describe the technique of propelling the kidney forwards with a hand on the patient's loin, and feeling the anterior surface of the kidney move into your other hand on the hypochondrium. Percussion note is resonant due to overlying bowel gas (remember: kidneys are retroperitoneal).

Kidney transplant
Smooth mass in either iliac fossa beneath a hockey stick-shaped scar. You may feel only one pole of the kidney. It is extraperitoneal and dull to percussion. Often a bruit is present.

Bladder
A very important skill in clinical practice but less often tested in exams. The bladder should be impalpable, and if you can detect it, the patient may have urinary retention. The bladder is suprapubic, extends superiorly in the midline, is smooth, and often tender in acute retention, and is dull to percussion when full of urine. If in doubt, perform a bladder scan and insert a urinary catheter.

Gall bladder
Rarely palpable. Remember Courvoisier's law: a palpable gall bladder in the presence of jaundice is rarely caused by gallstones. Where present, a gall bladder is palpated in the RUQ and is a rounded, focal swelling which can be detected on inspiration. Murphy's sign is useful clinically: as the patient breathes in, the inflamed gall bladder (cholecystitis) descends onto the examiner's hand causing the patient to catch their breath. Positive if LUQ is not tender.

Bowel
Sometimes palpable in constipated patients. Distinctively, stool-filled bowel can be dented by the examiner's hand.

Aorta
Just to left of midline above the umbilicus. More commonly palpable in slim patients. Should be pulsatile but not expansile.

Liver disease in the gastrointestinal examination
Signs of liver disease are a major feature of the GI examination. Be clear about the different clinical entities they represent.

Signs of chronic liver disease
(Stable, usually the result of long-standing hepatic insufficiency). Be able to explain the pathogenesis (e.g. gynaecomastia from oestrogen:androgen imbalance, spider naevi from reduced oestrogen metabolism). These are also signs of decompensated liver disease which are important to mention to the examiner:
- Spider naevi
- Gynaecomastia
- Palmar erythema
- Dupuytren's contracture
- Testicular atrophy
- Nail clubbing
- Cachexia

- Hair loss/thinning
- Oedema
- Bruising
- Hepatomegaly
- Portal hypertension.

Portal hypertension
Usually due to ↑vascular resistance in chronic liver disease (hepatic). Rarely acute, e.g. in Budd–Chiari syndrome (post-hepatic). Features include:
- dilated abdominal wall veins
- caput medusa
- splenomegaly
- ascites
- evidence of GI bleed.

Hepatic encephalopathy
An acute decompensation probably caused by hyperammonaemia (can be measured in blood), usually on a background of chronic liver disease. Causes include GI bleed, infection (especially spontaneous bacterial peritonitis), shunt (e.g. transjugular intrahepatic portosystemic shunt (TIPSS) procedure), diuretics, acute liver insult (e.g. alcohol binge). Features include asterixis ('liver flap') and altered consciousness:
- Grade 0: normal.
- Grade 1: 'soft' cognitive, sleep, or mood disturbance.
- Grade 2: disorientation especially in time, asterixis, lethargy.
- Grade 3: marked confusion and stupor.
- Grade 4: coma.

Clinical features more specific to alcohol misuse
- Withdrawal/delirium tremens (tremor, sweating, tachycardia).
- Parotid enlargement.
- Wernicke–Korsakoff syndrome.
- Features of other substance use: tar-stained fingers, injection tracks.
- Head and other injuries from falls.

Suggested routine for gastrointestinal examination

Around the bed space
Look for: fluid restriction sign, low-salt diet, nil by mouth (recent GI bleed), infusion (fluids, furosemide, electrolytes, parenteral nutrition, PPI).
  Observation of the patient: BMI and nutritional status (look for muscle atrophy, e.g. arms, thighs), skin and hair, tattoos or track marks (risk factor for hepatitis B or C), jaundice, conscious level (encephalopathy).

Examination
Ask patient to lift head off bed or cough (increase intra-abdominal pressure): often unmasks herniae, divarication of recti, abdominal masses.

Limbs
- *Asterixis*: ask patient to hold out arms in front and look for coarse myoclonic jerks seen in hepatic encephalopathy.
- *Hands*: clubbing (cirrhosis), palmar erythema (chronic liver disease), Dupuytren's contracture (chronic liver disease), koilonychia, leuconychia, Beau's lines (chronic illness).

- *Skin*: jaundice, pruritus (obstructive jaundice, uraemia).
- *Radial pulse*: rate and character. Hyperdynamic circulation in liver disease.

Face

Anaemia, scleral jaundice, xanthelasmata (PBC), glossitis, macroglossia (amyloid), aphthous ulcers (IBD).

Eyes

Scleral jaundice, xanthelasma, Kayser–Fleischer rings of Wilson's disease often mentioned but in practice only seen with slit lamp so do not say that you can see them with the naked eye.

Troisier's sign/Virchow's node: GI malignancy.

Chest

Look for spider naevi (in SVC distribution), gynaecomastia, Hickman line for parenteral nutrition, visible ribs in malnutrition.

Abdomen

Expose patient from xiphisternum to knees while preserving dignity with a bedsheet. Ask if the patient would like a chaperone. (See Fig. 50.2 for anatomy.)

- *Inspection*: look carefully for scars including posteriorly and in skin folds. Stomas? Remember ileal vs colon features (see ➔ Chapter 34).
- *Palpation*: always ask about pain first! Usually start with a light-pressure exploratory circuit of the quadrants to identify obvious abnormalities. Then palpate specifically for:
  - liver (start in RIF and move towards costal margin as patient inhales. If tense ascites, often only palpable laterally)
  - spleen (starting at umbilicus moving diagonally to left hypochondrium) and feeling for notch. Ask patient to roll to their right
  - kidneys: balloting or bimanually palpating within the renal angle
  - exclude bladder/kidney transplant
  - aorta.
- *Percussion*: percuss ~from sixth intercostal space downwards for liver, from umbilicus for spleen and remember percussion note over kidneys is resonant. Shifting dullness is important: identify a point between umbilicus and flank where resonant note becomes dull. Mark with two fingers. Ask the patient to roll away from your hand. Does the note over either finger change?
- *Auscultate*: liver/spleen rub, renal bruit (listen above umbilicus on both sides of midline, present in renal artery stenosis), bowel sounds (absent in ileus/postoperatively vs high-pitched tinkling/borborygmi in obstruction).

Lower limbs

Peripheral oedema, skin changes (pyoderma grenosum), hair loss, general muscle mass.

Other

Offer to: check hernial orifices, external genitalia in men and perform DRE and be able to explain what you are looking for (herniae, testicular atrophy, GI bleed or faecal impaction respectively)

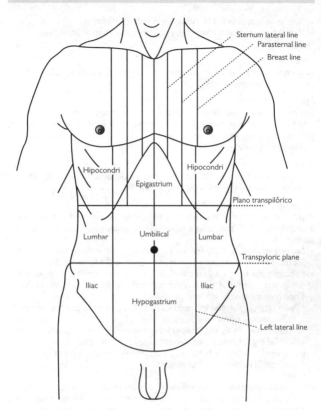

Sternum lateral line
Parasternal line
Breast line

Hipocondri

Hipocondri

Epigastrium

Plano transpilôrico

Lumbar   Umbilical   Lumbar

Transpyloric plane

Iliac   Ilíac

Hypogastrium

Left lateral line

Fig. 50.2 Surface anatomy of the abdomen. Reproduced from Henry Vandyke Carter – Henry Gray (1918) *Anatomy of the Human Body*, Bartleby.com: *Gray's Anatomy*, Plate 1220. Image is in the public domain.

Report your findings

'This is a 42-year-old gentleman who presents with vomiting and confusion. He has a number of peripheral stigmata of chronic liver disease including palmar erythema, spider naevi, and gynaecomastia. He was deeply jaundiced and asterixis was present. On examination of the abdomen the liver was smoothly enlarged eight fingers beneath the costal margin and was tender to palpation. Shifting dullness was present. In summary, this man has evidence of acute decompensation on a background of chronic liver disease. To investigate him further I would take a full alcohol history, perform a liver/viral screen and request a liver ultrasound looking for cirrhosis and the direction of portal flow.' (See Table 50.4)

Table 50.4 Patterns of findings

Stable chronic liver disease	Peripheral stigmata of chronic liver disease
	No encephalopathy
	Underlying causes: alcohol, IV drug use, diabetes, rarer causes (e.g. PBC), Wilson's disease
	Nutritional and fluid status
	Medications (spironolactone, diuretics)
Decompensated liver disease	Encephalopathy
	Jaundice
	Ascites
	Evidence of infection or GI bleed
	Evidence of chronic liver disease in background
Splenomegaly	Most common: chronic liver disease and portal hypertension
	Others:
	Myeloproliferative (pallor/purpura)
	Infectious (viral, malaria, endocarditis)
	Infiltrative (amyloid: macroglossia, cardiac failure)
Kidney transplant	Mass in iliac fossa beneath hockey stick-shaped scar
	Bruit (biopsy, stenosis)
	Cause of renal failure: diabetes, ADPKD, suprapubic catheter
	Previous dialysis (arteriovenous fistula, scars from lines or peritoneal dialysis catheter)
	Drug toxicity (steroids, tacrolimus tremor)
Crohn's disease	Aphthous ulceration
	Abdominal abscess or stoma
	Anorectal disease: fissure/tags
	Nutrition (?Hickman line)
	Non-GI manifestations include malabsorption, clubbing, joint or eye involvement
	Drugs (steroids)
Ulcerative colitis	Usually limited to colon
	Stoma
	Toxic megacolon acutely
	Associated with pyoderma gangrenosum (legs) and PSC (jaundiced?)
	Drugs (steroids)

Anticipate the following questions
- What are the main causes of cirrhosis in the UK?
- What are the causes of acute decompensation?
- How is hepatic encephalopathy managed?
- What other medical problems does alcohol misuse cause?

If you are doing really well
- What is the mechanism of gynaecomastia in liver disease?
- How is the severity of chronic liver disease graded?
- Name some rarer causes of cirrhosis.
- How is portal hypertension managed?

Others
- *Malabsorption*: wasting, ulcers, glossitis, nutritional status, Hickman line, oedema, bruising.

Neurological examination

History

Although we will focus solely on the neurological examination in this section, the reality of clinical neurology is that the diagnosis is often made primarily on the history with confirmation from the examination. For example, the potential causes to consider when examining a patient with weakness will be very different if the vignette brief is 'Please examine this patient who has experienced sudden-onset left-sided weakness' to one in which the brief is 'Please examine this patient who has gradually worsening weakness in both legs'.

Examination routine

There is no one correct way to perform the neurological examination. As most medical students will agree, neurology can be one of the most daunting specialties and the complexity of the examination undoubtedly contributes to this.[1] While examining a patient with a neurological disorder, try to localize the level of the lesion as you are going along. Students often display difficulty in eliciting reflexes. Make sure you practise on healthy colleagues so that you start to develop a sense of what is a normal reflex (and also develop confidence that you can actually find reflexes) and then try this on a range of patients on the ward. A good way to familiarize yourself with the appearance of abnormal signs is to watch neurologists examine patients online and look at images of abnormal findings (ℜ https://meded.ucsd.edu/clinicalmed/neuro2.htm, ℜ www.neuroexam.com/neuroexam/). In the OSCE environment, you are most likely to be asked to examine only a defined region (e.g. cranial nerves, upper limbs, or lower limbs). It is appropriate at the end of a limited examination to say that you would like to go on to examine the remainder of the nervous system.

General introduction

As with any patient, make sure that you introduce yourself properly (while doing this listen to their acknowledgement to see if there is an obvious disorder of speech), enquire as to whether they have any pain, and ensure their comfort and dignity throughout the examination.

General inspection

Look around the bed for signs of impaired mobility (wheelchairs, crutches, etc.), swallowing difficulties (nil by mouth signs etc.), visual difficulties (white stick, glasses, etc.), auditory difficulties (hearing aids etc.), or uneven gait (particular patterns of wear on the soles of shoes). Sufficiently expose the areas you have been asked to examine. Have a thorough general look at the patient and check for any asymmetry or obvious weakness (e.g. facial droop or decorticate posturing) and further clues (e.g. parkinsonian facies).

Reference

1. Pakpoor J, Handel AE, Disanto G, et al. (2014). National survey of UK medical students on the perception of neurology. *BMC Med Educ* 14:225.

Cranial nerve examination

I Olfactory

Ask about any changes in sense of smell (can be formally tested by odorant detection tests).

II Optic (mnemonic = ACFRO)

Test *acuity* using a Snellen chart. (NB: does the patient need to wear glasses?) Test *colour vision* to check for an optic neuropathy. Use the red end of a Neurotip™ to check for gross defects in colour perception and perform a detailed examination with Ishihara charts if required.

Map out *visual fields* (Fig. 50.3). Ask the patient to focus on the bridge of your nose at all times. Ensure you are in direct confrontation with the patient with your finger held equidistant between you both. Bring your finger systematically in from the edge of the visual field in all four diagonal quadrants with the patient covering each eye in turn. Test for visual neglect by holding both hands out wide and asking the patient which hand is moving while wiggling each set of fingers individually.

Test *reflexes*: pupillary reflex can be tested by shining a light into each eye in turn while looking either at the eye into which the torch is being shone (direct) or the other eye (indirect). Test for a relative afferent pupillary defect (RAPD) by 'swinging' the torch from eye to eye. A positive RAPD is relative dilation of one pupil when the torch is moved from the contralateral eye.

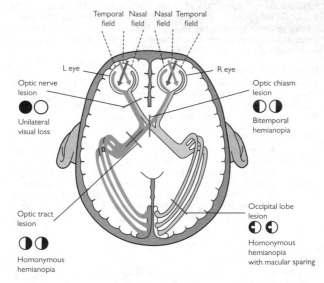

Fig. 50.3 Patterns of visual field loss. Reproduced with permission from Piers Page and Greg Skinner, *Emergencies in Clinical Medicine*, 2008, Oxford University Press.

Test the *accommodation reflex* by asking the patient to look at your finger and moving it in towards the patient's nose. A normal response is bilateral pupillary constriction.

Perform *ophthalmoscopy*: first of all look through the ophthalmoscope into each of the patient's eyes in turn from ~30 cm and check that the 'red reflex' is present (a normal sign—the absence of this can indicate cataracts or retinal pathology). Look carefully at the optic disc, checking for any swelling or cupping, and trace vessels out into the peripheral retina. Finally assess the macula. Compare both eyes.

III Oculomotor, IV trochlear, and VI abducens (eye movements)

Ask the patient whether they have double vision. Ask the patient to follow your finger with their eyes, keeping their head still, as you trace a large 'H' in front of them. Check that there is smooth, symmetrical tracking of your finger with both eyes. Notice if nystagmus occurs in any particular gaze position (a few beats of nystagmus at extreme peripheral gaze can be normal) and whether any eye fails to move in a particular position. Check for defects of saccadic eye movement by asking the patient to look rapidly from one hand to another while you hold your hands at both extremes of the lateral visual fields. Normal eye movements are shown in Fig. 50.4.

V Trigeminal

Test light touch in each of the three areas of trigeminal innervation (midpupillary line: lower jaw (mandibular branch, V3), cheek bone (maxillary branch, V2), and forehead (ophthalmic branch, V1)). Test power of jaw closure (feel contraction of temporalis and masseter) and jaw opening (pterygoids). Offer to test corneal reflex (touch the cornea with gauze, both eyes should blink but painful) and jaw jerk.

VII Facial

Ask the patient to smile, blow out their cheeks, and raise their eyebrows (NB: unilateral upper motor neuron facial weakness will spare the forehead but will not be spared in lower motor neuron).

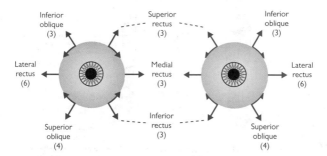

Fig. 50.4 Extraocular movements. Reproduced with permission from Brodal, Per, *The Central Nervous System* (5 ed.), 2016, Oxford University Press.

VIII Vestibulocochlear

Whisper a number in each of the patient's ears in turn and ask them to repeat that number (NB: does the patient use a hearing aid?). Perform the Rinne test. Strike a tuning fork, hold it initially in front of the patient's ear and then place the end opposite on the mastoid process. The Rinne test is positive if normal (i.e. air conduction louder than bone conduction). If the patient perceives the bone conduction loudest, that indicates either a conductive hearing loss or an ipsilateral sensorineural hearing loss (these can be distinguished by the following test). Perform the Weber test by striking a tuning fork and placing it in the centre of the patient's brow. Normally the patient should hear it equally in both ears. In conductive hearing loss, it is louder in the affected ear, whereas the reverse is true in sensorineural hearing loss.

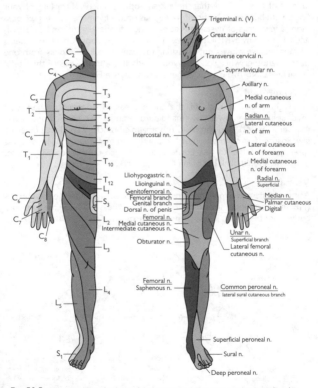

Fig. 50.5 Cutaneous distributions of dermatomes and corresponding peripheral nerves. Reproduced with permission from A. Arturo Leis and Michael P. Schenk, *Atlas of Nerve Conduction Studies and Electromyography* (2 ed.), 2012, Oxford University Press.

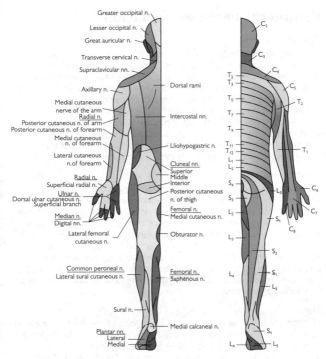

Fig. 50.5 (Contd.)

IX Glossopharyngeal, X vagus, XII hypoglossal (palate/tongue)

Examine for asymmetry of palate (IX) at rest and with the patient saying 'ah'. Offer to test gag reflex (sensory arm (IX) and motor arm (X)). Examine for wasting or fasciculations (if bilateral, think of motor neuron disease) of the tongue (XII). Ask the patient to protrude their tongue, press it laterally into the cheek against resistance, and wiggle it from side to side (XII). In unilateral palatal weakness, the uvula points away and the tongue towards the weak side.

XI Spinal accessory

Ask the patient to turn their head against your hand on both sides. This tests the contralateral sternocleidomastoid (i.e. a patient weak when turning their head left may have a right XI nerve palsy). Ask the patient to shrug their shoulders against resistance to test the trapezius.

Peripheral nerve examination

Gait assessment

Ask the patient (if able) to stand up and walk (make sure you follow them closely to ensure their safety). Assess their gait as they walk for a few steps before asking them to turn around and walk back to you heel-to-toe. Observe for specific patterns of gait disturbance and whether this is symmetrical or asymmetrical. Ask them to stand on their tiptoes and heels to assess flexor and extensor compartments of the legs. Assess limb girdle power by asking them to stand from a sitting position without using their arms. Test for Romberg's sign by asking them to stand facing you, get their balance, and then close their eyes. Be ready to support them if the test is positive! You are responsible for ensuring that your patient does not hit the ground.

Focused inspection

Look (and feel) for muscle wasting, particularly in the thenar eminence, hypothenar eminence, and between metacarpals in the hands and in the quadriceps (ask the patient to tense their leg to give yourself a better chance of seeing this). Look for evidence of fasciculations (particularly in large muscle groups). Look for contractures, tremors, and scars. Look for evidence of diminished sensation, such as burns or damaged skin (rarely neuropathic arthropathy) in the extremities. Look for any signs of risk factors or associated systemic disease that might predispose to neurological conditions as appropriate (e.g. tar-stained fingers, a vasculitic rash, or an irregularly irregular pulse).

Tone

Test for abnormal tone by moving each joint in the limb through all possible motions. This should be done both relatively slowly (feeling for parkinsonian rigidity) and quickly (feeling for a spastic catch from an upper motor lesion). In the lower limbs, gently roll the legs from side to side. In the case of normal tone, the foot should lag slightly behind the rotation of the leg. Specifically feel for cogwheel rigidity (associated with parkinsonism) in the wrist by rotating the hand in circles. Test for clonus in each lower limb in turn by asking the patient to relax their legs, gently rotating the heel and then jerking the foot briskly into plantarflexion. Up to 4 beats of non-sustained clonus may be normal. Remember that tone can be pathologically ↑ or ↓. Hypertonia is of two forms: upper motor neuron lesions of the pyramidal tract cause spasticity, which is a velocity-dependent ↑ in tone, catching when moved suddenly, whereas extrapyramidal lesions cause rigidity, which is velocity independent. In the arms, the best way to detect spasticity is with the pronator catch—flick the hand from pronation to supination, looking for a brief catch. In the legs, spasticity is best detected by quickly lifting the knee off the bed; watch the foot, which will lift off the bed if there is spasticity. Also look for clonus at the ankles by rapidly dorsiflexing.

Reflexes

Test each of the reflexes in Table 50.5.

Deep tendon reflexes should be elicited with a brisk motion, using the weight of the tendon hammer to generate the power of the strike

Table 50.5 Reflexes and their origins/locations

Reflex	Muscle, root, and nerve	Location
Upper limb		
Biceps	Biceps, C5–6, musculocutaneous,	Anterior elbow over biceps tendon
Supinator	Brachioradialis, C5–6, radial	Radial side of wrist ~8 cm proximal to thumb
Triceps	Triceps, C6–7, radial	Posterior elbow over triceps tendon
Lower limb		
Knee	Quadriceps, L2–4, femoral	~2 cm inferior to patellar
Ankle	Gastrocnemius/soleus, S1–2, tibial	Achilles tendon ~3–4 cm above heel
Plantar (Babinski)	Extensor hallucis longus, L4–5/ S1–2, tibial	Base of foot (see text)

($\otimes$ www.neuroexam.med.utoronto.ca/motor_6.htm). Compare reflexes at the same level between each limb, ensuring that you look at the muscle that will contract with the reflex, rather than just the movement of limb. If the reflex appears absent, ask the patient to clench their teeth just before you test the reflex (reinforcement/Jendrassik manoeuvre). Grade the reflexes as 0+ absent; ± present with reinforcement; 1+ reduced 2+ normal; 3+ increased without clonus; 4+ increased with clonus. Testing for presence of the Babinski sign should be conducted by firmly scratching with a thumb or blunt item (not the sharp end of a tendon hammer) from the heel, along the lateral side of the foot and then medially across the base of the toes. An abnormal response (extensor plantar response = upper motor neuron sign) is extension of the hallux (vs flexion normally) ± fanning of the other toes.

Power

Check for weakness by opposing each movement in the patient with your own. For example, for finger abduction, put your hand alongside the patient's and directly compare the strength of your own finger abduction with that of your patient (i.e. like for like). Isolate the muscle being tested and immobilize the proximal parts. Score the patient's power in each movement *while stabilizing the joint* using the MRC grading system.[1] Make sure that you do use sufficient strength yourself that the patient has to exert him- or herself to overcome you.

For each movement, try to think about the peripheral nerve and nerve root territory you are testing as you test that movement. Minimize your instructions to either push or pull to avoid confusion to the patient and to yourself. You will look more slick. (See Table 50.6 and Table 50.7.)

Table 50.6 Scoring power

MRC grade	Definition
0	No visible contraction
1	Visible trace of contraction
2	Movement with gravity removed (e.g. can flex knee with leg horizontal on bed)
3	Movement against gravity (but collapses with resistance)
4 (±)	Movement against resistance (4− low; 4 medium; 4+ high)
5	Normal power

Coordination

Hold your index finger ~ one arm's length in front of the patient. Ask the patient alternately to touch their nose and the tip of your finger. Look for any past pointing, intention tremor, or bradykinesia. Test for dysdiadochokinesia by asking the patient to rapidly pronate and supinate one hand in the palm of the other (demonstrate this to the patient). Test for cerebellar rebound by asking the patient to stretch their arms straight out in front of them and closing their eyes. Tell the patient to keep their arms where they are and then briskly push the arms downwards. A positive test is when the arms rebound above their initial position. Test coordination in the lower limbs by asking the patient to run the heel of one foot down the opposite leg and then lift the foot up to touch their leg again (heel–shin test). Repeat as quickly as possible.

Sensation

Test each of the modalities in Table 50.8.

Test for light touch, pin-prick, vibration, and joint position (proprioception) sense. Ensure that the patient's eyes are closed when testing all modalities. When testing proprioception, check that you are not supplying inadvertent cues by applying pressure to the skin of the sensitive finger pads. Test each joint at least three times. In general, test sensation from distal to proximal, since this is most likely to identify an abnormality quickly in the majority of cases. If an abnormality is detected, then systematically map out the extent of the sensory deficit. Adjust your method to suit: if you are looking for a mononeuropathy, test around the distribution of the nerve concerned; for a polyneuropathy, test distal to proximal (e.g. hallux, malleolus, leg, etc.); and for a root problem, test dermatomes. (See Fig. 50.5.)

Reference

1. Hahn AF, Bolton CF, Pillay N, et al. (1996). Plasma exchange therapy in chronic inflammatory demyelinating polyneuropathy. A double-blind, sham controlled, cross-over study. *Brain* 119:1055–66.

Table 50.7 Limb movements

Action	Muscle	Roots	Nerve
Shrug shoulder	Trapezius	C3, C4	Spinal accessory
Abduct shoulder	Supraspinatus, deltoid	C5, C6	Suprascapular and axillary
Flex forearm	Biceps	C5, C6	Musculocutaneous
Extend forearm	Triceps	C6, C7	Radial
Extend wrist	Extensor carpi	C5, C6	Radial
Extend fingers	Finger extensors	C7, C8	Posterior interosseous
Flex fingers	FDP and FDS	C8, T1	Median and ulnar
Abduct thumb	Abductor pollicis brevis	C8, T1	Median
Thumb to 5th finger	Opponens pollicis brevis	C8, T1	Median
Abduct 5th finger	Abductor digiti minimi	C8, T1	Ulnar
Abduct index finger	First dorsal interosseous	C8, T1	Ulnar
Flex hip	Iliopsoas	L1, L2	Femoral
Adduct hip	Hip adductors	L2, L3	Obturator
Extend hip	Hip extensors	L5, S1	Inferior gluteal
Extend knee	Quadriceps	L2, L3	Femoral
Flex knee	Hamstrings	L5, S1	Sciatic
Dorsiflex foot	Tibialis anterior	L5, S1	Deep peroneal
Plantarflex foot	Gastrocnemius	S1, S2	Tibial
Invert foot	Tibialis posterior	L4, L5	Tibial
Dorsiflex hallux	Extensor hallucis longus	L5, S1	Deep peroneal
Evert foot	Peroneus longus and brevis	L5, S1	Superficial peroneal

FDP/FDS, flexor digitorum profundus/superficialis.

Table 50.8 Testing modalities of sensation

Modality	Equipment	Spinal pathway tested
Light touch	Cotton wool ball	Anterolateral
Pinprick	Neurotip™	Anterolateral
Proprioception	None (flex and extend joint)	Dorsal columns
Vibration	Tuning fork	Dorsal columns

Nervous system: further examination

Clinically, every neurological patient should have at least a basic assessment of cognition, speech, and their functional status (i.e. ability to carry out activities important for daily life). In addition, if particular signs are detected on the general examination, the examiner should attempt to elicit some specific signs supportive of particular diagnoses.

Cognition

This is a discipline in its own right. There are multiple screening tools that can be used, such as the MMSE and MoCA (www.mocatest.org/).[1, 2] Cognitive defects may also be picked up during the general examination if the patient is finding it difficult to follow commands etc. As part of this, you should check for pathological primitive reflexes, including the snout, rooting and palmomental reflexes.

Speech

Test for receptive dysphasia by asking the patient to perform a three-step action (e.g. take this paper with your left hand, fold it in half, and place it on the table). Check for executive dysphasia by asking the patient to name common items (e.g. pen, watch, book, etc.). Test for defects in speech production at different levels within the palate by asking the patient to repeat particular phonemes (e.g. 'ga', 'ka', 'ma'; http://neuroexam.med. utoronto.ca/cranial_9_10.htm). Examine palate and tongue coordination by asking the patient to repeat the phrases 'baby hippopotamus' and 'British constitution'. Ask the patient to tell you about their day and assess their speech as they converse with you.

Parkinsonism

In addition to the general neurological examination, examine for the following signs:

- Resting tremor—ask the patient to put their hands on a pillow while counting backwards from 20.
- Cogwheel/lead pipe rigidity.
- Bradykinesia—ask the patient to open and close both hands quickly.
- Parkinsonian gait—flexed posture with short, festinating steps and turning en bloc.
- Postural instability—warn the patient what you are going to do, stand behind them and tug back quickly on their shoulders; Parkinson's patients typically fall like a 'beanpole' or take a few steps back (retropulsion).
- Micrographia—ask the patient to write several sentences.
- Parkinsonian voice—speak to the patient and assess whether they have a quiet, often monotonous voice.
- For extra marks, check for signs of atypical parkinsonism syndromes: vertical gaze palsy (PSP), cerebellar signs/postural drop (MSA), and spatial neglect (CBD).

Cerebellar

Most relevant signs are contained within the general examination, but in particular check for 'DANISH': dysdiadochokinesia, ataxia (head, trunk or limb), nystagmus, intention tremor, slurred or staccato speech and hypotonia. Past pointing and cerebellar rebound are also recognized features.

Functional

Arguably the most important assessment once the diagnosis is made. This can be done in many ways but can include timed walks, stair tests, and assessing the ability to dress, wash, make a cup of tea, etc. Are the current aids the patient has appropriate to their needs?

Life-threatening signs

If you find signs of a serious acute/subacute illness on general neurological examination, specific further examination may be necessary. If there are signs consistent with an acute/subacute progressive motor neuropathy, it is vital to check for respiratory compromise by measuring (and monitoring) forced vital capacity. If there are signs of an acute spinal cord syndrome, it is necessary to check for anal sphincter compromise. Concisely report your assessment as a list of positive findings and important negatives. Try to bring your findings together as a differential diagnosis.

Anticipate the following questions
- What are the causes, investigation, and treatment of strokes?
- Which MDT members will you involve in managing stroke patients?
- How can you differentiate between upper vs lower motor neuron lesions?
- What are the nerve roots for myotomes, dermatomes, and reflexes?

If you are doing really well
- What are the associations between area of blindness and area of pathology?
- What is RAPD and name types of pupillary responses?

Specific patterns of neurological deficit

Patterns of neurological deficit are associated with specific lesions (see Fig. 50.6).

Localizing the lesion

Much of neurological examination is directed at identifying the location of a potential lesion within the neuraxis. Throughout your examination you should consider whether the signs you identify fit with particular patterns. The main division within an examination of the peripheral nervous system will be between an upper and lower motor neuron lesion. Table 50.9 should help you think about your examination findings systematically:

References

1. Folstein MF, Folstein SE, McHugh PR (1975). "Mini-mental state". A practical method for grading the cognitive state of patients for the clinician. *J Psychiatr Res* 12(3):189–98.
2. Nasreddine ZS, Phillips NA, Bédirian V, et al. (2005). The Montreal Cognitive Assessment, MoCA: a brief screening tool for mild cognitive impairment. *J Am Geriatr Soc* 53(4):695–9.

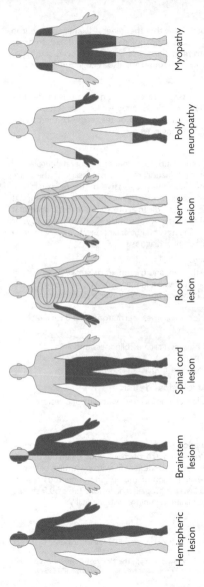

Fig. 50.6 Common patterns of neurological deficits. Reproduced from Aaron L. Berkowitz, *Clinical Neurology and Neuroanatomy: A Localization-Based Approach*, 2017, McGraw Hill.

Hemispheric lesion

Brainstem lesion

Spinal cord lesion

Root lesion

Nerve lesion

Poly-neuropathy

Myopathy

Table 50.9 Patterns of findings

	Lower motor neuron (LMN)	Upper motor neuron (UMN)	Sensory neuropathy	Mixed
Inspection	Fasciculations, wasting	Contractures	Burns, injuries	Fasciculations, wasting
Tone	↓	↑ ± clonus	↓	↑/↓
Power	↓	↓	↔/↓ (if pure)	↓
Reflexes	↓	↑	↓	↔/↓
Coordination[a]	↔	↔	(sensory ataxia—improves with patient observing movement)	↔/↓
Sensation	↔ (↓ if sensory nerves involved too)	↔ (↓ if spinal)	↓	↔/↓
Common patterns and causes[b]	Glove and stocking (e.g. MMN, GBS, CIDP, Charcot–Marie–Tooth). Single/multiple peripheral nerve, spinal root or plexus lesions	Symmetrical with sensory level (spinal—e.g. disc prolapse, tumour). Unilateral (cortical—stroke)	Glove and stocking (e.g. diabetes mellitus, folate/vitamin B12 deficiency, toxin, para-neoplastic, drugs etc.)	UMN and LMN signs (motor neuron disease, cervical myelopathy, vitamin B12 deficiency)

CIDP, chronic inflammatory demyelinating polyneuropathy; GBS, Guillain–Barré syndrome; MMN, multifocal motor neuropathy.

[a] Coordination can be difficult to assess in the presence of profound weakness.

[b] Become familiar with the distribution of nerves and nerve roots so as to localize lesions (➔ e.g. *Oxford Handbook of Neurology*, Chapter 2).

Obstetrics

Pregnancy is a very important time in a woman's life, so extra care and sensitivity is important when performing an examination of the pregnant abdomen. Building a good rapport early by simply congratulating them or asking them if they have thought of a name will help put your patient at ease!

As with any clinical examination, the following steps much be taken:
- Wash hands.
- Introduce yourself.
- Obtain informed consent—talk through what you are going to do.
- Expose: ask the patient to lie as flat as is comfortable for her and expose the abdomen ideally from pubic bone to xiphisternum.
- Pattern of examination is as follows:
  - Inspection
  - Palpation
  - Symphysis–fundal height (SFH)
  - Auscultation.

General well-being
- *Hands*: swelling, pallor, pulse, BP, capillary refill time.
- *Face*: jaundice, anaemia (conjunctiva), periorbital oedema.
- Leg or ankle oedema.

Abdominal inspection
- Position patient supine.
- Expose from the xiphisternum to the pubic symphysis.
- Abdominal distension consistent with appropriate gestation.
- Fetal movements seen.
- Surgical scars, e.g. appendicectomy, laparoscopy, previous caesarean section through Pfannenstiel incision (low transverse scar across the abdomen above the pubis).
- Signs of pregnancy:
  - Linea nigra: dark line from the xiphisternum to the pubic symphysis due to ↑pigmentation.
  - Striae gravidarum: stretch marks.

Palpation
- Ask about pain before starting.
- In a single pregnancy there should be two fetal poles (unless the head is deeply engaged, i.e. entered the pelvis).

Lie

Relationship between the longitudinal axis of fetus and mother. Feel either side of the uterus abdominally, and then the back and limbs of the fetus. The lie can either be:
1. *longitudinal* (resulting in either cephalic or breech presentation)
2. *oblique* (unstable, should ideally become either transverse or longitudinal)
3. *transverse* lying across the abdomen from left to right or vice-versa (resulting in shoulder presentation).

Feel the maternal abdomen to feel which side is the back (i.e. which side of the abdomen feels more full and similar to a smoother structure, e.g. back). This is compared to the other side, where limbs can be felt, including movements.

Presentation

Identify the anatomical part of the fetus that is closest to the pelvic inlet (cephalic, breech, or malpresentation, e.g. limb) and felt by placing thumb and fingers on either side of the presenting part.

Engagement

'How many 5/5th palpable?'

- Divisions for the fetal head into fifths ~1 finger width = 1/5th.
- If all of the fetal head is felt, that is '5/5ths palpable per abdomen'.
- If none of the fetal head is felt, that is '0/5th palpable per abdomen'.
- The head is engaged when the widest part (the biparietal diameter) has passed through the pelvic brim.

Symphysis–fundal height

- Palpate using ulnar border of left hand moving from sternum downwards.
- It is easier to feel for the fundus firmly first (see Fig. 50.7).
- Locate upper border of pubic symphysis.

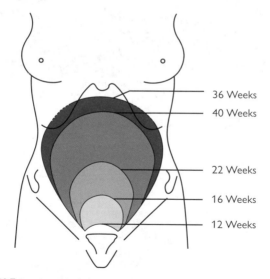

36 Weeks
40 Weeks
22 Weeks
16 Weeks
12 Weeks

Fig. 50.7 Location of fundus as pregnancy progresses. Reproduced with permission from Raine, Tim, et al, *Oxford Handbook for the Foundation Programme* (4 ed.), 2014, Oxford University Press.

- Place the tape upside down.
- Measure the distance in cm using a tape measure that should correlate with gestational age (± 2 cm).
- Plot as an 'x' on the customized growth chart.
- The SFH in cm should be the same as the gestation ±2 cm from 20 weeks onwards.

Auscultation

Once you have identified the lie of the fetus and where the back is, listen over the anterior shoulder of the fetus. Use some gel and a Sonicaid to listen for 1 min for the baseline heart rate which should usually be between 110 and 160 bpm.

To finish

- Wipe the gel away from both the patient's abdomen and the Sonicaid probe.
- Wash hands and thank the patient.
- Offer her help to sit back up.
- Summarize findings.

Gynaecology

There are three parts to a gynaecology examination:
1. Abdominal examination.
2. Speculum examination.
3. Bimanual vaginal examination.

The basic examination format is the same but as this is an intimate exam, it is vital that you take a professional approach and make your patient feel comfortable and at ease. It is also important to address any personal barriers you may have to performing the examination.

To start with
- Introduce yourself.
- Obtain informed consent for the examination.
- Get chaperone and equipment ready (e.g. speculum, gel ± swabs).
- Ensure the light at the examination table is working well, otherwise get a torch—*do not under any circumstances* use the torch application on your mobile device, even if you assure the patient that only the torch is in use.
- Ask the patient if she would like to go to the toilet to empty her bladder (making the examination more comfortable as there is less pressure on the bladder when the speculum opens or when you are performing a digital examination).
- Inform the patient that she can remove appropriate clothing behind a curtain and lie down on the examination couch with a sheet to cover herself.
- Wash hands and wear gloves.
- Check for whether she is ready for the examination, and enter the room/behind the curtain with the chaperone.

General inspection

Explain to the patient that the position she should be lying in is supine, with knees bent, heels brought up towards bottom, and then letting legs fall to either side of the bed. It is important to look out for other signs, which may be relevant to any gynaecological pathology. For example:
- Body habitus.
- Endocrine—goitre, skin changes such as acanthosis nigricans (velvety, hyperpigmented patches of skin which usually develop around the groin, neck and armpit, associated with obesity, insulin resistance suggestive of polycystic ovary syndrome (PCOS)).
- Secondary sexual characteristics—hirsutism, acne (suggestive of PCOS).

1. Abdominal examination

Make sure you ask about existing pain before starting. Like any examination, follow the normal routine: inspection, palpation, percussion, and auscultation. Important things to note include body hair distribution, scars, striae, tenderness, distention, masses, organomegaly, and inguinal lymphadenopathy.

2. Speculum examination

Inspection

Explain to the patient that the position she should be lying in is supine (flat), with knees bent, heels brought up towards bottom, and then letting knees fall to either side of the bed. Be aware of older women or women with restricted hip mobility. Draw back the cover sheet towards the suprapubic area to inspect the vulval area for:

- erythema
- ulceration
- warts
- lesions
- hair distribution
- scarring.

To ensure full visualization of the labia minora, clitoris, urethral orifice, and vaginal introitus (opening), use your gloved left hand and part the labia majora with your thumb and index finger. Ask the patient to cough to look for a prolapse or stress urinary incontinence.

Speculum procedure

1. Think about the size of the speculum needed and use lubrication.
2. Explain to the patient what you are going to do before proceeding.
3. Expose the introitus by spreading the labia from below using the left index and middle finger.
4. Gently insert the speculum at a 45° angle and pointing slightly downward using your right hand until at least half of it is inserted.
5. Gently rotate the speculum to a horizontal position and gently open the blades until the cervix is in view (the blades may not need to be fully opened).
6. Secure the speculum by turning the thumb nut.
7. Visualize the cervix and vaginal walls for any abnormalities, e.g. ectropion, cysts, polyps, and contraceptive coil threads (if you can't see the cervix, carefully draw the speculum back, reposition it, and try again).
8. Comment on whether the cervical os is open or closed (parous or nulliparous).
9. Perform any necessary tests, e.g. high vaginal swab, endocervical swab for culture and sensitivity, or cervical smear.
10. Withdraw the speculum slightly to clear the cervix and gently loosen the speculum to close the blades.
11. Continue to withdraw while rotating the speculum to 45°, avoiding contact with the vaginal walls.

3. Vaginal examination

Explain to the patient what you are going to do before proceeding. Using your gloved right hand, abduct your thumb and insert a lubricated index and middle finger into the vagina while flexing the remaining fingers into your palm. Initially, enter with your palm facing sideways and then rotate so it is facing upwards. Now, with your left hand press down on the lower aspect of the abdomen, so the uterus can be palpated bimanually. (See Fig. 50.8.)

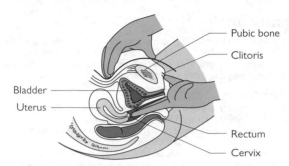

Fig. 50.8 Examination of the female reproductive system. Reproduced with permission from Raine, Tim, et al, *Oxford Handbook for the Foundation Programme* (4 ed.), 2014, Oxford University Press.

While placing two fingers into the vagina, examine the following in order:
- *Cervix*: consistency, tender, mobile, cervical excitation.
- *Uterus:* place your two fingers behind the cervix and press upwards to ballot the uterus between your fingers inside and hand on the suprapubic area.
- *Tilt*: check whether the uterus is anteverted or retroverted, the size of the uterus, whether it is mobile, smooth, and tender to ballot.
- *Adnexae*: these are both lateral fornices. Place the two fingers on the right side of the vaginal wall and using the left hand on the abdomen, try and ballot to check for masses or tenderness. Do the same with the left side.
- *Posterior vaginal wall*: feel for nodules and tenderness.
- Gently withdraw fingers and check glove for any blood or discharge.

To finish
- Cover the patient back up with a sheet once you have completed your examination.
- Thank the patient.
- Offer her help to sit back up.
- Offer the patient tissues—never wipe excess gel yourself.
- Close the curtain and allow the patient to dress in privacy.
- Inform her you will discuss the findings when she is dressed and back in the consulting room.
- Dispose of equipment correctly.
- Wash hands and summarize findings.

Ophthalmology

During your ophthalmology placement, ensure you acquire the following basic examination skills: history taking, visual acuity, visual field and colour vision testing, assessment of pupil reflexes, ocular motility, and fundus examination using the direct ophthalmoscope.

History station

Ophthalmic history taking may centre on a PC of visual loss in an OSCE setting. An efficient, focused history is required in these circumstances to determine the timing of onset, laterality, and whether associated with any other symptoms (headache, jaw claudication, flashes, floaters, etc. if acute visual loss; photophobia, epiphora, pain, itching, or reduced vision if red eye). Ask about precipitating/relieving factors, and timing to resolution if relevant.

Past ophthalmic history

Recent surgery, use of contact lenses, recurrent pathology (iritis, recurrent corneal erosion syndrome), known chronic ophthalmic disease (diabetic retinopathy/glaucoma), and current treatments (drops) are important to elicit.

Past medical history

The eyes are often affected by systemic disease. Maintain a high index of suspicion in immunosuppressed patients. Ask about vascular risk factors in the setting of acute vascular events (retinal artery occlusion). Topical drugs undergo significant systemic absorption: asthma/COPD, diabetics on hypo-glycaemic drugs, and those with ischaemic heart disease are at risk of ad-verse events with topical beta blockers. Likely longevity is important when determining the management of glaucoma and risk of blindness.

Family history

Certain disorders demonstrate Mendelian patterns of inheritance (retin-itis pigmentosa, retinal dystrophies, etc.) FHx of glaucoma (first-degree relative) confers ↑risk of glaucoma in any patient. Viral conjunctivitis may spread rampantly through households; ask about contacts.

Drug history

Establish what their current drop regimen is, whether they are able to phys-ically use their drops, who instils them, and ask about compliance ('Do you ever forget to use them?'). Ask about systemic drug use. Systemic beta blockers may reduce IOP. Chloroquine, fingolimod (MS), amiodarone (AF), and topiramate (epilepsy) may cause visual loss. Warfarin and use of alpha antagonists (tamsulosin) may render ophthalmic surgery more difficult, due to an ↑risk of bleeding or poor pupil dilation.

Social history

The DVLA has strict visual criteria for driving: vision must be 6/10 or better in the binocular state with a healthy binocular visual field. Patients with age-related macular degeneration, glaucoma, or diabetic retinopathy, for instance, may risk losing their driving licences (and independence).

Smoking is a vascular risk factor and may contribute to poor outcome (thyroid eye disease). Alcohol and smoking may cause a toxic optic neuropathy. Phosphodiesterase inhibitors for erectile dysfunction may cause photopsia (flashing lights). Digoxin and ethambutol toxicity may result in colour vision disturbances. Recreational drug use may be relevant (cocaine, amphetamines) as IV drug use ↑ the risk of endogenous endophthalmitis.

Examination

A basic ophthalmic examination involves visual acuity testing, confrontation visual fields, pupil responses, colour vision, ocular motility, inspection of the ocular surface with light source, red reflex, and fundoscopy. In many circumstances as a doctor (such as in general practice) this will need to be performed without use of a slit lamp.

Visual acuity testing

This is often documented poorly, yet it is medico-legally indefensible to omit it in patients with visual complaints. You should learn how to accurately measure distance and near acuity, and perform this throughout your career on patients in your care.

Distance acuity

Test each eye in turn with the appropriate spectacle prescription (best corrected visual acuity). Distance vision is measured with a Snellen chart, typically at 6 metres (see Fig. 50.9). Occlude one eye in turn and ask the patient to read to the smallest line visible. Record the number under the visible line as the denominator (e.g. 6/12: notating that patient can see from 6 metres what a person with normal vision can see from 12 metres). A pinhole corrects many forms of refractive error, and if patient cannot see 6/6, ask patient to look through pinhole and record this acuity. This is useful if a patient has forgotten their glasses.

Near acuity

Jaeger cards are often used, with letter sized denoted as N48–N4.5 (smaller number denotes smaller letter). Test each eye in turn, with reading glasses if appropriate and good lighting. Myopic patients have good unaided near vision but poor unaided distance vision.

Visual fields to confrontation

This is critical for identifying neurological visual field defects (from cerebrovascular disease, tumours, etc.). Sit opposite your patient at the same height. Ask them to cover one eye and the examiner covers the opposite one. Ask them to look at your pupil with the unoccluded eye and present fingers in each of the four visual fields at mid distance and present fingers in each of the four visual fields at mid distance, asking the patient to count how many you are holding up (make sure they maintain fixation on your eye). This objectively confirms the integrity of each visual field quadrant. Repeat for the other eye.

Pupillary reflexes

Note the pupil size in both eyes in ambient light conditions. Direct the light in one eye and observe the direct pupil reflex (same pupil) then the consensual pupil reflex (contralateral pupil), and repeat for the other eye. The Marcus–Gunn swinging flashlight test examines for a RAPD, a sensitive test of unilateral optic nerve or retinal disease. You should ask an ophthalmologist to demonstrate this as it is often done poorly, yet is a very important

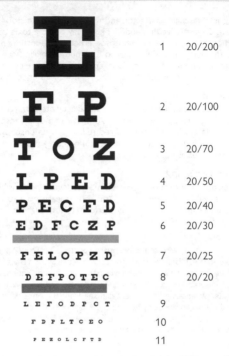

E	1	20/200
F P	2	20/100
T O Z	3	20/70
L P E D	4	20/50
P E C F D	5	20/40
E D F C Z P	6	20/30
F E L O P Z D	7	20/25
D E F P O T E C	8	20/20
L E F O D P C T	9	
F D P L T C E O	10	
P E Z O L C F T D	11	

Fig. 50.9 Snellen chart. Reproduced from 'Snellen chart' by Jeff Dahl – Own work by uploader. Licensed under CC BY-SA 3.0 https://commons.wikimedia.org.

objective clinical sign that should be performed on any patient with visual loss. The light is directed in the affected eye, before swinging to the un-affected eye, then back to the affected eye (if this pupil dilates in response to light, a RAPD exists). Test pupil response to accommodation (ask patient to look at a near target): both pupils should constrict as part of the accommodation response. (See Fig. 50.10.)

Common pupil abnormalities

Holmes–Adie pupil causes a unilateral tonically dilated pupil, often in young females. Near acuity is reduced due to impaired accommodation. Oculomotor nerve palsy may cause ptosis, reduced ocular motility (due to paralysis of four out of six extraocular muscles), and a non-reactive pupil. This may indicate a life-threatening intracranial pathology. Horner's syndrome results in unilateral subtle ptosis, miosis, apparent enophthalmos, and variably, anhidrosis due to interruption of sympathetic innervation to the eye. Pancoast's tumour (apical lung cancer) and carotid artery dissection are two pathologies that must be excluded in this patient group.

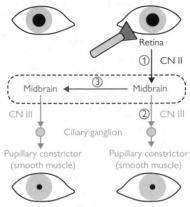

(a) Pupillary light reflex circuit

Retina
① CN II

Midbrain ←③— Midbrain

CN III ② CN III
Ciliary ganglion

Pupillary constrictor
(smooth muscle)

Pupillary constrictor
(smooth muscle)

Consensual pupillary reflex   Direct pupillary reflex

(b) Lesions affecting pupillary light reflex

| | (unilateral) lesion site | | |
	CN II ①	CN III ②	Midbrain (midline) ③
Ipsilateral stimulus			
direct response	×	×	√
consensual response	×	√	×
contrateral stimulus			
direct response	√	√	√
consensual response	√	×	×

Fig. 50.10 The pupillary light reflex is a simple reflex that is of great clinical utility. (a) Information regarding a change in luminance travels from the retina to the midbrain through the optic nerve. Within the midbrain, luminance information is processed by the pretectal nucleus and then passed on to the Edinger–Westphal nucleus, which contains preganglionic parasympathetic neurons that travel in the oculomotor nerve and ultimately control the pupillary constrictor muscle. Importantly, information crosses the midline within the midbrain so that a luminance change in one eye affects the pupils of both eyes. (b) The effects of three common lesions on the direct and consensual pupillary reflexes evoked by light flashed into each eye are illustrated. Reproduced with permission from Peggy Mason, *Medical Neurobiology* (2 ed.), 2017, Oxford University Press.

Colour vision

This is often examined with the Ishihara colour plates (although these are designed to test congenital red–green colour blindness). Each eye is tested in isolation and number plates are read consecutively, recorded as number of plates read over number presented (i.e. 14/17).

Fundoscopy

This is a key part of the neurological examination, and may be employed by examiners to distinguish candidates at finals. The eye clinic is the only place in the hospital with opportunities to perform dilated fundoscopy, and to receive feedback from an ophthalmologist.

It may be your only opportunity to learn or refine your technique before you qualify. You should aim to be able to examine an optic disc through an undilated pupil before the end of the placement. Practise, practise, practise is the only way to master this skill.

Three key tips: (1) get as close as you can with your ophthalmoscope, ~1 cm from the eye! (2) Ask patient to fixate at specific target to prevent ocular movement. (3) Dim room lights to maximize pupil size if not pharmacologically dilated.

Procedure

1. Introduction, consent, and instructions: '*May I examine the back of your eye? I am going to come quite close. May I put my hand on your head? Please look at the sign on the wall.*'
2. Switch ophthalmoscope on, adjust to medium-sized white light beam, keep the lens dial on 0 unless you need to dial in your prescription (on Welch Allyn, red numbers = myopic prescription, green = hyperopic).
3. Find the red reflex from 30 cm, and follow the red reflex in (this keeps light beam on the pupil), put your hand on patient's head with thumb on brow (to provide proprioceptive information), and get as close as physically possible to the ocular surface to maximize view. Approach 15° temporally to find the optic disc.
4. Find a retinal vessel and follow it. If two smaller vessels join to a larger one in the direction of movement, you are heading towards the disc, keep going (all retinal vessels originate at the optic disc).
5. When visualizing the disc, comment on margin (excludes disc swelling), colour (e.g. pallor), significant optic disc cup (glaucoma), and presence of new vessels (proliferative diabetic retinopathy).
6. Ask patient to look up, find red reflex and inspect retina, and do the same while asking patient to look right, down and then left (demonstrates systematic retinal examination).
7. Finally, ask patient to look at the light (this will bring the light beam onto the macula/fovea) and inspect for haemorrhages, exudates (diabetes), or scarring.

Ocular movements

In the binocular state, with the head kept still, ask the patient to track a target in the nine principal positions of gaze, and to report any double vision (diplopia). Ensure full abduction (abducens nerve—sixth cranial nerve), ability to look down and in (trochlear nerve—fourth cranial nerve), and adduction (oculomotor nerve—third cranial nerve). Complete third nerve palsy results in complete ptosis (paralysis of levator palpebrae superioris), fixed and dilated pupil, and eye looking down and out underneath the closed eyelid. Partial third nerve palsy may spare the autonomic features (pupil sparing) and suggests a microvascular cause such as diabetes/hypertension/vasculitis.

Orthopaedic examinations: general

General principles

Orthopaedic examination is an art, which can be learnt and mastered with practice. The focus should be on eliciting pertinent signs and the manner in which they affect the patient, which will aid in formulating a diagnosis and subsequently tailoring treatment plans. Patients should be respected, made to feel at ease, and their dignity should be preserved. The examiner should be aware that if the examination causes discomfort, the patient should be asked if they would like to proceed with the rest of the examination. Handwashing, introducing yourself, and explaining your role demonstrates professionalism and is likely to instil confidence in your patients. Communication with patients is vital so give them clear instructions on what you wish them to do and expose the region to be examined.

Equipment

A tape measure, goniometer (instrument to measure angles), and a tendon hammer are essential for orthopaedic examinations. Aids to functional assessment in a hand examination include a pen, comb, key, and coin.

Starting the examination

The examination starts from the moment that we encounter the patient. A plethora of information can be obtained by their general appearance, posture, and gait. Do they have a short limb, 'knock-knees', are they in pain, or not using a limb? Looking around the bedside for braces, walking aids, orthoses, and slings may help not only in establishing a diagnosis but also in understanding how the condition may disable the patient. Exposure of the joint to be examined must be done with clear instructions while preserving the patient's dignity. Both limbs should be exposed and examination should start with the unaffected limb for comparison.

Examination sequence

The commonest examination technique is derived from Apley's mantra of:
1. *Look* (inspection)
2. *Feel* (palpation)
3. *Move* (manipulation)
4. *Tests* (e.g. measure and gait for lower limb examination).

Having a systematic approach provides a repeatable and transferrable examination, which will pick up on important findings related to the diagnosis and the patient's disability.

Look

- *Observe*: front, back, side.
- *Shape and posture*: patient thin or obese? Spine straight/curved? Shoulders level? Abnormal limb posture? Flexed posture (assess for a fixed deformity on movement—look for deformity of three planes, compare with unaffected side.
- Wasting of muscle groups? (disuse, denervation). Swelling—diffuse (joint synovial fluid, blood, pus). Localized (ganglion, meniscal cyst).

- *Skin*: colour—pallor (ischaemia), blueness (cyanosis), redness (inflammation, infection, pain syndrome), purple (bruise/ecchymosis). Markings (wounds, scars, ulcers, sinuses). Quality—shiny (oedema, trophic change), abnormal creases (underlying fibrosis).

Feel

This is an exploration of anatomy and therefore should be communicated with your examiner (e.g. 'I am palpating the medial joint line of the knee between the medial tibial plateau and the medial femoral condyle while observing the patient's face, this does not appear to elicit pain'). Find landmarks and use them! Look at the patient's face to appreciate areas of tenderness.

- *Skin*: warm/cold (use the palm of your hand as more nerve endings/ sensitive), moist/dry.
- *Soft tissues*: lump (size, shape, surface, consistency, compressibility, fluctuation, mobility, illumination, percussion, auscultation), pulses.
- *Joint*: palpable effusion, synovial tenderness (inflammation/infection).
- *Tenderness*: correlating your anatomical landmarks with areas of tenderness gives you an idea of what the underlying structure/ problem is.

Move

Demonstration of movement makes communication clearer. Measurements should be carried out with a *goniometer* and both limbs compared. This can be compared with reference ranges for each joint.

- *Range of movement (ROM)*: in degrees. Starting at 0, anatomic position of joint (hyperextension is denoted by –ve degrees referenced from anatomical position). End range finishes when joint stops moving (e.g. ROM of −10° to 140° is a hyperextension of 10° and 140° flexion from the anatomical position).
- *Active*: patient moves without assistance. Functional degree of movement. Painful? Muscle power (MRC grade). Feel for crepitus (coarse and diffuse—joint, fine and specific—tenosynovial).
- *Passive*: examiner moves joint. Limited by pain and joint stiffness.
- *NB*: sometimes active movement cannot be performed due to limitations in understanding (young children/some neurological disorders).
- *Arthrodesis*: lack of active and passive ROM.
- *Degenerative joint/adhesive capsulitis*: limited active/passive ROM.
- *Tendon/muscle/nerve injury*: no active, only passive ROM.
- *Ligament laxity*: excessive ROM (hypermobility).

Special tests

These are discussed elsewhere and are used to elicit suspected abnormalities.

Measure

Length of limbs and muscle bulk can be measured using a measuring tape. It is vital when comparing limbs that the same fixed landmarks are used.

Gait

Involves two main phases: swing (40%) and stance (60%) (See Fig. 50.11 and Table 50.10.)

Further examination

Further examination of the joint above and below is essential to exclude referred pain (e.g. a patient with hip osteoarthritis presenting with pain referred to the knee). A complete neurovascular examination should be done to ascertain whether there is a true neurological deficit or if neurological symptoms are mimicking MSk symptoms. The MRC grading system is used to assess muscle strength.

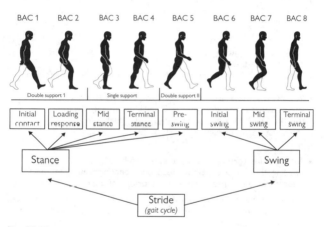

Fig. 50.11 Gait. Reproduced from Stöckel T. et al, The mental representation of the human gait in young and older dults. *Front Psychol.* 2015 Jul 14;6:943, under the CC Attribution 4.0 International license.

Table 50.10 Description of gait analysis

Gait	Description
Antalgic	Shortened stance phase (painful)
Spastic	Stiffed-legged (flexed hips and knees, equinus feet) 'scissoring' of legs
Foot drop	Equinus: in swing—peroneal nerve injury
High stepping	Foot drop, balance, proprioception
Waddling (Trendelenburg)	Trunk thrown from side to side—abductor weakness
Ataxic	Broad based, loss of balance

Upper limb examinations

Examination of hand

Look

Both upper limbs should be exposed to above the elbow. Place a pillow on the lap. Inspect hands with palms up, make a fist, turn to palms down and make another fist in this position. Ask to flex elbows and inspect olecranon fossa. Usual format of inspection for scars (surgery/trauma), sinuses.

Palmar aspect
- *Look*: skin colour, dry/moist, hairy/smooth, puckering and ridging of skin (Dupuytren's disease).
- *Swellings*: subcutaneous (dermoid cyst), tendon OA, ganglion at wrist.
- *Muscle wasting*: thenar eminence wasting (median nerve dysfunction).
- *Normal cascade*.

Dorsal aspect
- *Nails*: atrophy, 'pitting' (psoriatic arthropathy), 'grooved' nail, ganglion cyst at nail bed, subungual exostosis.
- *Swellings*: dorsal ganglion over wrist, RA nodules/gouty tophi (extensor surface).
- *Joint swelling*: metacarpophalangeal joint (MCPJ) plus proximal interphalangeal joint (PIPJ)—RA. Distal interphalangeal joint (DIPJ)—OA, PIPJ (Bouchard's nodes), DIPJ (Heberden's nodes), carpometacarpal bossing (OA mass).

Feel
- Temperature, texture of skin, and pulses felt.
- Swelling/thickening, subcutaneous tissue, tendon sheath, joint (each palpated for an effusion/tenderness), or one of the bones.

If a nodule is felt, flexion/extension of finger will ascertain if it is attached to underlying tendon. Does tendon glide freely or snap in extension (trigger finger)? Can a cord be felt or Garrod's pads on dorsal aspect of PIPJ (Dupuytren's)?

Move

Perform active movements then check additional passive movement. Active movements: clue from initial screening with palms up and making a fist may show 'lagging' finger. Thumb and each finger examined in turn.

Flexion and extension
Fingers:
- DIPJ = 0–80°.
- PIPJ= 0–100°.
- MCPJ = 0–40° of hyperextension to 90° flexion.

Abduction/adduction
MCP joints in extension relaxes collateral ligaments and allows maximal movement.

Thumb movements

To assess thumb movements with patient's palm up, hold hand flat on table. Ask to:
• 'stretch to the side'—extension
• 'bend thumb'—flexion
• 'point to the ceiling'—abduction (weak in median neuropathy)
• 'pinch my finger'—adduction
• 'touch your thumb to little finger'—opposition
• thumb behind plane of hand is retroposition.

Special tests

• *Muscles*: gross grip strength should be assessed by asking the patient to squeeze examiner's index and middle fingers:
  • *Flexor digitorum profundus (FDP)*: PIPJ held and immobilized in extension and patient asked to bend tip of finger.
  • *Flexor digitorum superficialis (FDS)*: grasp other fingers in full extension to inactivate FDP. FDP shares a common muscle belly. Isolate the MCPJ in extension of the finger that is being examined. Ask the patient to flex the finger. *NB*: little finger sometimes has no independent FDS. Index finger often has completely independent FDP therefore cannot separate mass action, FDS is tested with DIP in full extension and FDS flexed, patient asked to pinch against resistance—if unable then ?FDS rupture.
  • *Flexor pollicis longus (FPL)*: immobilize thumb MCPJ, ask to flex interphalangeal joint (IPJ).
  • *Long finger extensors*: ask to extend at MCPJs.

Intrinsics

• *Lumbricals*: flex MCPJ and extend IPJ.
• *Interossei*: Palmar ADduct and Dorsal ABduct ('PAD DAB').

Functional tests

This is the most significant part of the examination as it gives the examiner an idea of the disability caused. For the purposes of most examinations, props such as a key, coin, and pen are sufficient for a functional assessment. A series of tasks can be given to the patient to assess function and grip:
• *Precision*: 'Pick up a pin'.
• *End pinch*: 'Hold a card'.
• *Sideways pinch*: 'Holding a key'.
• *Chuck pinch*: 'Holding a pen'.
• *Hook grip*: 'Holding a bag handle'.
• *Span*: 'Holding a cup'.
• *Power*: 'Gripping a hammer'.

Pathology-specific tests

• *Hueston tabletop test*: demonstrates contractures of the PIPJ and MCPJ in Dupuytren's disease. Ask patient to place palm of the hand flat on the table top—if contractures exist, this cannot be performed.

Finger deformities
- *Boutonnières deformity*: damage to central slip causes proximal phalanx to button-hole through and cause a PIPJ flexion deformity. As central slip tear extends, the lateral bands displace palmar, further worsening the PIPJ flexion and causes secondary DIPJ extension.
- *Mallet finger*: flexion deformity of DIPJ. Injury to lateral slips leads to inability to extend DIPJ.
- *Swan neck deformity*: volar plate damage—PIPJ hyperextends and due to muscle imbalance → secondary DIPJ flexion.

See Fig. 50.12.

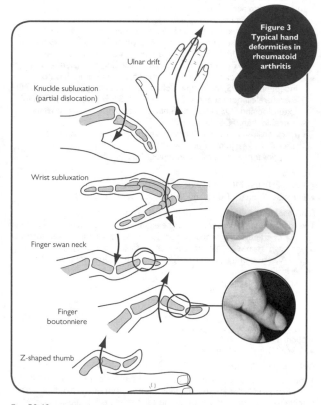

Figure 3
Typical hand deformities in rheumatoid arthritis

Ulnar drift

Knuckle subluxation
(partial dislocation)

Wrist subluxation

Finger swan neck

Finger
boutonniere

Z-shaped thumb

Fig. 50.12 Hand deformities in rheumatoid arthritis. Reproduced from www. arthritisresearchuk.org, Looking after your joints when you have arthritis Photographs reproduced from Marc C Hochberg et al, *Practical Rheumatology*, 3rd edition, 2011, Elsevier.

Further examination

Further examination of the wrist is essential to exclude referred pain. A complete neurovascular examination taking into account the possibility of carpal tunnel/cubital tunnel syndromes and Allen's test for vascular supply to the hand.

Examination of the elbow

Look

Both upper limbs should be exposed. Observe from front, back, lateral, and medial aspects of the elbow. Compare both sides. Usual format of inspection for scars (surgery/trauma), sinuses.

- *Front*: arms by side, elbows extended with palms forward. Normal carrying angle is 5–15° valgus. Look for cubitus varus or valgus. Ask to lift arms to shoulder height with elbows extended—look for '*gunstock deformity*'—varus deformity often results from previous childhood supracondylar fracture or a growth arrest on the medial side of distal humerus. NB: carrying angle can only be assessed once elbow is straight.
- *Side*: surgical scars.
- *Behind*: prominent olecranon bursa, swelling, rheumatoid nodules.

Feel

Anterior and lateral aspects of the elbow are best examined from the front, and medial and posterior from behind.

- *Front*: from lateral to medial, palpate the brachioradialis muscle, biceps tendon with lacertus fibrosus, brachial artery, and the median nerve.
- *Abnormal hard swelling*: myositis ossificans after elbow dislocation.
- *Biceps rupture*: '*hook test*' use finger to hook under tendon insertion— absent with more proximal muscle bulge.
- *Lateral*: palpate lateral supracondylar ridge, lateral epicondyle to common extensor origin (tender—lateral epicondylitis), and lateral collateral ligament. Extensor carpi radialis brevis (ECRB) and extensor carpi radialis longus (ECRL) are assessed with resisted wrist extension in neutral and radial deviation respectively. ERCB tenderness—tennis elbow.
- *Capitellar joint line*: tenderness → articular injury/osteochondritis dissecans.
- *Radiocapitellar joint line*: normal sulcus. Synovial hypertrophy—boggy. Fluid—fluctuant.
- *Radial head*: palpate while supinating and pronating at wrist. Feel for subluxation (congenital), crepitus (degenerative change) worsens with gripping of examiner's fingers during rotation.
- *Posterior*: feel for joint warmth. Tip of olecranon, medial and lateral epicondyles form a straight line with the elbow in extension and an isosceles triangle in 90° of flexion. If not normal—?previous injury. Palpate triceps insertion against resisted extension. Tenderness— partial tear. Inability to extend against gravity—complete tear. Palpate olecranon fossa in 30° flexion—loose body. Feel for rheumatoid nodules or olecranon bursa.
- *Medial*: palpate medial epicondyle to common flexor origin (tender medial epicondylitis), belly of pronator teres (*pronator syndrome*). Feel for ulna nerve behind medial epicondyle, subluxes in flexion in 10% of people.

Move

Perform active movements then check additional passive movement.

Active movements

- *Observe front—flexion and extension*: in sagittal plane with forearm supinated and fully extended. ROM −10° to 140°. Any more extension—?hyperlaxity. Reduced extension first sign of intraarticular injury.
- *Forearm rotation*: elbow flexed to 90°, arms adducted, start with thumbs pointing up. Supination 85°, pronation 85°.
- *Rotational deformity*: shoulder fully extended, elbow bent to 90° behind back, patient bends over. Observe from behind. Look for forearm asymmetry. If forearm not parallel to floor then internal rotational deformity of distal humerus (likely malunion of supracondylar fracture).

Special tests

- *Muscles*: strength in flexion/extension and supination/pronation can be resisted to test muscle groups.

Provocation tests

- *Lateral epicondylitis (tennis elbow)*: passive volar flexion of the wrist, elbow extension, and pronation. Tender lateral epicondyle.
- *Medial epicondylitis (Golfer's elbow)*: passive extension of the wrist and clenching of fist worsen symptoms. Tender medial epicondyle.
- *Impingement*: posterior (olecranon osteophytes/loose bodies)—just short of full extension—gentle rapid passive extension reproduces posterior pain. Anterior (coronoid osteophytes/radial fossa osteophytes)—just short of full flexion—gentle rapid passive flexion reproduces posterior pain.

Instability

- *Varus instability*: lateral collateral ligament (radial collateral plus lateral ulna collateral (LUC)).
- *Assess*: elbow flexed to 30° (unlocks olecranon and relaxes anterior capsule). Shoulder in full internal rotation—locks shoulder. Apply varus stress (under image intensifier)—radio-capitellar space increases.
- *Valgus instability*: ulna collateral ligament.
- *Assess*: elbow flexed to 30° (unlocks olecranon and relaxes anterior capsule). Shoulder in full external rotation—locks shoulder. Apply valgus stress (opening of joint/tenderness suggests injury).
- *Rotational instability*: lateral ulna collateral ligament—'*pivot shift*' similar to that in knee examination. Under image intensifier and GA, patient supine, elbow and shoulder at 90°. Fully supinate while holding hand and forearm. Slowly extend elbow applying valgus and axial compression. Elbow subluxation—dimple over radiocapitellar joint and prominence posterolaterally over radial head. At 45° ulna reduces with a 'clunk'.
- *Apprehension sign*: ask to rise from chair using arms to push up. May be reluctant due to instability. This creates axial load, valgus and forearm supination as above.

Examination of the shoulder

Look

Patient undresses to waist, scapulae should be visible. Observe from front, back, side, and axilla. Compare both sides. Look for slings or braces around the patient. Usual format of inspection for scars (surgery/trauma), sinuses.

- *Front*: prominence of acromioclavicular joint (ACJ) or sternoclavicular joint (SCJ)—degenerative/traumatic. Deformity of clavicle—previous trauma. Long head of biceps rupture—'Popeye' sign. Pectoralis major wasting or rupture (loss of anterior axillary fold).
- *Side*: surgical scars.
- *Behind*: prominent shoulder blade—malunion, osteochondroma, positional (static winging). Wasting of deltoid ('squared-off' appearance of shoulder)—axillary nerve injury/chronic shoulder pain. Hollowing of supraspinous and infraspinous fossa—supraspinatus and infraspinatus full-thickness cuff tears/suprascapular nerve lesion.
- *Axilla*: joint effusion.

Feel

Joint warmth, bony points

Palpate SCJ, clavicle, ACJ, acromion, subacromial margins, and margins of glenoid, bicipital groove.

Move

Active movements

Perform active movements then check additional passive movement. Movements are a combination of glenohumeral joint (GHJ), scapulothoracic joint (STJ), SCJ, and ACJ.

Observe front

- *Flexion and extension*: in sagittal plane. Flexion ROM 0–160°/170° (acromion limits movement). Extension ROM 0–40°.
- *Adduction*: not normally recorded.
- *External rotation*: arms by side and elbows at 90° of flexion. ROM 0–80°.

Behind

- *Internal rotation:* ROM limited by trunk getting in the way. Hence functional—how far behind one can reach with the tip of thumb (vertebral level T8, T5, etc.)—tests adduction and internal rotation combined.
- *Abduction*: referenced in coronal plane but does not correspond to plane of GHJ as scapula faces forwards by 30°. ROM 0–160°/180° in scapula plane. Stand behind and observe scapulae.
- *Scapular rhythm*: GHJ movement: STJ movement 2:1. More GHJ movement in lower range (90°), STJ in later range (60°). Isolate GHJ movement by fixing tip of scapula and acromion (abduction restricted to 90°). While assessing scapulothoracic rhythm, look for winging of scapula (from either injury to serratus anterior or to the long thoracic nerve).
- *OA*: full movement at STJ, little at GHJ.
- *Painful arc*: pain in midrange of abduction (70–120°)—cuff tear/ supraspinatus tendinitis.
- *ACJ arthritis*: pain at end range of abduction.

Special tests

Rotator cuff

- *Infraspinatus*: most powerful external rotation—elbow flexed to 90° power of external rotation assessed.
  - *Hornblower's sign*: complete tear, flex elbow and abduct shoulder to reach mouth (like sounding a hunting horn).
- *Infraspinatus and teres minor*:
  - *Drop sign*: arm passively maximally externally rotated then released if weakness falls 'drops' into internal rotation.
  - *Lag test*: examine from behind. Elbow at 90°, elevate 20° in scapula plane. Passively put in full external rotation. Patient asked to maintain position but drops into neutral rotation.
- *Supraspinatus*: abductor. Most patients with a tear can still initiate abduction using the deltoid. Shoulder elevated in plane of scapula (30°) forward from coronal plane. At 60° maximum tension of muscle fibres, internal rotation (reduced deltoid contribution), thumb down. Test resistance—*Jobe test*.
- *Subscapularis*: powerful internal rotator.
  - *Lift off test (most reliable)*: hand behind back and push examiner's hand away from small of back (reduced pectoralis contribution). Pain in shoulder may limit test. 'Lag' test pull hand away from back, ask patient to keep away from back—'lags' back—complete subscapularis rupture.
  - *Napoleon/belly press test*: hand on abdomen, patient pushes elbow forward (reduced pectoralis contribution).

Other muscle around shoulder

- *Deltoid*: tested in 90° abduction or by side of patient. Ask to forward flex (anterior), abduct (lateral), and extend (posterior) heads of deltoid.
- *Pectoralis major*: hands on waist and squeeze inwards—palpate muscle.
- *Latissimus dorsi*: downwards and backwards pressure of arm against resistance—palpate muscle.
- *Rhomboids*: hands on hips pushing elbows backwards against resistance—palpate muscle.
- *Serratus anterior*: patient pushes against wall with outstretched arm, fingers and palm pointing down—*scapula winging* observed (long thoracic nerve of 'Bell' palsy).
- *Trapezius*: patient shrugs shoulder against resistance.

Impingement tests

- *Neer's sign*: passively elevate the internally rotated shoulder in scapula plane while stabilizing the scapula. Pain 70–120°—downward pressure on scapula exacerbates.
- *Neer's test*: inject local anaesthetic into subacromial space and repeat manoeuver—positive if pain abolished.
- *Hawkins and Kennedy sign/test*: arm elevated to the horizontal and adducted by 10°. Subsequent internal rotation of the arm provokes pain. Can be repeated after local anaesthetic infiltration.

Acromioclavicular joint
- *Scarf test*: elevate arm to shoulder height and adduct arm across chest. Positive if pain occurs—ACJ arthritis.
- *O'Brien's test*: arm elevated to horizontal, adducted by 15° fully internally rotated. Patient asked to resist downward pressure on wrist, which causes pain. Less sensitive for ACJ OA, more sensitive for rotator cuff tears or SLAP (superior labrum, anterior to posterior) lesions.

Biceps tendon pathology
Long head of biceps (LHB), biceps pulley (in intertubercular groove), and insertion into supraglenoid tubercle (SLAP tears) cause pain.
- *Popeye sign*: bulky of biceps visible more distal in arm—LHB rupture.
- *Speed's test*: elbow fully extended, forearm supinated. Anterior shoulder pain on resisted elbow flexion—positive.
- *Yergason test*: taking the patient's hand as if to perform a handshake, elbow at side, 90° flexion. Resisted supination, not pronation, indicates biceps pathology.
- *Crank test*: shoulder abducted and elbow flexed to 90°. Resisted elbow flexion recreates pain.

Instability test
- *Sulcus sign*: inferior laxity on passive downward traction on the humerus in neutral rotation. If present in external rotation—rotator interval incompetence (coracohumeral and superior glenohumeral ligaments)
- *Load and shift tests*: stand behind patient. Stabilize scapula using thumb behind acromion and index finger on coracoid. Grasp proximal humerus close to the humeral head between thumb, and index and middle fingers. Passively move humeral head anterior and posterior to respective glenoid rims → pain/clicks—indicate rim damage/labral tears.
- *Apprehension tests*: patient seated or lying with shoulder at edge of couch.
  - *Anterior apprehension test*: shoulder abducted to 90° and elbow flexed to 90° with/without anterior pressure to back of humeral head and gentle external rotation → patient fears dislocation may occur, involuntary pectoralis major contraction = positive test.
  - *Posterior apprehension test*: horizontal adduction of internally rotated arm while axial load applied along humerus. If does not produce apprehension, maintain axial load and bring out of adduction and internal rotation → relocation of subluxed humeral head may occur.

Further examination
Further examination of the cervical spine is essential to exclude referred pain. Testing for generalized joint laxity using a Beighton's score is useful in cases of instability.

Spine examination

Look

Exposure to underwear, offer a blanket to keep warm or to preserve dignity if examination of the whole spine not required. Usual format of inspection for scars (surgery/trauma), pigmentation (neurofibromatosis), tufts of hair (spina bifida).

Observe

Front, back (coronal plane), and side (sagittal plane) and look for scoliosis (lateral curvature of the spine). 'Adam's Forward bend test'—patient bends forward and 'rib hump' may be seen.

Normally

Thoracic kyphosis (slight forward curve), lumbar lordosis (short backward curve). Abnormalities can occur as:
- kyphosis
- cervicothoracic (*ankylosing spondylitis*)
- thoracic (*Scheuermann's disease*, osteoporotic wedge fractures)
- loss of lumbar lordosis: protective paravertebral muscle spasm
- hyperlordosis: *spondylolisthesis, fixed flexion deformity of hips*
- assess shoulder asymmetry and pelvic tilt. If one knee flexed could be nerve root tension (flexing knee relaxes sciatic nerve).

Feel

- *Feel;* spinous process and interspinous ligament for steps.
- *Tenderness;* correlating your anatomical landmarks with areas of tenderness gives you an idea of what the underlying structure/problem is. 1—bony structures, 2—intervertebral tissues, 3—paravertebral muscles and ligaments. The vertebral level should be noted.

Move

All movements are performed actively by demonstrating/instructing. Passive movements can be performed at the end range of movement.
- *Cervical*: flexion, extension, rotation, lateral flexion.
  - *Spondylosis* (reduced flexion and extension).
  - *Cervical disc prolapse* (hold head to affected side, passive lateral flexion to contralateral side produces radicular pain).
- *Thoracic spine*: rotation (facet orientation and ribs restrict flexion, extension, and lateral rotation).
- *Lumbar spine*: flexion/extension (facet orientation restricts rotation).
  - Flexion measured on forward bend as 'fingers to knee, mid-shin, toes, etc. Is it smooth or hesitant?
  - Lateral flexion measured in similar manner.
  - Extension (support from behind, pain—*facet arthrosis*).
  - Rotation by fixing the pelvis.

Gait

Antalgic, neurological (broad based in *cervical myelopathy*), short legged (*compensatory scoliosis* as a result of leg length discrepancy). *A quick screening of lower lumbar nerve roots before walking may be useful*:

- *Squat* and get up (*L3*—quadriceps).
- Stand on *heels* (*L4*—ankle dorsiflexion).
- Stand on *one leg*—Trendelenburg (*L5*—hip abduction).
- *Tip toe* (*S1*—plantar flexion of ankle).

Special tests

Cervical spine

- *Spurling's manoeuvre*: narrows the involved neuroforamen (cervical radiculopathy). Axial pressure, hyperextend, lateral flexion, and rotated to affected side. Abduction of shoulder relieves pain.

Thoracic outlet syndrome

- *Adson's manoeuvre*: head extended and rotated to affected side, abduction of arm >15°—radial pulse obliterated.
- *Roo's manoeuvre*: shoulders abducted, elbows flexed to 90°—fingers actively and repeatedly flexed and extended—recreates tingling.

Cervical myelopathy

- *Lhermitte sign*: flexion of the neck precipitates 'lightning' or paraesthesia of lower limbs.
- *Upward plantar responses*.
- *Clonus*: at ankle/knee >3
- *Hoffman's sign*: flick DIPJ of index/middle finger. If thumb flexes—+ve test.
- *Inverted radial reflex*: finger flexion seen with brachioradialis tendon reflex.
- *Romberg's*: close eyes with feet together → unstable stance.

Lumbar spine

- *Sciatic stretch test*: with patient supine passively, raise the leg straight to 30–50°—ask about pain in back or down the leg. Lower the leg gently and passive dorsiflexion reproduces symptoms (*Lasegue's sign*). If patient sits up with knee straight (i.e. hip flexed at 90° then no nerve root tension). Can be done with patient sitting with knee flexed over the edge of the couch and actively extending each knee in turn ('*flip test*'). 'Crossover sign' is when the patient's symptoms are reproduced by a straight leg raise of the contralateral leg.
- *Bowstring test*: with patient supine, flex the hip and knee to 45°, then press on the popliteal nerve behind the knee, which recreates pain.

Measure

- *Rib cage excursion*: chest circumference in full inspiration and expiration ~difference of 7 cm. Reduced in *ankylosing spondylitis*.
- *Schobers test*: quantitative evaluation of lumbar spine flexion. Mark horizontal line at posterior superior iliac spines (PSIS) and second 10 cm above this. On forward flexion this distance should increase by at least 5 cm. Limitation by pain protection in *ankylosing spondylitis*.

Lower limb examinations

Examination of the hip

Look

Patient undresses to below waist and keeps underwear on to maintain dignity; offer a blanket for the supine part of the examination. Observe from front, back, and side. Compare both sides. Look for crutches or braces around the patient. Usual format of inspection for scars (surgery/trauma), sinuses.

- *Front*: muscle wasting. Can stand with feet flat on ground. Use blocks at this stage to correct leg length discrepancy. Palpate iliac crest to assess pelvic obliquity.
- *Trendelenburg's test*: originally described with examination from behind, it is best performed from the front. Place thumbs on each of the patient's anterior superior iliac spines (ASISs). Ask them to put their hands onto your forearms for balance. Ask to stand on one leg and bend other knee to 90° without flexing hip. This is repeated on the contralateral side. The sign is negative if the pelvis remains level; if the pelvis drops (due to abductor muscle weakness, painful hip, dislocation/subluxation of the hip or shortening of the femoral neck), this is a positive sign. As the pelvis is acting as a fulcrum, the opposite side drops if there is weakness. This can be remembered as 'the sound side sags'.
- *Trendelenburg lurch*: patient leans over the affected hip to shift body's centre of gravity in that direction.
- *Side*: surgical scars, posture, and presence of skin contractures.
- *Behind*: gluteal muscle bulk and presence or absence of scoliosis.

Gait

Ask the patient to walk—abnormal patterns of gait may be due to muscle weakness, compensatory adaptation to pain, or loss of motion.

Feel

Joint warmth: less specific as deeper joint.
Bony points: ASISs, ischial tuberosity, and greater trochanter.

Move

Perform active ROM then check additional passive movement.

- *Flexion*: patient supine and with knee flexed (prevents hamstring tightness), limited by soft tissues of abdomen and thigh. ROM 0–135°
- *Thomas's test*: a patient with a fixed flexion deformity at the hip compensates when lying on their back by arching the spine and pelvis into an exaggerated lordosis. The lordosis can be eliminated by flexing the contralateral hip. Ask the patient to flex both knees and hold them with their hands in a supine position. Then extend knee fully with a hand under their back on the contralateral side to eliminate the lumbar lordosis. The angle between the couch and the thigh demonstrates the fixed flexion.
- *Extension*: patient prone—not usually assessed. ROM 0–30°.
- *Abduction*: patient supine and pelvis stabilized with examiner's hand on opposite ASIS. ROM 0–45°.
- *Adduction*: patient supine and pelvis stabilized with examiner's hand on opposite ASIS. Abduct contralateral leg. ROM 0–30°.

- *Rotation in extension*: either supine with knee straight and patella used as measurement gauge or patient supine with knee flexed to 90°.
  - Internal rotation: ROM 0–40°. External rotation: ROM 0–60°.
- *Rotation in flexion*: earlier signs of hip pathology can be picked up in flexion. Supine with knee flexed to 90° (use tibia as protractor).
  - Internal rotation: ROM 0–40°. External rotation: ROM 0–50°.
- If internal rotation full in extension but reduced in flexion—anterosuperior femoral head pathology, common after avascular necrosis (*sectoral sign*).

Measure

Best done after movement because if a fixed deformity is present, the contralateral limb must be placed in a similar position for a comparison to be made.

- *Apparent*: from midline point in the body (umbilicus, xiphisternum) to medial malleolus.
- *True*: ideally centre of femoral head, i.e. axis of movement, however, no palpable landmark. Hence from ASIS to medial malleolus.
- *Galleazzi's test*: is shortening above or below the knee? Flex both knees to 90° and keep heels together. Look from side (femur) and front (tibia) to see where the discrepancy lies. If above the knee, a few lines can be drawn to determine if the discrepancy originates from above or below the trochanter.
- *Bryant's triangle*: point A—ASIS, point B – greater trochanter, point C is the intersection of a horizontal line from the ASIS and a vertical line from the greater trochanter. Compare both sides. Line from B to C shows supra-trochanteric shortening. Line from A to B shows amount of central dislocation compared to the other side.
- *Nelaton's line*: ASIS to ischial tuberosity. Greater trochanter normally lies below or on line. If above, then femur displaced proximally/supra-trochanteric shortening.
- *Schoemaker's line*: greater trochanter to ASIS continued onto the abdomen. If unilateral problem, then line intersects on the contralateral side; if bilateral, intersection is below the umbilicus.

Special tests

Impingement

- *Anterior impingement test*: patient supine, hip flexed to 90°, adducted and internally rotated. Positive if groin pain (labral tears).
- *Posterior impingement test*: patient supine at edge of couch, contralateral hip held flexed. Examiner fully extends, abducts, and externally rotates the examined hip. Test femoral neck against posterior acetabular wall.
- *FABER (Flexion Abduction and External Rotation) test*: ipsilateral foot placed on contralateral knee, 'figure of four' position. Push down on knee and contralateral ASIS. Pain from sacroiliac joint and posterior hip localize to different sites.
- *Ischiofemoral impingement test/HEADER (Hip Extension ADduction, External Rotation) test*: abnormal contact between ischium and lesser trochanter. Patient supine on edge of couch. Knee flexed to 90°, hip extended, adducted and externally rotated. Pain deep within groin/buttock.

Hip contractures
- *Ely's test (rectus femoris)*: patient prone, knee passively flexed, if tight then hip rises away from couch.
- *Ober's test (fascia lata/iliotibial band [ITB])*: patient lies on unaffected side, maximally flex both hips to flatten lumbar spine. Passively abduct the affected leg to 45° then into extension. If it does not fall into adduction and remains in abduction then ITB contracture.

Further examination
Further examination of the lumbar spine and knee is essential to exclude referred pain. A complete neurovascular examination should be done to ascertain whether there is a true neurological deficit or if neurological symptoms are mimicking MSk symptoms.

Examination of the knee

Look
Patient undresses to below waist and keeps underwear on to maintain dignity; offer a blanket for the supine part of the examination. Observe from front, back, and side. Compare both sides. Look for crutches or braces around the patient. Usual format of inspection for scars (surgery/trauma), sinuses.
- *Front*: look for alignment (genu valgum/genu varum) and shortening.
- *Side*: flexion/hyperextension deformities, recurvatum/procurvatum of tibia/femur.
- *Behind*: scars, bruising, swelling, Baker's cyst.

Gait
Ask the patient to walk—look for varus thrust (medial OA, lateral ligament laxity), valgus thrust (lateral OA, medial ligament laxity). Look at *foot progression angle* (angle of foot with an imaginary straight line (~10–15° external) and patella progression angle (0°) to assess rotational deformity.
- *Sat down*: assess patella height with legs hanging on edge of bed. Ask to extend knees to assess tracking (*J-sign* with patella moving centrally then subluxes laterally in full extension).
- *Supine*: scars especially arthroscopic and swelling better seen here. Quadriceps and calf wasting can be circumferentially measured from a fixed bony point (tibial tuberosity).

Feel
- *Joint warmth*: using palms of hands compare bilaterally.

Effusion
- *Ballottement test*: (massive effusion)—pressure on one side of knee is transmitted to hand on other side of knee.
- *Patellar tap test*: (moderate effusion)—hand over suprapatellar pouch to occlude press patella which bounces against trochlear.
- *Wipe/bulge test*: (small effusion)—suprapatellar pouch occluded. Stroke lateral gutter and watch fluid into medial gutter.
- *Palpation of joint*: with knee at 90° palpate along patella tendon, medial and lateral joint lines (?meniscal tear), femoral/tibial condyles, medial collateral ligament (MCL), and lateral collateral ligament (LCL), posterior aspect of knee (baker's cyst).

Move

Perform active movements then check additional passive movement.

- *Passive hyperextension*: by lifting both legs up by the ankles.
- *Extensor mechanism*: assessed by asking patient to 'straight leg raise'. Any deficit of full active extension which is passively correctable is known as an 'extensor lag'.
- If it appears as though there is a *flexion deformity* of the knee, place hand under knee and ask patient to push down. Passively try to straighten. If no movement—'fixed flexion deformity'.
- *ROM 0–150°*.

Special tests

Ligament testing

- *Anterior cruciate ligament (ACL) and posterior cruciate ligament (PCL)*: view both knees flexed to 90° from the side, look for *posterior sag* (PCL) injury by comparing the level of tibial tubercles.
- *Quadriceps active test*: if posterior sag noticed, fix the foot and ask patient to extend knee. If there is a posterior sag, the quadriceps pulls the tibial forward via the patella tendon.
- *Anterior and posterior draw tests*: knees flexed to 90°, check patient does not have painful feet and ask permission to lightly sit on feet to fix them. Then grasp tibia with both thumbs on tuberosity to pull tibia forward and backwards. Excessive movement backwards, positive posterior draw (PCL injury). Excessive movement forwards, positive anterior draw (ACL injury plus secondary restraints).
- *Lachman test*: most reliable for ACL. Grasp distal femur in one hand and with knee flexed at 20°, grasp the proximal tibia and try to displace anteriorly. If small hands, fix the patient's femur on the examiner's flexed knee. Note degree of displacement and feeling of 'end-point'.
- *Pivot shift test*: measures rotational component of ACL and recreates forces resulting in giving way when landing on a planted foot. With patient supine, grasp the tibia in both hands and keep ankle in examiner's armpit. With knee in full extension, apply internal rotation and valgus force with lateral hand (tibia subluxed anterolaterally) then flex to 20°—tibia reduces. Either obvious clunk (shift) or subtle (glide).

Medial and lateral collateral ligaments (MCL and LCL)

- *MCL*: hold leg above and below with knee in full extension, valgus force applied by pushing lower leg against lateral hand. If the knee opens up it implies a significant disruption to deep MCL and secondary stabilizers (cruciates, posteromedial capsule). Repeat in 20–30° flexion, which relaxes secondary restraints and allows assessment of superficial fibres of MCL.
- *LCL*: same as for MCL but apply varus stress. Less common and associated with a posterolateral instability.

Other tests

- *Dial test—postero-lateral corner (PLC) and PCL*: patient prone, knees and ankles together, maximum passive external rotation at 30° and 90°. PLC injury asymmetry at 30°. PLC and PCL injury asymmetry at 30° and 90°.

- *Apley's grind test (meniscus)*: patient prone, knee flexed to 90°, and axial rotatory force applied—*not performed*.
- *McMurray's test (meniscus)*: patient supine, knee flexed, one hand on top of knee, and one under the ankle. Varying degrees of compression from the top hand and rotation and flexion from the bottom hand to stress each compartment—*not performed*.
- *Patella glide (patella instability)*: knee slightly flexed, patella maximally moved side to side. If patella spilt into quadrants, should move one medially and two laterally; if does not, then lateral and medial retinaculum is tight respectively.
- *Clarke's test (patellofemoral joint pain)*: pressure over superior pole of patella and ask patient to contract quadriceps—*recreates pain—not performed*.

Examination of the foot and ankle

Look

Patient undresses to below waist and keeps underwear on to maintain dignity; offer a blanket for the supine part of the examination. Observe from front, back, and side. Compare both sides. Look for crutches, braces, orthoses, and footwear around the patient. Usual format of inspection for scars (surgery/trauma), sinuses.

- *Behind*: position of heel relative to the floor. The axis of the tibia compared to os calcis (*tibiocalcaneal angle* ~5° valgus). Achilles tendon swelling? Calf muscle bulk? Forefoot visibility (normally one and a half toes) 'too many toes' sign implies posterior tibialis tendon dysfunction. Ask patient to tip-toe (double heel raise). Assess gastro-soleus complex. If both heels in varus, posterior tibialis functioning well. If pes cavus consider *Coleman block test*.
- *Front*: ankle swelling—effusion/synovitis/osteophytes. Medial longitudinal arch—pes planus (flat)/pes cavus (↑arch). Midfoot deformity. Forefoot deformity—hallux valgus, hammer toe (single interphalangeal fixed flexion), claw toe (fixed flexion of both IPJs)
- *Skin and nail changes* (ulceration, pitting, etc.)
- *Plantar aspect of foot and between toes*: plantar keratoses and ulcers. Diabetic ulcers—under first, second, third metatarsal head and pulp of hallux.

Gait

Ask the patient to walk—disability, pain, and stiffness. Arthritic ankle—difficulty through rocker phase. First metatarsophalangeal joint (MTPJ) OA—difficulty with toe off.

Feel

Systematic and relate to underlying anatomy. Start at ankle and move distally.

Ankle

- *Medially*: swelling/tenderness—synovitis, posterior tibialis irritation, posterior tibial nerve compression, flexor hallucis longus snapping.
- *Anterior*: synovitis/effusion in notch of Harty (space medial to tibialis anterior).

- *Laterally*: tibialis anterior, long extensors, peroneus tertius.
- Anterolateral aspect of ankle joint—thumb pressure with plantar flexed foot—pushes hypertrophic synovium into joint. Then dorsiflex foot if pain worsens (positive *anterolateral impingement test*).
- Move to inferior tibiofibular syndesmosis—tender? Injury.
- *Squeeze test*: compression mid-calf level (compress tibia and fibula in coronal plane). External rotation of the foot with tibia stabilized anteriorly is an alternative.
- *Distal to joint line*: anterior talofibular ligament (70° to axis of fibula to talus). Anterior sinus tarsi—irritation of subtalar joint.
- *Posterior*: posterior to fibula—peroneal tendons, peroneal retinaculum, calcaneofibular ligament (deep). Achilles tendon (tenderness, thickening), bony swelling (*Haglund's deformity*). Passively plantar- and dorsiflex ankle while palpating Achilles tendon—if thickening moves, then from tendon not sheath.
- *Midfoot*: palpate from calcaneum (anteromedial tuberosity) to distal part of plantar fascia (plantar fasciitis/plantar fibromatoses)—worsened maximally dorsiflexing the great toe.
- Chopart's joints (talonavicular and calcaneocuboid)—tenderness crepitus. Between the two is the sinus tarsi (subtalar joint irritation). Assess other mid tarsal joints.
- First MTPJ: hallux rigidus. Metatarsal shafts—stress fracture.
- Second MTPJ: *Freiberg's disease*, synovitis.
- Tenderness between metatarsal heads, third webspace burning/paraesthesia radiating to toes—*Morton's neuroma*. Mulder's sign: reproduction of pain when squeezing the toes in a mediolateral direction and the production of a click by applying a dorsally directed pressure beneath affected webspace.

Move

Perform active ROM then check additional passive movement.
- *Ankle movement*: patient seated, test with knee flexed and extended.
- ROM 20° *dorsiflexion*, 40° *plantarflexion*.
- Passive movement assessed in forefoot in supination to exclude dorsiflexion at Chopart's and midtarsal joints. Inversion of heel to lock the subtalar joint will further isolate ankle movement. Cup the heel and rest sole of foot on forearm then assess movements.
- *Subtalar movement*: hold calcaneus with one hand and fix the talar neck with the thumb and index finger on the other hand. Apply varus and valgus stress to calcaneus. ROM 5° *valgus* to 5° *varus* with ankle in plantigrade position (foot 90° to tibia).
- *Inversion and eversion*: movement at subtalar, Chopart's and mid tarsal joints. Inversion 20° and eversion 10°.
- *Midfoot*: contribution to inversion and eversion assessed by fixing hindfoot. Also *abduction* and *adduction* 5° can be assessed this way.
- *First tarsometatarsal joint*: passive *plantar and dorsiflexion*—may contribute to hallux valgus.
- *Hallux*: dorsiflexion 80°, plantar flexion 40°. *Grind test*—axial load and torsion reproduces pain—hallux rigidus.

Special tests

Muscle testing

- *Tibialis posterior*: foot plantar flexed. Resisted inversion while palpating tendon behind medial malleolus.
- *Tibialis anterior*: maximum dorsiflexion and some inversion. Resisted dorsiflexion in this position while palpating tendon in front of medial malleolus.
- *Peroneus longus*: put foot in maximum plantar flexion and eversion. Ask patient to maintain position while examiner pushes foot inwards. Palpate tendons behind lateral malleolus.
- *Peroneus brevis*: foot placed in neutral position and resisted eversion performed.

Other tests

- *Coleman block test*: used in cavovarus foot. Plantar flexion of first ray is a result of sparing of peroneus longus. To move the lateral four metatarsals into plantigrade, the heel goes into varus. Coleman block test determines if hind foot varus is fixed or mobile. Block placed beneath foot with first ray not supported. If heel mobile, it goes into valgus. If fixed deformity, it remains in varus.
- *Thompson's test*: test for rupture of Achilles tendon, patient prone with feet dangling off edge of couch. Normally, the resting position with an intact Achilles is plantar flexion; if ruptured, the foot position is more neutral. Squeeze calf—if tendon intact, passive plantar flexion at ankle; if complete rupture, no response.
- *Anterior draw test*: used to test anterior talofibular ligament (ATFL) of lateral ligament complex. Grasp heel with one hand and distal tibia with the other hand. Attempt to translate heel anterior relative to tibia. Compare both sides—↑translation = ATFL laxity.

Paediatric examination

Paediatrics has been dubbed 'veterinary medicine' and for a good reason. How do you carry out a comprehensive examination in a population group that tend to start screaming when they see someone with a stethoscope (and not helped by some parents who insist on telling their children that they will get an injection if they do not behave)? One-third to one-half of children presenting to EDs are <5 years old, who can be especially challenging when they are fretful, tired and febrile.[1]

But the art—and the fun—of paediatrics is reinventing the examination at each encounter to get the clinical information you need. Watch paediatricians who have thought of whiz ways to get children to cooperate in the clinical exam (e.g. asking a child to 'flap your arms like a chicken!' to test shoulder abduction/adduction and nerves C5, C6, C7, and C8).

The key is to be opportunistic. If the baby who has presented was crying, but is now fast asleep, examine with the stealth of a panther, gently brushing the fontanelle to check if it is bulging or sunken, listening to the heart sounds and chest, and gently palpating the abdomen. If the heart rate, respiratory rate (always measure your own vital signs), and examination are normal (see Table 50.11 for normal values), you can be more reassured when the child starts crying again when you undress them to complete your examination (e.g. looking for rashes and looking in the ears and throat).

Also, see it from the child's point of view—you are a scary, large stranger. So get down to their level—paediatricians spend a lot of time crouching. Most examination of young children with stranger fear (6 months to 2 years) is best done on the parent's lap, where they feel more secure. Examining the child's teddy bear first might sound clichéd but it works. Distract them by asking them about who their favourite character from a Disney movie is or which football team they support. Remember that when children are ill, they often regress developmentally, so do not always expect age-appropriate behaviour.

Well/unwell

Alert (GCS has been adapted for children)? Capillary refill time (normal <2 sec)? Assess the child's nutritional status. Do they look like they are thriving, underweight, obese? Plot height, weight, and head circumference on a WHO growth chart. At the same time, you will be making a rapid assessment of development, with questions to parents/carers of the child's

Table 50.11 Paediatric normal values

Age (years)	Respiratory rate at rest (breaths/min)	HR at rest (bpm)	Systolic BP (mmHg)
<1	30–40	110–160	80–90
1–2	25–35	100–150	85–95
2–5	25–30	95–140	85–100
5–12	20–25	80–120	90–110
>12	15–20	60–100	100–120

function, covering, if required, the domains of gross motor, fine motor/vision, speech/language and social skills.

Respiratory

Ensure the parents remove the child's shirt as observation is key to observe the work of breathing. Does the child look blue (cyanosed), or more likely a pale grey? Remember, cyanosis is difficult to spot until oxygen saturations are <85%. Do they have an oxygen mask or nasal cannula in place? IV line (infection)?

Count the respiratory rate: be systematic and work from the nose to the diaphragm—nasal flaring, tracheal tug (use of accessory muscles), intercostal recession (rarer in babies and toddlers who have a more elastic ribcage), sternal recession, subcostal recession. Listen (from the end of the bed) for stridor (*inspiratory* upper airway problem) and if stridulous, approach with extreme caution. Also look for any scars, central lines, or ports (e.g. in CF) and at the hands for clubbing/anaemia.

Percussing

Percussing the chest is a useful sign in older children to spot consolidation or effusion but often difficult in toddlers and babies so is attempted infrequently in this age group. Percussion is essential if concerned about pneumothorax (hyper-resonance).

Auscultation

This should cover the same area as in adults, comparing each side. Listen for wheeze (*expiratory*), especially if prolonged, and crackles, and learn to distinguish these from transmitted upper airway sounds (very common in viral infections in children). Absent breath sounds (life-threatening asthma, pneumothorax).

ENT

Often counted as part of the paediatric respiratory exam. Leave this until last and ask someone to show you how to hold an otoscope and examine ears and throats—best done in older children at first while you gain confidence in what you are looking at.

Cardiac

Cyanosis, clubbing, central lines, scars as for respiratory examination. JVP difficult to assess in younger children because of anatomy (chubby necks). Growth and nutritional status important as the child pouring all her calories into coping with a large VSD will have little left over for normal growth.

Measure the heart rate, ask for a blood pressure

Assess peripheral pulses. The femoral and brachial pulses are easier to find in babies and toddlers—palpating the femorals is essential to rule out co-arctation of the aorta. Palpate for the apex beat—fourth intercostal space, slightly lateral to the midclavicular line from 0–7 years, then fifth intercostal space, midclavicular line. Palpate for a heave or thrill, as for adults.

Auscultation

Auscultate over the upper left sternal edge (pulmonary valve), lower left sternal edge (tricuspid valve), upper right sternal edge (aortic valve), and over the apex (mitral valve). Also, auscultate at the back between the scapulae in infants to pick up a murmur transmitted by a patent ductus arteriosus. Comment on any additional heart sounds (e.g. gallop rhythm, quality of the murmur (blowing, harsh)), systolic/diastolic, and grade any murmur detected. Examine elsewhere for signs of heart failure: sweaty, breathless, crackles at lung bases (pulmonary oedema), oedema (legs, sacrum), liver edge. There will likely be a history of poor feeding/growth.

Gastrointestinal

Observation as for respiratory examination, especially nutritional status. You can check the tongue, dentition, and look for ulcers at the end with the ENT exam, if performed. Inspect for scars, herniae, gastrostomy, colostomy/ileostomy, and peritoneal dialysis port. Ask the child to lie flat while you kneel down by the bedside. Explain what you are going to do—'If it hurts, just tell me to stop'. Auscultate for bowel sounds first, then look at the child's face as you palpate, as you would for adults. Palpate and assess for hepatosplenomegaly. Essential to start at RIF for these—large spleens can be missed in infants and toddlers because the mass is mistaken for the child tensing their abdominal muscles. Percuss size if necessary. Palpate for flank pain and renal masses. *Do not perform a rectal examination without a senior present*—this is rarely done in paediatrics and left to the senior/surgeons. If examining for fissures, ensure chaperone is present. Any boy presenting with abdominal pain should be assessed for testicular torsion but ensure a chaperone is present and this is best done by a doctor.

Genitourinary

Examining for trauma, abnormalities (e.g. hypospadias in boys, fused labia in girls), ambiguous genitalia, or for growth/endocrine problems. The *Tanner staging system* will be used to assess puberty in clinic (males: growth of penis, testes, and pubic hair; females: breast development, pubic hair). Examined when a senior is present and always ensure a chaperone is present.

Musculoskeletal

Use the *pGALS* (paediatric gait, arms, legs, and spine) exam to quickly but comprehensively screen for MSk disorders in children. Box 50.1 is a summary but see Arthritis Research UK's excellent teaching videos at ℘ www.arthritisresearchuk.org/health-professionals-and-students/video-resources/pgals.aspx.

Neurological exam

This can appear complicated for the simple reason that young children, or children with developmental delay, cannot follow commands. But you can still pick up a huge amount of information from simple observation. Paediatric neurology is a textbook in itself which you are advised to look up. Most healthy children with normal development over the age of 5 years will be able to understand and perform the normal adult neurological examination of upper/lower limbs and cranial nerves—but make it fun or they will get bored! And many children will tolerate fundoscopy, so have a go. You will have to adapt for younger children or those with developmental delay of any type, and rely more heavily on observing what a child can do. It is important to ask the parents about function and a knowledge of developmental milestones is essential (e.g. it is normal for a 6-month-old baby to be unable to sit unsupported but worrying at 12 months—see Box 50.2).

Box 50.1 pGALS examination

Screening questions
- Do you have any pain or stiffness in your joints/muscles/back?
- Do you have difficulty getting dressed without any help?
- Do you have any difficulty going up and down stairs?

Gait
- Observe walking. 'Walk on your tip-toes/walk on your heels.'

Arms
- 'Put your hands out in front of you.'
- 'Turn your hands over and make a fist.'
- 'Pinch your index finger and thumb together.'
- 'Touch the tips of your fingers with your thumb.'
- Squeeze the metacarpophalangeal joints.
- 'Put your hands together/put your hands back to back.'
- 'Reach up and touch the sky.'
- 'Look at the ceiling.'
- 'Put your hands behind your neck.'

Legs
- Feel for effusion at the knee.
- 'Bend and then straighten your knee.' (Active movement of knees and examiner feels for crepitus.)
- Passive flexion (90°) with internal rotation of hip.

Spine
- 'Open your mouth and put three of your (*child's own*) fingers in your mouth.'
- Lateral flexion of cervical spine—'Try and touch your shoulder with your ear'.
- Observe the spine from behind.
- 'Can you bend and touch your toes?' Observe curve from side and behind.

Reproduced with permission from Foster HE, et al., Musculoskeletal screening examination (pGALS) for school-age children based on the adult GALS screen. *Arthritis Care Research* 2006; 55(5); 709–716.

In all children, look for dysmorphic features, inspect the skin (for neurocutaneous disorders such as NF1), and inspect the back (for any spinal disorder such as spina bifida, kyphoscoliosis). If there is a wheelchair, what extra supports have been added (hypotonia)? Look for orthoses. Always observe gait in children able to walk and assess cerebellar function by asking them to walk heel-to-toe. In the younger child, observe movement, fixing and following (vision), and any response to sounds. You can find out loads by watching them play—Lego, a puzzle, leafing through a book. To assess upper and lower limbs, check tone (stiff, ↑; floppy, ↓). Check for head lag and ↓tone when pulling an infant gently to sit or holding them carefully on their chest and tummies (ventral suspension—ask to see these being done before trying them yourselves). Test reflexes, placing your finger or thumb between tendons and tendon hammer.

Box 50.2 Red flags for child development

Positive indicators
- Loss of developmental skills at any age.
- Concerns about vision (e.g. fixing or following an object).
- Hearing loss at any age.
- Persistently low muscle tone or floppiness.
- No speech by 18 months.
- Asymmetry of movements or other features suggestive of cerebral palsy (e.g. hypertonia).
- Persistent toe walking.
- Complex disabilities.
- Head circumference above the 99.6th centile or below 0.4th centile. Also, if circumference has crossed two centiles (up or down) on the appropriate chart or is disproportionate to parental head circumference.

Negative indicators
(What the child cannot do.)
- Sit unsupported by 12 months.
- Walk by 18 months (boys) or 2 years (girls).
- Walk other than on tiptoes.
- Run by 2.5 years.
- Hold object placed in hand by 5 months (corrected for gestation).
- Reach for objects by 6 months (corrected for gestation).

Reproduced from Bellman Martin, Byrne Orlaith, Sege Robert. Developmental assessment of children. *BMJ* 2013; 346:e8687.

In babies, assess primitive reflexes: Moro (sudden—but gentle!—head extension causes all four limbs to extend; goes by 4 months of age); grasp (both fingers and toes curl to grasp object touching palm or sole; goes by 5–6 months); rooting (head turns towards touch near mouth—to breast-feed; goes by 4–6 months); asymmetric neck reflex (or 'fencing'—the baby puts out the arm like a musketeer to whichever side head is turned; goes by 4 months); stepping (baby held upright will appear to step when feet touch surface; goes by 6 weeks of age).

Cranial nerves: use an object to see if child will fix and follow (II) and check pupillary reaction to light (III); assess eye movements with object or observe child looking around—symmetrical (III, IV, and VI)? Symmetrical smile/grimace (VII)? Startle/react to noise (VIII)?

To complete examination

Plot height and weight and head circumference on growth charts.

Causes of developmental delay
(See Table 50.12.)

Global delay
Everything is delayed. Usually apparent by 2 years of age. Associated with cognitive difficulties. 25% have no known cause.

Prenatal
- *Genetic*: Down's, cerebral dysgenesis, e.g. hydrocephalus.
- *Metabolic*: hypothyroidism, phenylketonuria .
- *Teratogenic*: ETOH, drugs.
- *Congenital infection*: rubella, CMV, toxoplasmosis.
- *Neurocutaneous syndromes*: tuberous sclerosis, neurofibromatosis.

Perinatal
- *Extreme prematurity*: intraventricular haemorrhage/periventricular leukomalacia.
- *Birth asphyxia*: hypoxic ischaemic encephalopathy.
- *Metabolic*: symptomatic hypoglycaemia, hyperbilirubinaemia.

Postnatal
- *Infection*: meningitis, encephalitis.
- *Anoxia*: suffocation, near drowning, seizures.
- *Trauma*: head injury.
- *Metabolic*: hypoglycaemia, inborn errors of metabolism.

Specific developmental delay
Motor
- *Causes*: cerebral palsy, congenital myopathy, spinal cord lesions, e.g. spina bifida, global developmental delay, idiopathic.
- *Hand dominance*: appears at 1–2 years/later therefore dominance before this time = abnormal (e.g. hemiplegia).
- *Late walking*: >18 months. *NB*: locomotor variants, e.g. bottom shuffling, commando crawling, may → acceptable delay.

Speech and language delay
- *Causes*: hearing loss, global delay, anatomical deficit, e.g. cleft palate/cerebral palsy → lack of palate coordination, environmental deprivation, normal variant/familial pattern.
- <20 words at 2 years → refer.

Autism
- Assessment of speech/language (history from mother).
- Interpersonal communication—pointing? Takes mother to what he wants? Eye-to-eye contact? Prefers to play on his own?
- Ritualistic/obsessive behaviour (spinning objects, rigidly ritualistic, dislikes changes in routine)?
- *Other traits*: dislikes crowded spaces/loud noise/having haircut.
- If neurological problems, then ask about obstetric history.

Reference
1. Downing A, Rugge G (2006). A study of childhood attendance at emergency departments in the West Midlands region. *Emerg Med J* 23(5):391–3.

Table 50.12 Developmental milestones

Age	Gross motor	Fine motor/vision				Speech/language	Social
		Draw	Brick	Cut	Beads		
6 weeks	Good head control—raises head to 45 when on tummy. Stabilizes head when raised to sitting position	Tracks object/face				Stills, startles at loud noise	Social smile (visual problem if not)
6 months	Sits without support, rounded back Rolls tummy (prone) to back (supine). Vice versa slightly later	Palmar grasp (5 months) Transfer hand to hand				Turns head to loud sounds Understands 'bye bye'/'no' (7 months) Babbles (monosyllabic)	Puts objects to mouth (stops at 1 year) Shakes rattle Reaches for bottle/breast
9 months	Stands holding on Straight back sitting (7½ months)	Inferior pincer grip Object permanence				Responds to own name Imitates adult sounds	Stranger fear (6–9 months–2 years) Holds and bites food
12 months	Walks alone (9–18 months) → 18 months is threshold for worry—i.e. Duchenne's MD, hip problems, cerebral palsy, etc.	Neat pincer grip (10 months) Casting bricks (should disappear by 18 months—persistence beyond this = abnormal)			2	Shows understanding of nouns ("Where's mummy?") 3 words (50% at 13 months) Points to own body parts (15 months), doll (18 months)	Waves 'bye bye' Hand clapping Plays alone if familiar person nearby Drinks from beaker with lid
18 months	Runs (16 months) Jumps (18 months)	To and fro (15 months)	4			Shows understanding of nouns ('Show me the xxxx') 1 to 6 different words	Imitates every day activities

(Continued)

Table 50.12 (Contd.)

Age	Gross motor	Fine motor/vision		Speech/language	Social
2 years	Runs tiptoe Walks upstairs, both feet/each step Throws ball at shoulder level	Vertical line Puzzles—shape matching is >2 years skill. Random effort <2 years. Turns several pages of book at a time	8	*Shows understanding of verbs* ('What do you draw with, what do you eat with?') 2 words joined together (50+ words)	Eats skilfully with spoon (2½ years)
2½ years	Kicks ball	Horizontal line		*Shows understanding of prepositions in/on* ('Put the cat on the bowl') 3–4 words joined together	
3 years	Hops on one foot for 3 steps (each foot) Walks upstairs, one foot per step; downstairs two feet per step	Circle Bridge ☐ ☐ ☐ (or train) Turns one page of book at a time	Griffiths beads Single cuts	*Understands negatives* ('Which of these is NOT an animal?') Understands adjectives ('Which one is red?')	Begins to share toys with friends Plays alone without parents Eats with fork and spoon Bowel control
3½ years			Cuts pieces	*Understands comparatives* ('Which boy is bigger than this one?' while pointing to middle-sized boy! Or draw circles to illustrate point)	
4 years	Walks upstairs/downstairs in adult manner	Cross Square (4.5 years) Triangle/person (5 years) 12 blocks Steps Big steps (5 years)	Small beads Cuts paper in half	*Understands complicated instructions* ('Before you put x in y, give z to mummy') Uses complex narrative/sequences to describe events.	Concern/sympathy for others if hurt Has best friend Engages in imaginative play, observing rules (4½ to 5 years old) Eats skilfully with little help Handles knife (at 5 years) Dressing and undressing

Source: http://mrcpch.paediatrics.co.uk/development/ by Christopher Kelly.

Written exams

Types of written exam

Throughout medical school you will be bombarded with different types of assessments—probably more so than your friends in other faculties. Although this may seem like a terrifying thought, it does actually provide a valuable motivation to stay on top of the curriculum as you go along. Do not end up cramming your revision into a few weeks before the end-of-year exams are due to begin. It is best to keep up with your workload! Assessments will take many forms from practical exams, to clinical OSCEs, to MCQ papers. This chapter will focus on the written exams that you are likely to encounter at medical school.

Why are written exams so important?

It may sound like a silly question, but passing exams allows us to:

- feel a sense of achievement and worth in terms of knowledge gained (needed to counter the stresses of medical school)
- build confidence
- gain a good ranking for job allocation
- possibly achieve honours or distinctions
- avoid the dreaded resits!

It is worth noting that not all medical schools have the same systems of examination:

- You will find that the quantity of subject material ↑ quite dramatically from your time at A2 level. The pass rate depends on the scoring system and most are standardized.
- Medical school is crazier than school and college with crazier workloads but also comes with crazier fun. Although it is used countless times, the phrase 'work hard, play hard' is fully adopted by every medic. It is a cliché for a reason!
- It is important to realize that while in school it may have felt like you were pitted against your peers, whereas at medical school your personal performance is all that counts. You are all in the same boat in a tough course whereby ~8% of students drop out within the first 2 years. So please help each other to succeed, practise, and become good doctors.

Key types of written examination

1. Multiple choice questions

MCQs involve a question with five possible answers to choose from. Each stem may also require a true or false answer. Some students feel that they are easy as the answer is right in front of you. However, others struggle with the process of elimination.

MCQs generally predominate in medical school summative exams, and so it is really important that you practise this type of question.

Example: which of the following statements about schwannomas is true?

a) They represent peripheral nerve tumours (T/F)
b) Treatment is excision (T/F)
c) They arise frequently in motor nerves (T/F)
d) They degenerate to malignancy (T/F)
e) The commonest presentation is a painless mass (T/F)

2. Extended matching questions

EMQs involve a clinical scenario with more than five options to choose from. This reduces the ability to guess an answer and it gets trickier to use the process of elimination.

Example: Medical School Council, example questions, EMQs ℘ www. medschools.ac.uk/MSCAA/examplequestions/Pages/EMQs.aspx.

3. Short answer questions

SAQs require the student sitting the examination to reproduce knowledge without having any options to choose from. The answers required are usually short as the name suggests and can be anything from a few lines to half a page. It is important to identify exactly what the question is asking to gain maximum marks.

Example: Medical School Council, example questions, SBAs ℘ www. medschools.ac.uk/MSCAA/examplequestions/Pages/SBAs.aspx.

4. Essay questions

These require the student to be able to answer all the points addressed in the question in an 'easy-to-read' and logical format. This can be quite tricky in a time-pressured examination and therefore it is a good idea to pre-plan an essay format or practise these questions (see ➲ p. 980).

5. Prescribing skills assessment (PSA)

The PSA is an important examination which has recently been introduced as either a summative or formative assessment in many UK medical schools. It tests a soon-to-be-doctor's ability to write new prescriptions and calculate drug dosages, among other skills, usually in the final year.

Positive and negative marking

It is important to find out whether your university marks its exams positively or negatively as this will sway how you answer the questions. Positive marking means that you will gain 1 point for answering a question correctly and 0 points for answering incorrectly. Whereas, negative marking means that when you answer a question incorrectly, a point is deducted. Therefore, if your exams are negatively marked you should avoid answering questions that you are unsure about. If not, guess away!

Formative vs summative

A fair number of assessments are classed as 'formative' where marks may not contribute to the end-of-year result. However, 'summative' assessments count towards your end-of-year mark (see Table 51.1).

General tips

Stay calm

If calm is not an adjective your peers would use to describe you, remember: it is possible to learn this skill. Remind yourself that there is always enough time and that rushing is not necessary. It is very important in medical school to learn how to switch off. Some possible ways to feel rejuvenated consist of exercising, meditating, listening to music, as well as participating in a social group. Being able to recognize when you are becoming stressed is an essential attribute—work on this first and then work out how to counter it. This will also hold you in good stead when you start life as a doctor.

Table 51.1 Formative vs summative exams

Formative	Summative
• May have a contribution to final mark	• Contributes to final mark
• Assessments take place throughout teaching modules in various forms	• Usually taken at the end of a teaching unit
• Allows pupils to improve by providing feedback/allowing the student to see if they are on track	• Used to reward achievement and possibly allocate students into quartiles/deciles for ranking
• Can be essays, presentations, posters, reflections, or sometimes practice MCQs/OSCEs	• Usually MCQ exams and OSCEs, although like formative examinations these can take any form

Be confident

Believing in yourself is really important. When you head into an exam, realize that there is nothing else you can do at that point, you have worked hard and you have the ability to pass the test—so get your head down, focus, and think positively. Confidence is important throughout medical school and when you begin practising as a junior doctor. If you are worried about a patient, speak up; if you think a drug has been prescribed wrongly, have the confidence to mention this to one of your team members. Medicine is about working together and using the opinion of everyone on the team to decide the correct management for the patient who is your priority.

Know that you are in the same boat as other medical students

No matter what people say or how they act, *everyone* at some point will experience the feeling of having no idea what they are doing and being totally and utterly lost—you are not alone although there will be plenty of times when you will feel isolated. Working together and chatting through worries and concerns is an important part of the medical school experience, just as much as all the fun times you will have with your colleagues!

The importance of exam technique

Developing a good exam technique is a valuable skill in medical school and the earlier you can decide what works best for you, the better. Knowing all the facts is only part of what is needed to pass an exam. If you can enter an examination room prepared, knowing exactly how you are going to answer the paper, you are more likely to stay calm and avoid stress (which only makes our brains cloudy). It will also help you to feel more confident about the task in hand. 'Exam technique' can be split into three stages: before, at the start, and during the examination.

Before

Know what type of exam you are about to sit

Find out about the types of questions and the exact content covered in this exam. All universities provide this for their examinations so remember to check far in advance. This will help you prepare your revision.

Practise all types of questions

Practise, practise, practise! Doing practice questions from textbooks, revision books, websites, and ones that you have made up with friends is a brilliant way of preparing. Do not leave this to the last minute as doing practice questions can reveal what you know well and where your deficiencies lie—not something you want to find out the night before an exam! It also allows you to feel confident when entering the examination room. Remember to ask around for older students' or lecturers' opinions on what type of practice question and resources would be most useful. There is often a range on offer and there is no point wasting your money on something that would be irrelevant. Some students start their revision using practice questions and identifying where deficiencies in their knowledge lie—and then revise those particular topics.

Start your revision early

Whether you are the type of student who does little and often throughout the year or the type to leave the majority of learning until the end, note that 4 weeks is not enough. Aim to have a revision plan sorted *at least* 2 months before any major exams—this gives you lots of time for revision preparation. Learning early makes life a lot easier but remember to have fun too. The best medical student works hard, is dedicated to learning and to their patients, but also knows exactly how and when to de-stress and relax. It is also handy to ask your peers for any tips or tricks that they can offer about the exam.

Know the length of the exam

This allows you to decide how much time you should spend on each question and will mean that you do not suddenly realize that you have only answered half the questions with 5 min to go! You can either plan beforehand how long you have per question, or just make sure that you have covered around half the questions by half time.

Get your equipment ready

Pens, pencils, rubbers, rulers, sharpeners, a watch—it is vitally important to turn up on the day with the correct equipment to sit your examination. No one wants to be walking into an exam and find out they have forgotten a rubber and their best pencil—preparation is the key to avoiding stress! If an exam is longer than 2 hours some students find that their concentration wavers and a sugar boost/hydration is helpful—so consider taking in some chocolate and a bottle of water. 2% dehydration may → around a 20% decrease in concentration! Also if you have a lucky charm or a mascot, do not forget it and do not be embarrassed—you will not be the only one bringing one! Make yourself as comfortable as possible.

Prepare your outfit the night before

This may not be something you feel you need to do, but some find that preparing everything the night before → a very clear and serene head in the morning!

Do NOT forget to set multiple alarm clocks to the correct time!

It is best to wake up early, have a light breakfast, take a shower to calm your nerves, and perform any other rituals you need to focus on the exam ahead. Never underestimate the amount of stress that exams may cause you and consequent mistakes that you are likely to make if you submit to the pressure.

Know how to get there, and get there on time

This sounds obvious, but it is best to double check your exam venue and make sure you know the route and how long it is going to take for you to get there. There have definitely been pre-exam scares and a last-minute dash to the correct venue a minute before an exam was scheduled to start. Some people prefer to arrive in *just* about time so that they can avoid last-minute 'stress-heads', but make sure you do not arrive late.

Go to the bathroom beforehand

You may want to use a toilet break to de-stress part way through an exam, but there is no point being half-way through a tricky section and being distracted by the call of nature.

At the start

Prepare your desk

Place your watch somewhere visible or note where the clock is, have your spare pencils and rubber handy, and make sure your desk does not wobble. Most examination centres require your student card for their identity check. Place it at the top corner of your table so the invigilators can see it without disturbing you during your exam.

Work out your timings and note them down

A great way to sit an exam well is to know what section you should be hitting at what time—or at least know when you should be half way through.

Fill in the details sheet and exam paper ASAP
This bit is a faff but you want to make sure it is done and dusted instead of wasting the first minutes of the written examination. There have been instances where candidates have forgotten to fill in their details which delays marking or may make your exam void.

Decide what sections to do first
Some students start at the front, others at the back, and others with certain sections—weird but something to consider! It is wise to spend the first couple of minutes inspecting the entire exam paper and start tackling the sections that you find easier. This way, you start building up your confidence and allow more time to answer the more challenging sections.

During

Ignore everyone else
A tip that applies to all of medical school, but especially during an exam. Do not worry about people who seem to be going faster than you or turning to a different part of the booklet. Just make sure you answer the questions on every page and do your own thing.

Slow and steady wins the race
Make sure you stick vaguely to those pre-planned timings. Do not rush through without thinking about a question, otherwise you will just have to completely redo it later! Calmly think through questions and if you are stuck, mark it so that you know to come back to it later before moving on.

Calm and confident
Try not to panic, you have done your revision and you have made it into medical school—much like everything else so far in your life, you will get through this too!

Read the question then read again
It is ever so important to know *what* the question is asking—many a mistake is made by misreading or misinterpreting questions. It may feel at times that you are meant to read their minds, but try to establish what exactly the question is trying to ascertain from you.

Eat food, drink water, use the toilet
If everything seems to be going wrong and you hit a brick wall, do something about it rather than giving up! Take a toilet break, have a sip of water or a bite of chocolate, or even take a step back to breathe. Your brain probably just needs a moment to regroup before focusing again.

Afterwards

Forget about it! Nothing you can do now, is there? Revise for the next exam and try to redeem yourself if you think you performed poorly. If you have finished all your exams, then simply celebrate, relax, and continue with your normal life which was put on hold during your revision period.

Multiple choice questions

What is an MCQ?

An MCQ is a question that asks the student to select the correct response from a list of four or five answers. A slight variation on this type of question is the SBA question. This type is slightly trickier and asks the student to select the 'best' or 'most appropriate' response, even though a few of the options may be partially correct and similar. MCQs generally predominate in medical school summative exams (especially in the first few years), and so it is really important to practise this type of question.

How should I prepare for MCQs?

- Do lots of practice questions—the more you do, the more familiar you will be with this style of questioning.
- Try to avoid learning straight facts and instead attempt to attach some understanding and meaning to the knowledge you acquire.
- Often MCQs ask the student to apply the knowledge they have learned to a particular scenario—quite tricky if you only have superficial knowledge of a subject!
- Decide how you want to answer the questions. Are you the type to go through quickly once then recheck your answers? Or do you prefer to answer the question once properly and then avoid returning to it?
- Work out how long you have per question.

How should I answer MCQs?

As with most things in medical school, it is important to work out *your own way* of answering an MCQ. However, here are some general tips:

- As with any question in a written exam, it is very important to read the question and then to establish *exactly* what it is asking (you may need to reread the question at this point). Misreading or misinterpreting the question is very common, especially in a time-pressured exam. This is where practice will help.
- Unless a particular answer jumps right out at you, using the process of elimination allows students to work their way calmly through questions. Do not be surprised if you find yourself playing ip-dip-doo between the last two answers though, this happens to everyone! An educated guess is an incredibly valuable tool, as long as your exam is not negatively marked.
- If you are really stuck, make a mark next to that question and leave it until the end of the exam—you just need some more time to mull it over at the back of your mind. Sometimes answering related questions to the topic that you are stuck on helps you to remember associated facts.
- Sometimes these questions can involve a lot of reading and so this is something you will need to prepare for. It is important to stay focused and relaxed to avoid having to reread the question numerous times.
- With SBAs, the trick is to not worry that more than three answers are correct which can be daunting, but to imagine yourself in that clinical situation, and work out what you would do initially or what is the most important thing.

- Establish a good pace for answering questions—it is important not to rush but also to avoid wasting time on a questions worth very few marks overall.
- Trust your instincts—often your gut instinct is going to be correct. Avoid changing too many answers after having completed the test. It is common to doubt yourself.
- Be on the lookout for double negatives, these can confuse anyone!
- Be on the lookout for flippant descriptions such as 'None of the above', 'Never', 'Always' which are usually the incorrect answers.
- Questions will often ask you to select the 'most likely' diagnosis or 'most helpful' investigation in a particular case, where more than one answer might be plausible. Try to narrow down the decision to the most plausible two or three answers when it is best of five.
- Remember, the answer is directly in front of you! You just have to spot them and there is a 50% chance of getting it right.

Example MCQ

Which cells produce insulin (true or false)?

a) Alpha   (F)
b) Beta   (T)
c) Delta   (F)
d) Theta   (F)
e) Gamma   (F).

Example SBA

A 72-year-old man has sharp, central chest pain which is worse when he inhales. His heart rate is 105 bpm, BP 120/70, and temperature is 38°C. His past medical history includes ischaemic heart disease with a recent myocardial infarction. What is the most likely cause of the chest pain (choose one)?

a) Acute coronary syndrome
b) Angina
c) Pulmonary embolism
d) Pericarditis
e) Ventricular rupture.

Answer: D (pleurisy with mild-grade pyrexia post recent MI).

Extended matching questions

What is an EMQ?

An EMQ is another type of question in which the correct answers are listed among incorrect answers on the page in front of you. It differs from an MCQ in that there are usually more than five options to choose from, often 10–14 options in an alphabetical list.

How should I prepare for EMQs?

- Work out how long you will have per question.
- Again, learn around the facts, memorizing words and facts will not help in these questions!

How should I answer EMQs?

- Work out the answer to the question before looking at the options.
- Use the process of elimination.
- Read the question to ensure you know what you are answering.
- If you are finding a question really tricky, mark it and then move on.
- Work out how long you have per question.

Example EMQ

EMQ options:
1. Angina
2. Aortic dissection
3. Gastro-oesophageal reflux disease
4. Non-ST elevation myocardial infarction
5. Pericarditis
6. Pneumonia
7. Pulmonary embolism
8. Shingles

For each of the following chest pain clinical scenarios, select the correct diagnosis.

A. A 75-year-old woman presents to the ED feeling sweaty and short of breath. On questioning, she reveals she feels as though something is constricting her chest but there is no pain. She is diabetic. ECG shows V1–V4 ST depression with raised troponin.

B. A 60-year-old obese lorry driver presents to the ED with 'awful burning' as well as sharp, central, and epigastric chest pain which began following a large meal. The ECG shows sinus rhythm.

C. A tall gentleman, with noticeably long arms and IHD, presents to the ED with severe chest pain, also felt between the scapulae. He begins to describe the pain and is noticeably SOB and subsequently collapses in his bed and becomes unresponsive.

Answers: A4 (silent MI in diabetics and elderly).

B3 (eating-related acid reflux).

C2 (connective tissue disorder/Marfanoid → poor collagen quality → dissection).

Short answer questions

What is an SAQ?
An SAQ is a question which carries a range of marks (usually 1–6) for a simple, concise answer. These questions can catch people out and it is very important to clarify how many points can be allocated for each question and exactly what the question is asking you to do. This type of question is less common than MCQs in medical school; however, you may still encounter them. It would be important to find out if your medical school will accept bullet-pointed answers, or prefers answers written in short prose.

How should I prepare for SAQs?
• There is no substitute for knowing your subject matter.
• As always: practise, practise, practise! This type of questions may be trickier to practise but a great way to work around this is to create questions with friends and you can try to answer each other's.
• Work out how long you have per question.

How should I answer SAQs?
• Always look at how many marks the question carries. This tells you exactly how many points need to be made and how much detail you will need to include in your answer.
• Read and reread the question to determine if it is asking for one answer or multiple answers. It is handy to underline important words so that you remember to answer all parts of a question (e.g. state/describe/list).
• Look out for whether the question is asking you to write in words, give a numerical answer, or even possibly to draw a graph or picture—people can often be caught out by this.
• The best SAQ answers are concise and simple. Waffling does not give you any extra marks, and may even cause you to lose time and marks if incorrect.
• Always attempt the question even if you are unsure to improve your chances of gaining some, if not all, marks.

Example questions
• Which hormones in the menstrual cycle rise between days 10 to 14? (3 marks.)
• Describe the features of the cells of the respiratory epithelium, name the type of cell, and explain why these features are necessary for its function. (6 marks.)

Essay questions

What is an essay question?

An essay question involves writing a concise but structured answer in prose to a given question. The answer sheets for these questions often only permit a certain space for your answer and so it is important to plan exactly how you are going to answer the question before you write anything on the page. You can use extra pieces of paper to map out thoughts or write bullet points as aide-memoires before writing the essay—this way, you will not forget any of your points and will have a structure. Essay questions in exams are time pressured and quite stressful, so it is important to practise this type of question beforehand.

How should I prepare for essay questions?

- Practise, practise, practise!
- Perfect your own essay format: think about a logical order to answering questions, including an introduction and conclusion, and a simple outline to follow.
- Work out how long you have to plan, to write, and to proofread your essay.
- Guess what questions could be answered with an essay and brainstorm ideas of what you could include—also a handy way to improve your knowledge throughout the year!
- Think about your essay format while doing essays which are not time pressured throughout the year—lots of preparation is needed before a stressful examination situation.

How should I answer essay questions?

- Use good examples to support any points that you make. Evidence is always needed to back up any point you make.
- Have an introductory and a concluding paragraph even if it is two sentences—this looks professional and will improve your mark.
- Spend a minute or two formulating a rough plan before you dive in. Having an essay plan is incredibly useful, you could try to use scrap paper to write down the important points to cover along with a reminder to write an introduction and conclusion.
- *Rules of three*: those who study the arts are more exposed to writing essays for their assessments. The general structure consists of the 'three Ps': three parts consisting of a paragraph for the beginning (introduction), middle, and end (conclusion) and dividing the middle into another three parts (e.g. objectives, methodology, results and discussion) or three paragraphs. Each paragraph should consist of three or four sentences with simple and succinct statements. There is no time or marks available for waffling.

Example essay questions

Describe the menstrual cycle, describe the pathophysiology driven by sepsis, explain the process of carcinogenesis, describe the role of the immune system in sepsis, etc.

Prescribing safety/skills assessment (PSA)

What is the PSA?

This is another nationwide mandatory requirement for final year clinical students looking at their ability to prescribe. The examination is online and involves MCQs and some SAQs. It will take place at some point during your final year (that is, if your medical school has introduced it). Topics covered include:
- writing a prescription for an example patient
- calculating medication doses
- adverse drug reactions
- data interpretation
- drug monitoring.

The specialities covered include medicine, surgery, elderly care, paediatrics, psychiatry, obstetrics and gynaecology, and general practice. The examination lasts 2 hours and you are allowed to use the online *BNF* or the paper version to answer the questions.

How should I prepare for the PSA?

- Find out when you will be taking it. The test requires at least a few weeks to prepare—knowing your date in advance will allow for this.
- Do the practice papers online. These practice papers vary in difficulty level and therefore it is very important to complete them all, at least a week before the real exam—there is lots to be learnt from these!
- Try to get access to prescribing modules online for practice.
- Get familiar with your *BNF*. You will use the *BNF* (either the online version or the book) during the exam and so the slicker you get at using it, the better you will ultimately do. This examination is very time pressured. Also a great tip is to work out which sections are on which pages— there are rather handy antibiotics and palliative care sections, as well as appendices at the end (e.g. drugs to consider in breastfeeding patients).
- Watch people prescribe and learn how to do this as soon as possible in clinical years. As soon as you become a doctor, you will be hounded by everyone to write up prescriptions; the more you have observed this as a medical student, the less scary it is as a doctor! Also, it will make this exam a lot easier.
- Summative vs formative? Find out (1) whether your medical school requires you to sit the PSA and (2) whether the results are formative or summative. It is crucial to be a good prescriber and therefore passing the PSA is very important, but it is nice to know whether the score is counted into your final year mark or not.

When you are in the exam

- Stick to your planned timings. It is very rare to find a student who tells you they had spare time in the PSA!
- Do not rush the calculations.
- Read the question properly. As with all other written exams, make sure you avoid making a mistake when reading the question.
- Use the *BNF* to its full advantage. Your life will be a lot easier if you start using and flicking through the *BNF* early on during medical school. There

are amazing chapters with lots of knowledge (e.g. the antibiotics chapter and the palliative care section)—learn where these are and the exam will seem a lot easier! At least you will know where to exactly find the relevant information when under immense pressure.

Example questions

- Will warfarin interact with amoxicillin?
  - Yes it will through the CYP450 pathway. Look up the warfarin 'inducers and inhibitors'.
- Write a prescription for a patient requiring rescue medication following an exacerbation of COPD:
  - Some things to consider include IV fluids, back-to-back 5 mg/2.5 mL salbutamol nebulizers (with at least four times daily maintenance doses), 500 mcg ipratropium bromide (Atrovent®) nebulizers four times daily, 40 mg PO prednisolone once daily for 5 days, 5 mL saline nebulizers PRN, antibiotics (doxycycline, amoxicillin, co-amoxiclav (Augmentin®) if exacerbation is caused by infective aetiology, etc.

PSA references

- Singer. Pocket Prescriber. CRC Press. 2015
- British National Formulary (BNF) and BNF for Children. www.BNF.org. Available in print, online and app

Resources for PSA

Aberdeen University	www.abdn.ac.uk/medical/electives/elective_information/download/73/Preparing_for_the_Prescribing_Safety_Assessment_plus_answers.pdf
British Medical Association	www.bma.org.uk/advice/career/applying-for-training/prescribing-safety-assessment
Prescribing Safety Assessment Guide for Foundation Doctors	www.yorksandhumberdeanery.nhs.uk/sites/default/files/remediation_training_guidance_for_trainees.pdf
Medical Schools Council	www.medschools.ac.uk/our-work/assessment/prescribing-safety-assessment

PSA question banks

PSA – sample questions	www.prescribingsafetyassessment.ac.uk/resources
Pastest	www.pastest.com/medical-student-prescribing-safety-assessment/exam/
On Examination	www.onexamination.com/exams/student/psa#QuestionBrowser
Prepare for the PSA	www.prepareforthepsa.com
Pass Medicine	www.passmedicine.com/student/index.php?gclid=EAlaIQobChMI1tGrpYr13QIVQed3Ch03cQ-KEAAYAiAAEgLpgPD_BwE

Other assessments

Reflective practice

Reflection is a task that will either plague you or carry you through medical school and much further beyond. If your case quickly begins to feel like the former, you are not alone. If you identify more with the latter, you already have the advantage. Whether you realize it or not, we are all constantly reflecting on our daily occurrences, whether professional or personal. Reflection can range from a passing thought about a minor experience, to a structured essay or formal meeting with a senior clinician.

What is it?

First consider what reflection is not; it is not a 'Dear Diary' entry. Your reflection should be structured around a well-recognized reflective cycle. While a 'Dear Diary' entry classically focuses on feelings towards a situation, a full reflective cycle delves into this and more. Second, consider what reflection is. In broad terms, a complete reflection should discuss the situation at hand, how you felt about it, what this means to you, and how you will use the knowledge gained from this experience. As you progress throughout medical school and your career as a doctor, your reflective skills will be further refined. Rather than reflecting solely on experiences, you may be asked to reflect upon a range of topics including minor procedures such as taking blood, medical journals, critical incidents, and more. A commonly used reflective cycle is the Gibbs cycle.

Why do I need to do it?

You will always have deadlines and assessments for written reflections, but this really is one of your most valuable tools for developing both professionally and personally. A robustly referenced reflective assignment will teach you a considerable amount about a subject you may otherwise have glossed over briefly in your subconscious mind. In many stages of your career, it will also be a method of evaluating you as a medical student and later as a doctor. Your reflections will be some of your only proof that you experienced something, and learned from it. Embracing this huge part of your learning experience can only help you now, later, and much later.

An example of a reflection

One such student chose anaesthetics, but because this was such a popular option, she was given the ICU. This placement required a structured reflective report at the end of it. She was required to summarize the job of an ICU consultant, research career paths to intensive care, and describe interesting experiences during the placement. She has now decided to pursue a career in intensive care, which goes to show that without the reflective assignment, she would have blindly whizzed through the placement, waiting for it to end. What a lost opportunity that could have been!

Presentations

By this stage in your academic career, you will have done too many presentations to count. The end of this learning tool is not in sight. Throughout medical school, you will have several presentations assigned to you. The majority of these, you will find, will be for the purpose of learning, rather than assessment. It is important to give each of these projects your full effort, regardless of their weight on your grades. You will go on to complete a range of types of presentations; however, the same underlying principles for all of these apply.

Types of presentations

The presentations you will be required to complete in medical school and your medical career will vary considerably. Some will seem easily manageable, and some may feel overwhelming at first. Here is a list of a few types that you will soon become very familiar with:

Small group presentations

One of the most common types of presentation that you will be assigned. If your medical course is split into preclinical and clinical years, you will always be a part of a small group during the preclinical years. Presentations are one of the many valuable learning tools you will use in these groups. You may be required to present these to your small group in subgroups or on your own. The topics of presentations here are generally focused around the course material; however, often the subject of your presentation may be entirely student selected.

Clinical group presentations

Another very common type of presentation in medical school. Throughout each of your clinical placements, you will be a part of yet another group. Because clinical placements are such a new environment with a new lesson to be learnt each day, you will have to be proactive about seizing this knowledge. Your group should be attached to a lead consultant who will help you structure this learning as much as possible. They may ask a different member of your group each week to present something you encountered on the ward during that time. Your topic may be anything from a simple case history, a review of a new medication, a common chronic condition, or management of a specific medical emergency. Again, this may be chosen by your lead consultant, or may be left up to you.

Research presentations

Occasionally, you will be required to take up some sort of research. However, some of the time, this will be a completely elected project in later years of medical school. As an assigned project, you may end up presenting your findings in front of your clinical group or the team on the ward. As an elected project, or an assigned project which you chose to take beyond the realms of medical school, a presentation is a huge achievement and a privilege.

These presentations may be at a local lunchtime meeting in the hospital department of your project's specialty (e.g. your project on asthma would be presented at the respiratory lunchtime meeting), or a poster presentation where you are required to summarize your project on a poster which is displayed at a conference, or potentially a formal PowerPoint presentation delivered to leading specialists at a national or even international conference. These are great for your CV! These are just a few of the types of presentations you will come across throughout medical school. Each of these is beneficial to you in several ways, and should be embraced with enthusiasm as large as your to-do list!

Why are presentations helpful?

Refining the art of a good presentation will enhance both your personal and professional skills. You will be doing them for the rest of your life, so you may as well start developing these skills now! Practising presenting in front of either a large or small group of people will help you firstly to develop confidence. Presenting in front of your peers feels different to presenting to leading medical professionals. Thus, being confident in yourself and your abilities early on is important. Secondly, presentations are a fantastically efficient way to deliver information. Not only this, but when you know that you will be in charge of this important task, your thorough preparation will teach you an impressive amount on the subject of your presentation.

Presentations related to research, whether at a local meeting or at an international conference, can have a huge, positive impact on your career. Applying for your very first job as a doctor happens through a points-based system. At this time, presentations specifically do not add points to your application; however, a project which is presented may go on to be published—which will add points to your application. Besides this, having a presentation (or two or three) looks fantastic on a CV and really puts you at an advantage. This shows future employers that you are keen and dedicated to the progression of the medical field. It's also a great way to learn a great amount about a specific topic in a specialty!

How to be a good presenter

If you are averse to public speaking, you are far from alone. Glossophobia—the fear of public speaking—remains the number one phobia. This means that people are more afraid of public speaking than spiders, darkness, heights, and even death! Do not feel as though you need to be the best presenter on your first day of medical school. You will be presenting often enough that this practice will eventually become slightly less daunting.

Here are some basic tips to help you be a good presenter

Speak slowly

When someone reads aloud, you will find that you need it to be read to you much slower than the speed at which you would read quietly to yourself. Present to others with this in mind. Do not read your presentation to yourself. Focus on speaking slowly, and then speak a little slower than that.

Speak clearly
This may sound obvious, but when you are nervous, speaking clearly can be a challenge. Avoid stumbling your way through your talk, or using too many 'umms' and 'aahs'.

Practise, practise, practise
There are few things more embarrassing than realizing in front of your audience that you have included the same slide twice. Practising can help avoid problems such as this, and keep you familiar with the words you will be speaking. It will also help you with timekeeping and rehearsing speaking slowly.

Know your stuff
Read around your topic. You may be asked questions afterwards, and knowing that you are prepared will help with both your presentation quality and anxiety. At the same time, however, be prepared to defend your sources. No matter how clever you sound, referencing a poorly recognized source is a sure-fire way to lose your credibility.

Know your own difficulties
If you suffer with something like dyslexia, try to accommodate for this to allow for a smoother presentation and to settle any worries you may have. You may want to practise a few more times to avoid having to read cue cards during your talk. Including more figures and visual aids, which you can discuss rather than written facts, may also be of help to you. Planning for potential presentation issues will help both yourself and your audience. Consider what you would do if the computer or presentation failed. Would you still be confident to deliver the presentation?

Be conscious of your appearance
Besides looking professional, make your best effort to be aware of how you appear to your audience. Try to stand up straight, avoid fidgeting, and make eye contact with your audience rather than your slides or cards.

Holding their attention
It is an art to be able to hold the attention of your audience throughout your presentation. You will have attended hundreds of lectures by the time you graduate and you will be able to appreciate what tactics do or do not work. The audience usually begin to lose interest or only remember the first 15–20 min of the presentation.

How to make a good presentation
Being a good presenter does not always mean that you will have a great presentation. If you are going to focus on a PowerPoint presentation, bear in mind the following things:

People like to know where they are going
Have you ever tried driving with someone who promises to get you to the destination, but only tells you where to turn about 3 metres from the turning point? Whether or not you drive, this is clearly an annoying position to be in. Do not let your audience feel this way! Having a slide dedicated to clearly laying out a plan for the rest of your presentation goes a long way, and shows that you are organized. Keep offering signposts. The more memorable lectures are the ones that answer the audience's questions before they have asked them because your presentation follows a logical structure.

People do not like to read and listen at the same time
Keep the words on your PowerPoint slides minimal. They should only be used as aide-mémoires. Your audience is also more likely to remember your slides if they contain succinct information only. Use them only to guide your topics of discussion. Your audience can only concentrate on a few things at once. They will not appreciate it if you are speaking while the presentation behind you is inundated with a plethora of words in tiny font and flying visual effects. There is such a thing as too much stimulation! Keep it simple and draw the attention to you as opposed to your slides.

People get bored by lack of change
A series of slides solely filled with words or with graphs is sure to quickly exhaust your listeners. Simply varying your methods of delivering information will keep your audience engaged and interested. Keep the font large, dark on light background, and easy to read (even from the back of the room).

Your audience will use your slides to organize their thoughts
Thus, if you clutter your slides, you clutter their minds. Simple, punchy, and succinct bullet points will be outstanding. Consider what 'buzzwords' to highlight to convey your principal messages clearly.

Keep your audience engaged
Asking an opening question to spark a debate is just one great way to allow an audience to participate in your presentation. You can also ask questions throughout the presentation. This will minimize the audience having to listen to just one voice during your presentation, while keeping them involved. Once again, your audience will be more likely to remember your presentation if you interact and immerse them into your topic.

Take note of others' good presentations
Learn their content and their style. Make notes on what you and the rest of the audience appreciated and things that did not work.

Essays

Essays are another type of assignment you will encounter throughout medical school. It is likely that you will have essays assigned to you much less frequently than reflective assignments and presentations, but you will find them to be equally important. You also may find that you are assigned essays much less often than your friends on other courses. For this reason, it is important to maintain basic essay writing skills, as you may eventually begin to feel out of touch with writing them.

Basic essay writing tips

Make a plan
The most difficult part of an essay is starting. Getting your sources together and making a plan is the best way to get past this barrier, while simultaneously setting yourself up for writing a well-structured essay. Examples include bullet points and mind maps.

Reference as you go along
Find out which referencing style your university uses, and make sure to reference your essay as you write it. Getting into this practice will save you from ending up with a horde of links at the end of your essay, which you will struggle to match to your statements. It will also save you copious time, which is so precious! Try and use resources such as EndNote™ which make it easier to keep a track of references. Library staff should be able to teach you how to use it, or else you can always learn through trial and error!

Spell check and grammar check
This may seem obvious, but you would be surprised to see that this is sometimes ignored by many, especially with the last-minute writers among us. You may also want to bear in mind that your essays will include many words that the spell-check program on your writing software will not recognize, such as hyperhomocystinuria or haematemesis. Also ensure your language setting on Microsoft Word is for English (United Kingdom) to avoid common spelling errors.

Be clear
No one is in your head but you. If you can deliver information clearly and efficiently, you are already on the path to a great essay. One way to enhance the clarity of your paper is to include subheadings. This allows your reader to follow the essay, knowing exactly where they are going.

Stop writing
You need to step away from the assignment and give your brain a break! Short frequent breaks will make you more efficient, as well as give you a fresh perspective when you return to your desk. Suddenly that run-on sentence your tired brain could not figure out how to fix is so obvious!

Do not be a last-minute writer

We all have (or identify as) that friend who does not start an essay until midnight before the due date. This reflects on your work and is extremely obvious to your assessors. Writing when you are tired allows for careless mistakes and only puts forward half of your best effort. You did not get into medical school by putting in minimal effort, so why start stumbling through unenthusiastically now?

Get feedback

Once you have finished writing, send your essay to a trusted friend or family member. A second opinion is always a good idea.

What not to do

There are many obvious things not to do in an essay, many of which are to ignore the above-mentioned basic essay writing tips. However, there are less obvious mistakes that can cost you. Here are a few of these:

Plagiarizing

It is actually really easy to accidentally plagiarize. Try to get out of the habit of switching words around, rather than collating information and delivering it in your own style. Luckily, most universities now require you to use proof-reading software which detects phrases that can be matched to both online sources as well as an archive of assignments submitted years before yours. This software should produce a percentage value which indicates the proportion of your essay that has been found to match other sources. You can then alter your essay to make it more appropriate before submitting your final draft.

Failing to see all the relevant points of view

No matter how thoroughly you cover one aspect of a topic, if you ignore the rest, you render your essay to a poor grade and possibly even a fail.

Straying from the topic at hand

This is also really easy to do. Discussing the adverse effects of smoking may lead you to researching COPD which leads you to the treatment of this disease and then onto a drug review of the newest inhalers and then inhaler accessories and on and on. There is nothing wrong with giving a good amount of background information, but make sure you can relate it to the original subject of the essay.

Evidence

There is a so-called hierarchy of evidence which is important to become familiar with, especially when writing a literature review of various sources of research on a topic. It is acceptable to use evidence of various clinical values, but be aware that the stronger your evidence, the stronger the basis of your essay. As you travel up the hierarchy there is an ↑ in quality of evidence and a ↓ in bias.

Dissertations

What is a dissertation?

Many students choose to intercalate (see ➲ Chapter 5). If you decide that this is the path you want to go down, you will be required to write a dissertation. Everyone has a vague idea of what it entails, but what exactly is a dissertation? We asked a few students how they would describe this subject, after having completed one:

- A dissertation is an extended formal project, which discusses a specific research question about a chosen topic.
- You can think of it as a very detailed essay. However, there are more differences than this. Here are a few:
  - An essay does not have to be about a study or research, but a dissertation is.
  - A dissertation is the conclusion of your studies. It provides in-depth information about what you have been studying, experimenting, and potentially discovering during the year (or longer for some). An essay, however, can be written about any topic at multiple points during your studies.
  - A dissertation is a write-up of a study for assessment. Essays can be an analysis, discussion, or even just a small review of literature.

How to choose a topic

The options are endless. Once you choose a field to intercalate in, that only just narrows it down. Many people can get lost at this first hurdle, but once you get past it, you will have already begun your journey. Your university may provide a list of interesting topics to intercalate in—choose wisely!

Here are a few tips to guide you:

- Think about what interests you and what will motivate you. You will be putting a lot of time and brainpower into this one project. If it does not interest you, you will put in less effort than is sufficient to excel. More so than this, spending an excessive amount of time on a topic you care very little about is agonizing!
- Talk to other people. Find out what other people are thinking of researching. Speak to people who have already completed a dissertation in your field. Obviously your research should be unique, but discussing other people's plans may point you in the right direction to help you figure out where to start.
- Consider the level of work already done on the topic. Do not do something that we already know everything about, because in simple terms, *what's the point*? Try to choose a topic that has a few gaps in the research. This way, you will provide yourself with a clearer plan, as well as be more likely to produce a project that will generate further interest.

How to form a research question

Now that you have chosen a broad topic, you have to get specific. What will your project look into? Again, make sure you are actually interested in answering the question you have come up with. Do not come up with something just to meet a deadline. Once you start, you have committed!

You can also discuss this with your supervisor(s). It is best to have an idea of what you want to research, rather than to set up a meeting only to ask 'So what should I do?' Show your supervisor that you have at least started to set up a path for yourself. Once you have an idea of this, look into papers to make sure that your question has not already been answered. Again, try to find a gap in the research, to make your project more impacting and worthwhile. Finally, be realistic. If you decide you want to enter into cancer research, for example, bear in mind that you probably will not find a cure to all cancers. But you can definitely make an important contribution to the field for you or others to build upon!

Importance of independent learning

You will generally be given an extended period of time to complete your dissertation. Resist the urge to procrastinate. Remember the future you is still you! Do not let future you feel stressed and pressured by the minimal time they have left, because present-day you could not face starting this huge task. You will need all the time you can get—whether it is used in the planning stage, meeting with your supervisor or colleagues, writing, or accommodating for setbacks. However, with all of this in mind, remember that you are only human, and humans need breaks too. If you feel like you have burnt out or are starting to go down that route, then stop. Only you can figure out your personal limitations. Sometimes it takes walking away from your project for a short period of time to feel ready to tackle it with some fresh ideas. No one will tell you to take a break. It takes the independence of knowing yourself and your abilities to be able to work well and efficiently. Never forget, your research and dissertation is not taught: it is yours. Use your knowledge, research, and dedication to help you complete an exemplary project.

What to do if you experience a setback

This can happen in a variety of ways, ranging from technical problems, logistic issues, and experiments going awry to simply realizing that your original plan is no longer valid or possible. Here is a short list of what you can do to deal with these:
- *Stay calm.*
- *Expect it:* research and experiments rarely go as planned. That is the nature of discovery. Many people before you have experienced setbacks, both big and small, only to work through them and achieve success.
- *Discuss it with your supervisor:* they will also be expecting some sort of blip in the plan. However, try another route up the same mountain before going to them.
- *Alter your plans as appropriate, with realistic goals.*
- *Report it in your dissertation, and discuss how you overcame it:* it is unlikely that everything you plan will turn out exactly as you had planned it. Your assessors will be more impressed by a report that is honest and unrelenting, than one that suspiciously states that everything was seamless and simple. Anybody who has conducted research will not be a stranger to the trials and tribulations of yielding positive data. Facing obstacles does not make you a researcher but finding solutions to those

obstacles demonstrates your creativity and ability to overcome those obstacles. There are countless researchers who may have spent years without obtaining positive data but at least they have demonstrated one possible way of not finding the answer. Negative results are still publishable in conference proceedings journals.

Role of your supervisor

Broadly speaking, the role of your supervisor is guidance, support, and advice. Try to meet with them or contact them regularly. They are there to guide your overall research, so use them to help point you in the right direction. Do not be afraid to approach them. Generally, they have taken up this role because they are interested in the subject matter and are more than happy to provide this support role. However, do not ask them technical questions or issues that you could potentially figure out on your own.

What to do if your supervisor is less than helpful

Some people have trouble with their supervisors, whether it is due to them being difficult to access, less receptive to your questions or a clash of visions and personality, etc. Firstly, some people actually have two supervisors. Try not to keep either of them out of the loop, but if you find that one is being more helpful and invested in your success, approach them for support initially. Secondly, use this as an opportunity for learning. Unfortunately, you will find yourself outside your comfort zone at times, but this does lend itself to valuable learning opportunities. Embrace this and know that at the end of it, you will have gained another useful skill. Formal complaints really should be a very last resort. Remember, even if you do not always see eye to eye, they are experienced academic professionals and are granted the role of supervisor for a reason. If you believe that your case is exceptional and is having a negative impact on your project, discussing the matter with the course organizers is an option. Possible outcomes include mediation, reassigning you to another supervisor or research department, or a new project altogether (e.g. library project, audit, or grant proposal).

Writing a proposal

A proposal is exactly what it sounds like: proposing what you intend to research for your dissertation. Most proposals include a small literature review, your goals for the research, the reason for your motivation, and why it is important or worthwhile. You may also want to include a timeline to map out your general goals. This will show that you have been planning thoroughly and realistically.

The planning stage

Everyone does this differently, but it is definitely much easier to start with a plan than to dive head first into a blank document. It may help to jot down the general structure of your dissertation first. Here is a suggested one:
- Title, including your details, name of supervisors, and department.
- Introduction.
- Literature review.
- Methods including any technical details, e.g. any equipment used.
- Results.

- Discussion including limitations and suggestions for future studies.
- Conclusion.
- References.
- Appendix (e.g. raw data if deemed necessary).

Write as you go along. This especially applies for your introduction and literature review, as these should not typically change much. This makes the barrier of starting much easier. Once you have a general structure, start to jot important points, then expand on these points. You may refer to other dissertations to inspire a structure. Just ensure that you do not plagiarize, and make sure to reference anything you use. But it is more than fine to read around for inspiration.

Referencing

If you cannot back it up do not claim it as yours unless it is genuinely your own idea. You will be challenged, so make sure you have a reputable source for anything you report. Reliable information can generally be found in well-recognized papers and journals. When considering using a source, think to yourself: 'Could this stand in a debate on the topic?' If you are really unsure about a source you want to use, you can ask your supervisor what they know about its validity. Remember to be extensive. If you have not come up with the specified information yourself, you must back it up. Do not forget to include references of any images, figures, and tables that you have not made yourself. Some images and graphs may be susceptible to copyright issues so ask for written permission prior to its inclusion within your dissertation and reference correctly. You can also use references to direct your reader to more information. This will keep your word count down, as well as keeping your report focused on your work.

Some final advice

Writing a dissertation can be very daunting at many and possibly all stages of the task. This is normal, and everyone experiences this feeling. However, try to bear in mind the number of people before you who have done it, and the number of people after you who will do it. Other students have had your supervisor and have made it work. You are just as equipped as they are, and your dissertation is yours! Make it the best you possibly can!

Part 6

Career planning

Making decisions

Early career investment

Medical school presents numerous opportunities for students to gain further experience in a field of medicine that they find interesting. This includes either clinical or research placements that are assessed and form part of the course, to opportunities that are voluntary, such as essays and prizes. You may not know it at the time, but these selected components may be pivotal early experience that may shape your future career.

Base hospital selection

In some large medical schools, there may be a choice of teaching hospitals to use as your 'base' for 3 years. Each base hospital is linked with its own selection of surrounding district general hospitals and primary care facilities. Your base hospital selection will likely be influenced more by where you live, or would like to live, rather than any specific educational requirements at the time of selection. Of course, if one base hospital has a particular department that you wish to work in, or is renowned for a specialty that you are intrigued by, you may consider it an advantage to be placed there.

Student selected components

(See ⮕ Chapter 56.) Student selected components (SSCs), or modules (SSMs), are programmed opportunities for student selected clinical placements. A medical degree may allow opportunities for three or four SSCs (typically of 1 month's duration). You can either select placements in areas of career interest, to gain further insight or simply because you find the subject matter of interest, or you may select an SSC to fill a gap in the medical curriculum. You may select an SSC to address an area of weakness in your clinical knowledge or skills, based on past performance in assessments, for example. It is typical to require a supervisor report at the end of an SSC, and you may be required to write a case report on a particular patient with a literature review.

Elective

(See ⮕ Chapter 55.) Your medical elective is a unique and treasured time in your undergraduate training; it is likely you have been anticipating it from the start of medical school. There is a world of possibilities, both in terms of destination and in the content of your placement. If your budget allows, considering splitting your elective to allow you to visit two destinations (developing world and developed world), and consider experiencing more than one specialty (medical and surgical). You may be able to undertake a short research project, but ensure you can complete it in the short time that you have, and ensure your supervisor has a strong publication record to minimize risk of disappointment. Read elective reports catalogued in the medical school, and browse online elective reports for reviews on placements and practical tips in organizing your elective.

Intercalated degree

(See ➲ Chapter 5.) There is a huge variety of intercalated degrees available, and they present a wonderful opportunity to step off the undergraduate conveyor belt, explore a subject matter in depth, undertake research, augment your CV for the remainder of your career (you will reap the rewards throughout), and enjoy another year at university. Intercalated Masters degrees are now available, which you are only awarded on qualification from medical school. It is possible to intercalate at an external institution, usually only if that course is not offered locally. Funding may be available, and some universities will heavily subsidize course fees for intercalating students as an incentive. External funding may also be available, such as the Wolfson Scholarship (℘ www.wolfson.org.uk/funding/education/intercalated-awards). An extra year is largely irrelevant in the long term, but the rewards are constant, cumulative, and lasting. Ask existing students about the course you are considering undertaking so you can gain a firm idea of the content, advantages, and challenges—and, of course, the process of application. Some full-time research degrees (Master in Research) may offer a range of established supervisors and basic science projects. You are likely to lean towards the subject matter that you are most interested in, but be reassured that the skills learnt are often generic and easily transferable to other fields should your career and research interest change in the future.

Project option/research placement

Some medical schools require students to undertake a compulsory research or audit project during the latter half of clinical school, in a subject matter of their choosing. This is a wonderful opportunity to get work published, provided you are organized and can find a suitable supervisor and project that may be undertaken within the specified time period. The work completed may be of sufficient standard for presentation at national level, and you may go on to undertake further projects with your supervisor later, depending on whether you stay local to the unit for the remainder of medical school or beyond. The medical school may have a list of established supervisors to choose from, who are likely to suggest particular projects that are suitable for the period of time that you have. The reputation and output of the supervisor, experience of recent medical and research students, and profile of the group may influence your decision to join them for this period.

Prizes

Prizes are an excellent way to distinguish yourself: they stay on your CV indefinitely, and will look impressive in future job applications, indulge your interest in a subject, and usually come with some cash. There are a huge number of prizes available, either administered internally by the medical school, or offered externally by charities, Royal Colleges, Royal Society of Medicine, etc. Some, such as the Duke Elder Prize in Ophthalmology, are well publicized and recognized at interview. Entering such competitions is a statement of commitment to the specialty in itself, even if you do not win.

How to choose a specialty

A medical degree can be used a springboard to a vast range of careers. Although exciting, this degree of choice may be somewhat paralysing. Choosing a medical career is a complex decision, influenced by personality/character traits, personal attributes/skills, life aspirations, experience, and your personal circumstances—all of which may evolve and some of which may conflict. Then of course there is the nature of the job, the workplace environment, and the competition for training places to consider. The NHS is changing faster than ever, and it is incredibly important that when you are considering a future career, you take into account the likely changes within the bigger picture of healthcare provision and how they may impact on the working pattern and environment in your chosen specialty.

Career planning is not an entirely logical or linear process, but is influenced by many internal and external factors, and there is no set time when it should consciously take place. Many students feel under pressure to make an early decision, and feel concerned when others seem settled on a specialty choice, but research has shown that early aspirations is a poor indicator of an individual's final career destination in medicine. It is natural for career aspirations early in medical school to be influenced by changing life circumstances and priorities, which of course are not always predictable! Knowledge and understanding of what you enjoy and where you thrive in the workplace can only come with experience, and this information should guide you as you work on developing your career over the years. Career planning is not about a one-off decision, but is an evolving, fluid process.

You may have colleagues who feel they have had a clear idea of their career from a very early stage: do not worry about this. Many successful clinicians were not sure of their career as a medical student, and instead enjoyed their training, were patient, and waited to make an informed decision later on. Although the Modernising Medical Careers programme has meant that decisions do need to be taken earlier, there is an increasing move towards flexibility in the early stages of specialist training (*Accreditation of Competencies Framework*) which is good news for the many junior doctors who are less certain about their intended specialty. If you are currently unsure as to a specialty choice, there are many resources that may help you to narrow it down, but no magic 'sorting hat' to match you to your 'perfect' specialty. There is no right or wrong specialty for you, simply better or worse fits.

Career certainty and uncertainty

Medical students (and junior doctors) may fall into three main categories of career certainty:

The certain: 'I know exactly what I want to do'
It can be helpful to have a clear idea of the career you wish to pursue. Early insight will help you tailor your opportunities to your interests, even as an undergraduate. Evidence of an early commitment to a specialty can be beneficial when competing for a place on some of the more sought after training programmes, neurosurgery or cardiothoracics, for example.

However, outside of the most competitive specialties this demonstration of early commitment is not necessary, as most of the requirements for a competitive portfolio can be covered generically, with commitment to a specialty being addressed closer to the time of competitive selection. It is of course extremely common for even the most focused and driven individuals to have a change of plan at some stage during the training process. If you have accumulated a lot of experience (e.g. audit projects, research, and presentations) in one particular specialty and then have a change of heart, that experience is still valuable, and likely to be looked upon as valid when applying for a different specialty.

The fairly certain: 'I have a pretty good idea of what I want to do'

This is probably the most common position: e.g. considering yourself a physician, a surgeon, or a GP with a reasonable degree of certainty—but having not yet identified a subspecialty interest. This is fine: core-training programmes mean that for many career pathways, the detail of the final specialty choice can be deferred for a few years after foundation training. For example, if you wanted to pursue medicine but were not sure of a specialty, you would apply for core medical training, aim to pass your MRCP examinations, and understand that you will have around 18 months to choose your medical specialty (such as gastroenterology, haematology, etc.) after starting core training. The exceptions to this are those specialties with run-through training programmes, such as neurosurgery, ophthalmology, and obstetrics and gynaecology, which therefore require, in general, an earlier commitment. In addition to this, the recently introduced Accreditation of Competencies Framework has brought ↑flexibility to early training pathways.

The uncertain: 'I don't know what I want to do'

Depending on what stage you are at, it may be absolutely fine to not know what you want to do. However, it may be a good idea to do a little bit of work now to ensure that the decision you eventually make is a well-informed one. Discuss your career uncertainty with your educational supervisor, or an individual within the medical school designated to provide medical careers guidance. You may find using careers tools and questionnaires helpful (see ➔ 'Where to find out more …' p. 1007). These generally aim to help you crystallize your understanding of yourself—strengths and weaknesses, values, drivers, and personality. Although the use of such tools will not provide you with an immediate answer to your specialty choice conundrum, it helps move you forward in the decision-making process and can help define the type of work and environment where you are likely to thrive. Combining this improved 'self-knowledge' with focused research into your current shortlisted specialities (e.g. taster weeks, discussion with trainees and substantives in a specialty, Strengths, Weaknesses, Opportunities, and Threats (SWOT) analyses, etc.) will help guide you towards one of the more certain categories mentioned earlier.

Personal traits

It is interesting that while, in general, we often assume that specialties tend to attract similar personalities, there is no clear evidence that particular personality types are likely to be found in certain specialties. There may be an aspect of conditioning within a speciality (your personality may adapt or even evolve to function effectively in the clinical environment you are in). One way in which personality typing can be useful when looking at speciality choice is that it can often predict particular aspects of a speciality that may be challenging for a given personality type.

Some doctors feel a 'calling' to a particular specialty, perhaps because of a powerful personal experience. More likely, you will tend to gravitate towards specialties that stimulate your interest at medical school and tend to play to your personal strengths, as you see them. For example, if you are a natural communicator with patients, enjoy continuity of care, and the challenge of difficult discussions, a specialty such as oncology may be naturally appealing. It is not that a certain personality type cannot work effectively within a certain specialty, but that certain specialties may present a more comfortable working environment for a given individual. Dealing with acutely ill patients in the resuscitation unit may be thrilling and stimulating for some doctors, but cripplingly stressful for others.

For another individual, the prospect of ongoing responsibility for patients may feel suffocating, making a career that requires continuity of care unpleasantly stressful. Perceiving a specialty as competitive may deter some doctors from pursuing it as a career, as they may consider their academic record insufficient for the purpose of selection. If this is the case, seek advice from your supervisor or medical careers advisor; this may be entirely erroneous and it would be unfortunate to make such an important decision on the basis of rumour or assumption. It is also worth considering how geographically flexible you are prepared to be, as there is a significant geographical variation in competition ratios within specialties across the UK

Job traits

Clinical jobs can vary tremendously in terms of the nature, intensity, variety, predictability, and continuity of the workload. The combination of these characteristics in each specialty is likely to become more important the more senior you become. These aspects of the job may not be obvious when you are a medical student, focused on the scientific and clinical aspects of each specialty, but they are very important when deciding on a medical career. Take time to observe, or ask about, the following factors when on any clinical placement:

Clinical variety

Consider the variety of patients you will see in particular specialties (age and sex), the nature of clinical problems (acute vs chronic), the variety of clinical work, outpatient consultations, ward work, and operating/procedures.

When considering whether you might enjoy a specialty where breadth of knowledge is required (GP, emergency medicine, etc.) consider if you are happy to cope with the flip side of variety, which of course is ↓depth of knowledge. Similarly, in order to become an expert in a field and especially in a practical specialty, it is necessary to perform procedures repeatedly, which while highly rewarding for some, may spell boredom for others.

Shift pattern/intensity

Emergency medicine, general medicine, anaesthetics, and surgery involve full shift work and unsociable shift patterns, during your years of training and beyond. Consider your other priorities, and seek advice from current trainees/consultants to gain insight into how they maintain their work–life balance. On the whole, there tends to be greater flexibility with job planning after training is completed.

Continuity of care

Some clinicians value the long-term involvement with patients such as in primary care, endocrinology, renal medicine, and psychiatry. However, others value not having ongoing responsibility for patients when they leave work, such as in anaesthetics or emergency medicine.

Predictability of the workload

Some specialties such as emergency medicine, trauma surgery, or transplant surgery may have an unpredictable workload compared to specialties such as dermatology, urology, or general practice where the workload is likely to be more predictable.

Dealing with life and death

This is a reality in acute care: emergency medicine, intensive care medicine, general medicine, care of the elderly, or surgical specialties (vascular surgery, neurosurgery, cardiothoracic surgery). It may stimulate some doctors yet paralyse others. You may feel that you prefer not to deal with life-threatening situations and would prefer a specialty that is unlikely to encounter them (dermatology, ophthalmology, etc.).

Length of training

General practice is currently the shortest post-foundation training programme, at 3 years to completion of training. Many GPs are now developing a specialist interest (GPwSI), either by further focused training and experience after their certificate of completion of training or perhaps after coming into GP training from another specialty (paediatrics, O&G etc.) There is an increasing move towards delivering care in the primary care setting, and a GP with specialist knowledge and training can be a very useful asset. A specialty with a long training programme, such as plastic surgery, ophthalmology, or paediatrics, may be off-putting for some, although a run-through training programme guarantees geographical stability for a period, which has obvious advantages if you wish to settle down. Refer to postgraduate training websites if you are unsure about the duration of training in each specialty.

Interest in subject

A medical career is long, and you will spend much of your waking time devoted to doing it or reading about it! It is important therefore to opt for a career which is likely to sustain your interest for many years to come.

Advances in technology

Although new technologies are likely to change the way we practise medicine and interface with patients in every specialty, there are clearly some specialties that will be more at the cutting edge for this. New techniques, emerging technologies, breakthroughs in basic science (stem cells, gene therapy, etc.), your thirst for research, or simply engaging with the changes to clinical practice in a progressing field may be more relevant to ophthalmology or cardiology than, say, psychiatry or general practice.

Opportunities for research

Many specialties present opportunities for research. However, in some it is almost compulsory (cardiology, oncology) or the competition for jobs is such that it is often required. Take advice on this from senior trainees or consultants within the specialty.

Portfolio careers

Many doctors develop a 'portfolio career'—pioneered among GPs, this is now a pattern of working seen more broadly across the specialties. Some examples of ways that doctors add diversity to their clinical careers include medical education, medical journalism, business, medico-legal practice, and management.

Problem-solving

This is an integral part of a career in medicine. Are you more of an analytical problem-solver, perhaps attracted to the more cerebral specialties where diagnosing provides a challenge, such as neurology, infectious diseases, general medicine, etc.? Or do you enjoy the challenge of a practical problem, such as might be found in theatre deciding how to reconstruct a section of anatomy in plastic surgery?

Pay

Basic consultant pay scales are the same across the specialties, but there is clearly more scope in some specialties for generating income from private practice. Most partners in general practice currently earn more than the basic consultant's salary. Although this probably will not be your main consideration when choosing a specialty, if it is particularly important to you, you should take earning potential into account.

Life aspirations

Clearly there are many things to take into account when planning your career, not least your aspirations for life outside of medicine. The majority of doctors do not have family commitments at the time they make their specialty choice, and it can be very difficult to decide whether to go for something which may prove challenging at a later date if juggling family commitments, or to make a 'compromise' decision before it is actually needed.

Again, there are no right or wrong answers, but it is possible to work flexibly in any specialty, although the part-time training route is better established in some than others. Take time to sound out senior colleagues and trainees in the specialty who appear to be managing to balance work and family commitments. There will usually be a lead within each Local Education and Training Board (LETB) for less than full-time training and a discussion with this individual ahead of time may be useful. If geographical location is very important to you, e.g. your partner has a job tied to a specific location, then having a 'plan B' specialty that is less competitive, such as general practice, may be a sensible option. If you are determined to go for something highly competitive such as neurosurgery or ophthalmology, you may have to compromise on location in order to secure a training post. Competitive specialties tend to stay competitive throughout, even at consultant level—again, you may have to be prepared to go where the jobs are. The location of your family and friends may be pivotal in where you wish to work, and you may have to account for this in your choice of career. You may wish to spend time working abroad, either in the developed or developing world. Taking time out of a training programme is often possible but requires a lot of early planning and organization (12–18 months in advance). You may already have identified an organization you wish to work with.

Role models

You are likely to come across individuals who stand out and are in some way inspirational to you. Being inspired by an individual is a perfectly valid reason to be initially attracted to a specialty, although it is important to attempt to deconstruct the basis of this appeal: what is it about this role model that is so inspiring? Do they have exceptional surgical skills, is it their ability to lead a team, their capacity for analytical thinking, or their interaction with patients? Identifying the traits that have stood out for you can be an important part of crystallizing your own values, but the attributes identified may not necessarily be specialty specific, so it is important not to assume they are. This is where spending some time on written reflection around your observations and thoughts can be particularly useful.

Strategies for the undecided

Choosing a career involves consideration of some or all of these complex factors, but it is also important to allow time and space for creative thinking before important decisions are made. Doctors tend to be very good at getting things done and being efficient, and the benefits of carving out some 'empty time' may not be immediately apparent. However, if you reflect on when and where you have your most creative ideas, it is likely to be when you are in the shower, or out on a walk, rather than when you are sitting at a desk writing a list of 'pros and cons'. Give your brain the chance to think creatively—make sure you are not constantly on the go! If you are undecided on your career, seek out as many opportunities for discussion as possible. This may be with trainees, or substantives in the specialties you are interested in, your educational supervisor/tutor, or a careers counsellor at your university. Chat to people who know you best both inside and outside of medicine.

Such conversations are likely to bring you progressively closer to understanding your unique set of values and strengths, and which specialties may provide a good fit for you.

There are several tools that you might find useful, yet none are overarching. The Myers–Briggs Type Indicator is a popular tool to characterize personality types, often used in industry, leadership, or team working contexts. It may be helpful in identifying how you think, express yourself, and respond to your environment—and therefore which clinical context may be naturally more challenging to you. It may provide valuable insights. Formal use of this tool requires an investment of time and money as the completed questionnaire needs to be fed back and discussed with you by a trained Myers–Briggs practitioner. However there are simpler versions available based on the original theory which you may find useful (e.g. in Anita Houghton's book '*Finding Square Holes*'; see ➜ 'Where to find out more …' p. 1007).

The Sci59 is an online questionnaire which attempts to identify your most suitable specialties based on responses to 130 questions. This is not evidence based but may be a useful starting point for considering or rejecting career possibilities for those who are completely stuck. Its recommendations are based on responses from individuals already established within the different medical specialties.

The SWOT analysis is a useful way of structuring your thoughts around a particular event or process. It can be a useful tool to look at a proposed career path, particularly if you have already done some work on self-assessment. For example, if you were considering general practice as an option, armed with your insights from self-assessment exercises, you might want to sit down with a local GP trainer and work through a SWOT analysis together. This gives you a framework to consider your strengths and weaknesses in the context of the opportunities and threats of the rapidly changing primary care landscape.

Top tips

1. Choosing a medical career is not a simple logical choice, and there is no tool which will tell you the answer.
2. Make the best of your opportunities and use your clinical placements to ask the key questions on careers that are most important to you.
3. Networking by talking to people (at work, even informally) will help you collect perspectives to make a well-informed decision.
4. Be positive. Choosing a career is an exciting process. You will find many specialties fulfilling, and there is not a single correct answer.
5. There is always a way out! Rest assured that even if you have decided your speciality since the age of 10, made the wrong choice of specialization down the line, or want to leave the field altogether to pursue an entirely different career, there is always a way out and back in again.

Where to find out more ...

Websites

- ℘ Specialtytraining.hee.nhs.uk—the official site for details on the specialty selection process. Competition ratios for the different specialties, person specs.
- *Accreditation of Transferable Competencies Framework*—introduces more flexibility into early medical career pathways and guides those who wish to switch to a different specialty: ℘ http://www.aomrc.org.uk/reports-guidance/accreditation-of-transferable-competences-0914/.
- *The Gold Guide*—useful information on practical details of specialty training such as time out of programme, inter-deanery transfer, and less than full-time training: ℘ https://www.copmed.org.uk/gold-guide-7th-edition/the-gold-guide-7th-edition.
- *BMJ Careers*—career news, features, and events: ℘ https://www.bmj.com/careers/careers.
- *Sci59*—if you are a BMA member, you can access this tool via the BMA website: ℘ https://www.bma.org.uk/advice/career/applying-for-training/sci59-medical-specialty-psychometric-test.
- *National Institute for Health Research*—for information about academic career pathways: ℘ https://www.nihr.ac.uk/funding-and-support/funding-for-training-and-career-development/training-programmes/integrated-academic-training-programme/integrated-academic-training/academic-clinical-fellowships/.
- *Alternative roles for doctors. Ideas of jobs where a medical degree and clinical training or experience are valued.* ℘ https://www.healthcareers.nhs.uk/explore-roles/doctors/career-opportunities-doctors/alternative-roles-doctors.
- *Royal College* websites often have useful career information and many organize annual career events for students and foundation doctors: ℘ www.rcpsych.ac.uk; www.rcseng.ac.uk.
- *The NHS Careers* website has recently replaced the excellent NHS medical careers website: ℘ www.healthcareers.nhs.uk.
- *Myers–Briggs personality type tool*: ℘ www.myersbriggs.org/my-mbti-personality-type/mbti-basics.
- *Faculty of Medical Leadership and Management* provides advice and guidance on medical leadership in the UK: ℘ www.fmlm.ac.uk.

Books

- Lim D (2011). *How to Get a Specialty Training Post: The Insider's Guide.* Oxford: Oxford University Press.
- Elton C, Reid J (2012). *The ROADS to Success*, 3rd ed. Postgraduate Deanery for Kent, Surrey and Sussex. Available free as an ebook at ℘ www.cmec.info/wp-content/uploads/2011/07/Roads-To-Success1.pdf
- Houghton A (2005). *Finding Square Holes.* Carmarthen: Crown House Publishing.

Article

- Goldacre MJ, Laxton L, Lambert TW (2010). Medical graduates' early career choices of specialty and their eventual specialty destinations: UK prospective cohort studies. *BMJ* 340:c3199.

Getting ahead

Making contacts

It can be very helpful to have a mentor or senior peer who takes an academic or pastoral interest in your career throughout medical school.

Many universities will allocate a clinical supervisor or tutor who is available for informal advice or more structured assistance where necessary. They will also provide a reference for your job application and will be the first point of contact for any pressing issues with the medical school. It is important that you maintain a good working relationship with your tutor otherwise they will not have much to go by except for your academic records. You may wish to forge your own links, perhaps within a speciality of your interest. Be clear with yourself why you are doing this; people will be able to detect obsequiousness a mile off, but will respond much better if you have a clear goal such as becoming involved in a research project.

How to make contacts?

Informal

If you wish to make yourself known within a clinical specialty, a good place to start is with the ward team. Get to know the junior trainees and the registrars, and make an effort to attend clinics, ward rounds, or theatre sessions. You may identify a particular area of interest and approach the consultant with ideas for an audit, case review, or literature search. Taking the initiative is very much encouraged, noticed, and supported. Similarly, many specialities have nurse specialists who are a mine of useful information and may also be able to suggest suitable fields for study (and critically know how to gather this information). Remember that your interests can extend beyond the clinical curriculum, e.g. you may wish to get to know people with similar religious/political/sporting/social inclinations.

Student societies

Many medical schools will have medical student societies for those with a particular interest, e.g. in surgery or paediatrics. Local and informal meetings may be a good introduction. If your medical school does not have such a society, why not start your own with the help of the student union? Ask a consultant to act as your patron or director and approach your student union, your members, organizations, and companies for funding. This will show great initiative. If these are going well, why not join with similar societies at other medical schools or form a national society for medical students interested in the same subject matter? Social media is an easy of way of gaining interest and publicizing events/causes.

Websites/Internet fora

There are a number of online sites where like-minded (and frequently diametrically opposed) medical professionals exchange views and information. Be mindful of GMC guidance on doctors' use of social media.

National societies

Most specialities are keen to engage trainees and medical students from an early stage in their career. Check their websites for free/reduced conference registration, student-focused meetings, and funding opportunities.

Conferences

National conferences are a great way to meet people within a specialty. Student participation is greatly encouraged yet remains relatively rare. Medical students who present posters or oral presentations stand out (for the right reasons) and are spared from the more direct lines of questioning afterwards! Organizing your own conference will make you stand out, but do not underestimate the amount of work and responsibility involved. You will need to find funding (often from medical industry, perhaps ask a friendly consultant to make an introduction on your behalf), a venue, and facilitate registration, catering, etc. The most rewarding part of conference organization can be choosing a suitable programme and your 'fantasy line-up' of speakers. You will be amazed by the good will shown to such endeavours and many eminent people will offer their services for free.

Charities, volunteering, and patient groups

Getting involved from the patient's perspective can be truly eye opening, and your involvement will be encouraged. You may start with voluntary or fundraising work and then take a more active role in committee management. Most charities have a medical advisor, why not start early? There is a misconception that medical students can only do some good after graduating as a doctor. In fact, society in general will be keener to help ambitious and righteous students who have the time and energy to invest in making a positive change. Once you start working, it becomes more difficult to dedicate your precious free time to big events.

Extracurricular activities

Leaving home and going to university opens up a panoply of new opportunities, of which you should take full advantage. Many medical students continue an existing interest at a higher level, e.g. sports or music, or try something entirely new. However, unlike many other undergraduate courses, the demanding and rigid scheduling of the preclinical and clinical courses does not accommodate other activities easily. A Classics student may be able to spend two entire days each week playing university-level rugby and fit in self-directed learning around this, but the medical student timetable is generally full from 9 a.m.–5 p.m., Monday to Friday (and at some medical schools, Saturday too!).

This is not to say that it is not possible to do both things well. Medical schools are rightly proud of the extracurricular achievements of their students. The selection committee have chosen you to act as an ambassador for the university and in return, you will be expected to contribute to your university, much like helping them to help you. A good doctor is someone with the skills required to take a step back from medicine to see the bigger picture, not to mention the direct benefits of having other interests outside of work. This guide is not intended to explain the variety of extracurricular activities available to you at medical school but to offer some tips for how to succeed in medicine *and* something different.

> **Paraphrased advice from an Oxbridge medicine tutor, last millennium**
>
> *'Of medicine, rowing, socializing, and relationships, many can do two things well, some can do three things well. It is very rare to manage all four.'*

Time management

You will need to be extremely organized and make good use of your time in order to fit in medicine with other interests. It may be a good plan to get an idea of your workload and how you cope with it before committing to too many different activities. Bear in mind that many medical students have not had to apply themselves too onerously in order to achieve top marks at high school. It can be a shock at medical school to find that life is harder, that you are no longer top of the class, and there is no alternative to hours of bookwork. Anatomy, for example, cannot be deduced from native wit or basic principles, and instead requires diligent learning.

Scheduling

If you know from the outset that you are committed to playing football at university level, and that this will require a full day off midweek to travel to games, it is worth being upfront with your tutors from the start. You may be able to swap tutorial groups or practical classes in order to accommodate this. In addition, being honest will be more highly regarded than simply failing to turn up. Remember that students must sign in for many lectures and practicals and that your absence may be noted. If you really do have to miss sessions, approach a friend in advance and ask them to take notes on your behalf and spend time filling you in afterwards. Offer something in return. If you do not understand the content you have missed, ask your tutor to spend some time going over it. Continuing to meet deadlines and performing well in written work will be evidence that you are not neglecting your studies and may make others more inclined to be helpful towards you.

Like-minded individuals

Taking part in university-wide activities means that your colleagues will study subjects other than medicine. They may not appreciate your workload or inflexible timetable, nor be willing to accommodate it. Taking part in medical school societies has the advantage that everyone else does what you do. Sharing an interest can → spending quality time with the next best thing to family, fostering long-term friendships, becoming less homesick, and creating a sense of belonging away from home.

Priorities

If you do find yourself missing hours of study during the week in order to play the piano, you may need to sacrifice your free time at the weekend in order to catch up. What you should not neglect, however, is good-quality sleep, exercise, diet, and your well-being! Remember to find joy in the things that you decide to invest time into. You only have one shot at going to medical school so make the most of your time inside and outside your studies. You may be surprised at finding out your hidden interests and passions but you will only be able to recognize them if you put yourself out there.

Niche interests

You may think that you are the only person with an interest in early medieval music or the plays of Christopher Marlowe. This is unlikely to be the case. Why not start your own society? Using social media it is easy to make contacts, and you may be able to get funding from the university or medical school. Showing such initiative does not harm your CV either as it demonstrates your multiple interests, wholesome personality, leadership, and teamwork skills. Society members may not study the same subject but your shared interests may just spark an ever-lasting friendship with people from all walks of life.

Voluntary work

Many students do voluntary work, particularly in preparation for medical school applications. Your clinical experience may expose you to particular areas worthy of your time such as care homes or hospices. Working with the homeless offers valuable experience with those with substance misuse/addictions.

There are ample opportunities advertised by the volunteering centres at your university and in town. There will always be something for you to do and somewhere to make a positive influence. Volunteering and helping out has also been demonstrated to help with mild depression and offering a sense of personal satisfaction, purpose, and identity. Medical students tend to be altruistic and righteous but many feel disheartened by believing that they can only help others after graduating as a doctor. 'Caring' skills are extremely valuable and until recently neglected by most courses. Remember though that being a successful doctor will make you a valuable member of society and you should prioritize your studies.

Funding

There will be a number of small grants and prizes available through medical school or university to support those performing in extracurricular activities at a high level, e.g. to cover the cost of music tuition or sports training camps. A successful applicant is likely to be someone who also performs well academically.

Potential conflicts

Remember that medical students represent the profession, even in non-medical environments. Medical practitioners should not allow their own political, moral, or religious beliefs to influence patient care. This is not to say that you should not be politically or spiritually active in your free time, but use common sense in avoiding potential conflicts.

Social media

You should interact with others online in the same way that you would face to face and remember that you are representing the medical profession even when 'off duty'. Read the GMC guidance on social media (℅ www.gmc-uk.org/guidance/ethical_guidance/21186.asp).

Remember also to use discretion when deciding which photos of you may be seen by others.

Sex, drugs, drink, and fast cars

Familiarize yourself with the GMC standards expected of medical students (℅ www.gmc-uk.org/education/undergraduate/professional_behaviour.asp).

Excessive alcohol and recreational drug use are not uncommon among medical students. Remember, however, that these are fitness to practise issues, even before you have qualified. GMC guidance for undergraduates refers explicitly to:

- drink driving
- alcohol use that impairs work or affects the working environment
- dealing, possession, or use of recreational drugs, even if there are no legal proceedings.

There is also clear guidance on the help available to those with true substance addiction (℅ www.gmc-uk.org/education/undergraduate/26665.asp) with responsibilities both on the part of the medical school and the student. Most undergraduate recreational drug use, however, is not in the context of addiction so use common sense. If you have concerns about substance misuse by a fellow student, you should share them.

Alcohol

'Social' drinking is an important part of undergraduate life for many people, a chance to relax after hard work and have fun. Moderate drinking is a perfectly acceptable behaviour in both medical students and doctors. However, you need to be aware of the associated issues (habit forming or high-risk behaviours, liver damage, ↑risk of some cancers, cardiovascular risk, cognitive impairment). Remain mindful of Department of Health guidance: do not regularly exceed 2–3 units/day for both sexes (i.e. 1 bottle of wine = 10 units, 1 pint of beer = 2.5–3 units).

Drinking societies

Once an integral part of university life, they are increasingly falling out of favour, particularly with the authorities. This is one of the more ugly faces of undergraduate socializing, encouraging binge drinking, dangerous and disrespectful behaviour, and peer pressure to misbehave. Again, remember that you are representing the medical profession—hard to do when you are 12 pints down, naked, and strapped around a tree because your friends find it hilarious.

Recreational drugs

The use of *all* recreational drugs is taken very seriously by medical schools and the GMC. Do not take the risk! If you have a genuine addiction, be brave, be honest with yourself, imagine your career ahead of you spanning four decades, and seek help early. Your university's occupational health department can offer you advice and refer you to an appropriate specialist counsellor.

Smoking

Doctors are allowed to smoke. Most hospitals are smoke free so it will be a struggle to nip out for a quick one during a 12-hour shift. Cigarette smoke is very pervasive and the smell will stay on your breath and in your hair and clothes when seeing patients. Imagine telling a non-smoker they have lung cancer when you smell of Benson and Hedges. This harmful habit is often started early in life (e.g. at university) and is very hard to break. The addiction is more powerful than years of studying blackened lungs in pathology or atheromatous vessels. The sensible approach is never to start.

Driving offences

In the fitness to practise declaration, medical students/doctors must list any driving offences (other than where a fixed penalty notice has been accepted and paid). Drink driving is likely to result in a fitness to practise hearing.

Safe sex

Even as a medical student you have a responsibility towards promoting public health and safe behaviour. For this reason you should set an example in your sex life, and encourage others to do the same. There are multiple options including barrier contraception, devices, and medicines to avoid STIs as well as unwanted pregnancies. More information is available from your GP or the university occupational health department.

Importance of logbooks

Logbooks form a proof of procedural/surgical experience and they are essential, particularly if you plan on pursuing a surgical specialty. When you eventually apply for postgraduate clinical posts (medical or surgical), you will be required to prove the statements you make. Systematic recording of surgical procedures is a requirement of the Intercollegiate Surgical Curriculum Programme (ISCP). A logbook of surgical experience may be of interest to your clinical/educational supervisors when your progress is assessed during medical school. later, surgical logbooks are important for annual appraisals of training (ARCPs), revalidation, and continuing professional development.

What to record

It is important to record the following details of all procedures:
- Date of procedure.
- Hospital.
- Procedure.
- Elective/emergency.
- Laterality (left or right).
- Hospital number (no identifiable patient details otherwise).
- Your role in the procedure:
  - P: primary surgeon.
  - PS: primary surgeon, supervised.
  - A: assisted.

Operation note

You should enter key details about the operation itself: was there anything that describes the complexity of the procedure, or any complications? This will add to the demonstration of your surgical experience.

Where to record it

Traditionally, logbooks were paper based and entered manually, and later, on a spreadsheet. Electronic, online logbooks are now available which have many advantages:
- Automatic backup of data (so that you cannot lose it).
- Automated analysis:
  - Tabulation of surgical numbers.
  - Surgical progress over time.
- Built-in audit facility: automated surgical outcome data.

There is a pan-surgical web-based logbook available for use by medical students, administered by the Royal College of Surgeons Edinburgh (⅏ www. elogbook.org/logbookclient/registration or www.surgeon-logbook.com).

Top tip

Start today! Record all surgical procedures you are involved in, using an online surgical logbook. This will establish good habits early, and allow cases you contribute to as a medical student to form part of your career record.

Reflective practice

Implicit in medicine is the concept of life-long learning. Reflective practice is one method that assists with this continuous cycle of learning. It provides a way of breaking down experiences, both clinical and non-clinical, to help evaluate one's own practice and to identify learning outcomes as well as areas for development and improvement. You will experience many things throughout your career, some more significant than others. Reflecting on your experiences will also assist you in developing coping mechanisms and prepare you for recurrences.

Why do I need to reflect?

Reflective practice is widely used during undergraduate and postgraduate training programmes as experiential learning. It is found at all levels from student to consultant level and is becoming increasingly important in the process of revalidation. In addition to traditional modes of assessment, reflective practice is now being incorporated into training programme assessments as a way of demonstrating particular competencies and to prove personal professional development. Exams and assessments aside, it can be used to formalize your thoughts, establish your own strengths and weaknesses, and therefore adapt your individual actions and learning needs.

What do I reflect on?

We all reflect daily. Any situation which makes you think after the event has occurred can be included in reflective practice. Some situations may be more pertinent and meaningful to you than others. There are situations which make you feel good or pleased, those which make you feel upset or worried, those which analyse a significant event, those which demonstrate a void in your knowledge, and those which make you feel improvements or changes are possible. These are just a few examples of scenarios which can form the basis of a reflective piece.

How do I reflect?

Reflective practice can be done individually or with your peers, other colleagues, or your supervisors. It can take the form of case-based discussions or informal conversations. It can also be done more formally in writing which often helps cement thoughts and feelings. It is useful to practise writing these from an early stage and to find your own preferred structure. Below are some subheadings and questions (with example answers) which you may want to consider during reflective practice:

1. *A brief introduction*
- What is this reflection focusing on?
- Why do you want to talk/write about this situation?

Example: 'Good communication with patients is vital. This reflection focuses on the importance of tailoring an explanation of a diagnosis to a patient.'

2. *The scenario itself*
- What happened?
- What was the situation?

Keep this concise and be sure to anonymize any patient information.

Example: 'I saw an elderly patient who was hard of hearing in clinic. I needed to explain their diagnosis of osteoarthritis so that they would understand the condition and management options.'

3. Your performance

- What did you find easy?
- What did you find difficult?
- How did you feel?
- What were your thought processes?

Example: 'I found it easy to describe the condition clearly and concisely without using medical jargon. I used a plastic model of a knee joint as a visual aid to help with this. The patient understood and was grateful for the explanation I provided. This made me feel pleased. I found it more difficult to explain a clear management plan as there were still blood tests and radiographs pending. I feel I could have appeared more confident in my delivery of the options available and could have simplified the plan.'

4. Learning achieved

- What did you learn?
- Why is this relevant?

Example: 'I learned that it is important to communicate and tailor the explanation of a condition to each patient as an individual. In this situation, I used a visual aid in the form of a model to help with the explanation as the patient was hard of hearing. Others may prefer all the specific details and figures of their condition while others may prefer just an outline. This is particularly important as I will be seeing patients of all ages and backgrounds.'

5. Learning needs

- Is there anything you would do differently?
- What are your further learning needs?
- Why are these important/relevant?
- How and when will you complete the learning cycle?

Example: 'Giving leaflets to patients or signposting them to further resources and information is always good practice and I could have given this patient a leaflet to take home at the end of the consultation. I would also like to improve my confidence in discussing the management options with patients to help gain their trust. I understand that this may come with time but I could also address this learning need by asking my senior or supervisor to observe me during my next consultation so that they can give me feedback on my performance.'

Resource

BMJ: ℬ www.bmj.com/content/336/7648/827.

Finding projects

What field or specialty?

If you are fortunate enough to have a clear career ambition, this will not be a difficult choice. You may score valuable CV points with a short extracurricular project which displays your enthusiasm for a given specialty. If you are in the undecided majority, you may be guided instead by a particular doctor with whom you have developed a good rapport, or a specific clinical or scientific question you wish to answer. You should bear in mind the following points:

1. Who will supervise the project?

You will need a mentor to oversee and direct your work. If you have developed a good relationship with a doctor on the wards, do not be afraid to ask if they have any suitable projects. Alternatively, they may be able to recommend a colleague.

2. How much time will it take?

Remember that extracurricular projects must not affect your performance in mandatory courses and you should only commit to something you can do in your spare time before the deadline. Be realistic; you will not be able to access the case records of 5000 patients or master a complicated bioinformatics programme without a dedicated full-time stint.

3. What skills do I have to offer?

In many instances you may find your most valuable assets are spare time and enthusiasm, and most projects will not require any particular skills at the outset. However, if you have a passion for computer programming or database management you should make this known and tailor the project towards these areas.

4. What skills will I gain?

You may well be asked at interview what you have learned from a given project. Be prepared to discuss specifics (such as the complication rate following ileal conduit formation or the cost–benefit analysis of IV compared to PO paracetamol), as well as more generic or transferrable skills such as scientific writing, critical analysis of literature, and time management.

5. What is my goal?

You should have a clear aim of what you wish to get out of an extracurricular project. Some supervisors will have a dataset they wish to gather, or want to know an answer to a specific question; however, these aims may not be of immediate benefit to you. Make sure that you have something to show for your efforts, such as authorship of a paper, a poster presentation, or a talk at a local meeting.

Some starting suggestions

Clinical
- A clinical audit that 'closes the loop'.
- Data-gathering exercise. This could be clinical (e.g. the incidence of herpes zoster among rheumatology patients treated with rituximab or a case series of children with nephroblastoma), or subjective (e.g. a patient satisfaction survey following cataract surgery).
- Clinical protocol, e.g. the hospital-wide guidance on how to manage diabetic ketoacidosis or outpatient paracentesis.

Management
- Quality improvement. Are there any aspects in which your department could perform better and how could this be achieved? What supporting data is required?
- Service review, e.g. the impact of a breathlessness intervention service on readmissions in patients with COPD.

Academic
- Literature review or meta-analysis (e.g. what is the evidence in support of a particular intervention)?
- Book/chapter writing. Many doctors are involved in writing textbooks or handbooks and would be only too pleased to delegate some of this.
- A focused basic science project.

Communications and education
- Educational video, e.g. how to break bad news, or a clinical demonstration of knee examinations.
- Social media, such as a website or forum to discuss issues relevant to medical students or share information. Be aware of GMC guidance for responsible use of social media (℞ www.gmc-uk.org/Doctors__use_of_social_media. pdf_51448306.pdf).
- A patient information leaflet (e.g. 'What you need to know about eczema').

Finding funding
Limited funding may be available via:
- individual specialty organizations (℞ www.money4medstudents.org/bursaries-and-grants)
- your medical school
- your college (where applicable)
- your supervisor (if they have a research grant of their own).

Clinical audit

Clinical audit is a tool used to evaluate performance against an existing standard or criteria (e.g. NICE guidelines), and is an important part of quality improvement and management. Most clinical departments will be required to audit a number of outcome measures on a regular basis. Audits invariably require a degree of data collection, and as a result medical student involvement is both encouraged and mutually beneficial.

What is the audit cycle?

A clinical audit should:
- select an area to evaluate (e.g. waiting time for hip replacement surgery)
- compare current performance against objective guidelines (e.g. 18-week target)
- identify areas for improvement
- suggest and implement changes to facilitate this (such as a streamlined referral pathway)
- re-audit the same measure following these changes to show any outcome improvement.

This is known as the *audit cycle*, and the aim of any audit should be to 'close the loop'. (See Fig. 54.1)

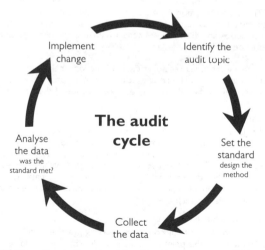

Fig. 54.1 The audit cycle. Reproduced from http://www.nature.com/bdj/journal/v217/n7/images/sj.bdj.2014.861-f1.jpg.

How to get involved

Identify a department in which you have a particular interest, or colleagues with whom you have established a good rapport. A good place to start would be to ask the junior doctors in that team; some of them may already be involved in clinical audit and would be glad to supervise you and happy for your help. Alternatively, email the consultant in charge of departmental audits and management issues. Ask for a suitable measure to audit; many departments will have a long list of outstanding projects. Choose one that will be manageable for you in the time available. Be very clear on what it is that you are auditing before you start.

Identify the standards against which you will be comparing your data (usually NICE guidelines or similar). Audits are part of clinical governance and some are more political than others. Some audits are related to funding and will always be given more priority. If you are given a re-audit that has been done for several cycles, then it is probably best to request the previous reports and presentations to ensure that you are conducting the audit correctly and in a similar fashion.

Data collection

Take plenty of time at the outset to decide what data you need to collect. You will need a list of patients for inclusion; this data is likely to be provided by a data manager, the audit department, or secretaries. You then need to decide what pieces of information you need to collect for each patient (demographics, date of referral, date of surgery, GP surgery, complications, etc.). There is nothing more frustrating than finding something vital has been missed and having to access 50 sets of notes again to find it. Create a pro forma template on which you will collect data and ask someone to check it before you start.

> Be aware of the rules regarding data protection: make sure to check which computers you should use, ask for an encrypted data stick, and know what (anonymized) data may be taken outside of the hospital.

Data analysis

You should define your inclusion criteria, show how many patients were identified, how many notes were accessed, and demographics of the data set. Your main outcome is the performance against the objective measure (i.e. 85% of patients had hip replacement surgery within 18 weeks of referral). You should then identify reasons why 15% of patients did not receive treatment in this time (cancelled by patient, staff shortage, administrative hurdles in referral process, etc.).

Implement change

It may be beyond your remit to change working practices within a department! However, at this point in the audit cycle, changes should be implemented to improve performance within a given measure, e.g. more space allocated in orthopaedic theatres or a computerized referral process.

Re-audit

After changes have been implemented, the data collection should be repeated after an appropriate interval (usually 3-6 months) to evaluate any improvement. Realistically you are unlikely to be involved throughout the entirety of the audit cycle and someone else may re-audit.

How to showcase your contribution

It is very useful for your CV to show involvement in a clinical audit. You may wish to submit a formal report of your findings to the department, or even present your data at a clinical directorate meeting. Being able to show evidence of involvement in quality improvement activities such as audit will stand you in good stead.

Quality improvement projects

These are very similar to auditing with the main difference of reviewing your data collection, sampling a smaller population, and implementing changes as well as reviewing its impact far more frequently (e.g. weekly).

Audit vs research

Audits and research are not the same thing but both contribute to clinical governance. Audits look at whether your hospital met set and defined standards in terms of clinical practice. These standards may have been set by local, regional, or national bodies. Conversely, research looks for new knowledge, discoveries, and inventions. See Table 54.1 for other differences.

Table 54.1 Audit vs research

Audit	Research
Measures whether targets are being met	Creating new information, sometimes with very little pre-existing knowledge
Set against defined standards	Guided by a hypothesis/theory
Retrospective	Either retrospective or prospective
Does not involve live subjects	May include live subjects (e.g. animals or human)
Ethical approval not required	Ethical approval required if human or animal subjects involved

Further reading

NHS England. *Clinical Audit*: ℘ https://www.england.nhs.uk/ourwork/qual-clin-lead/clinaudit/.
Royal College of Obstetrics & Gynaecology. *Understanding Audit*. Clinical Guideline Advice No. 5. ℘ www.rcog.org.uk/globalassets/documents/guidelines/clinical-governance-advice/clingov5understandingaudit2003.pdf.
Hexter AT. *How to Conduct a Clinical Audit: A Guide for Medical Students*. National AMR. ℘ www.southampton.ac.uk/sias/resources/howtoseries/howtoclinicalaudit.page.

Medical research

When starting out at medical school it is easy to become awestruck by how much there is to 'know'. However, as one progresses, it becomes apparent that what is unknown is an equally daunting prospect. Medicine is full of controversies and uncertainties in the management of even the most common conditions.

It is medical research that pushes forward these limits of our understanding, with the aim in doing so of improving patient care. This is acknowledged directly by the GMC which states: 'Research involving people directly or indirectly is vital in improving care and reducing uncertainty for patients now and in the future, and improving the health of the population as a whole.'

Many students will experience research as part of their medical degree, and a proportion will go on to become leading academics of the future. While those that follow a focused research career are the minority, it is becoming increasingly recognized that all doctors should be able to engage with research, for instance, facilitating patients of theirs who wish to participate in studies.

What research is and is not

Research is about discovering new concepts. Both the processes of research and the potential results may have adverse consequences (e.g. an adverse reaction to a drug in a trial, or finding the Huntington disease mutation in a sequencing study). As a result, there are strict ethical and procedural frameworks in place to minimize risks. While certain 'Eureka!' moments and individuals have become ingrained in our collective psyche—the discovery of the double helix, or penicillin—the reality is that the majority of the development of new knowledge is the sequential result of persistent hard work, often among teams of collaborators.

Levels of research evidence

There is a quantitative hierarchy of levels of evidence to signify the quality of the study (Fig. 54.2). For instance, the data is more likely to be applicable to your practice if a new treatment has been demonstrated to be more effective against the current gold standard treatment in a randomized controlled trial with patients (level 1) as opposed to one expert claiming it is without any testing (level 5 opinion). Conducting research that has a high level of evidence will also attract more positive attention, funding, and job opportunities in research.

Medical research and evidence-based medicine

Medical research and the practice of evidence-based medicine are intrinsically linked. Evidence-based medicine utilizes the outputs of research to enable decisions to be made on the most robust available evidence. In contrast, it is medical research that generates this evidence. It is not uncommon for the conclusion of systematic reviews to highlight '*more research is needed*'.

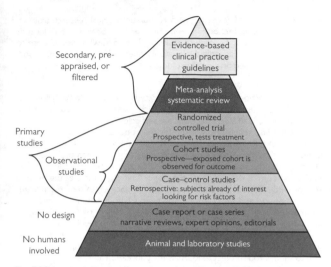

Fig. 54.2 Levels of clinical evidence. Reproduced from wikimedia under the Creative Commons Attribution-Share Alike 4.0 International license.

Audit and service evaluation

Audit and service evaluations are performance measures and while they often use overlapping methodologies with research, they do not generally have the same risk of adverse events.

Research careers

A range of opportunities are now available to undertake and get involved with medical research, many of which are part of formal 'academic programmes'. While such programmes offer great opportunities and structure they are not the only way. Alternative schemes to that of England are available in the devolved nations:

- National Institute for Health Research: ℘ www.nihrtcc.nhs.uk/intetacatrain.
- Wales Clinical Academic Track WCAT: ℘ www.walesdeanerg.org/index.php/wcat.html.
- Academic Training Northern Ireland Medical & Dental Training Agency: ℘ www.nimtda.gov.uk/speciality-training/information-for-speciality -trainees/spec-academic/.
- Scottish Academic Training (SCREDS): ℘ www.nes.scot.nhs.uk/education-and-training/by-discipline/medicine/specialty-training/scottish-academic-training-(screds).aspx.

Some students may know they wish to pursue medical research from an early stage in medical school; others, however, only begin to consider it as they come close to or become consultants. How and when you choose to undertake research is an individual matter influenced by experience, opportunities, luck, and personal circumstances.

Research at medical school

Many medical schools offer the opportunity to intercalate a Bachelor's research degree (usually a BSc) during which students complete a specific research project and study a specific area of science.

A few medical schools now also offer the opportunity to combine a PhD with medical training as part of an MB PhD programme. It is also often frequently possible to pause medical training (e.g. between preclinical and clinical years), to undertake further research as a stand-alone degree (e.g. PhD). Sometimes, depending on the opportunities available at the medical school, a BSc may be upgraded to a Master's (MSc) which requires a longer research period and dissertation. However, Oxbridge students have their intercalated degree automatically upgraded to a Master of Arts (MA) upon graduating. It is not infrequent that graduate entries to medical school have considerable medical research experience. This time will not only teach you valuable skills about research but will offer a plethora of opportunities for you to submit your project to journals for publication and international conference presentations.

Foundation Programme

A number of Academic Foundation Programmes offer a 4-month research rotation as part of the 2-year Foundation Programme, with the intention of giving trainees more experience of research.

Specialist training

Academic clinical fellowships (ACFs)

These posts incorporate both clinical and research training (usually a ratio of 75% to 25%) and give trainees the opportunity to develop research ideas and skills to support an application for a research training fellowship or an application for a place on an educational programme (→ a higher degree).

PhD

The PhD is seen as the key foundation for an academic career. PhDs typically take around 3 years to complete during which students undertake rigorous scientific research which they then submit as a thesis. A number of specific fellowship schemes are available for doctors (e.g. MRC, Wellcome, and NIHR Clinical Research Fellowships).

MD

Similar to a PhD, MDs require the completion of a detailed research thesis. These are often more clinically orientated and may be completed in 2 years, sometimes alongside clinical training. PhDs are increasingly favoured over MDs for those wishing to pursue a research career.

Other opportunities: Masters degrees

A huge range of Master's programmes are available for doctor to enable further research experience. Many are orientated towards part-time or distance learning facilitating learning alongside formal training programmes. Some specialist training programmes themselves incorporate a Master's degree.

Other options include a 1-year MRes (Master of Research) which is a Master's degree that places more weighting on research as opposed to attending lectures. MPhil (Master of Philosophy) is considered as half of a PhD and usually lasts for 1 year.

Clinical lectureships

Similar to ACFs but at more senior training grades, and usually post PhD these programmes offer part clinical and part research training.

Post CCT

A range of fellowship opportunities are available to enable doctors to establish themselves as academic leaders. In general, research-active clinicians are predominantly employed by universities, while holding honorary contracts with NHS providers.

Clinical fellowships (CFs)

A range of stand-alone fellowships variably including research are often available. In some cases these may be linked with specific studies (e.g. in supporting a clinical trial)

Out of programme research (OOPR)

The term given to doctors who spend time in research, outside of their specialist training programme. This may be to complete a personal research fellowship, but it may be for independently arranged research experience to gain more experience prior to returning to clinical training or applying more formally for other schemes and awards, such as a PhD. (See Fig. 54.3.)

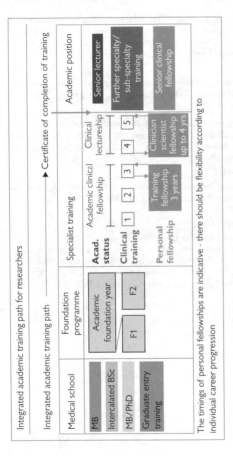

The timings of personal fellowships are indicative – there should be flexibility according to individual career progression

Fig. 54.3 Overview of academic posts in the UK. Reproduced with permission from NIHR, www.ukcrc.org.

Types of research

Just as careers in medicine can be very diverse, so can medical research. Different types of research may suit different types of individuals. Consequently, students should not be put off by a single bad experience (e.g. 'I didn't enjoy my BSc project in X's lab, so I won't enjoy a research job').

Laboratory research

For many, the image of medical research is a researcher wearing a white coat, sitting by a bench, pipette in hand. While laboratory research does make up a considerable proportion of medical research, it is only one of several areas. Within laboratory research diverse ranges of techniques may be used, making even this extremely variable. As technologies develop, laboratory scientists increasingly require a range of skills from bench work to advanced computing. Bear in mind that this type of research usually takes a much longer time until completion, compared to clinical projects. In return, your work is likely to be published in a journal with a higher impact factor than clinically orientated journals.

Clinical research

This involves research which interacts directly with patients and can range from drug trials and development of new devices, to qualitative assessments of patient experiences.

- *Epidemiological studies*: often look at the bigger picture studying the health of populations.
- *Translational research*: is a popular term at the moment and applies to the application or 'translation' of laboratory discoveries into clinic. As technologies facilitate ↑speeds of analysis, this process is becoming more two way, so-called 'bench to bedside and back again' medicine and research.
- *Other types of research*: include medical education research, health systems, and health technology research.

Funding medical research

(See ⟶ Chapter 5.) Medical research is expensive (a UK clinical trial costs ~£9000 to recruit one patient, so a trial powered to included 300 patients would cost ~£2.7 million). Research involves not just the direct costs of the experiments (e.g. reagents) but also salaries of researchers, institutional overheads, insurance, university fees, etc. As a medical student undertaking a BSc, many of these will be provided for by the supervisors' funding; however, when applying for fellowships (e.g. for PhD), it is important to find out what is and is not covered (e.g. fees).

Funding comes from one of three main areas:

Government

The government funds research through three main streams: the Medical Research Council, the National Institute for Health Research (NIHR, part of the NHS), and directly from the Department of Health.

Charities
The Wellcome Trust is the UK's largest non-governmental funding of scientific research. National (e.g. Cancer Research UK) and local (e.g. Great Ormond Street Charity) medical charities also provide a significant proportion of funding and have a range of schemes supporting medical students/ doctors in training to undertake research.

Industry
The majority of drug trials will be funded by pharmaceutical companies. In addition, various companies also sponsor research and career development through a range of schemes and opportunities for funding research among doctors and medical students (e.g. funding PhD research training fellowships).

Why do research

In addition for the medical need for research there are lots of other reasons for wanting to undertake or get involved with research and pursuing a research career. Some do it because of sincere passion, some do it to jump through hoops in an attempt to improve job prospects, and some do it out of sheer curiosity.

Eureka! Finding out new things

Discovering something new, particularly when it has the potential to improve lives, is a pleasurable experience on to which some researchers become hooked. There is a sense of achievement and an adrenaline rush when your hard work has been accepted for publication and embraced by your peers all over the world. Though ground-breaking advances may be rare, even smaller contributions in your field of expertise can carry with them a strong sense of satisfaction.

Personal development

Research requires a range of skills, some distinct (e.g. certain methodologies), but many which complement and overlap with those needed to be a good doctor. Like medicine, successful research requires good teamwork, time management, and leadership/management skills. Working in a research environment is often a great time to develop and refine these skills outside the traditional hierarchies of clinical practice.

Lifestyle

Researchers often have a degree of autonomy and flexibility in managing their workload which is distinct, and often envied by pure clinicians. Similarly, there are many opportunities to network and travel nationally and internationally. Undertaking medical research also enables links and interactions with a wide range of individuals and experts in a range of disciplines and areas, which in itself is often very rewarding.

Career progression

Undertaking research simply to 'fill a box' on an application form is not a good reason; however, research experience itself will often help in applications for both clinical and non-clinical jobs.

Challenges to undertaking research

Research is rarely straightforward and when pushing the boundaries of knowledge, a number of challenges and obstacles may arise and these may include:

Red tape

Large volumes of often necessary red tape may distract you from the research itself. This is often, but not always, important for safeguarding patients and public.

Ethics

You are expected to conduct your research ethically as per the guidelines published in *Good Practice in Research* by the GMC.[1] If using live subjects, whether animals or patients, you must seek permission to conduct the study at your centre from the local ethics committee. Each university, medical school, and hospital ought to have their own ethics committee who tend to meet up once a month to discuss research methodologies. The time to approval may take weeks to months and you will be likely to alter your methodology several times during the process. Filling out the application form can sometimes take hours and days but it is essential to be transparent, ethical, and uphold patient safety/animal rights at all times.

Methodology issues

Clinicians tend to get used to a fast turnaround of tests (e.g. FBC) but many research techniques, particularly if novel, are often less well refined, take longer, and require extensive optimization before results are generated. Unless the methodology for your research project has been validated in a prior study, you are more likely to have to develop a new methodology altogether since your research is novel. There is no guarantee that your methodology will be flawless and problems may only be noticed down the line, which consumes much time, money, manpower, and resources.

Competition and politics

Research is a competitive environment and the difference between being 'first' and just behind in making a discovery can be profound. Much like countries at war, the same mentality is sometimes observed between research departments and universities. While many researchers are becoming more open to the idea of collaboration to overcome resource limitations, many are still sceptical and would rather not share the credit with a competing institution.

Challenges of research careers

For those considering developing a research career there are a number of additional challenges to be faced. Researchers need to maintain their funding and may have less secure positions. Salaries vary and there are full-time research positions available but most medical researchers are also practising clinicians. It is after all the clinicians who are able to identify a problem within healthcare or patient management that drives the need for solutions through research.

Lack of funding

There is only so much information a research project can yield before more resources, staffing, and costly technology become necessary to advance the study. There have been many cases where research studies will suddenly halt due to a lack of funding. The options are to then either apply for further funding and delay the end date of the study or publish whatever data you have managed to collect so far.

Subjects

If your research involves animal models or patient participation, then this may become a rate-limiting step to obtaining results. You are required to obtain informed consent (both verbal and written) from patients who have the right to drop out of the study at any time. Animal models may not be able to consent but you are required to undergo formal training into their appropriate treatment and some models are genetically modified that may → issues such as costs and availability.

Level of evidence

There are five levels of evidence with one being the highest level.[2] Research departments are under tremendous pressure to churn out high-quality studies with a high level of evidence in order to build a reputation, research profile, and obtain more funding to propel further and larger studies. You may be asked to fill in a research grant proposal[3] to obtain funding.

Bias

This is a term for a systematic error which deviates from a true finding. For instance, the researcher may influence the results to favour a finding, albeit incorrect. There may also be bias with respect to choosing your study cohort (rather than achieving true randomization), incorrect data collection and interpretation, patients forgetting personal details when interviewed, etc. Bias ought to be unexpected and put down to the 'human factor' as opposed to being intentional. It should also be accounted for in publications.

References

1. General Medical Council. *Good Practice in Research*: ℘ www.gmc-uk.org/guidance/ethical_guidance/5992.asp.
2. Oxford Centre for Evidence-based Medicine. *Levels of Evidence* (March 2009): ℘ www.cebm.net/oxford-centre-evidence-based-medicine-levels-evidence-march-2009.
3. The Writing Center, University of North Carolina at Chapel Hill. *Grant Proposals*: ℘ writingcenter.unc.edu/handouts/grant-proposals-or-give-me-the-money.

Generic research skills

There are now numerous documents, including the 'Gold Guide', outlining generic research competencies for different posts. Generally these include the following:

General research skills

Critical appraisal

Before looking for something 'new', understand what is already known. This includes a detailed search of the existing literature and a critical review of what is published.

Developing research questions

The key to the majority of research is testing a hypothesis.

Data interpretation and statistics

Often key to interpreting and designing studies is a good understanding of medical statistics.

Developing research proposals and grant applications

Sustaining funding is crucial for any research to progress.

Research ethics and governance skills

Ethics and law

Such as applying for ethical approval, ensuring the relevant laws and regulations (e.g. Animal [Scientific Procedures] Act, Human Tissue Act or Data Protection Act) are adhered to.

Understanding research integrity and intellectual property

'*Knowledge is power*', attributed to Francis Bacon, highlights the importance of understanding the consequence of research discoveries.

Research communication skills

Writing and publishing

If you do not publish it, from the perspective of the rest of the world, it has not been done. There is an inherent obligation to publish the results of studies and this in itself requires a specialist set of skills. You are expected to communicate a principal message as succinctly and effectively. As the old idiom goes: '*publish or perish*'.

Presentation and teaching skills

Researchers are expected to be good at presenting their work in presentations and sharing their knowledge through teaching and conferences. It is an art to be able to convey your principal message within minutes to an audience with varying skills and experiences.

Networking skills

Many discoveries are the result of collaborations and, as with most careers, networking skills are often key to this.

Ethics and research governance

Research involving human subjects carries with it potential for harm. Unfortunately, there are many examples in history where medical research has caused more harm than good. Consequently, a number of guidelines, regulatory procedures, and laws have been developed to assess and appropriately manage such risks, two of which are:

The Declaration of Helsinki

A set of ethical principles for human research, first published by the World Medical Association in 1964 and last updated in 2013. This was developed from the Nuremberg Code (1946), the first set of internationally agreed guidelines of research involving people that was produced following the unethical experiments carried out by Nazi doctors.

Good Clinical Practice

Good Clinical Practice (GCP; ℘ www.gov.uk/guidance/good-clinical-practice-for-clinical-trials) is a set of internationally recognized ethical and scientific quality requirements that must be followed when designing, conducting, recording and reporting clinical trials that involve people.

Other laws relevant to research

These include the Data Protection Act and the Human Tissue Act, which regulates the use of human tissues in research and the Animal (Scientific Procedures) Act, which regulates scientific experimentation using animals. Some core principles outlined by the GMC can be seen in Box 54.1.

Ethical review

A key component to ensuring research fulfils these principles is for it to be assessed by an independent ethical review committee. NHS research is reviewed by the NHS Health Research Authority and can be accessed through a centralized Integrated Research Application System (IRAS; ℘ www.myresearchproject.org.uk/).

Research governance

This refers to the structures which ensure that research is carried out to the ethical and other standards required, for instance, abiding by the Human Tissue Act.

Box 54.1 Core principles of most guidelines (GMC guidelines)

- Scientific validity of research.
- Protecting participants from harm.
- Consent.
- Confidentiality.
- Honest, integrity, abiding by law.

Tips for getting involved in research

When wanting to get involved in research there are a number of questions to ask yourself:

Why do you want to do research?

Is it to find out more, is it 'for the CV', is it because of a specific patient?

What do you want to get out of the research?

Do you want a taster, a publication, and/or to learn a method?

How much time do you have?

Are you looking for a full project for a degree, are you looking for a summer vacation project, or something to do in the evenings/weekends? Other opportunities include committing some of your time during your elective and special study module (SSM) towards research.

Does the research match your other interests?

If you want to be a cardiologist, doing a project in neuroscience might not be the most appropriate for your long-term career aims.

What methodologies are you interested in and think you will enjoy?

If you get motion sick looking down a microscope or the thought of animal experiments turns your stomach then pick something else!

Consider location and what is available

Different centres and universities have different expertise and different patient cohorts and so it is important to consider what is available where, and how that affects your choice. For instance, if you are interested in X disease of the left testis then you might need to move to a centre specializing in that condition.

Look around and be open to opportunities and consider them when they arrive

Sometimes the best opportunities are not the ones you 'plan' for. If you hear of an opportunity, explore it, and then decide whether you think it is appropriate for you. Just because it is not your 'ideal' project, it does not mean it might not be excellent. These often turn out to be the best! Departments are always looking for keen students to train and help out with projects, whether that is recruiting participants or collecting data, you may initially find it difficult to make contact. The best solution is to send the departmental secretary an email with your intentions, interests, and CV. Other platforms include UROP (Undergraduate Research Opportunities Programme) whereby departments advertise research opportunities and are actively seeking students to help out.

Choose a good supervisor

(See ➋ Chapter 5.) In order to undertake research you will need someone with experience to guide and support you such as a supervisor. This should be someone who has expertise in your area of interest and who can also invest their time (or their team's time) in supporting you.

Talk to lots of potential supervisors

The more people you talk to, the more options you have and the more you will get a sense of which project might work well with you. Just because they are considered a deity in their area does not mean that they will be the best choice for a supervisor. If they do not reply to you/find time to meet with you, they probably will not be able to invest in you as an individual, so do not feel discouraged and find someone else. There will always be someone to support you—your job is to find them.

Not all projects work out

Do not get disheartened if one fails or does not yield positive or expected results—another project might be different. It is sometimes worth having more than one strand to a project.

Keep up with technology

Much research is dictated by the available technology (e.g. next-generation sequencing), so it is important to keep up with advances. Increasingly, good computer skills are vital for good research and its presentation.

Get some mentors

A mentor differs from a supervisor in that they are separate and independent from your day-to-day working

'But I haven't got any publications'

At a junior level, applicants are assessed on their potential, so it is not essential to have publications, though it may help. Publications often take time to come through. Discuss with your supervisors how best to optimize your chance of publications. Yet, you must be prepared to hear that the study may not be ready for publication, may need more work before being published, and may not feature your contribution in the final publication.

Believe in yourself!

Some people think they are not 'clever enough' to do research if they have not done any previous research at medical school. This is a fallacy. The most important thing is a good idea, good support, commitment, and enthusiasm. Everyone loves a good leader so you have the power to persuade others to share your vision. Much like any job, this is where you sell your skills, abilities, and ideas. If you can put this together, then anyone has a good chance of being successful.

Writing up research

A popular adage goes that the only bad research is unpublished research. While research offers medical students a number of transferrable skills that do not need a publication to validate them, you could be left with nothing concrete to show for hours of effort.

Another school of thought is that bad, incomplete, or unnecessary research is harmful or distracting to the field. In general, you should aim to finish each piece of research that you undertake with some form of report; this need not be a submission to a journal—in many cases the limited scope of your work would be better suited to an abstract, poster, or oral presentation.

Publications in job applications

Note the following guidance for publications to be awarded points in the Foundation Year application process:

- A maximum of 2 points are awarded for publications (compared to 5 for undergraduate/postgraduate degrees or 43 for medical school performance).
- You need to be a named author but not necessarily the first author.
- Publications under review or still in progress will not be considered.
- Publications must have a PubMed ID (PMID), and the link you include with the PMID must lead directly to evidence of your article with one click. This is relevant for example where your work is published as an abstract at a conference, and where one click will not lead directly to your own work. In this case, the publication will not be scored.

Where should you aim to submit your work?

Your supervisor will advise on this. A good outcome would be if your work formed a part of a larger study already underway in the group, in which case your contribution may be acknowledged with 'middle authorship'. Unless you have spent a significant period in research (i.e. a summer studentship or intercalated BSc), first authorship may not be realistic. Short, stand-alone projects may be more appropriately submitted to conference proceedings as poster or oral presentations. There may also be local opportunities to present your work (e.g. medical student fora or regional meetings). There is no harm in aiming high with the choice of journal. The comments of editors and reviewers can be extremely valuable in improving your submission for next time (though a thick skin is required!)

Who are you writing for?

In science writing, one should assume that the audience will be scientists but not specialists in the field.

How should the report be structured?

Most journals have very strict guidelines on word count, formatting, and sections to be included. This information is available via the relevant homepage under 'Author instructions'. In general, a scientific paper should comprise the following sections:
1. Title and author information.
2. Abstract (usually 250–300-word summary).
3. Introduction.
4. Methods.
5. Results.
6. Discussion (including limitations and future work).
7. Conclusion.
8. References.
9. Figures, tables, and legends (these are usually uploaded separately or featured at the end of your submission).
10. Acknowledgements.

Title and author information

Often the source of much discussion, but your supervisor will decide upon the order of authors. Their academic affiliations should be attributed correctly, and a designated 'corresponding author' should be identified and contact details included. Elsewhere in the manuscript, one should include any conflicts of interest (e.g. funding which could be viewed to introduce bias) and each author's specific contribution.

Abstract

(See ➲ pp. 96–7.) This is the section that will be most widely read (and many editors will make a decision based on this) and available to everyone via PubMed. Hence it is important to make it punchy! In about 250 words, you should aim to introduce the field, and describe the context and importance of your work. You should then outline your research question and mention the methods used before summarizing your findings, your interpretation of them, and why they are important. The principal finding of your study will need to be peer reviewed by experts in the field and deemed worthy to compared to the existing medical literature.

Introduction

This is often the hardest section to get right, and counterintuitively best left until last when you have a clear aim of the purpose and context of your work. A good introduction should introduce the non-specialist reader to your field, briefly summarizing the existing and relevant literature. You should then outline the gaps in existing knowledge, or current difficulties pursuing these investigations, and how you plan to address them.

Methods

Often placed towards the end of the manuscript, and more for reference than for reading from beginning to end. The aim here is to provide sufficient information that someone else could replicate your work and see similar results.

If, for example, your work involves a literature search, you should outline the search engine, the search terms, exclusion criteria, the date accessed, etc. Basic science work should include explicit information about reagents (e.g. manufacturer) and protocols. The statistical tests (e.g. paired student t-test) and software (e.g. SPSS, Microsoft Excel) used should be described. This is also the section where ethical approvals should be detailed.

Results

Many readers will skip straight from the abstract to the results and figures. This should be broken down into manageable sections, each with a sub-title outlining the major content (e.g. 'The lungs contain a diverse immune cell repertoire' or 'Demographics of study participants'). You should state the results in a factual way without too much interpretation/discussion at this stage.

Discussion

This is the section where you are free to interpret your data and the in-sights they offer. You should outline the strengths of your methodology to support your findings, and similarly acknowledge any potential flaws or weaknesses. Finally, having introduced the field and the current position of research in the introduction, you should finish here by describing how things have changed in light of this piece of work and what further studies are required.

Conclusion

This consists of one paragraph with three to four sentences stating the purpose of your study and the principal findings. Many people who access your publication will be most interested in reading your conclusion at first glance before deciding to read the entire manuscript. You do not have to be too specific with conveying your findings within this section but you must offer the general gist succinctly.

References

This section is more important than a simple bibliography may seem. Many readers will be directed to other papers from your introduction. Referencing a paper in your manuscript constitutes a 'citation' and scientists monitor how many times their work is cited. In fact, it is in this way that scientific journals earn their impact factor; e.g. *Nature* has an impact factor of about 40, meaning that the articles published in it were cited on average 40 times in the last year.

There are different formats of citing references, which the journal in question will dictate. Software for storing, organizing, and formatting references will save you a lot of time and effort at this stage. Make sure you read the submission guidelines carefully since every journal has their unique formatting style for references.

The common options include Harvard (mentioning the author and year of publication within the main text) or Vancouver (chronologically numbering all references when first used in the main text). EndNote™, for instance, is a simple and popular program (⌕ www.endnote.com).

Figures and legends

Figures usually form the scientific nub of the paper (i.e. the concrete evidence of the work you have done and the raw data). Some thought should be given to making your figures look attractive, uncluttered, and easy to interpret. Consistency of formatting and appearance is also important. You will spend many painful hours moving boxes around a page before you achieve adequate figures! Some journals have preferred types of figures (e.g. dot plots rather than bar graphs which may 'hide' data). Figure legends should give an explicit description of the data shown in each figure, describing the symbols/formatting uses.

Acknowledgements

This is where the authors thank and describe contributions from other people who are not listed as authors. For example, John Brown gave valuable feedback on the manuscript, Sarah Smith gave reagents X and Y, and so on.

How do I submit my paper?

Virtually all manuscript submission now occurs electronically. Details and uploading facilities are available on the journal's homepage.

What happens if my paper is rejected?

Unfortunately, this is the most likely outcome for most submissions and you should be prepared for this. There is no room in journal editing for sentimentality or recognition of the huge amount of work involved in preparing a manuscript. Where possible, you should seek feedback from the editor or reviewers. A common response is that your work would be better suited to a more specialist (i.e. lower-impact factor) journal. Individual reviewers, usually experts in the field from all parts of the world, may offer more specific feedback, e.g. highlighting weaknesses in methodology or discrepancies in data interpretation. Although bruising, this objective and anonymous feedback is often extremely helpful and leads you to improve your manuscript before sending it elsewhere.

Persevere!

Most manuscripts are not accepted by the first journal to which they are submitted, and even then only after various revisions have been made. Prepare yourself for a lengthy and sometimes frustrating process, but do keep on trying! Once your work is accepted for publication, there is no other sense of satisfaction and pride like it.

Medical student prizes

Why should you bother?

Applications for junior doctor posts increasingly rely on standardized forms instead of face-to-face interviewing. Any outstanding achievements that you can add to your CV will help set you apart from other candidates. The current job application form does not award points for medical school prizes (although academic trainees may list them in the 'Academic Achievements' section). However, your referees will have access to this information and may use this in their appraisal of you. Also, subsequent job applications are likely to recognize medical school prizes.

What prizes are available?

This will vary considerably according to your medical school and you should consult your local intranet for details. However, a number of prizes (particularly those offered by individual specialty societies) are awarded on a national basis.

Examination performance

A number of prizes are awarded to students based on their performance in formal examinations, both at undergraduate and clinical school level. You do not apply as such, and the news will usually come as a pleasant surprise to you. Prizes such as these showcase your achievements compared to your entire academic year and as a result are rightly regarded as prestigious.

Poster or oral presentations

Many local and (inter)national meetings at which students and trainees present posters or oral presentations offer prizes for the best work. Such awards recognize the quality of the work presented, the manner in which it is presented, and the initiative required to undertake the project in the first place. Presenting your work in written or oral form should be the ultimate aim of any extracurricular projects you take on in medical school.

NB: the current Foundation Year application scheme no longer allocates points for presentations, no matter how prestigious (🖰 www.foundationprogramme. nhs.uk/pages/home/how-to-apply)

Electives

Many medical schools offer prizes for the best elective reports, including the chance to present your work at hospital-wide meetings. A number of funding opportunities exist from specialist groups (e.g. the Renal Association or the Association of Anaesthetists), for students seeking to undertake their elective in these fields. Awards such as these are competitive and as a result are also considered as prizes.

Specialist prizes

A number of opportunities are available both locally and nationally to recognize excellence in a particular area. For example, your medical school may have an endowment to fund an annual essay competition in the field of Psychiatry or Paediatric Surgery. Prizes such as these require initiative and time to enter but may be less competitive than other, more widely publicized awards. Similar opportunities exist at a national level (℅ www.money4medstudents.org/competitions-and-awards).[1]

Summer studentships

A number of bursaries are offered for summer studentships, usually to undertake a period of basic or clinical research within the UK. Like elective bursaries, these awards are competitive and are considered as a medical student prize. Useful sources of information:

- Wellcome Trust: ℅ www.wellcome.ac.uk/Funding/Biomedical-science/Funding-schemes/PhD-funding-and-undergraduate-opportunities/WTD004448.htm.
- Biochemical Society: ℅ www.biochemistry.org/Grants/SummerVacationStudentships.aspx.
- University College London: ℅ www.ucl.ac.uk/ich/education/vacation_studentships.
- Undergraduate Research Opportunities Programme (UROP): may be available at your university.

Outside of medicine

Medical students may receive awards to recognize their achievements and contributions to fields outside of medicine, e.g. sports, music, or voluntary work. While still very commendable, they are unlikely to carry as much weight as prizes awarded for excellence in medicine. However, referees may use this information in their account of you.

Reference

1. Maruthappu M, Sugand K (2013). *Medical School: An Applicant's Guide.* Cardiff: Doctor's Academy.

How to critically analyse a research paper

Critiquing papers is an essential skill as a scientist, researcher, and clinician since you can only be expected to provide optimal, judicious, and evidence-based care to your patients if you have reviewed the justification yourself. As part of your intercalated BSc written exams, you may be expected to conduct a critical appraisal of a well-known journal publication. To critique a paper is challenging since you ought to challenge everything, from the key messages addressed in the abstracts, the methodology, data collection and analysis, limitations, and inferences. This is what ultimately distinguishes between high- and low-quality research. A handy checklist for systematically reviewing any piece of research is listed in Table 54.2

Table 54.2 Checklist

Title	
Is the title appropriate and clear?	☐
Is the article published in a reputable/high-impact factor journal?	☐
Are the authors well regarded in the field of study?	☐
Abstract	
Does the abstract provide a concise overview of the research?	☐
Does the abstract highlight the research question, as well as the method used to address it?	☐
Are the main findings provided as well as recommendations or conclusions?	☐
Introduction	
Is the literature review relevant, balanced, and up to date?	☐
Does the literature review/authors highlight a need for this current piece of research?	☐
Is a focused and relevant study question/aim expressed?	☐
Methods	
What type of study design was chosen? Is it the *most suitable* to answer the research question?	☐
Are there limitations/problems/bias with this study approach?	☐
Is the study sufficiently powered? Are the study subjects generalizable?	☐
Have ethical concerns been appropriately raised and addressed?	☐
Have the study methods been justified, and described in enough detail to allow replication?	☐
If the method is based on standard protocols, have adequate references been given?	☐

Table 54.2 (Contd.)

Have the statistical methods been specified, with a rational for the choice? Are they *appropriate*?	☐
Results	
Do the results make sense with regard to the study method used?	☐
Were the statistical analyses performed correctly?	☐
Have tables and figures been labelled clearly and appropriately (including legends)?	☐
Are they easy to interpret? Do they represent the data collected?	☐
Have any gaps in data gathering/processing been accounted for?	☐
Discussion/analysis	
Have the results obtained been interpreted *objectively* and *appropriately*?	☐
Are the results discussed in light of points raised in the literature review?	☐
Do the authors needlessly speculate or consistently refer to unpublished data?	☐
Were the results obtained statistically significant? Are they clinically/biologically so?	☐
Are study strengths as well as limitations discussed?	☐
Were the study objectives met (i.e. did they answer their research question)? If not, why?	☐
Have new insights or recommendations for practice been made based on this research?	☐
Have the authors highlighted suggestions for future research?	☐
Conclusion	
Has the key message(s) been summarized and succinctly relayed?	☐
Has there been an objective assessment of the study?	☐
References	
Are the papers cited appropriately?	☐
Do the authors cite their own publications needlessly?	☐
Have any conflicts of interest or financial disclosures been reported?	☐

Further reading

Centre for Evidence Based Medicine, University of Oxford. Critical appraisal tools: ℘ www.cebm.net/critical-appraisal/

University College London. Critical appraisal of a journal article: ℘ www.ucl.ac.uk/ich/support-services/library/training-material/critical-appraisal

University of Cambridge. Critical appraisal resources: ℘ https://library.medschl.cam.ac.uk/research-support/critical-appraisal-resources/

Special study modules

Since 2003, it has been a GMC requirement that medical schools allocate one-quarter to one-third of course time to SSMs (also known as student selected components (SSCs)). There will normally be two or three SSM periods each academic year, lasting 4–8 weeks each. You will be able to choose from a list of standalone projects covering many different specialities and disciplines (noting that you may not get your first or indeed second choice). Usually a consultant or lecturer will oversee each SSM.

Why do SSMs?

- *Transferrable skills*: SSMs encourage self-directed learning, independent thinking, and critical evaluation of data.
- *Specialist skills*: you may learn how to undertake a formal literature review, a database search, or master a laboratory technique.
- *CV points*: if you choose wisely and your project goes well, your work may culminate in a poster presentation or even in a journal publication.
- *Beyond the curriculum*: the clinical school schedule cannot cover every speciality in depth in 3 years. SSMs are a great opportunity to explore a specialist interest that is not covered elsewhere in the curriculum.

Which SSM to choose?

If you have a burning desire to specialize in plastic surgery or public health, the choice of a relevant project may be easy. For the majority of you, how-ever, bear in mind the following:

- *Supervision*: look for a project that offers adequate but not excessive supervision. Laboratory projects, for example, will rely on someone to help you learn new techniques whereas literature reviews or audits will require you to be more independent.
- *Output*: what will you get out of this? A small but defined project offering a realistic goal such as a poster presentation or authorship on a paper or protocol may be more valuable to you than a more expansive or nebulous project.
- *Developing career interests*: if you don't have a specialty in mind, SSMs are an opportunity to explore an area not fully covered elsewhere in the curriculum.
- *Time frame*: will you realistically achieve your goals in the given time? This should not interfere with your core studies.
- *Skills*: if you are IT literate, setting up a database of liver transplant patients may be just the SSM for you.
- *Enjoy it*: SSMs should give you freedom, both intellectually and from the rigid timetabling of clinical school. Although it sounds obvious, try to choose a project that will not feel like a slog.

Electives

Electives: overview

A medical elective usually takes place during the latter years at medical school prior to graduating. It is an opportunity to try something different and pursue an area of study in which you are particularly interested. Many students also use the elective as an opportunity to travel abroad. The duration of the elective varies between medical schools but you will typically have between 6 and 8 weeks. It is possible to achieve many things in this time but the best electives are those that are planned carefully and well in advance.

Sources of information

Think broadly about the sources of information that are available to help guide your decision-making.

Medical school

Your medical school may be able to provide you with examples of previous students' elective choices, sometimes including other students' project reports.

Other students

Speak to students from previous years; they may have contact details or suggestions of places where they did their electives.

Hospital staff

Talk to hospital staff including consultants and other senior doctors. They may have supervised students on previous electives or have contacts in their field of expertise around the world.

Online

The Internet is a vast resource that may help you to find the contact details of specific institutions or directories of organizations. Remember, however, that smaller, more remote institutions in the developing world may not have websites—to find these, you may need to rely upon word of mouth.

Types of elective

Most medical schools will permit a wide range of different types of elective. The emphasis is on what you can learn and gain from the time rather than where it is spent. Possible types of elective include:

Hospital placement

Many students choose to undertake their elective based in a hospital. This may range from a large teaching hospital in the US to a small rural hospital in Africa.

Community project

Particularly for those students considering a career in general practice, you may decide that you would like to spend your elective working in a community-based setting. For example, you may choose to be based at a homeless shelter in inner city London, with a community HIV/AIDS programme in Africa, or with a maternal health project in Bangladesh.

Non-governmental and missionary organizations
A number of non-governmental and missionary organizations take students for elective placements.

Specific medical student organizations
Some organizations such as the International Federation of Medical Students' Associations (IFMSA) exist specifically for medical students and offer a range of elective projects and exchange programmes.

Expedition medicine
Perhaps you have a passion for climbing, skiing, or diving? You could undertake an elective in expedition medicine, mountain medicine, dive medicine, aviation and space medicine, or with the 'flying doctors'.

> **Top tip**
> Refer to the *Oxford Handbook of Expedition and Wilderness Medicine*, by Johnson et al. (2nd ed, 2015, Oxford University Press) for more information on this vast field and which opportunities to look out for.

Clinical placement
Many students choose to undertake a clinical placement as part of their elective. Think imaginatively about which clinical area you would like to be based in. It is also important to do your research carefully. If you have a specific area in mind, make sure you find an institution where this specialty is available.

Research project
Some students choose to carry out an audit or research project during their elective period, often alongside a clinical placement. This can range from a qualitative study to a laboratory-based project, a quantitative study, or an audit of existing guidelines. If you are going to be carrying out a research project, it is particularly important to plan ahead. You will need to put together a research proposal and are likely to need to apply for ethical approval (see ⤳ Chapter 54 for more advice).

Funding
Many organizations provide funding for medical students and it may be possible to pay for the whole enterprise this way. As well as saving money, elective bursaries often take the form of awards and prizes which can be helpful for your CV later on.

Electives: setting objectives and funding

Where to start

Before you make any decisions, take a few moments to think through what you want to get out of your elective. With careful planning, it is often possible to achieve multiple things in the same elective period.

Taking a break

Being a medical student can be exhausting and many see their elective as a 'break' from studying. Some electives are more tightly organized than others but it is certainly possible to build in sun, sea, and sand if you wish.

Travel experience

It can be difficult to travel for long periods of time during medical school whether because of finance or course commitments. This can be your opportunity to see the world.

Career development

Although it is difficult to gain much from research over such a short period, simpler projects could be completed during the elective period. It is also an opportunity to network with doctors from other specialties and institutions.

Try a new specialty

No medical school claims to rotate all students through every medical and surgical specialty. This can be a problem if you have a passing interest in ophthalmology or plastic surgery but have never had any formal experience. The elective can be your opportunity to explore potential career options.

Demonstrating commitment to specialty

If you have an idea which specialty you would like to pursue, the elective is a further opportunity to develop your 'commitment'. If you are less certain, but want to think strategically, find an elective that is applicable to multiple potential specialties. For example, an elective working in a clinic for pregnant women with HIV could be considered as commitment to genitourinary medicine, obstetrics and gynaecology, infectious diseases, or public health.

Questions to ask yourself

Do you have a particular location in mind?

Perhaps there is a country you have always wanted to work in? Would you rather stay in the UK or go abroad? Do you want to go to a developed or developing country? Do you want to be in an urban or rural area?

Do you have a particular area of interest?

For example, you might have particularly enjoyed your paediatrics placement, you might want to learn more about malaria, or you might want to explore life as a cardiac surgeon.

What is your budget?

While there are sources of financial support available, some options are inevitably more expensive than others.

Do you want to travel alone or with friends?
While some students will want to travel independently, it may be more important for you to travel with others. Electives can be isolating if you are by yourself but you will be less independent travelling as part of a group.

Do you have foreign language skills?
It is clearly preferable for you to be able to communicate with patients and staff in your chosen location. Speaking the local language is not always a prerequisite but you should think carefully about this communication challenge. 'Crash courses' in medical Spanish are popular for students intent on travelling to South America.

What time of year will you be travelling?
Consider the climate of the country you are considering at a given time of year.

Sources of funding

There is a wealth of opportunities available to students requiring funding for their medical elective. Planning early is important here so apply in plenty of time to give yourself the highest possible chance of securing a bursary or grant. If you are fortunate to secure a grant, make sure you send a letter of thanks and a copy of your elective report.

Local
There may be sources of funding open only to students from your medical school. There may also be funding available in your local area through charitable trusts or local companies.

National
These grants are open to all students across the UK and are likely to be competitive, so it is particularly important to plan your application carefully. Do not be put off by perceived competitiveness, though, as they are often underwhelmed by the number of high-quality applications. Make a decision that balances the effort required, potential reward, and likelihood of success. There are useful websites for this including ℘ www.trustfunding. org.uk.

Specific
Some sources of funding are available specifically for certain fields (e.g. paediatrics, obstetrics), and there are specific grants available for women in medicine and for mature students. Look at the royal colleges and specialty associations as most will offer elective awards.

Applying for funding

Make your application stand out
Being enthusiastic and original in your application will help to make your form stand out. This is not something to complete a day before the application deadline—prepare well in advance and ask others to read it critically first.

Ensure that your application is clear

State your aims and objectives and rationale for doing the project and include a copy of your research proposal. If possible, explain the impact of your project either on your career or the wider community. Funding bodies want to feel that they are supporting projects that will have the greatest possible impact.

Justify all the costs you state

Include a breakdown of costs including flights and accommodation. Ask for what you need but economize as far as possible. Funding bodies want maximum reward for their money—projects that are good and economical are most likely to be funded.

Confirm your arrangements

Ensure that the arrangements with your host institution are confirmed, and attach a copy of your application form or approval letter. The more organized your project appears to be the harder it is for it to be turned down by funders.

Choose a referee

You may be asked to provide a referee for your application, so ask someone who knows you well. Exuberant personalities write enthusiastic references!

Prepare your CV

Applications may require you to include a CV so make sure you have prepared this ahead of time.

Travel arrangements

The key message regardless of where you are planning to go on your elective is to start making travel arrangements well in advance. The Foreign Office website has advice about areas of the world that are unsafe and not recommended for travel.

Passport and visa

Remember that your passport must be in date for at least 6 months from the date you return from your travels. Check whether the country you are visiting requires a visa. You may need to organize this in advance and make arrangements to travel to the relevant embassy in the UK. Alternatively, you may be able to arrange a visa online.

Insurance

This should cover health, possessions and flight cancellations. Specific policies are available for medical students travelling on electives. Some insurance companies will provide cancellation cover in case you fail an exam and are unable to go on your elective. Others will cover the need for repatriation following illness abroad or sustaining a needle-stick injury. If your elective is in a country within the European Union, you should complete the Department of Health European Health Insurance Form, EHIC. This form is available online and will provide you with free emergency healthcare should this be required. It is still important to arrange travel insurance to cover ill health and any treatments that become necessary.

Medical indemnity

This is an important part of the organization for your elective. Contact your defence union to find out whether they will cover you during your elective. If not, they will be able to advise you about which organizations are likely to provide cover. This issue is particularly important for students travelling to the US and Canada; check with your institution whether indemnity cover is provided through them. It is important to remember that the same professional codes of conduct apply to you on your elective as they do as a medical student in the UK. Do not perform procedures or provide care to patients that you would not be confident or competent to perform in the UK.

Health checks

Some countries require you to undergo a medical assessment (sometimes including a CXR) before you travel. You will need to arrange for this to be done privately well in advance of travel. A travel clinic should be able to arrange this for you as well as any vaccinations that are required for your elective destination.

Flights

Remember that some airlines and travel operators offer student discounts on flights. It is advisable to book as early as you can, particularly if you intend to travel during the peak season.

Looking after your health abroad

Before you go

Book yourself in to a travel clinic or with your local student health service at least 3 months in advance—you may require a number of vaccinations over a period of weeks. They will be able to advise you about the specific risks and conditions found in the areas you will be travelling to. The National Travel Health Network and Centre (NaTHNaC) website provides detailed information and advice (℘ www.nathnac.net).

Vaccinations you may require in addition to the UK national schedule include:

Hepatitis B

You should already have been vaccinated against hepatitis B before starting at medical school, but the current Department of Health guidance suggests that a single booster should be given 5 years after the primary vaccination course.

Yellow fever

Particular areas of endemicity include South and Central America and Africa.

Typhoid and paratyphoid

These infections are most prevalent in low-income areas of the world with poor sanitation and lack of access to clean water. Typhoid is particularly common in Asia, as well as parts of South America and Africa. Rare outbreaks have been reported in Europe.

BCG

No longer part of the national schedule so if you have not received a BCG vaccination against TB you should consider this if travelling to an area of ↑risk (Asia, Africa, Central and South America).

Meningitis

Meningitis C vaccination is currently part of the UK National Vaccination Schedule. However, travellers visiting at-risk areas for meningococcal disease are advised to receive the quadrivalent ACW125Y vaccine.

Hepatitis A

Students at greatest risk of hepatitis A infection will be those visiting areas with poor sanitation. Vaccine and immunoglobulin are available.

Japanese B encephalitis

This is endemic in parts of Asia and the South Pacific so consider vaccination if travelling to these areas.

Rabies

You should consider rabies vaccination if you are travelling to an area in which rabies is present and you will not be able to access immediate post-exposure treatment (particularly in rural, undeveloped areas).

HIV

If you are travelling to a country with high rates of HIV infection and you will be working in a clinical capacity, it may be advisable to take HIV PEP with you. You can buy a 3- or 7-day pack that could be used in case of an emergency while you seek medical help at a specialist unit. The antiretroviral drugs used will vary. The key is to use appropriate precautions, particularly in areas of high HIV endemicity. When performing procedures or observing in theatre, always wear gloves, goggles, mask, and gown. If you are at risk, start taking your prescribed HIV PEP medications, and get yourself to a hospital with an HIV centre as soon as possible. The Department of Health has a useful website with information about HIV postexposure prophylaxis.

Malaria

The first step in preventing malaria is avoiding bites. Wear trousers and long sleeves after dark, and use an insect repellent containing DEET. Take an insecticide-treated bed net with you (you may not be provided with one in your accommodation, and those provided often have holes in them!). Ensure that you tuck your bed net in all around underneath the mattress. If required for the area you are travelling to, ensure you arrange to take a supply of antimalarial prophylaxis with you. A range of options are available depending on where you are travelling to (and therefore local resistance patterns).

Pre-existing medical conditions

If you have any pre-existing medical conditions, make sure you make an appointment with your GP to ensure that you have all the necessary advice and medications you need before you travel. Check whether there are any restrictions on whether you can take any of the medications you require out of the UK. If you have diabetes and require insulin, remember to get a letter from your GP explaining the reason for taking needles and syringes abroad.

While you are away

Traveller's diarrhoea

This is a common problem faced by travellers but there are a few tips to help reduce the risk. Remember to drink only boiled or bottled water, avoid ice in drinks, avoid salad and fruit (unless you peel it yourself), and ensure that food you eat is cooked.

Road safety

The biggest threat to your safety abroad is trauma resulting from a road traffic accident. You would always wear a bike helmet and seatbelt at home, so do not forget to do so when on your elective.

Useful sources of information

There are a vast number of useful resources available to help you plan your elective.

Websites

- The BMA medical electives website has useful information regarding planning your elective: ℜ https://www.bma.org.uk/advice/career/going-abroad/medical-electives.
- The Medics Travel website provides a range of information and resources for planning your elective: ℜ www.medicstravel.com.
- The International Federation of Medical Students' Associations (IFMSA) organizes an electives programme with a range of projects and exchanges: ℜ www.ifmsa.org.
- The WHO Medical School Directory provides a comprehensive list of medical schools you can apply to: ℜ www.who.int/hrh/wdms/en/.
- If you are looking to work with a non-governmental organization, check out the World Association of Non-Governmental Organizations (WANGO) directory: ℜ www.wango.org.
- The Department of Health's 'Fit for travel' website offers a range of advice on travelling abroad: ℜ www.fitfortravel.nhs.uk/home.aspx.
- The Foreign Office offers an 'A to Z' by country with detailed travel advice for each destination: ℜ www.gov.uk/foreign-travel-advice.
- The National Travel Health Network and Centre (NaTHNaC) website provides detailed, up-to-date information on recent clinical updates and the vaccinations required for travel to each country in the world: ℜ https://travelhealthpro.org.uk/.

Books

Mark Wilson, *The Medic's Guide to Work and Electives Around the World* (3rd ed, 2009, CRC Press), contains an extensive directory of contact details for institutions around the world, and is available at most medical school libraries.

Career planning

Foundation Programme applications

The application is fairly simple but requires you to make decisions that will shape the start of your career. Hence, it is worth giving it some thought and setting time aside to ensure it is completed correctly. There is an element of lottery to the application system, as the number of students choosing to apply to different deaneries and different jobs will fluctuate each year. However, all programmes are designed to give you the skills needed to progress beyond foundation and the vast majority of people really enjoy their foundation jobs, regardless of whether it was their first choice or their 191st. In addition, most people find that the foundation years fly past, so do not be afraid to try somewhere new or something different. This era signifies a new chapter of your life.

Types of application

Standard applications

Anyone wanting to become a junior doctor in the UK must apply to the Foundation Programme via the Foundation Programme Application System (FPAS). This application requires the submission of evidence of your academic achievements by both you and your medical school. It also requires you to rank the geographical areas (known as deaneries, or Units of Application) in which jobs are available, and then the jobs within an area, in order of preference.

Academic applications

If you wish to undertake or explore a career in medical research or medical education you can also apply for Academic Foundation Programme (AFP) posts. This application must be in addition to the standard non-academic application.

Linked applications

If you want to ensure that you will be placed in the same deanery as another applicant, most usually a partner, then it is possible to link your applications together. However, be aware that once linked it is impossible to unlink the applications, and that you will both be ranked according to the lower overall score. Some Units of Application treat linked applications in different ways when it comes to job allocations, so find out what rules apply in your preferred deaneries.

Timeline of applications

The exact dates vary from year to year and can be found online.
- *September*: registration opens and indicative programmes can be viewed online.
- *October*: website enables submission of applications—do not miss this!
- *February*: final programmes become available to view online.
- *March*: primary list allocation—most people are told their deanery and situational judgement test (SJT) score.
- *April*: deadline for submission of job preferences and jobs for the primary list are allocated.
- *May–July*: reserve list applicants are allocated to jobs.
- *August*: start work as a Foundation Year 1 (FY1) doctor.

Submitting your online application

Find out the window for submitting your application as soon as possible and then submit early—you can guarantee the website will be overloaded on the last day. At the very latest, try to submit a full 3 days before the deadline. If you are going to be out of the country (e.g. on elective), make sure you have Internet access at the required time. If you do not submit your application on time you will not be able to start the Foundation Programme alongside your peers. There are no exceptions, for anyone or anything. It is worth checking that your files of supporting documentation are downloadable from different computers. If the UK Foundation Programme Office (UKFPO) cannot access your documents then they will not be considered; there will be no opportunity to resend. Similarly, check that any PubMed IDs for publications link directly to the full article. More than one click and UKFPO will not go hunting for them and they will not count. (See Table 56.1.)

Educational performance measure (EPM)

The EPM has three components:

1. Your decile ranking

Your decile is decided by your medical school, which will rank you against your peers according to your grades up to the point of application. If you fall in the top decile (10%) you will be awarded 43 points, 2nd decile 42 points and so on, with those in the 10th decile receiving 34 points. As you can see, there is only a 9-point difference between the top and bottom scores, so try not to feel too stressed if you receive a lower ranking.

2. Any publications

Up to 2 points are available for publications. To count, the work must have been undertaken while you were at medical school, have a PubMed ID, and you must be a named author (not a collaborator). Keep alert during your degree for opportunities to become involved with research and publications. Ask your tutors if they have any projects you could become involved in, or consider writing up a case report if you come across an interesting patient. Not only will this strengthen your Foundation Programme application, it will provide you with experience in an important part of modern medicine.

Table 56.1 Components of the application

Component	Maximum points available
Situational judgement test	50
Educational performance measure	50
(Decile ranking)	(43)
(Publications)	(2)
(Additional degrees)	(5)

3. Any additional degrees

Previous degrees and intercalated degrees are worth extra points. If you have more than one additional degree, choose the one worth the most points. A guide to the points system is given on 🔊 http://www. foundationprogramme.nhs.uk/ but look up individual degrees.

Situational judgement test

The SJT is a 140 min long exam that aims to test your problem-solving skills in a series of work-related scenarios. Questions 1–47 ask you to rank five responses to a given situation, while for questions 48–70 you must select the three most appropriate of eight possible responses. You should answer from the perspective of an FY1 doctor, and choose based on what you *should* do (not necessarily what you would do, or what you might have seen others do!). The test is held twice in each application year (in early December and in early January). Your medical school will tell you which sitting you have been entered into and you can only take the test once.

Top tips

Time management

This exam is tight for time so calculate in advance how long you have to spend on each question and set yourself targets for various time points. Do not be falsely reassured by the practice tests! In previous years, students have felt the actual exam had more text to read and was harder to complete in the time available. There is no negative marking, so it is vital to answer every question.

Key knowledge

Some questions require an understanding of people and hierarchies that you may not have come across as a medical student. Try to find out about the role of educational supervisors and the correct order in which to seek help. For example, as an FY1 you should normally approach the registrar and then consultant in your own team first, rather than approaching a different team. Other topics to brush up on include rules regarding diabetes, seizures, the DVLA, and the rare occasions when it is appropriate to breach patient confidentiality.

Practice tests

There are two official practice tests available and you should take both of them. It is possible to complete them online, but as the actual SJT will be paper based it is best to print out the papers. This will allow you to familiarize yourself with the printed format and practise filling in the answer sheet, which can be confusing the first time around.

Books and courses

Although various books and courses exist, they are not advised. Aside from being expensive, they are not created by those that write the actual SJTs and thus are based on guesswork. In many, the questions provided have shorter text, which prevents you from practising the timing component. Most people agree there is an element of luck to this test, and it is perhaps not worth spending too much time (or money) preparing.

Sample SJT question

One of the nurses, Jill, has undermined your decisions several times, and has twice called you incompetent in front of patients and staff. More recently, a FY1 colleague told you that you should not allow her to speak to you like that. You have not had feedback from any other team members to indicate that there are any problems with your performance.

Rank in order the appropriateness of the following actions in response to this situation (1= most appropriate; 5= least appropriate).

A. Continue to ignore Jill's comments.
B. Inform the nurse in charge about Jill's comments.
C. Find Jill when she is on a break and ask what her concerns are with you.
D. Inform your consultant about Jill's comments.
E. Ask other FY1s if they have had similar problems with Jill.

Reproduced from UKPFO website: ℳ www.sjt.foundationprogramme.nhs.uk/sample.

Ranking jobs within a deanery
Whatever your deanery, you are likely to have a considerable number of jobs to rank, so start the process early. Studying a map of the area enables you to mark the different hospitals on the map so you can see them in relation to one another and the transport systems. Printing out a list of the jobs and cutting them up can help with physically re-arranging and comparing the various options.

Useful resources

- Applicant's handbook for FPAS (ℳ www.fpas.nhs.uk).
- For further information on the SJT and to access the practice papers go to ℳ www.sjt.foundationprogramme.nhs.uk.

Sample SJT question answer: DEBCA

Rationale
This question requires you to see that Jill is behaving unprofessionally and to understand this could have a negative effect on the team. In many SJT questions your first action should be to speak to the person offending. The best first move is to inform your consultant (D) who is in a position to investigate and take action as required. The next best option would be to talk to the other juniors (E) so that they can also recognize it as unprofessional behaviour and report anything relevant to the consultant. Although telling the nurse in charge (B) is not a bad thing to do, it is ranked lower down as your consultant would be a better person to undertake this. While talking directly to the person causing the issue (C) is often a good starting place, it is likely to result in further tension and an unfavourable interaction. However the worst approach listed would be just to ignore Jill's comments (A) as the situation would persist.

Academic Foundation Programme

Academic career pathways

The AFP will, for many doctors, be their first exposure to clinical research, and it may be that you wish to return to pure clinical medicine after this period. However, it is important to remember that the majority of academic doctors carry out research and teaching alongside their clinical work, and that it is not always necessary to choose one over the other. While specifics regarding training pathways alter with time and within different countries (NB England, Wales, and Scotland all have their own pathways. See the UK Foundation Programme website for a more detailed overview of the current schemes), for those considering remaining in academia long term, the following sections will provide a brief overview of the current pathway in England.

Specialist training (ST)

A natural path to take after an AFP is to apply for an Academic Clinical Fellowship within your specialty of interest. They are 3 years long (i.e. ST1–ST3), and while mostly clinical in nature, they will have ~25% of time allocated for academia. Like the AFP posts, the first year will focus on developing clinical experience, with the aim of the second and third year allowing you to determine an area to undertake a MD/PhD, and to apply for funding. While this may seem like a daunting task, you will certainly receive help and guidance from experienced clinical researchers who have successfully made this transition.

Training fellowship

Once successful in gaining funding, you will undertake a 'training fellowship', which will comprise the project that will hopefully lead to the award of a MD/PhD. While the inherent level of clinical medicine within this period will vary depending on your project, most doctors will continue to have protected clinic time to ensure skills are maintained/developed.

Academic clinical lectureship

Once you have completed your MD/PhD, you can apply for a clinical lectureship post (up to 4 years in length). This will allow you to complete your clinical training, alongside carrying out postdoctoral research. This stage will also likely require you to obtain your own funding via bodies such as the Wellcome Trust, the Medical Research Council, Cancer Research UK, etc.

Senior lectureship/consultant

Completion of your clinical training will then allow you to apply for consultant and senior lectureship positions. If you wish to continue in research, then grant applications and sourcing of funding will be an ever-present part of the job.

Career taster weeks

As a foundation doctor, it is important to think hard about your likely career so that you can tailor your efforts to what is required to get a job in that specialty. Time is shorter than you think: within 18 months, you will apply for core/specialty training and in doing so, you will likely have chosen the bearing of your training: medicine, surgery, general practice, or one of the specialties. The earlier you decide, the more efficient your efforts will be towards forming a competitive application by considering relevant Royal College examinations (MRCP, MRCS, etc.), conducting teaching, and undertaking research and audits. However, be reassured that many of the essential skills required at selection for jobs are generic. Specialty-specific achievements are more relevant to more competitive specialties (plastic surgery, neurosurgery, ophthalmology, etc.).

Career tasters

The UKFPO allocates 5 days per year for foundation trainees to 'taste' a selected specialty. Prior to the Modernising Medical Careers programme, trainees could spend as long as they desired as SHOs, sampling careers until they were certain of their decision. This is no longer possible under the modern system of postgraduate medical training. You will only have the opportunity to sample three or four specialties as a foundation doctor before you apply for core/specialist training, not necessarily in the specialties of your interest. Taster weeks can therefore be very helpful in examining a specialty with the sole purpose of considering whether it is the career you wish to pursue. It can also provide you with a way to demonstrate commitment to, and insight into, a specialty during the selection process. This is the most difficult step; once you know what you want, you can plan.

What to ask about on taster weeks

Ask a variety of people, including both trainees and consultants. Do not worry about approaching them to ask these sorts of questions; on the whole, people generally thoroughly enjoy talking about their stories, work, and experiences. Ask the questions that really matter about your considered specialty:

- The best and the worst aspects of the job.
- Work–life balance (and option for less than full-time training).
- Career satisfaction.
- Likely changes to the speciality over the next 30 years.
- Opportunities for clinical/basic science research.
- The need for a higher research degree.
- Opportunities for working abroad/developing countries.
- Ask registrars what it is like being a trainee in their deanery (the nature and intensity of the work, the nature of exams, morale, quality of training).
- Ask consultants how they see their work, and if there are any regrets.
- Why do trainees leave the specialty? What do trainees struggle with?
- What are the attributes of a successful trainee?

Seek advice and support in building an appropriate CV for job applications:
- Are there any research projects/audits you can become involved in?
- Ask registrars about the process of application and interviews—this will present a clear idea of what you need to do.
- Ask about mandatory skills courses, and those that are recommended on entry to the specialty.
- Ask about scientific meetings, presentations, prizes, and exams—which are worth working towards at your stage?

Top tips

1. *You need to take the initiative*: discuss the need for a taster week early with your educational supervisor (ES) so that it can be planned appropriately (at least 6 weeks' notice is required). Your ES may help to identify a suitable contact in the relevant department.
2. *Negotiate a timetable*: for the week with the departmental lead overseeing your taster week. Ensure your timetable is suited to your needs, has clearly defined objectives, and will be most helpful in answering your questions. Ensure you have some 1:1 time with a senior clinician to discuss issues that you consider important and relevant to the specialty.
3. *Write a reflection on your experience*: this will help to organize your thoughts, consider what you have seen and heard, and form a useful record for your supervisor and for yourself on your journey to your chosen career path.
4. *Inspect the register of established tasters*: local to a foundation school. This may simplify the organizations of your taster week.

Resources

- ℘ www.foundationprogramme.nhs.uk
- ℘ www.foundationprogramme.nhs.uk/pages/home/your-career-path/resources
- ℘ www.careers.bmj.com/careers/advice/view-article.html?id=20000642
- ℘ www.careers.bmj.com/careers/advice/A_general_practice_taster_programme_for_foundation_doctors
- ℘ www.careers.bmj.com/careers/advice/view-article.html?id=20012762

General references

Funding

Examples of Royal College travel grants:
- ℘ www.rcplondon.ac.uk/research/funding-and-awards/travelling-fellowships-and-bursaries
- ℘ www.rcseng.ac.uk/surgeons/research/awards-and-grants/travel-awards
- www.rcsed.ac.uk/fellows-members/awards-and-grants.aspx
- ℘ www.rcpsg.ac.uk/membership/supporting-your-career/awards-and-scholarship.aspx
- ℘ www.rcophth.ac.uk/professional-resources/awards-and-prizes
- ℘ www.rcog.org.uk/en/careers-training/awards-grants-prizes

Royal Society of Medicine grants:
- ✆ www.rsm.ac.uk/prizes-awards/other-prizes-and-awards.aspx

US-UK Fulbright Commission:
- ✆ www.fulbright.org.uk

Examples of research funding websites:
- ✆ www.mrc.ac.uk/research/international
- ✆ www.mrc.ac.uk/funding/science-areas/global-health
- ✆ www.wellcome.ac.uk/Funding/Biomedical-science/Funding-schemes/PhD-funding-and-undergraduate-opportunities/index.htm
- ✆ www.wellcome.ac.uk/Funding/Biomedical-science/Funded-projects/Major-initiatives/Major-Overseas-Programmes/index.htm

Conference Of Postgraduate Medical Deans (UK): A Reference Guide for Postgraduate Specialty Training in the UK
- The Gold Guide: ✆ www.hee.nhs.uk/2014/06/04/the-gold-guide-fifth-edition-is-now-available

General Medical Council advice on time out of programme
- ✆ www.gmc-uk.org/doctors/approval_out_of_programme_post.asp

Volunteering opportunities abroad
- Médecins Sans Frontières (MSF)/Doctors Without Borders: ✆ www.msf.org.uk/work-overseas

- Voluntary Service Overseas: ✆ www.vsointernational.org

Projects Abroad
- ✆ www.projects-abroad.co.uk/volunteer-projects/pro/medicine-and-healthcare/#medicine

A useful list of other organizations that medics can volunteer for can be found on the MSF site:
- ✆ www.msf.org.uk/other-organisations-working-overseas

British Medical Association's guidance on working abroad
- ✆ www.bma.org.uk/developing-your-career/career-progression/working-abroad

Volunteer toolkit
- ✆ www.hee.nhs.uk/wp-content/blogs.dir/321/files/2014/03/2312-HEE-Toolkit-for-evidence-v8-Whatever-design-update.pdf

Good Clinical Practice
- ✆ www.crn.nihr.ac.uk/learning-development/good-clinical-practice

Index